Intraepithelial Neoplasia of the Lower Genital Tract

For Churchill Livingstone

Commissioning Editor: Lucy Gardner
Copy Editor: Laura Wilson
Project Controller: Sarah Lowe
Design Direction: Sarah Cape

Intraepithelial Neoplasia of the Lower Genital Tract

Edited by

David Luesley MA MD FRCOG

Reader in Gynaecological Oncology,
University of Birmingham;
Honorary Consultant Obstetrician and Gynaecologist,
City Hospital NHS Trust,
Birmingham, UK

Joe Jordan MD FRCOG

Birmingham Women's Hospital,
Queen Elizabeth Medical Centre,
Edgbaston, Birmingham, UK

Ralph M. Richart MD

Professor of Pathology in Obstetrics and Gynecology,
Columbia University College of Physicians and Surgeons,
New York, USA

CHURCHILL LIVINGSTONE
EDINBURGH HONG KONG LONDON MADRID MELBOURNE NEW YORK AND TOKYO 1995

CHURCHILL LIVINGSTONE
Medical Division of Pearson Professional Limited

Distributed in the United States of America by Churchill
Livingstone Inc., 650 Avenue of the Americas, New York,
N.Y. 10011, and by associated companies, branches and
representatives throughout the world.

© Pearson Professional Limited 1995

First published 1995

ISBN 0-443-04964-5

British Library Cataloguing in Publication Data
A catalogue record for this book is available from the British
Library.

Library of Congress Cataloging in Publication Data
A catalog record for this book is available from the Library of
Congress.

The
publisher's
policy is to use
**paper manufactured
from sustainable forests**

Printed in Singapore

Contents

1. The normal anatomy and histology of the cervix, vagina and vulva   1
   T. P. Rollason

2. The pathology of cervical neoplasia   19
   Ralph M. Richart, Thomas C. Wright

3. Vulvar intraepithelial neoplasia   37
   Catherine M. McLachlin, Christopher P. Crum

4. The epidemiology of cervical neoplasms   49
   Melissa R. Krone, Nancy B. Kiviat, Laura A. Koutsky

5. Costs and benefits of cervical screening   61
   S. Wilson, C. B. J. Woodman

6. Immunology of the lower female genital tract with emphasis on genital infections   71
   Per-Anders Mårdh, Marius Domeika

7. Viral infections and lower genital tract neoplasia   83
   H. Kitchener

8. The application of molecular biology to the detection of HPV infection   95
   J. R. M. Ellis, L. S. Young

9. The etiology and natural history of vulvar dysplasia   111
   Vicki V. Baker

10. Vulval and multifocal intraepithelial neoplasia   121
    Rashna Chenoy, David Luesley

11. Vulvar warts: clinical and subclinical   133
    Alex Ferenczy

12. Cytokine therapy of lower genital tract neoplasia   155
    Richard Cirelli, Paul Rockley, Stephen K. Tyring

13. Vaginal intraepithelial neoplasia   169
    Alberto Lopes, John M. Monaghan, Greg Robertson

14. Minor cytological abnormalities   177
    Mahmood I. Shafi

15. Management of cervical intraepithelial neoplasia   185
    J. A. Jordan

16. Human papillomavirus testing: major advance or scientific hoax?   197
    Richard Reid, J. Thomas Cox

17. CIN in pregnancy   221
    Patrick G. Walker

18. The abnormal smear in postmenopausal women   231
    M. E. L. Paterson, D. W. Sturdee

19. Psychological aspects of the investigation and treatment of abnormalities of the cervix   241
    I. E. Doherty, P. H. Richardson

20. Adenocarcinoma-in-situ and related lesions   251
    John Cullimore

21. Cervical disease in HIV-infected women: prevalence, pathogenesis, detection, and treatment   263
    Thomas C. Wright

22. Early invasive cervical carcinoma   277
   Edgardo L. Yordan, George D. Wilbanks

23. A critical appraisal of screening and diagnostic techniques   293
   W. P. Soutter

24. Retinoids in differentiation and prevention of malignant transformation   309
   Nadine Darwiche, Luigi M. De Luca

25. Oncogenes in cervical neoplasia   325
   Laure Aurelian

26. Role of the male partner in the carcinogenic process   341
   R. Barrasso

27. Concurrent genital infections recognized at colposcopy   349
   Jorma Paavonen

Index   357

Contributors

Laure Aurelian PhD
Professor, Department of Pharmacology and
Director, Virology/Immunology Laboratories,
University of Maryland School of Medicine,
Baltimore, Maryland, USA

Vicki V. Baker MD
Associate Professor of Obstetrics, Gynecology and
Reproductive Sciences and Director of
Gynecological Oncology, University of Texas-
Houston Health Science Center, Houston, Texas,
USA

Renzo Barrasso MD
Director, Colposcopy Unit, Department of
Obstetrics and Gynaecology, University Hospital
Bichat, Paris, France

Rashna Chenoy MD
Senior Registrar, North Staffordshire General
Infirmary, Stoke-on-Trent, UK

J. Thomas Cox BS MD
Director, Gynecology Clinic and Consultant in
Colposcopy Health Services, University of
California, Santa Barbara, Santa Barbara,
California, USA

Christopher P. Crum MD
Associate Professor of Pathology, Harvard Medical
School; Director, Division of Women's and
Perinatal Pathology, Brigham and Women's
Hospital, Boston, Massachusetts, USA

John Edward Cullimore MD MRCOG FRCSEd
Consultant Gynaecologist, Princess Margaret
Hospital, Swindon, Wiltshire; former Research
Fellow, Birmingham and Midland Hospital for
Women, Birmingham, UK

Nadine Darwiche PhD
Post-Doctoral Fellow, Differentiation Control
Section, Laboratory of Cellular Carcinogenesis and
Tumor Promotion, National Cancer Institute,
NIH, Bethesda, Maryland, USA

Luigi M. De Luca PhD
Head, Differentiation Control Section, National
Cancer Institute, NIH, Bethesda, Maryland, USA

Ingrid E. Doherty MSc
Chartered Clinical Psychologist, West Lambeth
Community Care NHS Trust, Directorate of
Mental Health, South Western Hospital, London,
UK

Marius Domeika PhD MD
Researcher, Institute of Clinical Bacteriology,
Centre for STD Research, Uppsala University,
Uppsala, Sweden

J. R. M. Ellis PhD MSc
CRC Postdoctoral Research Fellow, CRC Institute
for Cancer Studies, University of Birmingham
Medical School, Birmingham, UK

A. Ferenczy MD
Professor of Pathology and Obstetrics &
Gynecology, McGill University and The Sir
Mortimer B. Davis Jewish General Hospital,
Montreal, Quebec, Canada

J. A. Jordan MD FRCOG
Birmingham Women's Hospital, Queen Elizabeth
Medical Centre, Edgbaston, Birmingham, UK

Henry C. Kitchener MD FRCOG(Glas)
Consultant Gynaecologist, Aberdeen Royal
Infirmary, Foresterhill, Aberdeen, UK

Nancy B. Kiviat MD
Professor of Pathology, University of Washington, Seattle, Washington, USA

Laura A. Koutsky PhD MSPH
Associate Professor of Epidemiology, Center for AIDS and STD, University of Washington, Seattle, Washington, USA

Melissa R. Krone MS
Research Scientist, Center for AIDS and STD, University of Washington, Seattle, Washington, USA

Alberto De B. Lopes MB ChB MRCOG
Gynaecological Oncology Fellow, Regional Department of Gynaecological Oncology, Queen Elizabeth Hospital, Gateshead, UK

David Luesley MA MD FRCOG
Reader in Gynaecological Oncology, University of Birmingham; Honorary Consultant Obstetrician and Gynaecologist, City Hospital NHS Trust, Birmingham, UK

Catherine M. McLachlin MD
Assistant Professor, Department of Pathology, Victoria Hospital and The University of Western Ontario, London, Ontario, Canada

Per-Anders Mårdh PhD MD
Professor and Head of Institute of Clinical Bacteriology; Head, Centre for STD Research, University of Uppsala, Uppsala, Sweden

John M. Monaghan MB FRCSE FRCOG
Director, Gynaecological Oncology Services, Queen Elizabeth Hospital, Gateshead; Senior Lecturer in Gynaecological Oncology, University of Newcastle upon Tyne, Newcastle upon Tyne, UK

Jorma Paavonen MD PhD
Associate Professor, Department of Obstetrics and Gynecology, University of Helsinki, Helsinki, Finland

Michael Paterson MD FRCOG FRCSEd
Consultant Obstetrician & Gynaecologist, Northern General Hospital, Sheffield, UK

Richard Reid MD
Director, Gynecologic Endoscopy, Crittenton Hospital, Rochester; Assistant Professor, Wayne State University School of Medicine Ob/Gyn, Detroit, Michigan, USA

P. H. Richardson PhD
Senior Lecturer in Psychology, Division of Psychiatry and Psychology, United Medical and Dental School of Guys and St Thomas' Hospital, London, UK

Ralph M. Richart MD
Professor of Pathology in Obstetrics and Gynecology, Columbia University College of Physicians and Surgeons, New York, USA

G. Robertson MBBS MRCOG FRACOG
Gynaecological Oncology Fellow, Royal Hospital for Women, Paddington, Sydney, NSW, Australia

Paul Rockley MD
Instructor, Department of Internal Medicine, University of Texas Medical Branch, Galveston, Texas, USA

Terence P. Rollason BSc MB ChB FRCPath
Consultant Gynaecological Pathologist, Birmingham Women's Services Trust; Senior Clinical Lecturer, University of Birmingham, Birmingham, UK

Mahmood I. Shafi MB BCh DA MRCOG
Senior Registrar and Subspecialty Trainee in Gynaecological Oncology, City Hospital NHS Trust, Birmingham, UK

Pat Soutter MD MSc FRCOG
Reader in Gynaecological Oncology, Royal Postgraduate Medical School, Hammersmith Hospital, London, UK

David W. Sturdee MD FRCOG
Consultant Obstetrician and Gynaecologist, The Solihull Hospital, Solihull, UK

S. T. Tyring MD PhD
Professor of Dermatology, Microbiology and Immunology and Internal Medicine, University of Texas Medical Branch, Galveston, Texas, USA

Patrick Walker MD FRCOG
Consultant Obstetrician and Gynaecologist, Royal Free Hospital NHS Trust, London, UK

George D. Wilbanks MD
Chairman, Rush-Presbyterian—St Luke's Medical Centre, Chicago, Illinois, USA

Sue Wilson BA
Deputy Director, Centre for Cancer
Epidemiology, University of Manchester,
Manchester, UK

C. B. J. Woodman MD MRCOG MFPHM
Professor of Cancer Epidemiology, University of
Manchester, Manchester, UK

Thomas C. Wright MD
Associate Professor of Pathology, College of

Physicians and Surgeons of Columbia University,
New York, USA

Edgardo Yordan MD
Associate Professor of Obstetrics and Gynecology,
Rush Medical College, Chicago; Director of
Gynecologic Oncology, Rush-Presbyterian—St
Luke's Medical Center, Chicago, Illinois, USA

Lawrence S. Young PhD MRCPath
Professor, CRC Institute for Cancer Studies,
University of Birmingham Medical School,
Birmingham, UK

Preface

Cervical cancer is still a major global health problem with striking geographical variation. In the underdeveloped world, established and advanced disease constitute the bulk of the problem, whereas in those more developed countries—especially those with screening programmes—there has been a decline in mortality from invasive disease. Whilst this could be ascribed to aspects of health promotion, screening and other socioeconomic factors, inevitably it has resulted in a sharper focus on preinvasive disease.

Cervical cancer and its preinvasive counterparts provide an ideal opportunity to investigate the malignant process—the long-term objectives being first to understand, then to intervene and finally to prevent. This activity could be seen as "missing the point" and a potential waste of resource and effort, as the far more pressing health care problem—"the unseen part of the iceberg"—is the huge scale of invasive disease that annually claims hundreds of thousands of lives in the underdeveloped parts of the world. This philosophy is both superficial and misguided. The intense, multidisciplinary research effort addressing the most basic problems posed by preinvasive disease offers the best opportunity of addressing the problems posed by established disease by both early intervention and prevention.

Dysplasia of the lower genital tract—and of the cervix, in particular—can also be seen as a major health care problem in the developed world. Considerable resources are annually consumed in the detection and treatment of cervical intraepithelial neoplasia. As all health care systems become more cost conscious, the scale of this problem in real terms has mushroomed. It is patently obvious that not all women who have an abnormal cervical smear will die of cervical malignancy, similarly not all those with pre-invasive disease of the vulva and vagina will succumb to vulvar or vaginal cancer. What we cannot offer at present is a logical and rational approach to care based upon sound scientific observation. However, the work has been done, is being done and will continue to be done. The results will be available and should be applied to what we believe should be a system of health care sensitive and adaptable to new data.

This book represents a multidisciplinary approach to the problems we perceive. That this area of medicine is multidisciplinary cannot be disputed, and our attempts to bridge the disciplinary interfaces, we feel, will bring the scientific aspects of research into sharp focus for clinicians and the clinical aspects into focus for the bench scientists. One of the challenges presented by multidisciplinary multiauthorship is to achieve a meaningful structure, whereby one chapter necessarily builds upon those before it. We feel that there is a discernible direction, although each contribution easily stands alone as well. The rapidly evolving molecular disciplines have been brought into the text in an integrated, rather than "add-on", fashion. This gives this exciting area much more meaning, especially for those coming mainly from a clinical background. Furthermore, what up until now may have seemed to be a rather loose knit of science, epidemiology, pathology and clinical medicine has been brought together in a way which now seems obvious to the point whereby one might quite plausibly question why they were never seen so objectively.

Those who have contributed are well-recognized experts in their own fields yet also open minded enough to see their own particular areas as part of the whole. The substance of their texts reflects this attitude along with a crispness of delivery and clarity of thought. No textbook can ever be truly up to date; the gestation of such works prevents this. Nevertheless, we feel that it is as contemporary as is possible, and also that each contributor has presented their topic in state-of-the-art format with ample direction for the future.

David Luesley
Ralph Richart
Joe Jordan

1. The normal anatomy and histology of the cervix, vagina and vulva

T. P. Rollason

CERVIX

GROSS ANATOMY

The cervix is the most caudal portion of the uterus and protrudes into the upper vagina. It measures 2.5–3 cm in length in the adult multigravida. It is divided from the uterine corpus by a fibromuscular junction termed the internal os. The vagina is fused circumferentially to the cervix dividing it into an upper, supravaginal and a lower, vaginal portion. These portions are of approximately the same length. The cervix is normally angulated downward and backward. The shape of the cervix is highly variable. The nulliparous cervix has a circular os and a diameter of approximately 2.5 cm. The multiparous cervix is larger and more protruding and has a transverse, slit-like external os. The reflections of the vaginal epithelium around the sides of the cervix constitute the vaginal fornices. The vaginal portion of the cervix (portio vaginalis) is divided into anterior and posterior lips, the anterior is shorter and projects lower than the posterior.

The cervical canal connects the uterine isthmus (internal os) with the external os. This is an elliptical cavity showing longitudinal ridges (plicae palmatae) composed of epithelium and connective tissue. The canal has a maximum diameter of approximately 7–8 mm. It is approximately 3 cm long and is flattened anteroposteriorly. The use of the terms anatomic and histological internal os relates to the difference seen in the position of the macroscopic os and the histological point at which the epithelium changes from isthmic endometrial to endocervical. These terms have little clinical relevance.

The supravaginal portion of the cervix is separated anteriorly from the bladder by the parametrial connective tissues which also extend to the sides of the cervix and between the layers of the broad ligaments. Posteriorly the supravaginal cervix is covered with peritoneum which continues down over the upper vaginal wall and is reflected onto the rectum forming the pouch of Douglas (rectouterine pouch).

The cervical stroma is made up of fibrous, muscular and elastic tissue. Fibrous tissue predominates, with smooth muscle located mainly in the endocervix.[1] At the isthmus smooth muscle and fibrous tissue are present in approximately equal proportions and in concentric arrangement, making up a functional sphincter.

The arterial supply of the cervix is derived from descending branches of the uterine arteries[2] which pass to the lateral walls along the superior margins of the paracervical ligaments (transverse cervical ligaments or cardinal ligament of Mackenrodt). These ligaments together with the uterosacral ligaments, which attach the supravaginal portion of the cervix to the second to fourth sacral vertebrae, are the main source of fixation and support. The ligaments consist largely of fibrous tissue with smaller amounts of smooth muscle. The uterosacral ligaments appear to be the main ligaments holding the uterus in an anteverted position. The lateral ligaments appear to provide most general support. The ureter runs downwards and forwards within the parametrium some 2 cm from the cervix.

The venous drainage parallels the arterial system but communications exist between the cervical vessels and venous supply of the neck of the urinary bladder. The lymphatics have an origin both in the mucosa and deep in the fibrous

1

stroma.[3] These systems collect into two lateral plexuses in the isthmic region and produce four efferent channels running towards the external iliac and obturator nodes, the hypogastric and common iliac nodes, the sacral nodes and the nodes of the posterior wall of the urinary bladder.

The cervical nerves derive from the superior, middle and inferior hypogastric plexuses of the pelvic autonomic system. The nerve supply is largely limited to the endocervix and deep ectocervix accounting for the relative insensitivity of the portio vaginalis.

HISTOLOGY

'Original' (native) squamous epithelium

The vaginal portion of the cervix is lined by stratified squamous, nonkeratinizing epithelium (Fig. 1.1). This epithelium is replenished by proliferation of basal cells every 4–5 days during reproductive life. Maturation may be accelerated by estrogens and inhibited, at the midzone of the epithelium, by progestagens.[1,4] In adult life this epithelium is fully mature and glycogen laden due to estrogenic stimulation. This is also the case in early postnatal life under the influence of maternal estrogen. In postmenopausal women the epithelium undergoes atrophy with thinning, loss of differentiation and loss of glycogen. In the premenopausal female the epithelium is of similar appearance to that of the postmenopausal woman. During pregnancy superficial maturation is lost under the influence of elevated progesterone.

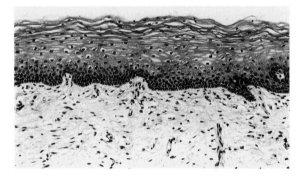

Fig. 1.1 Ectocervical squamous epithelium showing small, dark, basal cells, midzone basketweave pattern and flattened cells of the superficial zone.

It is usual to divide the ectocervical epithelium into three zones: basal, midzone and superficial. The basal zone is composed of one or two layers of cylindrical or elliptical cells approximately 10 μm in diameter. These have scant cytoplasm and nuclei oriented perpendicular to the underlying basal lamina (basal membrane) which is well demonstrated by electron microscopy or immunohistochemical staining with antilaminin. The cells of this layer are actively dividing. The lower few layers of the midzone contain larger cells than the basal layer with more cytoplasm, often termed parabasal cells. In normal epithelium mitoses are seen in these cells as well as the basal layer but with less frequency. Glycogen synthesis occurs in this layer. The upper midzone or intermediate cell zone is composed of nondividing, glycogen-rich cells which show a gradual increase in cytoplasm with increasing height. The overall pattern of this zone is often termed 'basketweave'. Nuclear size is constant from this level to the surface. The cells of the superficial zone show flattening and an overall cell diameter of approximately 50 μm. The nuclei are small and pyknotic and the cytoplasm glycogen-rich and eosinophilic. Keratinosomes are evident on electron microscopy. The epithelial surface is cornified and on electron microscopy a complex surface pattern of microridges is present; together these are believed to help prevent trauma to the underlying layers and stop infective agents entering the deep epithelium. Under some exogenous stimuli keratinization occurs above the superficial cells; this is represented by a dense, eosinophilic layer of variable thickness (Fig. 1.2). It is due to a relative increase in cell cytoplasmic keratin production. The keratinized cells are most commonly anucleate.

The atrophic epithelium of postmenopausal women (Fig. 1.3) shows little or no surface epithelial maturation and absent or sparse stromal papillae (rete pegs are not normally seen even in the mature cervix). These papillae are finger-like extensions of vessels and stroma into the epitheliun.[5] Occasional squamous epithelial cells showing a large solitary vacuole, leading to a 'signet-ring' cellular appearance are common in the ectocervical epithelium (Fig. 1.4). Occasionally this cell pattern becomes dominant.[6] The cause of this change is uncertain but it appears

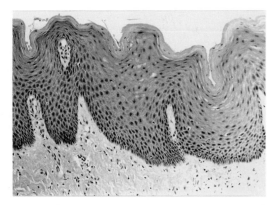

Fig. 1.2 A dense band of hyperkeratosis is seen above the stratified squamous epithelium.

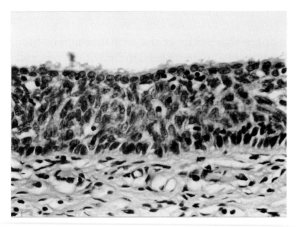

Fig. 1.3 The squamous epithelium is composed of small, dark, basal-type cells, the pattern of simple epithelial atrophy.

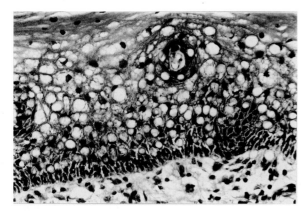

Fig. 1.4 Vacuolated squamous ectocervical cells. The epithelium contains numerous vacuolated squamous cells. This is a normal variant and the architecture of the epithelium is essentially preserved.

entirely benign. Similar changes may be seen in cervical intraepithelial neoplasia.

Dendritic Langerhans' cells are seen in the cervical epithelium as in the vulva (see the section on vulvar histology below). Their role in the development of malignancy is unclear but they appear reduced in number in smokers.[7]

'Original' (native) columnar epithelium

The endocervical columnar epithelium is composed of a single layer of mucin-secreting columnar cells. These cells have basally placed round or oval nuclei and uniform, slightly granular cytoplasm filled with mucin droplets (Müllerian mucinous epithelium). The secretory cells appear to undergo cyclical synthesis, secretion and exhaustion under β-adrenergic control.[8] Acidic and neutral mucins are produced with acidic predominating. The relative proportions of different mucins vary with the menstrual cycle. Sialomucins increase relative to sulfomucins in the preovulatory phase of the cycle but fall after ovulation and postmenopausally, when sulfomucins predominate.[9,10] Secretion appears to be both apocrine and merocrine in type.

Occasional nonsecretory cells with cilia are present which probably play a role in mucin movement. Solitary neuroendocrine cells may also be identified on specific staining.[11]

On two-dimensional sections the endocervix appears to show surface epithelium and underlying tubular elements. Whilst the endocervical surface epithelium is often referred to as a mucosa and the tubular elements as glands, neither is actually true. The surface epithelium, and epithelium of the underlying structures, has no associated submucosa and is a simple epithelium, not a mucosal surface. Fluhmann[12] demonstrated conclusively that the endocervical 'glands' are actually deep, cleft-like infoldings of the surface epithelium (Fig. 1.5) with numerous blind secondary outpouchings. The complex pattern of these crypts leads to their histological appearance as isolated tubular glandular units. The epithelium of the crypts is identical to that of the surface whereas true glands have different epithelium in their ductal elements from that in their secretory portions. Although occasional crypts may be

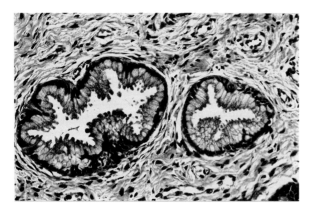

Fig. 1.5 Endocervical crypts. The infolding seen is common as is the apical 'snouting'. The cytoplasmic pallor is due to the content of intracellular mucin.

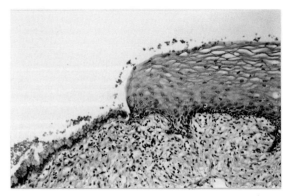

Fig. 1.6 The squamocolumnar junction is evident in the center of the picture where the stratified squamous epithelium changes abruptly to a monolayer of columnar cells.

more than 1 cm deep the maximum depth in well-oriented secretions is closer to 8 mm (mean 3.4 mm).[13]

It is usually stated that the endocervical epithelium has an origin in the subcolumnar reserve cells[14] and that mitoses are not seen in the columnar epithelium in normal conditions. In fact subcolumnar reserve cells are difficult to see even at the ultrastructural level and in the experience of the author mitoses are seen, though infrequently, in normal endocervical epithelial cells and may be quite frequent in circumstances of increased cell turnover, e.g., active inflammation.

The endocervical epithelium, as well as crypt infolding, also shows coarse mounds or cushions called rugae which present on either lip of the cervix.[1] This pattern fuses with the longitudinal 'arbor vitae' in the canal (the plicae palmatae previously referred to). There is a further fine grouping of folds to produce pendulous areas resembling bunches of grapes.[15] The basic single surface subunit is the villus which is usually ovoid and between 0.15 and 1.5 mm in diameter.

Squamous metaplasia and the transformation zone

The squamocolumnar junction (SCJ) of the cervix is the point at which the endocervical columnar epithelium meets the ectocervical stratified squamous epithelium (Fig. 1.6). This is not a fixed point throughout life. The understanding of the changes that occur at the SCJ throughout life is fundamental to an understanding of the processes leading up to tumor formation in the cervix.

Before puberty, the SCJ is located at, or close to, the external os of the cervix. This point is often called the 'original' SCJ. The junction is a sharp one. In fact, however, the term 'original' SCJ in these circumstances is usually a misnomer as in 75% of infants there is evidence that there is squamous metaplastic epithelium rather than true 'original' squamous epithelium at the SCJ.[16] This phenomenon is discussed further in relation to the congenital transformation zone (see below).

Under the influence of increasing ovarian hormones at puberty there is an increase in the size of both the corpus and cervix. This leads to eversion of the cervix which is more marked anteriorly and posteriorly than at the sides. The endocervical epithelium then comes to lie on the vaginal portion of the cervix. This endocervical epithelium appears red and rough and is often clinically termed an erosion (incorrect as no ulceration is present) or an ectopy (ectropion). It is common for the everted endocervical epithelium to have a blunt papillary pattern of epithelial folding and a prominent subepithelial chronic inflammatory cell infiltrate (Fig. 1.7). This pattern, despite being termed a papillary erosion or papillary cervicitis, is a physiological condition and not a disease process. This zone of eversion is most extensive in women under 20 years of age and

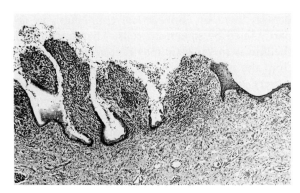

Fig. 1.7 Simple 'papillary cervicitis'. This is a normal variant. Tongue-like papillae are seen arising from the endocervical epithelium adjacent to the squamocolumnar junction.

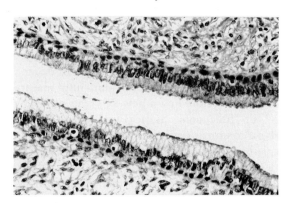

Fig. 1.8 Reserve cells. Beneath the endocervical crypt epithelium can be seen an almost regular layer of small dark reserve cells showing little cytoplasm and no differentiation.

following the first pregnancy. It is usually more extensive on the anterior lip of the cervix.

The zone of eversion is exposed to the reduced pH of the vagina and it appears to be this stimulus which leads to the series of changes which follow and culminate in replacement of the everted endocervical epithelium by more resilient squamous epithelium. Two major mechanisms are suggested; the first appears to be direct ingrowth of the adjacent squamous epithelium of the portio. Tongues of squamous epithelium growth beneath the adjacent columnar epithelium and expand between the endocervical mucinous cells and the basement membrane.[17] The endocervical cells are gradually displaced upwards, degenerate and are sloughed. It is unclear how important a role this mechanism has, some arguing that it is the more important,[17,18] others that it is of minor or no relevance.[15]

The second process is usually called squamous metaplasia but the process is not a truly metaplastic one, metaplasia being the replacement of one adult, differentiated epithelium by another of different type. Fluhmann[12] termed the process in the cervix squamous prosoplasia, possibly a better term. In the first part of the process small, nondifferentiated, cuboidal reserve cells with large nuclei appear beneath the columnar epithelium (Fig. 1.8). These usually appear first on the upper, more exposed parts of the villi and superficial crypts. The origin of these reserve cells has been contentious. It has been argued that they arise from a preexisting population of inconspicuous reserve cells beneath the columnar cells (first proposed by Mayer[19]), from the columnar cells themselves,[12] or from stromal,[20,21] or circulating mononuclear[22] cells. The latter now seems certainly not the case.[23] The reserve cells proliferate to produce a layer several cells thick (reserve cell hyperplasia); at this stage the columnar cells remain as a complete or incomplete surface layer. Electron microscopically these reserve cells resemble the parabasal cells of the ectocervical epithelium.[14,17] The multilayered reserve cells then begin differentiation to clearly squamous cells with increasing amounts of eosinophilic cytoplasm but without surface maturation and with little intracellular glycogen and a now incomplete persisting surface columnar cell layer (incomplete or immature squamous metaplasia) (Fig. 1.9). The

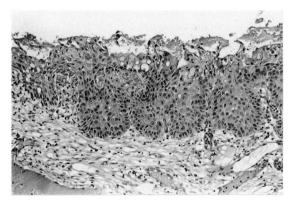

Fig. 1.9 There is a layer of persisting endocervical cells above the squamous epithelium, so-called immature squamous metaplasia.

proliferation of reserve cells and later squamous differentiation tends to obliterate the spaces between the 'villi' of the zone of eversion. Finally, all of the surface columnar cells are shed or degenerate and the squamous epithelium fully matures. There is therefore now a new SCJ (the 'physiological' or 'functional' SCJ) (Fig. 1.10). The zone where columnar epithelium has been converted to squamous is termed the 'transformation zone'. Viewed alone at the end of the process of metaplasia, the transformation zone epithelium may be indistinguishable from the native ectocervical epithelium.

The process of metaplasia may extend into the shallower underlying crypts for their full depth and obliterate them, but usually the crypts either persist, lined by endocervical epithelium, or are partly lined by squamous cells. That surface epithelium is metaplastic may therefore be deduced from the presence of underlying crypts, as there is very little overlapping of crypts by 'original' squamous surface cells. The openings of the crypts may still be evident on the cervical surface of the transformation zone but the squamous proliferation may lead to their blockage; this produces the very common 'Nabothian follicles'. These are in reality mucus retention cysts of the crypts due to continued mucin production, with cystic dilatation related to lack of mucin drainage. The cysts may rupture leading to a local macrophage response, sometimes with associated inflammation. It has been recently recognized that simple

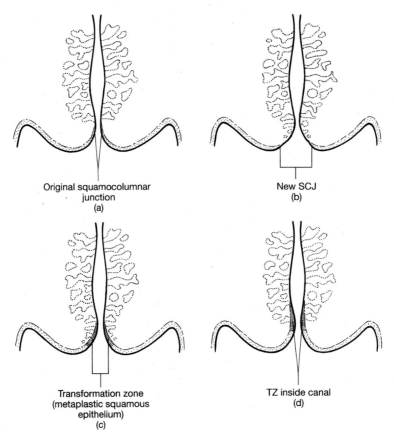

Original squamocolumnar
junction
(a)

New SCJ
(b)

Transformation zone
(metaplastic squamous
epithelium)
(c)

TZ inside canal
(d)

Fig. 1.10 Alterations in the transformation zone in adult life. (a) Prior to the menarche. (b) Eversion of the endocervix under the influence of ovarian hormones. (c) Squamous metaplasia converts the everted columnar epithelium to more resilient squamous. (d) With the fall in ovarian hormonal stimulation at the menopause the eversion is reversed and the SCJ passes into the lower canal.

Nabothian cysts may extend through most of the cervical wall. In these cases the cervical wall may appear replaced by mucin-filled cysts up to 1 cm diameter.[24] These retention cysts are lined by benign endocervical cells, often flattened and without mitoses. There does not appear to be any premalignant potential though histological confusion with minimum deviation adenocarcinoma is possible.

Whilst, as previously indicated, cervical eversion and thus squamous metaplasia are most marked during adolescence and pregnancy the process continues throughout adult life and all stages of the processes described above are commonly seen in cervical biopsy specimens. Interestingly there is evidence that the transformation zone of virgins is larger than that of sexually active young women of the same age.[15,25] After the menopause the shrinkage of the cervical stroma causes 'retraction' of the SCJ into the endocervical canal. The process of squamous metaplasia is not a reversible one and the canal is then lined in its lower portion by squamous epithelium. Reserve cell hyperplasia in the canal is often extensive in the postmenopausal patient particularly when atrophic changes are prominent in the stratified squamous epithelium. The reasons for this are obscure.

Rarely, apparently at any age, there may be sebaceous glands beneath the ectocervical epithelium. This has been suggested to be due to trauma, surgery or inflammation.[26]

The congenital transformation zone (CTZ)

The CTZ is essentially a zone, originally of endocervical epithelium, which undergoes squamous metaplasia in late intrauterine or early extrauterine life. It appears to be related to metaplasia in a zone of endocervical epithelium which passes onto the portio under the influence of maternal estrogen and is replaced by squamous epithelium when the estrogenic stimulus declines. Alternatively, it may be that the CTZ is formed in a similar manner to essentially identical zones seen in diethylstilbestrol-exposed women,[27] i.e., due to incomplete conversion of the early cuboidal epithelium of the vaginal anlage at the upper (uterine) end to squamous epithelium followed by gradual squamous replacement in late intra-

uterine and extrauterine life. This second theory does not explain, however, the downgrowths of epithelium which must relate to preexisting crypts; these can really only be explained on the basis of a previous endocervical eversion.

The histological features of the CTZ in a typical case are a thinned epithelium with shallow, fine (but blunt ended) epithelial downgrowths sometimes with squamous 'eddies' at the base, low or absent epithelial glycogen and a very fine layer of surface keratinization (Fig. 1.11). The epithelium gives the impression of being immature in its lower half, but maturing abnormally rapidly to keratinization over a few cell layers. No nuclear pleomorphism is seen and the adjacent stroma appears normal. Parakeratosis may be seen and variant patterns can be identified which show some epithelial thickening rather than thinning. The junction with the 'normal' ectocervical squamous epithelium is sharp and, when seen in the adult, the CTZ is usually separated from the SCJ by a zone of more typical 'adult' type squamous metaplasia. The low glycogen, thin epithelium, etc. may lead to a colposcopic impression of cervical intraepithelial neoplasia.

Pixley[16] has shown that, even in utero, after 36 weeks gestation 75% of fetuses actually show a zone of metaplastic squamous epithelium adjacent to the truly 'original' endocervical surface epithelium (he termed this the 'original' metaplastic epithelium). The admixture of mature and immature metaplastic patterns with endocervical epithelium in this zone was highly variable and was

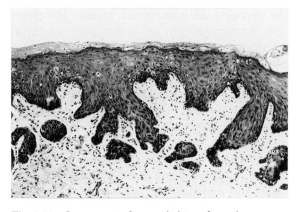

Fig. 1.11 One pattern of congenital transformation zone. Fine, irregular epithelial downgrowths are seen without underlying crypts. The surface is keratinized.

seen at all gestational ages. Before 30 weeks gestation the 'original' transformation zone was flat without intraepithelial vascular projections. This pattern could be identified through infancy and childhood in 40–50% of cases. Whilst it is still not clear how this relates to the CTZ seen in the adult it seems highly likely that the CTZ represents the end result of the earliest stages of metaplasia, which Pixley suggests are an integral part of organogenesis at this site. He demonstrated that the original transformation zone could pass in a small proportion of patients well onto the vaginal surface, this is certainly also true of the CTZ.

Cervical changes during pregnancy

Under the stimulus of gestational hormones the cervix softens and enlarges. This is due to increased vascularity and stromal edema. Acute inflammatory changes are also commonly seen in the superficial stroma. In late pregnancy there is accumulation of large amounts of extracellular glycoprotein and collagen disruption leading to further softening, facilitating dilatation etc. in labour. Decidualization of the stroma under pro-gestational effects is common in the superficial stroma. It may be patchy or diffuse and affects both the endo- and ectocervix. Some degree of decidualization occurs in more than one-third of pregnant women and takes some weeks to disappear after delivery.[28]

Macroscopically, decidual foci appear as raised, vascular nodules and colposcopically they may closely resemble invasive carcinoma. Histologically the stromal cells are indistinguishable from decidualized endometrial cells, being large and pale with clearly defined cytoplasmic margins and large, round, monomorphic nuclei. Very occasionally foci of decidualization may be seen in the absence of pregnancy or obvious endometriosis; usually in association with progestagen therapy.

As indicated previously, very extensive zones of cervical eversion are classically seen in pregnancy and immature metaplasia and reserve cell hyperplasia are extensive. This is most striking in primigravida. True erosions may be seen also, usually immediately adjacent to the portio squa-

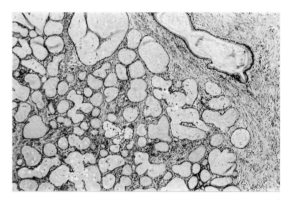

Fig. 1.12 Simple glandular hyperplasia in the form of 'tunnel clusters'. Numerous small and dilated, mucin-filled crypts are seen with flattened, nonatypical epithelium (normal crypt epithelium for comparison to upper right of picture).

mous epithelium.[28] Microglandular hyperplasia (see below) is often very florid and may produce visible protrusions into the endocervical canal.

Simple glandular hyperplasia (tunnel clusters, adenomatoid proliferation)

This very common condition consists simply of a localized proliferation of small and cystic, crowded endocervical crypts (Fig. 1.12). It usually occurs some distance into the endocervical canal rather than around the SCJ. Two variants have been described[12] but this is an unnecessary complication. The epithelium is often attenuated or flattened. Squamous metaplasia is often seen above the proliferated crypts. These foci appear to be more common on the posterior cervical lip.[29] The condition is entirely benign and the only danger lies in histological overdiagnosis as malignancy. Its cause is unknown. It may be a reaction to blockage of the superficial crypt lumen[27] or a regressive phenomenon. The term 'tunnel clusters' has been commonly used for these foci and is preferable to 'adenomatoid' or 'adenomatous' hyperplasia which suggest a tumorous process.

Mesonephric remnants and hyperplasia

Mesonephric remnants are common in the lateral wall of the cervix (Fig. 1.13). Whilst stated to be found in 8% of cervices,[30] personal experience suggests that this is an underestimate. Occasion-

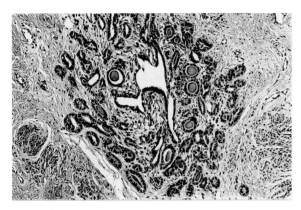

Fig. 1.13 Simple mesonephric remnants. The mesonephric duct can be seen in the center of the photograph, surrounded by small mesonephric tubules showing typical, dense, eosinophilic secretions.

ally these remnants appear unduly prominent and extensive, a condition termed mesonephric hyperplasia. Recently such simple hyperplasia has been divided into three patterns: lobular, diffuse and pure ductal types.[31] Lobular hyperplasia is the commonest pattern and shows rounded tubules in poorly defined lobular aggregates. The diffuse type may look very worrying and be mistaken for adenocarcinoma. The ductal type shows large ducts with epithelium which often forms micropapillae. This form may be misdiagnosed as cervical intraepithelial glandular neoplasia. All of these patterns are entirely benign, though they may, in very rare cases, be associated with mesonephric carcinoma.

Diffuse laminar endocervical glandular hyperplasia

This condition is simply a hyperplasia of the superficial (inner third) endocervical crypts producing a discrete layer sharply demarcated from the underlying cervical stroma.[32] An inflammatory cell reaction may be seen but no desmoplastic stromal response is evident. The condition is completely benign.

Microglandular endocervical hyperplasia (MEH)

Whilst very common in women with no excess hormonal stimulation, this condition appears to be related (in its more florid forms) predominantly to progesterone stimulation, most commonly due to oral contraceptive use and less frequently to pregnancy, where it may be very extensive.[33] On some occasions it appears to be stimulated by estrogen alone. It is typically seen in young women but does occur postmenopausally. In some cone biopsy series it has been seen in almost 30% of cases.[33] The lesion may occasionally produce the macroscopic appearances of a polyp, erosion or even a carcinoma.[34]

Microscopically MEH may be sessile or polypoid. It consists of aggregated, closely packed, predominantly small, round glands. Typically the stroma is hyalinized and contains a marked acute and chronic inflammatory cell infiltrate (Fig. 1.14). Polymorphs are also seen in the gland lumina. Solid and reticular variants are described.[35] The lining cells are usually cuboidal and contain small, regular nuclei, sometimes with glycogen vacuoles. Mitoses are uncommon. Cellular vacuolation may be prominent. This condition may be confused with clear cell or other adenocarcinomas, particularly those MEH variants with nuclear pleomorphism,[35] but it is itself benign.[36] Immunohistochemistry can help in differentiation of atypical MEH variants and carcinoma in the rare cases where difficulties arise.[37]

Epithelial metaplasias and endometriosis

Tubal metaplasia

This is a common condition, present in almost a

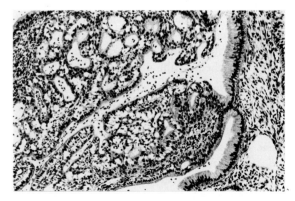

Fig. 1.14 Microglandular endocervical hyperplasia. Numerous small crypt outpouchings are seen clustered around the central crypt. Inflammatory cells are numerous and the endocervical cells appear vacuolate.

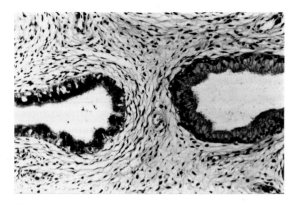

Fig. 1.15 Tubal metaplasia. To the left of the photograph is a normal endocervical crypt. The crypt to the right shows tubal-type ciliated cells. The cells appear hyperchromatic but no true atypia is evident.

third of all cervices in cone biopsy and hysterectomy specimens.[38] Essentially, it consists of replacement of the endocervical epithelium by ciliated, nonciliated and peg cells, as seen in the tubal epithelium (Fig. 1.15). It may occur within variant glandular patterns such as MEH. No atypia is seen and mitoses are very sparse. There is an undoubted association of tubal and endometrioid metaplasia (see below) with previous cervical surgery, particularly cone biopsy.[39] It occurs most commonly in deep crypts of the upper endocervix but also in superficial crypts and surface epithelium. In postconization specimens the changes tend to occur at the SCJ.

Whilst tubal metaplasia is entirely benign it may cause problems in histological diagnosis. Particularly when inflammatory changes are superadded it may be mistaken for cervical intraepithelial glandular neoplasia.[40] Immunohistochemical staining with HMFG1 and carcinoembryonic antigen (CEA) may help in the differentiation.[41,42]

Endometrioid metaplasia

This is usually seen in association with tubal metaplasia and is essentially the replacement of the endocervical mucinous epithelium by endometrial-type cells. Both tubal and endometrioid metaplasia may lead to considerable problems in cytological intepretation and differentiation from glandular neoplasia.

Intestinal (goblet cell) metaplasia

This is very rare[43] and, as goblet cells are common in high-grade cervical intraepithelial glandular neoplasia (CIGN), it is a diagnosis that should be made with caution.

Endometriosis

Cervical endometriosis (i.e., organized endometrioid glands and stroma) probably occurs in around 4% of cervices[30] but is undoubtedly more common at the SCJ after previous surgery or trauma.[39] It may be divided into superficial and deep variants. The superficial variant is rarely associated with endometriosis elsewhere in the pelvis. On the ectocervix it appears as small blue or red nodules, usually a few millimetres in diameter. Exfoliated cells in cytological preparations, as with tuboendometrioid metaplasia, may lead to an erroneous diagnosis of glandular neoplasia.

VAGINA

GROSS ANATOMY

The vagina extends from the vestibule to the uterus, lying dorsal (posterior) to the urinary bladder and ventral (anterior) to the rectum. According to Ulfelder & Robboy[44] it is probably of paramesonephric (Müllerian) duct origin caudally to the level of the hymen with urogenital sinus epithelium replacing paramesonephric epithelium to the level of the ectocervical os.

The long axis of the vagina forms an angle of more than 90° with that of the uterus. The vaginal length is approximately 7 cm along the ventral wall and 9 cm along the dorsal. The upper third of the vagina is supported by the levator plate and rectal attachment, the middle third by the pelvic diaphragm and inferior aspect of the cardinal ligaments and the lower third by the pelvic and urogenital diaphragms and the perineal body. These three 'compartments' define to a large extent tumor spread and disease localization. They also demarcate to some extent the lymphatic drainage systems, though divergent views are expressed in the literature on the vaginal lymphatic system. Lymphatic vessels are extensive in the superficial subepithelial tissues and anastomose in a deep perivaginal plexus in the adventitia. According to Plentl & Friedman[45] (as summarized by Fu & Reagan[46]) the lymphatics of the anterior vaginal wall drain into the lymph nodes of the lateral pelvic wall or vesical nodes, whereas the lymphatics of the posterior vaginal wall drain into the deep pelvic, rectal and aortic nodes. The lymphatics of the vaginal vault drain into the lateral and posterior pelvic nodes, as do those of the cervix. The lymphatics from the central portion of the vagina merge into lateral collecting trunks, which usually drain into the superior gluteal nodes. The lymphatics of the distal vagina anastomose with the lymphatics of the vestibule and drain into the femoral nodes. The vaginal lymphatics may also anastomose with those of the uterine cervix, urinary bladder and rectum.

The vaginal blood supply is derived from the vaginal artery which arises from the uterine or adjacent internal iliac artery and anastomoses with the uterine, inferior vesical and middle rectal arteries. It also anastomoses with the azygos artery. The veins collect into lateral channels which communicate with the uterine, vesical and rectal veins and eventually reach the internal iliac vein.

Only small numbers of nerve fibers penetrate the tunica propria of the vagina and terminate in the epithelium. No Paccinian or Meissner's corpuscles are seen in the muscularis and tunica propria. Most fibers supply the muscularis and adventitia.

The vagina only has a serosal aspect at the proximal, posterior margin where it borders the cul-de-sac. Elsewhere the adventitia is confluent with the endopelvic fascia.

HISTOLOGY

The vaginal wall has three layers: adventitia, muscularis and 'mucosa'. The 'mucosa' is in fact a simple squamous epithelium and no true mucosa and muscularis mucosa is seen. The vaginal surface shows folds or rugae composed of epithelium and connective tissue with intervening furrows. Numerous transverse rugae are seen throughout the vagina and there is one anterior and one posterior longitudual furrow.

The surface epithelium of the vagina is a stratified squamous epithelium similar to that of the ectocervix. It is nonkeratinizing and glycogenated. In the reproductive years the epithelium is 150–200 μm in thickness. The basement membrane is thin and histologically the epithelium undulates due to the rugal pattern. No subepithelial glands are seen. Lubrication of the vagina is probably simply by cervical secretions and transudation across the epithelium.[47] The epithelium can be divided on the basis of the cellular characteristics into different levels, as for the cervix (see above). Epithelial thickness varies both with age and to some extent with the menstrual cycle.[48] The greatest thickness is found between days 7 and 17 of the cycle corresponding with greatest glycogen content. In the postmenopausal and premenarchal woman the epithelium is very thin.

The superficial lamina propria, immediately beneath the epithelium, is loose, myxoid and may contain occasional somewhat pleomorphic triangular or stellate cells.[49] This subepithelial myxoid zone is also present in the cervix and vestibular area[50] and may play a part in the development of benign vaginal polyps[51] and embryonal rhabdomyosarcomas. This zone is more prominent in infants and children. Scattered lymphocytes are often seen near the epithelial base and even lymphoid aggregates may be seen in the absence of disease.[52]

The deeper lamina propria shows variably condensed connective tissue, generally loosely textured but becoming more condensed in its deeper parts. It contains elastic fibers and is highly vascular with numerous lymphatics also present. Beneath the lamina propria are inner circular and outer longitudinal muscle coats.

VULVA

GROSS ANATOMY

The vulva consists of the mons pubis, the labia majora and minora, the vestibule of the vagina, the hymen, the great vestibular (Bartholin's) glands, the clitoris, the bulbs of the vestibule and the external urethral orifice. Skene's glands and the minor vestibular glands also open into the vestibule.

The labia

The labia majora are paired cutaneous folds which become more prominent at puberty due to the deposition of subcutaneous fat, increase in skin melanin pigmentation and development of hair on their lateral aspects. They terminate in the mons pubis anteriorly and the perineal body posteriorly and form the lateral boundaries of the pudendal cleft. Development of pubic hair may be divided into five stages:[53] (1) no pubic hair, (2) sparse hair on the labia majora and on the mons pubis in the midline; (3) increase in hair on the mons pubis and thickening of the hair; (4) extension to all but the lateral corners of the 'adult' pubic triangle and further thickening; and (5) normal adult pattern with extension to the inner thighs.

Age of attainment of an adult pattern varies greatly (between 12 and 17 years of age in normal individuals).

The size of the labia majora varies with age, race and parity.[54] Asymmetry is not uncommon. During pregnancy or hormone therapy labial pigmentation may increase.[55] In the postmenopausal woman there is a gradual decline in density of hair follicles[56] and reduced pigmentation. Overall labial size also reduces somewhat with loss of subcutaneous fat and poor muscular tone. The introitus tends to gape. The infant vulva reflects maternal hormonal stimulation for approximately 4 weeks after delivery[57] with increased labial pigmentation, clitoral prominence, etc.

The labia minora are thin folds of hairless skin without subcutaneous fat and lie between the labia majora on either side of the vaginal and urethral openings. They are separated from the labia majora by the interlabial furrows. Anteriorly they divide to a rather variable degree into medial and lateral arms which pass respectively behind and in front of the glans of the clitoris to produce the anterior clitoral prepuce and the posterior clitoral frenulum. Posteriorly the labia minora fuse to form a transverse fold, the frenulum of the labia or fourchette, behind the vagina. Pigmentation of the labia minora also becomes more pronounced at puberty when the skin becomes rugose.

The mons pubis (mons veneris) forms a cushion of hair-bearing skin anterior to the labia and clitoris and covering the pubic symphysis. It becomes prominent at puberty due to the deposition of subcutaneous fat and hair growth.

The vestibule and hymen

The vestibule extends from the clitoris to fourchette and forms the cleft between the labia minora. Within the vestibule are the openings of the vagina, urethra and the ducts of Bartholin's and the minor vestibular glands which become active at puberty. The minor vestibular glands are tubular, mucin-secreting glands. Bartholin's glands are small, paired, rounded bodies lying in the deep tissues of the posterior aspect of the labia majora. The ducts of Bartholin's glands are approximately 2.5 cm in length and open onto the vestibular surface on its posterolateral aspect. The glands consist of lobular aggregates of mucin secreting acini the cells of which have clear, vacuolated cytoplasm and basal nuclei. The main duct is lined by transitional type epithelium in its deep portion but this changes to stratified squamous epithelium as the orifice is approached.[58]

The hymen is a thin, incomplete membrane of connective tissue at the junction of the vestibule and vagina. It is reduced by regular coitus to a series of small tags around the vaginal orifice — the carunculae myrtiformis. Around puberty the hymen thickens somewhat but the orifice increases in size.

Clitoris

The clitoris is composed entirely of erectile tissue covered with thinly keratinized squamous epithelium. It is situated in the midline anteriorly. Attached to the lower surface of the lateral urogenital diaphragm and ischiopubic rami are the crura of the clitoris which are covered by muscle. These crura extend anteriorly to form the corpora cavernosa and fuse beneath the pubis at the subpubic angle to form the body of the clitoris. Between the crura and the vaginal opening are two erectile tissue masses termed the vestibular bulbs, these are attached to the urogenital diaphragm and pass forwards around the urethra to form a fused slender erectile tissue band on the ventral surface of the clitoris. Engorgement of these vestibular bulbs during sexual arousal narrows the opening of the vagina.

The urethra

The urethra runs downwards and forwards from the internal urethral orifice, embedded in the anterior wall of the vagina. It passes through the pelvic floor and perineal membrane and ends at the urethral orifice, anterior to the vaginal opening and posterior to the clitoris. It is approximately 4 cm long.

The urethral mucosal aspect shows longitudinal folds; the posterior fold pushes into the lumen leading to a crescentric cross–section. The proximal urethra is lined by transitional epithelium identical to that of the bladder. The distal urethra is lined by nonkeratinizing squamous epithelium which makes up the majority of the lining. At the external urethral meatus the epithelium is keratinized. The lamina propria is made up of loose vascular connective tissue with numerous veins, resembling erectile tissue. The muscle coats are divided into an outer striated muscle layer and an inner smooth muscle layer. The outer layer makes up the external urethral sphincter. The fibers of the external sphincter are oblique and circular. In the middle third the wall is completely surrounded by muscle; in the upper and lower thirds the posterior wall contains little striated muscle. The inner smooth muscle layer is continuous, circular and oblique and fuses with the detrusor. In the lower third of the urethra there are gland groups on either side of the lumen. These possess common ducts which open at the lateral aspects of the external urethral orifice. These ducts are termed Skene's ducts (paraurethral ducts). The urethral epithelial lining is under the influence of ovarian hormones and the epithelial cells undergo cyclical changes similar to those seen in the vagina.[59] In the postmenopausal years the urethral epithelium undergoes atrophic change.

Blood, lymphatic and nerve supply

The arterial supply of the perineum comes from branches of the internal iliac and femoral arteries. The femoral artery in the femoral triangle gives off the superficial and deep pudendal arteries and the internal pudendal artery leaves the internal iliac and passes through the greater sciatic notch and lesser sciatica foramen to enter the anal triangle of the perineum posteriorly. Venous drainage mirrors the arterial supply. The vaginal and vulval veins appear to be very progesterone sensitive[60] in that varices are commonest in pregnancy and often form in the first trimester (arguing against a purely mechanical cause). Varices in the nonpregnant may undergo cyclical changes with the menstrual cycle.

Lymphatic drainage is to regional lymph nodes in the groins. These drain to deep pelvic nodes and ultimately to para-aortic nodes. The drainage is bilateral with the labia minora draining to both ipsi- and contralateral nodes.[61–63]

THE HISTOLOGY OF THE VULVAR SKIN

Epithelium

The vulvar epithelium is of keratinized, stratified squamous type. The epithelium may be divided into four layers: basal, prickle cell, granular and horny (Fig. 1.16). The basal layer consists of tall, darkly staining cells which are applied closely to the basement membrane. Mitoses are found largely in this layer. Those mitoses that appear higher are often seen on deeper sectioning to be associated with the tips of dermal papillae. The basement membrane is a homogeneous band 0.5–1.0 μm thick which is rich in mucopolysaccharides. It is seen clearly on periodic acid-

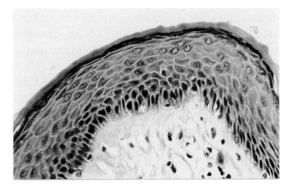

Fig. 1.16 The keratinizing squamous epithelium of the labia majora is shown. The four epithelial layers — basal, prickle, granular and horny — can be seen.

Schiff staining. It should not be confused with the electron micsoscopically visualized basal lamina which is a true membrane only 35–45 nm thick.

Immediately above the basal layer the keratinocyte differentiates to produce the larger, polygonal cells of the prickle cell layer where intercellular bridges are prominent. The keratinocytes then flatten and broaden with cytoplasmic, eosinophilic, keratohyalin granules — the granular layer. Above this the cells lose their nuclei and become intensely eosinophilic due to keratinization. The skin of the labia and clitoral frenulum has relatively inconspicuous granular and horny layers. Epithelial turnover time is probably between 59 and 75 days.[64] The skin on the medial aspects of the labia minora is often described as a mucosal surface; this is incorrect as it has no submucosa. It is however devoid of granular and horny layers (and therefore nonkeratinized) and is hormone sensitive,[59] undergoing the same series of changes with the menstrual cycle as those seen in the vagina.

Within the vulvar epithelium are three cell types which are not keratinocyte derived: the melanocyte, the Langerhans cell and the Merkel cell. The melanocytes lie predominantly in the basal layer of the epidermis. They are between one-tenth and one-fifth as common as keratinocytes.[65] These cells produce the pigment melanin. They are best demonstrated by the dopa reaction, silver impregnation or by immunohistochemical staining with anti-S100 antibody. As well as sunlight, the production of melanin is under the influence of hormones though the nature of this effect is unclear. Melanocytes appear to transfer melanosomes to keratinocytes by active phagocytosis of melanocyte dendrites by keratinocytes. Both estrogens and progestagens increase melanin pigmentation of the vulva.

Langerhans cells are bone-marrow-derived cells with extensive elongated cell processes (dendritic cells). They are intimately concerned with the body's immune system and act as antigen-presenting cells[64] and in activating T-cells. They express a range of surface antigens including Fc and C3 receptors and appear approximately one-fifth as frequent as squamous cells on the vulva. They occur throughout the epithelial thickness but are usually evident as high-level clear cells on H and E staining. They can be demonstrated by impregnation with gold chloride or by immunostaining with anti-OKT6. They do not react to ultraviolet light. They may occasionally be seen in the dermis. Merkel cells are neuroendocrine in origin and are found singly or in clusters in or just above the basal epithelium. They too have dendritic processes and they are intimately associated with nerve fibres via Merkel cell – neurite complexes.[64] They may act as paracrine regulatory cells and are thought to function as mechanoreceptors.

Dermis and adnexal structures

The dermis is divisible into the papillary portion which projects between the epithelial ridges (rete ridges) and the deeper reticular dermis which extends to the subcutaneous fat. The papillary dermis contains fine collagen fibers passing at right angles to the surface. The collagen in the reticular dermis lies parallel to the surface and is coarse. Elastic fibres and vascular and lymphatic plexuses are also present.

The labia majora and mons pubis contain numerous hair follicles with associated sebaceous glands and are rich in apocrine sweat glands. Eccrine sweat glands are also present. Occasionally modified sweat glands in the form of breast tissue are seen in the labia majora, which is at the extreme caudal end of the milk line.

Eccrine sweat glands are tubular glands with a basal coil from which a duct leads through the dermis directly into the epidermis. They comprise three segments: a secretory portion (Fig. 1.17), intradermal duct and intraepidermal duct (Fig. 1.18). The secretory portion makes up half of the basal coil which lies at the junction of the dermis and subcutaneous fat or at the lower border of the dermis. The secretory portion shows only one layer of distinct cells, of two types, clear and dark, with an outer layer of myoepithelial cells. Clear cells produce aqueous material and glycogen, dark cells sialomucins. The intradermal duct has two layers of small, basophilic epithelial cells. The intraepidermal portion is spiral, with a lining of migrated dermal duct cells (one inner, two to three outer).

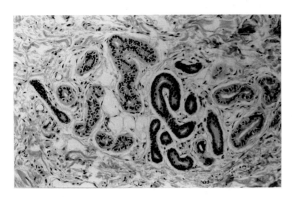

Fig. 1.17 In the center of the picture is the basal coil of an eccrine vulvar sweat gland. The paler staining elements make up the secretory portion. Light and dark cells cannot be clearly defined here.

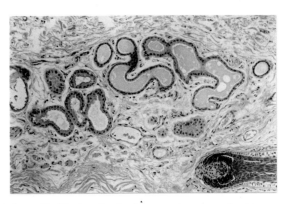

Fig. 1.19 The basal coil of an apocrine sweat gland is seen adjacent to the base of a hair follicle. Even at this magnification the apical secretory 'snouts' of the apocrine cells can be seen to the left of the picture.

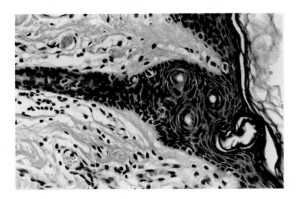

Fig. 1.18 The intraepidermal eccrine duct is clearly shown spiralling to the surface.

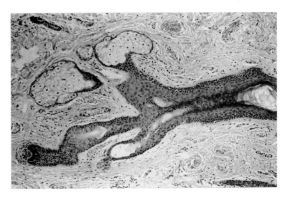

Fig. 1.20 Lobules of a sebaceous gland are seen opening into a hair follicle. The peripheral basophilic cells are not well seen at this magnification but the lipid-rich vacuolated cells are clearly evident.

Apocrine glands, together with hair and sebaceous glands, derive from the hair germ. The duct usually ends in a pilosebaceous follicle above the sebaceous duct. These glands are also tubular with lining cells which undergo decapitation secretion. There are again three gland segments, as in eccrine glands. The basal coil lies in the subcutaneous fat and is composed purely of secretory cells (Fig. 1.19). The secretions are sialomucins.

The labia minora are usually hairless and without sweat glands but sebaceous glands are present, particularly anteriorly near the clitoris; this is the only site other than the areola of the nipple where sebaceous glands are present without hair follicles in the female. Sebaceous glands usually have several lobules which open into a common duct lined by stratified squamous epithelium and, on the labia majora, thence into the pilosebaceous follicle (Fig. 1.20). The sebaceous lobule consists of a peripheral layer of basophilic cuboidal cells with, internal to this, lipid-rich vacuolated cells. These cells disintegrate to produce the gland secretion (holocrine secretion). Sebaceous glands are well developed at birth but atrophy after a few months. At puberty the glands again enlarge.

The detailed structure of the hair follicle is not pertinent to this chapter but reviews are widely available.[64]

REFERENCES

1. Krantz K E. The anatomy of the human cervix, gross and microscopic. In: Blandau R J, Moghissi K, eds. The biology of the cervix. Chicago: University of Chicago Press, 1973; p 57.
2. Gustafson R. The vascular, lymphatic and neural anatomy of the cervix. In: Jordan J, Singer A, eds. The cervix. London: Saunders, 1976; p 50.
3. Reiffenstuhl G. The lymphatics of the female genital organs, 1st edn. Philadelphia: J B Lippincott, 1964.
4. Koss L G. Diagnostic cytology and its histopathologic bases, 3rd edn. Philadelphia: J B Lippincott, 1979.
5. Kolstad P, Stafl A. Atlas of colposcopy, 2nd edn. Baltimore: University Park Press, 1977.
6. Kupryjanczykj J, Kujawa M. Signet ring cells in squamous cell carcinoma of the cervix and in non-neoplastic ectocervical epithelium. Int J Gynecol Cancer 1992; 2: 152–156.
7. Barton S E, Maddox P H, Jenkins D, Edwards R, Cuzick J, Singer A. Effect of cigarette smoking on cervical epithelial immunity: a mechanism for neoplastic change? Lancet 1988; 2: 652–654.
8. Whitaker E M, Nimmo A J, Morrison J F B, Griffin N R, Wells M. The distribution of β-adrenoreceptors in the human cervix. Quart J Exper Physiol 1989; 74: 573–576.
9. Wakefield E A, Wells M. Histochemical study of endocervical glycoproteins throughout the normal menstrual cycle and adjacent to cervical intraepithelial neoplasia. Int J Gynecol Pathol 1985; 4: 230–239.
10. Gilks C B, Reid P E, Clement P B, Owen D A. Histochemical changes in cervical mucus-secreting epithelium during the normal menstrual cycle. Fertil Steril 1989; 51: 286–291.
11. Fetissof F, Berger G, Dubois M P et al. Endocrine cells in the female genital tract. Histopathology 1985; 9: 133–146.
12. Fluhman C F. The cervix uteri and its diseases, 1st edn. Philadephia: J B Saunders, 1961.
13. Anderson M C, Hartley R B. Cervical crypt involvement by intraepithelial neoplasia. Obstet Gynecol 1980; 55: 546–550.
14. Gould P R, Barter R A, Papadimitriou J M. An ultrastructural, cytodynamical and autoradiographic study of the mucous membrane of the human cervical canal with reference to subcolumnar cells. Am J Pathol 1979; 95: 1–16.
15. Singer A, Jordan J A. The anatomy of the cervix. In: Jordan J A, Singer A, eds. The cervix. London: J B Saunders, 1976; p 13.
16. Pixley E. Morphology of the fetal and prepubertal cervicovaginal epithelium. In: Jordan J A, Singer A, eds. The cervix. London: J B Saunders, 1976.
17. Feldman D, Romney S L, Edgcomb J, Valentine T. Ultrastructure of normal, metaplastic and abnormal uterine cervix: use of montages to study the topographical relationship of epithelial cells. Am J Obstet Gynecol 1984; 150: 573–688.
18. Ferenczy A, Winkler B. Anatomy and histology of the cervix. In: Kurman R, ed. Blaustein's pathology of the female genital tract, 3rd edn. New York: Springer-Verlag, 1987; p 141.
19. Mayer R. Die Epithelentwicklung der cervix und Portio vaginalis uteri. Archive Gynaekologica 1910; 91: 579–586.
20. Song J. The human uterus: morphogenesis and embryological basis for cancer. Ilinois: Thomas, 1964.
21. Lawrence D W, Shingleton H M. Early physiologic squamous metaplasia of the cervix, light and electron microscopic observations. Am J Obstet Gynecol 1980; 137: 661–671.
22. Singer A, Reid B L, Coppleson M. The role of peritoneal mononuclear cells in the regeneration of the uterine epithelium of the rat. Aust NZ J Obstet Gynecol 1968; 8: 163–170.
23. Morris H H B, Galter K G, Sykes G, Casemore V, Reason D Y. Langerhans cells in human cervical epithelium: an immunohistochemical study. Br J Obstet Gynaecol 1983; 90: 400–411.
24. Clement P B, Young R H. Deep nabothian cysts of the endocervix. A possible source of confusion with minimal-deviation adenocarcinoma (adenoma malignum). Int J Gynecol Pathol 1989; 8: 340–348.
25. Coppleson M, Reid B, Singer A, Sullivan J. Quoted in: Jordan J, Singer A, eds. The cervix. London: Saunders, 1976; p 88–89.
26. Robledo M C, Vasquez J J, Contreras-Mejuto F, Lopez-Garcia G. Sebaceous glands and hair follicles in the cervix uteri. Histopathology 1992; 21: 278–280.
27. Anderson M C. The cervix, excluding cancer. In: Female reproductive system, 3rd edn. London: Churchill Livingstone, 1991; p 47.
28. Johnson L D. Dysplasia and carcinoma-in-situ in pregnancy. In: Norris H J, Hertig A T, Abell M R, eds. The uterus. Baltimore: Williams & Wilkins, 1973; p 382.
29. Segal G H, Hart W R. Cystic endocervical tunnel clusters. A clinicopathologic study of 29 cases of so-called adenomatous hyperplasia. Am J Surg Pathol 1990; 14: 895–903.
30. Brown L J R, Wells M. Cervical glandular atypia associated with squamous intraepithelial neoplasia: a premalignant lesion. J Clin Pathol 1986; 39: 22–28.
31. Ferry J A, Scully RE. Mesonephric remnants, hyperplasia and neoplasia in the uterine cervix: a study of 49 cases. Am J Surg Pathol 1990; 14: 1100–1111.
32. Jones M A, Young R H, Scully R E. Diffuse laminar endocervical glandular hyperplasia: a report of seven cases. Am J Surg Pathol 1991; 15: 1123–1129.
33. Nichols T M, Fidler H I C. Microglandular hyperplasia in cervical cone biopsies taken for suspicious and positive cytology. Am J Clin Pathol 1971; 56: 424–429.
34. Wilkinson E, Dufour D R. Pathogenesis of microglandular hyperplasia of the cervix uteri. Obstet Gynecol 1976; 47: 189–195.
35. Young R H, Scully R E. Atypical forms of microglandular hyperplasia of the cervix simulating adenocarcinoma: a report of five cases and review of the literature. Am J Surg Pathol 1989; 13: 50–56.
36. Jones M W, Silverberg S G. Cervical adenocarcinoma in young women. Possible relationship to microglandular hyperplasia and use of oral contraceptives. Obstet Gynecol 1989; 73: 984–989.
37. Young R H, Clement P B. Tumorlike lesions of the uterine cervix. In: Clement P B, Young R H. Tumors and tumorlike lesions of the uterine corpus and cervix. New York: Churchill Livingstone, 1993; p 1.

38. Jonasson J G, Wang H H, Antonioli D A, Ducatman B S. Tubal metaplasia of the uterine cervix: a prevalence study in patients with gynecologic pathologic findings. Int J Gynecol Pathol 1992; 11: 89–95.

39. Ismail S M. Cone biopsy causes cervical endometriosis and tubo-endometrial metaplasia. Histopathology 1991; 18: 107–114.

40. Jaworski R C, Pacey N F, Greenberg M C, Osborne R A. The histologic diagnosis of adenocarcinoma-in-situ and related lesions of the cervix uteri. Cancer 1988; 61: 1171–1181.

41. Brown L J R, Griffin N R, Wells M. Cytoplasmic reactivity with the monoclonal antibody HMFG1 as a marker of cervical glandular atypia. J Pathol 1987; 151: 203–208.

42. Rollason T P, Byrne P, Williams A, Brown G. Expression of epithelial membrane and 3 fucosyl-*N*-acetyllactosamine antigens in cervix uteri with particular reference to adenocarcinoma-in-situ. J Clin Pathol 1988; 41: 547–552.

43. Trowell J E. Intestinal metaplasia with argentaffin cells in the uterine cervix. Histopathology 1985; 9: 551–559.

44. Ulfelder H, Robboy S. The embryologic development of the human vagina. Am J Obstet Gynecol 1976; 126: 769–776.

45. Plentl A A, Friedman E A. Lymphatic system of the female genitalia. Philadelphia: W B Saunders, 1971.

46. Fu Y S, Reagan J W. Development, anatomy and histology of the lower female genital tract. In: Pathology of the uterine cervix, vagina & vulva. Philadelphia: W B Saunders, 1989; p 21.

47. Sedlis A, Robboy S J. Diseases of the vagina. In: Kurman R J, ed. Blaustein's pathology of the female genital tract, 3rd edn. New York: Springer-Verlag, 1987; p 97.

48. Gregoire A T, Kandil O, Ledger W J. Glycogen content of human vaginal tissues. Fertil Steril 1971; 27: 64–68.

49. Elliot G B, Elliot J D. Superficial stromal reactions of the female genital tract. Arch Pathol 1973; 95: 100–101.

50. Clement P B. Multinucleated stromal giant cells of the uterine cervix. Arch Pathol Lab Med 1985; 109: 200–202.

51. Rollason T P, Byrne P, Williams A. Immunohistochemical and electron microscopic findings in benign fibroepithelial vaginal polyps. J Clin Pathol 1990; 43: 224–229.

52. Schmidt W A. Pathology of the vagina. In: Fox H, ed. Haines & Taylor Obstetrical and gynaecological pathology, 3rd edn. Edinburgh: Churchill Livingstone, 1987; p 146.

53. Tanner J M. Growth at adolescence, 2nd edn. Oxford: Blackwell, 1962.

54. Krantz K E. The anatomy and physiology of the vulva and vagina. In: Philipp E E, Barnes J, Newton M, eds. Scientific foundation of obstetrics and gynaecology, 2nd edn. London: Heinemann, 1977; p 65.

55. Parker F. Skin and hormones. In: Williams R H, ed. Textbook of endocrinology. Philadelphia: W B Saunders, 1981.

56. Barman J M, Astore J, Pecoraro V. The normal trichogram of people over 50 years. In: Montagna W, Dobson R L, eds. Advances in biology of skin, vol IX, Hair growth. Oxford: Pergamon Press, 1969.

57. Dewhurst J. Quoted in: McLean J M. Anatomy and physiology of the vulval area. In: Ridley C M, ed. The vulva. Edinburgh: Churchill Livingstone, 1988; p 57.

58. Rorat E, Ferenczy A, Richart R M. Human Bartholin gland, duct and duct cyst. Arch Pathol 1975; 99: 367–374.

59. McLean J M. Anatomy and physiology of the vulval area. In: Ridley C M, ed. The vulva. Edinburgh: Churchill Livingstone, 1988; p 39.

60. Gallagher P C. Varicose veins of the vulva. Br J Sexual Med 1986; 13: 12–14.

61. Iversen T, Aas M. Lymph drainage from the vulva. Gynecol Oncol 1983; 16: 179–189.

62. Figge D C, Tamimi H K, Greer B E. Lymphatic spread in carcinoma of the vulva. Am J Obstet Gynecol 1985; 152: 387–394.

63. Philipp E E, Barnes J, Newton M. Scientific foundations of obstetrics and gynaecology. London: Heineman, 1977; p 118.

64. Lever W F, Schaumberg-Lever G. Histology of the skin. In: Histopathology of the skin, 3rd edn. Philadelphia: Lippincott, 1983; p 8.

65. Cochran A J. The incidence of melanocytes in normal skin. J Invest Dermatol 1970; 55: 65–70.

2. The pathology of cervical neoplasia

Ralph M. Richart   Thomas C. Wright

INTRODUCTION

Virtually all neoplasms of the cervical squamous and endocervical epithelium arise as a consequence of human papillomavirus (HPV) infection (see Refs 1–4 for recent reviews). Cervical intra-epithelial neoplasia (CIN), vaginal intraepithelial neoplasia (VAIN), vulvar intraepithelial neoplasia (VIN), perianal intraepithelial neoplasia (PAIN), penile intraepithelial neoplasia (PIN), and their invasive counterparts contain elements of the HPV genome which can be identified using standard molecular techniques, such as filter in-situ hybridization (FISH), dot or slot blot hybridization, Southern blot hybridization, or in situ hybridization.

It has long been known that cervical neoplasia rarely, or never, occurs in virgins and that its clinical pattern is that of a sexually-transmitted disease. Recently,[5] it was reported that there is a very strong correlation between the number of sexual partners a woman has had and the risk of infection with HPV. The fact that the risk is step-wise and is associated with other risk factors for cervical cancer confirms the importance of the number of sexual partners in a woman's risk of developing an HPV-related lesion of the genital tract.

The epidemiological data linking HPV with lower anogenital tract epithelial neoplasia have been reviewed.[6] The most important features are as follows: (1) the vast majority of women with CIN have concurrently detectable HPV DNA and the rate is substantially higher than in controls; (2) HPV detection is associated with a 10-fold or greater risk of cervical neoplasia; (3) in high-grade CIN lesions the relative risk of neoplasia asso-

ciated with HPV is 40; (4) the proportion of CIN apparently attributable to HPV infection is about 90%; (5) women who are HPV DNA positive and Papanicolaou (Pap) smear negative have an increased risk of developing CIN within the first 1–2 years of follow-up; and (6) the risk of progression of HPV-related lesions may be correlated with the viral type.

These data support a 'central, causal role' for HPV in epithelial neoplasia of the lower anogenital tract and complement the vast amount of clinical, morphological, and molecular data which support the same conclusion. It is generally assumed that the initial HPV infection in the genital tract epithelium requires that the virus be in the form of a complete virion — that is, a central core of DNA surrounded by its protein coat. HPV is a DNA tumor virus that has a double-stranded, tightly coiled, circular genome of about 8000 Da.[7,8] When the capsid protein is fully formed, it forms an icosahedral structure. A complete virion measures approximately 55 nm in diameter. The mechanism of attachment of the virus and the early phases of its infection are not understood.

HPVs are named by number and are numbered according to their order of discovery. More than 66 different types have been identified and type based upon their hybridization homology. Of these, more than 20 infect the male and female lower anogenital tract (Table 2.1).

It has recently become clear[9] that HPVs can be divided into three groups: those of low or no oncogenic potential, those of high oncogenic potential, and those of intermediate oncogenic potential. The low oncogenic potential group includes HPV types 6, 11, and the 40 s other than 45; the intermediate oncogenic potential group

Table 2.1 Anogenital human papillomaviruses

HPV type	Disease association	Oncogenic association
6	Condyloma accuminata Low-grade dysplasias Laryngeal papillomas	Rarely malignant
11	Condylomata acuminata Low-grade dysplasias Laryngeal papillomas Conjunctival papillomas	Rarely malignant
16	CIN 1–3 Bowenoid papulosis Bowen's disease Cervical, vulvar, and anal cancers	Malignant
18	CIN 3; rarely CIN 1–2 Cervical cancers	Highly malignant
31	CIN 1–3, cancers	Malignant
33	CIN 1–3, cancers	Malignant
35	CIN 1–3, cancers	Malignant
39	Bowenoid papulosis	Rarely malignant
41	Condylomata and cutaneous flat warts	Benign
42	Flat condylomata Bowenoid papulosis	Benign
43	Low-grade dysplasias	Benign
44	Condylomata acuminata	Benign
45	Condylomata/CIN/cancers	? Highly malignant
51	CIN 1–3, cancers	Malignant
52	Condylomata acuminata CIN 1–3, cancers	Malignant
53	Genital HPV	?
54	Genital HPV	?
55	Genital HPV	?
56	Condylomata acuminata CIN 1–3, cancers	? Highly malignant
57	Genital HPV	?
58	Genital HPV	?
59	Genital HPV	?

includes types 31, 33, 35, 51, and 52; and the high oncogenic potential group includes types 16, 18, 45, and 56. In the high oncogenic potential group, type 16 is distinguished from types 18, 45, and 56. These last three types appear to have the highest oncogenic potential as they are underrepresented in CIN lesions and overrepresented in cancers.

The suggestion that CIN 1 and flat condyloma be grouped together as low-grade CIN[10] (or cytologically as low-grade squamous intraepithelial lesion (SIL)[11]) and that CIN 2 and 3 be grouped together as high-grade CIN (or cytologically as high-grade SIL) was based on molecular, biological, and clinical evidence that favors such a grouping. In studies of HPV types in low-grade and high-grade CIN lesions,[12] it was found that

there was substantial heterogeneity in the low-grade CINs. Nineteen percent of the low-grade lesions contained HPV types 6 or 11; 29% types 16, 18, or 33; and 19% 'novel types.' Twenty-two percent had more than one HPV type identified. In contrast, high-grade CINs contained types 16, 18, or 33 in 88% of the lesions, and only 7% were associated with multiple HPV types.

It has been thought for more than 20 years that intraepithelial neoplasia (IN) as it occurs in the male and female lower anogenital tract is a continuum of change which, in the cervix, begins with CIN 1 (mild dysplasia), progresses through CIN 2 (moderate dysplasia), and CIN 3 (severe dysplasia/carcinoma-in-situ), and ends with invasion.[13,14] It is clear from recent molecular studies, however, that, although the concept of a continuum is useful clinically and histologically, the changes which begin with HPV infection and end with invasive cancer occur in a step-wise, not in a continuous, fashion and that discrete events can be identified which profoundly change the biology of these diseases.

When the virus enters the nucleus, it may remain there in a latent form or it may produce an active, replicative infection in which the number of viral particles increases substantially during the life-cycle of the epithelial cell until the cell, containing large numbers of complete virions, is exfoliated at the cell surface. This productive infection is associated with viral cytopathogenic effects (CPE), and it is these CPEs which create the typical histological and cytological changes which the pathologist can recognize as being due to a productive HPV infection and which are generally designated condyloma, flat condyloma, or CIN 1, depending on the configuration and site of the lesion (Fig. 2.1).[15–17]

It is instructive to discuss the pathological changes which occur in the lower genital tract in terms of latent HPV infection, productive HPV infection, and IN.

LATENT INFECTION

There is relatively little direct information concerning latent infection of the epithelia with HPV. It is assumed that the epithelial cells are infected by the virus but that viral replication

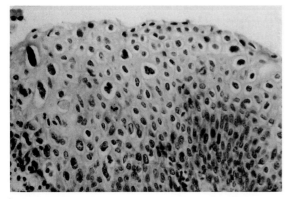

A

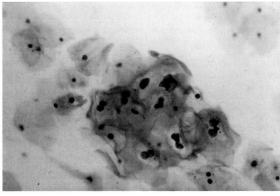

B

Fig. 2.1 The cytopathic effects of an HPV infection that can be detected either in **A** histological specimens, or **B** cytologic specimens include perinuclear halos, multinucleation, hyperchromatic nuclei, and irregular outlines.

does not occur except as a single copy duplication during the cell's normal replicative cycle. It is assumed that the epithelium can be infected latently because a significant number of patients can be identified as producing low levels of HPV DNA in the absence of a clinical lesion or morphologically identifiable CPE.[18–21] Clinical observations of sexually inactive women who have no clinical or cytological evidence of HPV-related changes but who develop such changes following immunosuppression are highly suggestive of the presence of epithelial cells containing latent virus particles which became productive when the immunological controls on viral replication were relaxed.[22,23] Similar observations of HPV changes which occur during pregnancy and regress follow-

ing pregnancy suggest that the concept of HPV latency is valid.[24]

Is it important to stress that the hallmark of a latent infection is that there are no clinical, colposcopic, cytological, or histological changes which identify that the host is infected with HPV. The only way the latent infection is discovered is through screening with highly sensitive molecular probes or by biological inference when lesions develop in the absence of an obvious source of a new HPV infection. The concept of HPV latency is important clinically, as it has been used as a justification for extensive — and, oftentimes, harmful — treatment of histologically normal-appearing mucosa. Paradoxically, it has also been used as a justification for not treating low-grade CIN, as latent virus cannot easily be eradicated. It is important to remember that the goal of therapy is to eradicate lesions and not to treat HPV DNA. If a latent virus remains latent, then the woman or man would appear not to be at risk for the subsequent development of genital-wart-related cancer. If the virus becomes reactivated, then it will produce CPE, and it will be possible to identify the activation. Therefore, although biological latency clearly occurs, it appears be an irrelevant issue when considering therapy and follow-up of HPV-related lesions.

The concept of histological, cytological, or molecular biological latency must be differentiated from the concept of the subclinical lesion which has been defined in several different ways. Small, papillary projections on the medial aspects of the labia and around the introitus are sometimes referred to as subclinical lesions, as are the small macules and papules which occur on the HPV-infected penis.[20,25,26] Similarly, some authors have used the term 'latent infection' or 'subclinical infection' to describe the atypical transformation zone in the cervix of women who are cytologically negative. This clinical concept of subclinical HPV infection is taken to mean any lesion which cannot be detected by visual inspection or a Pap smear but is identified using other techniques to be HPV-related. If the cell is latently infected and the virus only replicates one time with each cell division, it will not produce CPEs, and there is no available technique with which to identify specific cells which are HPV infected. HPV DNA positive/Pap smear negative patients can be identified by inference as being HPV infected, but it is impossible to identify individual cells which are latently infected, as molecular probe technology is insufficiently sensitive to detect such a low copy number in individual cells. Hence, the pathologist or cytologist is left with being able to identify as being HPV infected only those cells which contain CPEs or which contain a sufficiently large number of viral particles to be detected by in-situ hybridization for HPV DNA or RNA. For all practical purposes, this is limited to individual cells with a minimum of 10–50 copies per cell.[27]

SCREENING FOR SUBCLINICAL OR LATENT HPV INFECTIONS

Screening by colposcopy, cervicography,[28] acetic acid application, or visual inspection has produced a literature in which it has been stated that there is a high rate of apparent HPV infections which are not detected by cytology or conventional screening techniques. These studies all rely upon histology as the gold standard, and it has been argued that subtle histological and cytological changes are associated with latently infected epithelia which do not have fully developed CPE and which are not detected by cytology. Investigators have suggested that cytology may have a false-negative rate as high as 80% and that the prevalence of lower vaginal, introital, and labial HPV infections may be as high as 15–20% in certain populations.

The best example of these putative subclinical latently infected epithelia are the symmetrical micropapillary projections which are commonly seen on the medial aspects of the labia, around the introitus and in the region of the hymenal ring (Fig. 2.2).[26] This region of the female genital tract appears commonly to contain areas of papillomatosis, acanthosis, parakeratosis, and mild variation in nuclear size and shape commonly accompanied by small but uniform perinuclear halos (Fig. 2.3). This constellation of changes has commonly been diagnosed as being HPV-related. Such lesions are uniformly negative using in-situ hybridization for HPV DNA, and such patients, when tested for the presence of HPV DNA in the genital tract using slot blot or Southern blot techniques or even

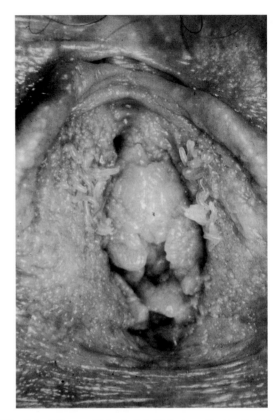

Fig. 2.2 Micropapillomatosis labialis presents as symmetric micropapillary projections that develop on the medial aspects of the labia.

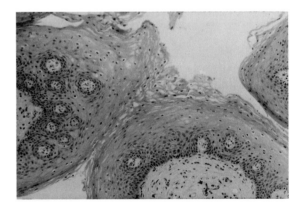

Fig. 2.3 Biopsies of micropapillomatosis labialis contain papillomatosis, acanthosis, and parakeratosis but lack the characteristic cytopathic effects associated with HPV infections.

the highly sensitive polymerase chain reaction, have no higher rate of detectable HPV DNA than do appropriately chosen controls. Micropapillomatosis vulvae appears to be a normal anatomical finding in many women which is sometimes accentuated due to the presence of monilia or other vaginitidies. It is important to note that micropapillomatosis labialis uniformly lacks the full constellation of cytological and histological alterations which consitute HPVs' CPE. Without such changes, such 'lesions' are almost always pathologists' diseases rather than patients' diseases.

Similarly, the extraordinarily high prevalence of HPV infections and the extraordinarily high false-negative rate of cytology reported in many cervicographic studies strongly suggest that the problem is not cytological false negativity but histological overdiagnosis.[29,30] Some of the photomicrographs accompanying articles on this subject serve to confirm that this is probably the case. In our consultation material, we commonly review biopsies taken as a result of cervicographic or colposcopic screening of the cervix which have been interpreted as containing CIN 1 or a higher grade lesion. It is our general experience that the vast majority of such histological diagnoses in patients with negative Pap smears are in error and that the changes are, in fact, squamous metaplasia, reparative processes, or other alterations which produce mild cytological changes but do not contain the typical CPE required for the diagnosis of an HPV-related lesion. If clinicians are to use magnification techniques for screening and to rely upon the histopathological diagnoses of biopsies taken from colposcopically or cervicographically abnormal areas, it is incumbant upon them to be certain that the pathologist is rendering an accurate diagnosis on the submitted biopsies, particularly if positive biopsy diagnoses are associated with negative Pap smears in 20% of the cases or more. Under such circumstances, we believe it is appropriate to evaluate the accuracy of the pathologists' diagnoses and to use in-situ hybridization for HPV DNA to quality control the diagnoses (see below).

CERVICAL INTRAEPITHELIAL NEOPLASIA

CIN has classically been divided into three grades — CIN 1, CIN 2, and CIN 3 — corresponding to the old terminology of mild dysplasia, moderate dysplasia, and severe dysplasia/carcinoma-in-situ, respectively.[13] The CIN terminology was promulgated to foster the idea of a continuum and, particularly, to abrogate the concept of a two-stage disease process — a benign dysplasia and a precancerous carcinoma-in-situ. Recent molecular evidence, however, suggests that the development of cervical cancer from precursor lesions occurs in a series of discrete steps and that a conceptually more accurate representation of the biologic potential of the lesions would be obtained by dividing the disease process into two, rather than three, stages. These have been designated low-grade CIN and high-grade CIN, based upon a number of criteria which will be outlined below.[31] This roughly corresponds to the low-grade SIL and high-grade SIL which was proposed as the Bethesda classification for cytological diagnoses.[11] However, the Bethesda classification must be based on somewhat more arbitrary criteria, as the sample is cytological rather than histological and as some of the characteristic changes can only be detected in histological sections.

Low-grade CIN

Low-grade CIN lesions are classically well differentiated and can be identified due to the presence of the typical CPE of HPV. Papillomavirus, when it infects a mucous membrane epithelium and produces a productive infection, uniformly produces an alteration in the growth pattern and cytology of the epithelial cells. The cytological changes in low-grade lesions are a result of the development of nuclear polyploidy, which is one of the most characteristic CPEs.[32] Any deviation in the normal amount of DNA in a population of cells is referred to as heteroploidy. The two most commonly encountered types of heteroploidy are polyploidy and aneuploidy. Polyploidy is defined as even multiples of the normal amount of DNA and is found physiologically in a number of human tissues, including the liver, cerebellum, corpus luteum of pregnancy, and the Arias-Stella reaction of the endometrium. It is also found as one of the characteristic features of productive HPV infections.[32] Aneuploidy is defined as an abnormal amount of DNA or abnormal chromosome number which is not an even multiple of the haploid number. Aneuploidy is generally believed to be a rather specific marker for cancer or a cancer precursor in the absence of prior treatment with chemotherapeutic or radiotherapeutic agents, both of which might produce confusing cytologic alterations.

HPV appears to interfere with the normal conduct of mitosis in productively infected cells and to interfere with cytokinesis. As the nuclear DNA content doubles in preparation for mitosis, polyploidy results in those cells which fail to complete mitosis successfully. Multinucleated cells commonly occur, and the degree of polyploidization increases through multinucleation. When this mechanism is understood, it can readily be appreciated that CIN 1 lesions are recognizable due to the effects of polyploidization on the cell population. All heteroploid epithelia contain nuclei which vary in their size, shape, staining, and chromatin distribution pattern. This constellation is generally referred to as cytological atypia. As polyploidization and cytological atypia appear

to be a constant accompaniment of a productive HPV infection in the cervical mucous membrane, they should be considered to be a *sine qua non* for the diagnosis of an HPV-related lesion. As the mechanism of polyploidization is through multinucleation, the presence of multinucleated cells should also be viewed in the early stages of this disease process to be a *sine qua non* for an HPV-related diagnosis. The other effects include an increased mitotic rate (which will generally lead to an increase in mitotic figures) and koilocytosis (the degenerative change of the cytoplasm which histologically is seen as a perinuclear halo (Fig. 2.1)). The full CPE of HPV in the early productive infection include an increased mitotic rate, multinucleation, cytological atypia, and koilocytosis (Fig. 2.4). These changes may be

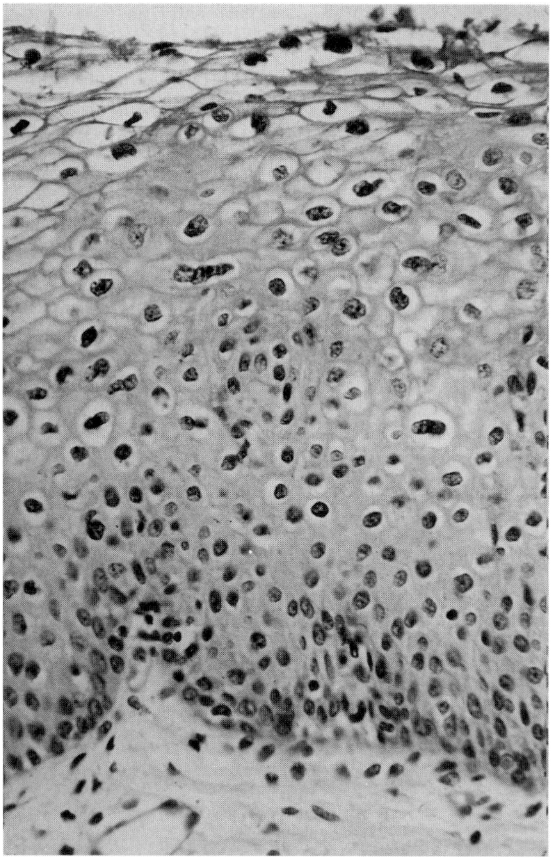

Fig. 2.4 Low-grade CIN lesion with extensive HPV cytopathogenic effects, including nuclear enlargement and hyperchromaticity, multinucleation, and perinuclear halos.

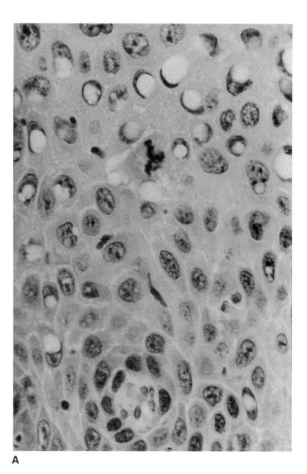

A

Fig. 2.5 Abnormal mitotic figures detected in CIN lesions. **A** Tripolar mitotic figure that can be detected in low-grade CIN lesion.

accompanied by parakeratosis or hyperkeratosis and, if the lesion is acuminate, by papillomatosis as well.

The mitotic figures in low-grade CIN lesions either have a normal morphological appearance or contain two types of abnormal mitoses — one referred to as a tetraploid dispersed metaphase and the other as a tripolar mitosis (Fig. 2.5A).[33-35] Both tetraploid dispersed metaphases and tripolar mitoses are seen in association with polyploidy and are not diagnostic of an aneuploid, precancerous change.

A number of authors have studied the histological/cytologic changes which are predictive of an HPV-related infection by using in situ hybridization for HPV DNA as the standard against which to calibrate the morphological changes

which occur in the uterine cervix.[36-40] The authors of these studies are uniformly in agreement that the only consistent criterion which serves to distinguish the HPV-related lesion from a reparative, metaplastic, or other benign process which may mimic HPV CPE is cytological atypia. Hence the histopathologist must, when distinguishing between HPV-related lesions and those changes which can mimic HPV CPE, be a skilled cytologist and must apply cytological criteria at the histological level. The fact that cytology is a somewhat arcane skill may account for the difficulties which appear to be encountered when making accurate diagnoses of low-grade CIN and distinguishing true HPV-related changes from the myriad of other changes which superficially appear to be similar. The way to make the right diagnosis

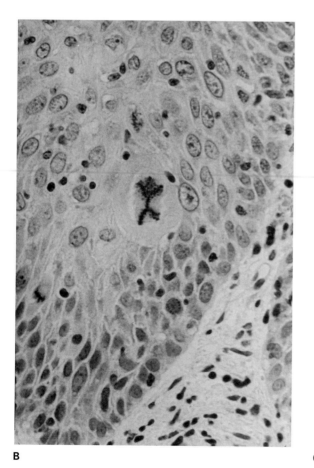

B

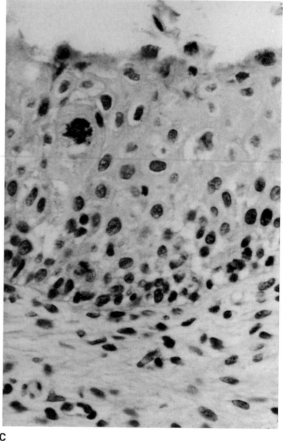

C

Fig. 2.5 Abnormal mitotic figures detected in CIN lesions. **B** Abnormal mitosis diagnostic of an aneuploid lesion.
C Highly abnormal mitosis with extensive disorganization of chromosomes diagnostic of an aneuploid, high-grade CIN lesion.

consistently is to insist upon finding at least two — and preferably three — of the changes (e.g., multinucleation, nuclear atypia, and koilocytosis) which are generally found in association with HPV infections and to apply in situ hybridization as a quality control procedure in the laboratory.

In situ hybridization

In situ hybridization for HPV DNA can be applied using standard commercially available kits and can be helpful in identifying, in the aggregate, those biopsies which contain human papillomavirus. It has now been reported by a number of authors that, although a wide range of HPV types can be identified as infecting the female genital tract, the majority of HPV-related lesions

of the cervix are HPV 16, 18, 31, 33, 35, 51, or 56. HPV types 6 and 11 — low- or no-oncogenic risk types — appear, contrary to some prior publications, to constitute less than 10% of the flat, acetowhite HPV lesions of the cervix.[3,39,41] In addition, a substantial number of other known HPV types, as well as a number of novel HPV types, produce cervical infections with the same cytopathogenic effects as do the known viral types. It appears to be well established that if a productive infection occurs in the cervix, sufficient virus will be assembled to be detectable by in-situ hybridization using the commercially available kits (Fig. 2.6).[42–44] These kits will detect approximately 30–50 viral copies per cell. Although not all of the cells will contain large numbers of viral copies, at least some cells generally will do so,

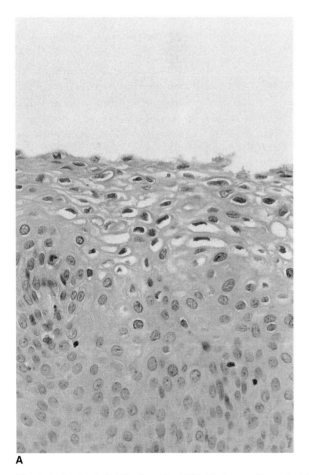

A

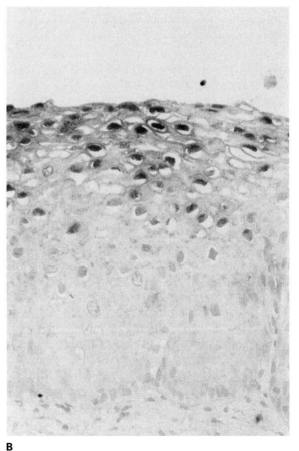

B

Fig. 2.6 In situ hybridization of a CIN 1 lesion performed with a commercially-available biotinylated probe for detecting HPV 16/18. Blue staining nuclei containing HPV 16 or 18 DNA are present in the superficial layers of the lesion, confirming that this is an HPV-related lesion. **A** H&E stained section. **B** In situ hybridization.

and those cells will be detectable using in situ hybridization. Their detection requires, however, that the in situ kit contain a probe which is specific for the viral type to be identified or one which cross-hybridizes with that type under the conditions used. The two available kits contain only probes to seven viruses: HPV types 6, 11, 16, 18, 31, 33, and 35. These types are the most prevalent ones found in cervical infections and sometimes cross-hybridize with other prevalent viruses, leading to a relatively high detection rate using these kits.[37,45]

In order to optimize the sensitivity of in situ hybridization, it is necessary to fix the tissues in neutral-buffered formalin. Acidic fixatives, such as Zenker's or Bouin's solutions, degrade the DNA and result in a greatly diminished signal strength so that the proportion of cases in which HPV DNA can be detected is reduced substantially.[46]

When in situ hybridization is applied to neutral buffered formalin-fixed cervical biopsies, most authors agree that approximately 80% of low-grade CIN lesions contain detectable HPV DNA. As these studies have been performed by pathologists with a special interest in gynecological pathology and cervical neoplasia, it is assumed that these detection rates can be used as a standard against which other laboratories might measure their diagnostic skills.[36] As the number of viral copies generally decreases with increasing grade of intraepithelial neoplasia, the application of in-situ hybridization to high-grade lesions generally results in a diminished proportion of cases being detected as positive for HPV DNA, whereas acuminate warts — which characteristically have a high number of HPV copies per cell — will generally have a higher rate of positivity than even the low-grade CIN lesions. Table 2.2 is a summary of the positivity rates compared to the

histological grade of the lesion in CIN and VIN cases. These percentages have now been confirmed by a number of authors and may prove useful in laboratories' evaluation of cervical, vaginal, or vulvar biopsies.

Using in situ hybridization, it has generally been found that epithelia which have histological changes not thought to be HPV related will be positive for HPV DNA using in situ hybridization in less than 3% of the cases. The striking difference between the 80% positive rate in those lesions which contain typical HPV CPE and the 3% positive rate in those which do not and the consistent finding that the most important criterion in distinguishing HPV from non-HPV-related lesions is cytological atypia strongly argue that cytological criteria must be adhered to rigidly in order reproducibly to distinguish HPV from non-HPV, even at the histological level.

Koilocytosis

The inconsistent use of the term 'koilocytosis' is a major cause of diagnostic confusion. To most clinicians, the term 'koilocytosis' connotes an HPV-related lesion. The gynecologist will almost uniformly infer from the term 'koilocytosis' or 'koilocytotic atypia' that the pathologist wishes to imply that this change has been caused by HPV. In contrast, pathologists use those terms inconsistently. Some mean to imply, when the term 'koilocytosis' is used, that the lesion is HPV related, whereas others use the term 'koilocytosis' to designate a cell in which a perinuclear halo is present.[15–17,47] It is critical that gynecologists know if their pathologist or cytologist uses the term 'koilocytosis' to imply an HPV-related change or if they are using purely morphologic criteria under which the term 'koilocytosis' may be used for any lesion in which perinuclear halos are found.

Perinuclear halos are found in normal squamous metaplasia, in the normal epithelium of the introitus and hymeneal ring (see the discussion of micropapillomatosis labialis above), and in a number of infectious and reparative processes, including trichomoniasis, moniliasis, and post-therapeutic reparative processes. It would be useful if a general agreement could be reached that

Table 2.2 Relationship between HPV type and histology. Note absence of low oncogenic risk HPV types in intraepithelial neoplasia

Diagnosis	% HPV Positive			
	6/11	16/18	30s	Other
Low-grade CIN	22	34	34	10
High-grade CIN	0	65	33	2
Vulvar condyloma	0	100	0	0
High-grade VIN	91	0	8	0

the term 'koilocytosis' would be used only if an HPV-related change is thought to play a role in the process, but until such uniformity of terminology and definitions is agreed upon, it is incumbant on clinicians to know the criteria that their pathologist uses to make a diagnosis of koilocytosis. If it is meant to imply an HPV-related lesion, it is clear that the term 'koilocytosis'[40] should only be used when there is not only a perinuclear halo but cytological atypia as well. As significant cytological atypia is required for a diagnosis of HPV infection and is its most important diagnostic feature, this simple agreement would go a long way towards eliminating the confusion brought about by the inconsistent use of the term 'koilocytosis.' Finally, it should be noted that koilocytosis is a descriptive term and is only one of the morphologic features associated with HPV infection. It should never be used as a diagnostic term or as a substitute for the conventional terms accepted for HPV-related lesions.

High-grade CIN

In high-grade CIN lesions there is an increased mitotic rate, an increased degree of cytological atypia, increased numbers of mitoses in the upper and middle third of the epithelium, and a high degree of disorganization of the epithelium (Fig. 2.7). 'High-grade CIN' is a term which

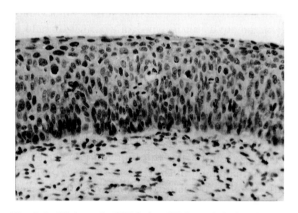

Fig. 2.7 High-grade CIN lesion. High-grade lesions have a high degree of cytologic atypia, mitoses in the middle and upper thirds of the epithelium, and a high degree of disorganization.

should be restricted to those lesions which the pathologist believes are true precursors to invasive cancer.[31] The clinician should be able to infer from the diagnosis of high-grade CIN that in the pathologist's opinion the lesion is a true cancer precursor (i.e., intraepithelial neoplasm) and not a productive HPV-related change of uncertain biological potential. One event which has been **posited** as distinguishing a productive HPV infection from a cancer precursor is the continued production or overproduction of the proteins encoded for by the E6/E7 open reading frames of high or intermediate-oncogenic risk viruses. The E6/E7 region of HPV is the major transforming region of the virus and, when expressed within a host cell, produces a variety of cellular changes.[48–51] When expressed in conjunction with an activated ras oncogene in vitro, this region causes transformation of cultured human cervical epithelial cells, and it is believed that it subsumes the same role in vivo.[52,53] Although the mechanism of action of the proteins encoded by the E6/E7 region are not fully understood, it is known that E6 binds to a protein called p53, which is important in regulating cell proliferation.[54] Similarly, E7 binds to the retinoblastoma gene product, RB or p105, an important tumor-suppressor protein which is also thought to play a critical role in regulating cell division.[55–58] Inactivation or destruction of p53 and pRB secondary to binding by E6 and E7 encoded proteins could theoretically result in unchecked cellular growth.

These molecular events (in conjunction, most certainly, with other unknown events) result in a less well differentiated, poorly growth regulated, highly mitotically active epithelium which contains abnormal cell divisions and is aneuploid. One of the characteristics of aneuploid cell populations is that they are highly cytologically atypical. Aneuploidy is routinely accompanied by abnormal mitotic figures which can readily be recognized by the experienced pathologist. These include two-group and three-group metaphases, multipolar mitoses in excess of three, highly abnormal mitotic figures, and coarsely clumped chromosomes (Fig. 2.5B,C). The counterpart of these changes in the interphase nucleus is a highly abnormal chromatin distribution pattern.

If pathologists can identify abnormal mitotic figures of the types just described in tissue sections, they can be assured that this is an aneuploid lesion and can reliably diagnose it as a high-grade CIN with the implication that this lesion will, if not removed and the patient lives long enough, progress to invasive cancer.

The distinction between low-grade and high-grade CIN

It is apparent that the low-grade CIN lesion can be identified based on the typical cytopathogenic effects of HPV and can be diagnosed as such with a reasonable degree of reproducibility, provided strict criteria are fulfilled. However, it must be pointed out that in the initial infection the CPE of all the HPV types which effect the cervix are indistinguishable one from the other and that it is impossible, at the light microscope level alone, to distinguish a low-grade CIN lesion associated with low- or no-oncogenic risk HPV types from a low-grade CIN lesion which is produced by the high- or intermediate-oncogenic risk viral types. It is impossible, based on a histological examination of a cervical biopsy alone, to predict what a low-grade lesion's course will be, i.e., will it regress, persist, or progress.

If, on the other hand, a high-grade lesion is diagnosed, based upon a high degree of disorganization, a high degree of cytological atypia, mitoses in the upper levels of the epithelium or, most importantly, the presence of abnormal mitotic figures, then it is possible to infer that this is an aneuploid lesion, is a true cancer precursor, and will, if not treated, have the potential to develop into invasive cancer.

Colposcopic observational studies of CIN lesions over time have demonstrated that high-grade lesions often begin this development as a small focus within a low-grade lesion.[58,59] The small focus of high-grade CIN then gradually expands and replaces the low-grade lesion. This transition from a low-grade to a high-grade CIN occurs as a monoclonal event within an HPV-infected epithelium. Studies of the biology of HPV infections in culture and model systems suggest that a key molecular event in the progression of a benign, low-grade lesion to a high-grade lesion is either a structural change in the HPV genome or a change in the regulation of the E6/E7 open reading frames that results in an over expression or inappropriate expression of the E6/E7 encoded transforming proteins.[53] Unfortunately, although the histological appearance of fully developed high-grade lesions is known, the histological correlates of the monoclonal events that change a benign HPV infection into a premalignant high-grade lesion are unknown. Even if the histological correlates were known, the degree of sampling that would be required to find such a monoclonal event at its earliest stages would preclude its being observed in the majority of cases. Therefore, in the absence of the histological changes, such as the presence of abnormal mitotic figures, which identify a high-grade lesion, the pathologist can conclude only that the epithelium is infected with HPV but cannot exclude that the monoclonal event which initiates the change to a true precursor lesion has occurred.

Clinical relevance

Fortunately, the use of modern therapeutic approaches to HPV-related lesions obviate the need to distinguish between high-grade and low-grade lesions. The clinician's role — having received a diagnosis of an HPV-related lesion — is to rule out invasive cancer and to treat the lesion based on its size and distribution.

The recent introduction of the loop electrosurgical excision procedure (LEEP) has greatly simplified the diagnosis and therapy of CIN, as the colposcopist need only identify the atypical transformation zone, use LEEP to remove it in its entirety, and await from the pathologist the decision as to whether invasion is or is not present.[60-64] It is extremely important that the clinician deal with a pathologist and cytologist who clearly understands the pathogenesis of HPV-related lesions, who knows how to distinguish HPV-related lesions from their mimics, and who knows how to tell cancer from not cancer. It is also important to understand the histological and cytological changes related to HPV and to understand the mechanisms through which they occur, as this helps refine the diagnostic criteria which are used and leads to a greater understanding of the nature of the disease process. However, at a practical level, the fine distinctions discussed above are not terribly important, provided the clinician can rely upon the skills of the pathologist to determine whether an HPV-related lesion is present and to tell cancer from not cancer.

Microinvasion

Microinvasive carcinoma of the cervix is a clinical entity which was originally described in 1947 by Mestwerdt.[65] There are currently two working definitions which are widely used. One, promulgated by the Society of Gynecologic Oncologists in the US, defines microinvasive carcinoma as 'one in which neoplastic epithelium invades the stroma in one or more places to a depth of 3 mm or less below the base of the epithelium and in which lymphatic or blood vessel involvement is not demonstrated'.[66] A more recent definition ratified by the International Federation of Obstetricians and Gynecologists is as follows:[67]

Stage Ia: Preclinical carcinoma of the cervix that is diagnosed only by microscopy.

Stage Ia1: Minimal microscopically evident stromal invasion.

Stage Ia2: Lesions detected microscopically that can be measured. The upper limit of the measurement should not show a depth of invasion of more than 5 mm taken from the base of the epithelium, either surface or glandular, from which it originates. A second dimension, the horizontal spread, must not exceed 7 mm. Larger lesions should be staged as Ib.

Irrespective of which definition is used (the authors prefer the SGO's), it should be realized that the definition of microinvasive carcinoma is empirical. It is derived from prospective clinical studies in which patients were treated with radical hysterectomy and pelvic lymph node dissection, then followed for 5 years until the clinical outcome was known.[68-72] The clinical outcome was then correlated with a number of histological features which could be measured or clearly defined, and a constellation of histological characteristics were chosen such that patients who had them could be assured that their risk of metastasis and death, if treated by simple hysterectomy, was less than or equal to the risks of a more radical treatment procedure, i.e., radical hysterectomy and lymph node dissection. In practice, the SGO definition has served the gynecologic community extremely well, as there are very few patients with metastatic disease whose cervical cancers have 3 mm or less of stromal penetration measured from the basal lamina and lack lymph vascular space involvement.[65] In patients with 3–5 mm of invasion, the metastatic rate is about 5%.

From the published data it is clear that, for squamous cell cancer of the cervix, there is an easily applied set of criteria which distinguish patients at risk for metastases from those who are not at risk. The problems arise when these criteria are applied by the general community of pathologists to specimens removed and submitted for histological examination. It is the experience of the authors and others who receive consultation slides that a diagnosis of microinvasive carcinoma of the cervix is commonly in error. The overwhelming majority of the errors are made in overdiagnosing CIN as microinvasion, but in a smaller percentage of cases, patients with frankly invasive cancer are underdiagnosed as microinvasive carcinoma. The best documented study of the error rate in the diagnosis of microinvasion was published by members of the Gynecologic Oncology Group. In their study, all diagnoses of microinvasion were reviewed centrally. The authors found that 50% of the time the diagnosis of microinvasion was in error.[72] In 45% of the cases, the referee pathologists diagnosed only CIN in sections originally diagnosed as microinvasion, whereas in 5% they diagnosed frankly invasive cancer. As a result of this study, it has been suggested that a formal review of every diagnosis of microinvasive carcinoma be made to be certain that the diagnosis is made accurately and that the patient is not over- or undertreated for her disease.

The most common cause of a misdiagnosis of microinvasion is overinterpretation of tangentially cut tongues of epithelium or gland involvement by CIN. Highly inflamed cervices containing CIN with an irregular basal lamina are also commonly overdiagnosed as microinvasion. One of the best ways of avoiding an inaccurate diagnosis due to poor orientation and tangential cutting is for the clinician to orient the punch biopsies at the time they are taken by placing them on a piece of lens paper or hard-surfaced brown paper towel, such that the plane of the epithelium is perpendicular to the plane of the paper support. If the biopsies are placed in fixative on a piece of paper, they tend not to curl during the fixation process. They have only a single flat surface, and if that flat surface is embedded down by the pathologist or the technician, tangential cutting is minimized. If cone biopsy specimens or LEEP specimens are submitted for pathology, they should be opened fresh and either pinned out flat or placed in capped, perforated, plastic cassettes prior to being fixed. Even when great care is taken to achieve optimal tissue preparation, the differentiation of micro-invasive carcinoma from CIN or invasive cancer may be difficult, and the pathologist and clinician should carefully monitor the diagnosis and be certain that it is properly made.

A diagnosis of microinvasive carcinoma of the endocervix is occasionally rendered but is wholly inappropriate. There are no published empirical series which have provided the background information necessary to establish microinvasive adenocarcinoma as an entity. Unlike squamous neoplasia, endocervical neoplasms appear not to have a microinvasive phase, as metastases can occur early in the process of invasion and are unpredictable. Therefore, lesions of the endocervical epithelium should be diagnosed as either adenocarcinoma-in-situ or adenocarcinoma, and a diagnosis of microinvasive carcinoma of the endocervix should not be made.

ADENOCARCINOMA AND ADENOCARCINOMA-IN-SITU

It would appear that endocervical adenocarcinoma-in-situ and invasive adenocarcinoma are etiologically related to HPV, just as are the squamous lesions of the lower genital tract. Most of the adenocarcinomas and adenocarcinomas-in-situ are associated with HPV types 16 or 18, with the vast majority being HPV 18 related.[73-76] In contrast to the SILs, however, the histological features of a productive viral infection phase in the endocervical epithelium have not been described, and endocervical epithelial infections with low- or no-oncogenic risk viruses have not been reported. Endocervical neoplasms, in their in situ phase, can be diagnosed by virtue of the disorderliness of the epithelium, the cytological atypia, and the increased mitotic rate (Fig. 2.8). However, some reparative and regenerative processes and endocervical metaplasia may mimic endocervical adenocarcinoma-in-situ, and the histological distinction between the two is sometimes difficult. This difficulty is contributed to by the fact that some endocervical adenocarcinomas-in-situ and invasive adenocarcinomas are minimally deviated from their normal appearance, and the cytological alterations may consist of minimal chromatin clumping and an enlarged nucleolus, despite evidence for deep invasion into the cervical stroma. Therefore, the histopathologist may sometimes overdiagnose a reparative process as neoplasia and sometimes underdiagnose neoplasia as a reparative process or miss the changes all together due to the minimal alterations which can sometimes be present. Unfortunately, HPV DNA in situ hybridization, using commercially available kits is not particularly helpful in these cases as the viral copy number appears, in general, to be lower in glandular lesions than in productively infected squamous lesions and is usually below the limits of sensitivity of this method. HPV appears uniformly to be integrated into the host DNA in adenocarcinomas rather than occurring in an episomal form, as commonly takes place in the squamous epithelia.[77] As the same viral types which infect the squamous epithelium infect the endocervical epithelium, it is not surprising that there is sometimes concordance between the two lesions, requiring the clinican who detects any HPV-related lesion to examine all potential sites of HPV infection and rule out neoplasia.

Among the invasive adenocarcinomas, a number of morphological subsets have been described. These include minimal deviation adenocarcinoma (or adenoma malignum), classical endocervical type adenocarcinoma, endometroid carcinomas, clear cell types of carcinoma, mesonephric carcinoma, mixed types, and the villoglandular type.

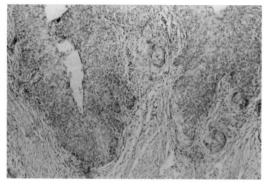

A

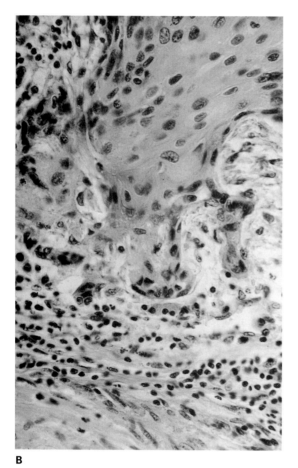

B

Fig. 2.8 Microinvasive carcinoma of the cervix. **A** Multiple small tongues of microinvasive squamous cell carcinoma have broken through the basement membrane and invade into the stroma. **B** A characteristic feature of these lesions is increased cytologic differentiation in the invasive component.

The adenoma malignum, or minimal deviation adenocarcinoma, is, as the name implies, an extremely well differentiated glandular cancer which mimics normal endocervical glands, both in cytology and in pattern. The distinguishing features which allow the pathologist to differentiate normal endocervical variants from cancer include irregularities of the glandular shape, mild cytological changes including an increase in nucleolar size, the presence of mitotic figures, glands extending beyond the plane of the normal endocervix, and obvious signs of invasion such as perineural infiltration.[78] These minimal deviation tumors are commonly missed in biopsies, and the pathologist must have a high index of suspicion. If clinicians suspect invasive carcinoma based on clinical findings, they should alert the pathologist to that possibility so that attention is paid to these difficult-to-diagnose lesions.

The conventional endocervical adenocarcinoma does not generally present a diagnostic problem, except in those cases in which it is difficult to distinguish adenocarcinoma-in-situ from invasive adenocarcinoma. Adenocarcinoma-in-situ is, by definition, a change which is confined to the epithelium of the endocervical glands and which occurs in a distribution which is the same as the endocervical glands. Cribriforming, or a gland-in-gland pattern, is one of the constellation of features associated with adenocarcinoma-in-situ or adenocarcinoma, but when it occurs in the context of a normal gland distribution pattern, the diagnosis of adenocarcinoma-in-situ can generally be made with confidence (Fig. 2.9**A,B**). This requires, however, that a conization be performed to rule out invasive adenocarcinoma, and that the entire involved endocervix be examined microscopically. When areas which significantly deviate from the usual endocervical gland pattern or obvious tongues of invasion are found, the diagnosis of invasive carcinoma can be made.

An unusual, but important, morphological pattern seen in adenocarcinomas is the villoglandular carcinoma, a recently recognized morphological variant in which the neoplastic endocervical epithelium is thrown up into villoglandular folds.[79] The importance of this variant is that is carries an extremely good prognosis.

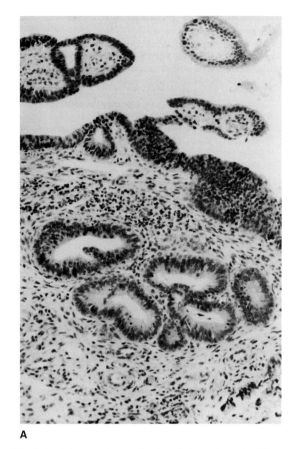

A

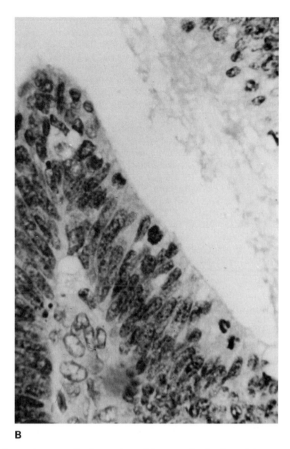

B

Fig. 2.9 Adenocarcinoma-in-situ of the endocervix. These neoplasms have cytologic atypia and increased mitotic activity. **A** Dark-staining glands with increased mitotic rate. Note for comparison one piece of normal endocervix in right upper corner. **B** Highly atypical nuclei and large number of mitoses characteristic of adenocarcinoma-in-situ.

SMALL-CELL CANCER

Small-cell cancers of the cervix are rare variants of squamous cell cancers thought to be derived from a common progenitor cell and typically included with the APUDoma group of neuroendocrine small cell cancers. It appears to be related principally to HPV type 18, although, as with the endocervical adenocarcinomas, a small proportion of the small cell cancers contain HPV 16 or no identifiable HPV.[80] The identification of this morphological variant is important because of its poor prognosis. The criteria which are used are similar to those used for small cell cancers in other parts of the body.

REFERENCES

1. Wright T C, Richart R M. Review: Role of human papillomavirus in the pathogenesis of genital tract warts and cancer. Gynecol Oncol 1990; 37: 151–164.
2. Galloway D A, Holmes K K, Koutsky L A. Epidemiology of genital human papillomavirus infection. Epidemiol Rev 1988; 10: 122.
3. Reid R, Lorincz A T. Should family physicians test for HPV infection? J Family Practice 1991; 32(2): 183–188.
4. Cobb M W. Human papillomavirus infection. J Am Acad Dermatol 1990; 22: 547–566.
5. Lev C, Bauer H M, Reingold A et al. Determinants of genital human papillomavirus infection in young women. J Nat Cancer Inst 1991; 83: 997–1003.
6. Schiffman M H. Commentary: Recent progress in defining the epidemiology of human papillomavirus infection and cervical neoplasia. J Nat Cancer Inst 1992; 84: 394–398.

7. Pfister H. Papillomaviruses: General description, taxonomy, and classification. In: Salzman N P, Howley P M, eds. The papovavirdae, vol 2. New York: Plenum, 1987: pp 109–139.

8. Broker T R. Structure and genetic expression of papillomaviruses. Obstet Gynecol Clinics North Amer 1987; 14: 329–348.

9. Lorincz A T, Reid R, Jenson A B, Greenberg M D, Lancaster W, Kurman R. Human papillomavirus infection of the cervix: Relative risk associations of 15 common anogenital types. Obstet Gynecol 1992; 79: 328–337.

10. Richart R M. Clinical commentary: A modified terminology for cervical intraepithelial neoplasia. Obstet Gynecol 1990; 75: 131–133.

11. National Cancer Institute Workshop. The 1988 Bethesda System for reporting cervical/vaginal cytologic diagnosis. JAMA 1989; 262: 931–934.

12. Lungu O, Zun W Q, Felix J, Richart R M, Silverstein S, Wright T C. Relationship of human papillomavirus type to grade of cervical intraepithelial neoplasia. JAMA 1992; 267: 2493–2496.

13. Richart R M. Natural history of cervical intraepithelial neoplasia. Clin Obstet Gynecol 1968; 10: 748.

14. Friedell G H. Carcinoma, carcinoma-in-situ, and "early lesions" of the uterine cervix and the urinary bladder: Introduction and definitions. Cancer Res 1976; 36: 2482–2484.

15. Meisels A, Roy M, Fortier M, Morin C. Condlyomatous lesions of the cervix: Morphologic and colposcopic diagnosis. Am J Diag Gynecol Obstet 1979; 1: 109.

16. Meisels A, Fortin R, Roy M. Condylomatous lesions of the cervix: II Cytologic, colposcopic and histopathologic study. Acta Cytol 1977; 21: 379–390.

17. Meisels A, Roy M, Fortier M et al. Human papillomavirus (HPV) infections of the cervix: The atypical condyloma. Acta Cytol 1981; 25: 7–16.

18. Ferenczy A, Mito M, Nagai N et al. Latent papillomavirus and recurring genital warts. New Engl J Med 1985; 313: 784–788.

19. MacNab J C M, Walkinshaw S A, Coriner J W et al. Human papillomavirus in clinically and histologically normal tissue of patients with genital cancer. New Engl J Med 1986; 315: 1052–1058.

20. Schneider A. Latent and subclinical genital HPV infections. Papillomavirus Report 1990; 1: 2–5.

21. Nuovo G J. Correlation of histology with human papillomavirus DNA detection in the female genital tract. Gynecol Oncol 1988; 31: 176–183.

22. Halpert R, Fruchter R G, Sedlis A, Butt K, Boyce J G, Sillman F H. Human papillomavirus and lower genital neoplasia in renal transplant patients. Obstet Gynecol 1986; 68: 251–158.

23. Vermund S H, Kelley K F. Human papillomavirus in women: Methodologic issues and role of immunosuppression. In: Kiely M, ed. Reproductive and perinatal epidemiology. Boca Raton: CRC Press, 1990: pp 143–168.

24. Pastner B, Baker D A, Orr J W. Human papillomavirus genital tract infections during pregnancy. Clin Obstet Gynecol 1990; 33: 258–267.

25. Ferenczy A, Richart R M, Wright T C. Pearly penile papules: Absence of human papillomavirus DNA by the polymerase chain reaction. Obstet Gynecol 1991; 78: 118–122.

26. Bergeron C, Ferenczy A, Richart R M, Guralnick M. Micropapillomatosis labialis appears unrelated to human papillomavirus. Obstet Gynecol 1990; 76(2): 281–186.

27. Nuovo G J, Richart R M. Human papillomavirus: A review. In: Mishell R, Kirschbau T H, Moorow C P, eds. Yearbook of obstetrics and gynecology. Chicago: Year Book Medical Publishers, 1989: p 297.

28. Szarewski A, Cuzick J, Edwards R, Butler B, Singer A. The use of cervicography in a primary screening service. Br J Obstet Gynecol 1991; 98: 313–317.

29. Spitzer M, Krumholz B A, Chernys A E, Seltzer V, Lightman A. Comparative utility of repeat Papanicolaou smears, cervicography and colposcopy in the evaluation of atypical Papanicolaou smears. Obstet Gynecol 1987; 69: 731–735.

30. Rehder K E, Blyther J G. Cytology and cervicography compared to cytology alone for human papillomavirus detection. Colposcopy Gynecol Laser Surg 1988; 4: 1–7.

31. Richart R M. A modified terminology for cervical intraepithelial neoplasia. Obstet Gynecol 1990; 75: 131–133.

32. Fu Y S, Huang I, Beauderon S et al. Correlative study of human papillomavirus DNA, histopathology and morphometry in cervical condyloma and intraepithelial neoplasia. Int J Gynecol Pathol 1988; 7: 297.

33. Fujii T, Crum C P, Winkler B et al. Human papillomavirus infection and cervical intraepithelial neoplasia: Histology and DNA content. Obstet Gynecol 1984; 63: 99.

34. Fu Y S, Braun L, Shat K U et al. Histologic, nuclear DNA, and human papillomavirus studies of cervical condyloma. Cancer 1983; 52: 1705.

35. Winkler B, Crum P C, Fujii T et al. Koilocytotic lesions of the cervix: The relationship of mitotic abnormalities to the presence of papillomavirus antigens and nuclear DNA content. Cancer 1984; 53: 1081–1087.

36. Richart R M, Nuovo G J, HPV DNA in-situ hybridization can be used for the quality control of diagnostic biopsies. Obstet Gynecol 1989; 75: 223–226.

37. Felix J F, Wright T C. Comparison of in-situ hybridization and PCR for detecting HPV in lesions clinically suspicious for condylomata accuminata. Int Acad Pathol Annual Meeting, 1991.

38. Nuovo G J, O'Connell M, Blanco J S et al. Correlation of histology and HPV DNA detection in condyloma acuminatum and condyloma-like vulvar lesions. Am J Surg Pathol 1989; 13: 700–706.

39. Franquemont D W, Ward B E, Anderson W A, Crum C P. Prediction of "high-risk" cervical papillomavirus infection by biopsy morphology. Am J Clin Pathol 1989; 92: 577–582.

40. Ward B, Burkett B, Peterson C et al. Cytologic correlation of cervical papillomavirus infection. Int J Gynecol Pathol 1990; 9: 297–305.

41. Bergeron C, Barrasso R, Beaudenon S, Flamant P, Croissant O, Orth G. The multiplicity of HPV types detected in 181 cervical biopsies as related to histologic finding (Proc Papillomavirus Workshop, 1990, Heidelberg). p 286.

42. Nagai N, Nuovo G J, Friedman D, Crum C. Detection of papillomavirus nucleic acids in genital precancers with the in-situ hybridization technique. Int J Gynecol Pathol 1987; 6: 366–379.

43. Richart R M, Nuovo G J. HPV DNA in-situ hybridization can be used for the quality control of diagnostic biopsies. Obstet Gynecol 1989; 75: 223–226.

44. Nuovo G J, Richart R M. A comparison of slot blot, Southern blot, and in in-situ hybridization analysis for

HPV DNA in genital tract lesions. Obstet Gynecol 1989; 74: 673–679.

45. Nuovo G J, Richart R M. A comparison of Biotin and 35-S based in-situ hybridization methodologies for detection of human papillomavirus DNA. Lab Invest 1989; 61: 471–476.

46. Nuovo G J, Richart R M. Buffered formalin is the superior fixative for the detection of HPV DNA by in-situ hybridization analysis. Am J Pathol 1989; 134: 837–842.

47. Koss L G, Durfee G R. Unusual patterns of squamous epithelium of the uterine cervix: Cytologic and pathologic study of koilocytotic atypia. Ann NY Acad Sci 1956; 63: 1245.

48. Storey A, Pim D, Murray A et al. Comparison of the in vitro transforming activities of human papillomavirus types. EMBO J 1988; 7: 1815–1820.

49. Phelps W C, Yee C L, Mungei K et al. The human papillomavirus type 16 E7 gene encodes transactivation and transforming functions similar to those of adenovirus E1A. Cell 1988; 58: 539–547.

50. Kanda T, Furuno A, Yoshiike K. Human papillomavirus type 16 open reading frame E7 encodes a transforming gene for rat 3Y1 cells. J Virol 1988; 62: 610–613.

51. Bedell M A, Jones K H, Laimins L A. The E6–E7 region of human papillomavirus type 18 is sufficient for transformation of NIH 3T3 and rat 3Y1 cells. J Virol 1987; 61: 3635–3640.

52. Matlashewski G, Schneider J, Banks L et al. Human papillomavirus type 16 DNA cooperates with activated ras in transforming primary cells. EMBO J 1987; 6: 1741–1746.

53. DiPaolo J A, Woodworth C D, Popescu N C et al. Induction of human cervical squamous cell carcinoma by sequential transfection with human papillomavirus 16 DNA and viral harvey ras. Oncogene 1989; 4: 365–399.

54. Werness B A, Levine A J, Howley P M. Association of human papillomavirus types 16 and 18 E6 proteins with p53. Science 1990; 248: 76–79.

55. Dyson N, Howley P M, Munger K, Harlow E. The human papillomavirus 16 E7 oncoprotein is able to bind to the retinoblastoma gene product. Science 1989; 243: 934–937.

56. Barbosa M S, Edwards C, Fisher C et al. The region of the HPV E7 oncoprotein homologous to adenovirus E1A and SV40 large T antigen contains separate domains for Rb binding and casein kinase II phosphorylation. EMBO J 1990; 9: 153–160.

57. Hollingworth R E, Lee W-H. Tumor suppression genes: new prospects for cancer research. J Nat Cancer Inst 1991; 83: 91–96.

58. Richart R M. Colpomicroscopic studies of the distribution of dysplasia and carcinoma in situ on the exposed portion of the human uterine cervix. Cancer 1965; 18: 950.

59. Coppleson M. The origin and nature of premalignant lesions of the cervix uteri. Int J Gynecol Obstet 1970; 8: 539.

60. Bigrigg M A, Codling B W, Pearson P, Read M D, Swingler G R. Colposcopic diagnosis and treatment of cervical dysplasia at a single clinic visit: Experience of low-voltage diathermy loop in 1000 patients. Lancet 1990; 336: 229.

61. Luesley D M, Cullimore J, Redman C W E et al. Loop diathermy excision of the cervical transformation zone in patients with abnormal cervical smears. Br Med J 1990; 300: 1690–1693.

62. Prendiville W, Cullimore N S. Large loop excision of the transformation zone (LLETZ). A new method of management for women with cervical intraepithelial neoplasia. Br J Obstet Gynecol 1989; 96: 1054–1060.

63. Mor-Yosef S, Lopes A, Pearson S, Monaghan J M. Loop diathermy cone biopsy. Obstet Gynecol 1990; 75: 884–886.

64. Wright T C, Gagnons S, Richart R M, Ferenczy A. Treatment of cervical intraepithelial neoplasia using the loop electrosurgical excision procedure (LEEP). 1991; 79: 173–178.

65. Mestwerdt G. Probe exzision und kolposkopie in des fruhdiagnose des portiokarcinoms. Zentralblatt fur Gynakologie 1947; 4: 326.

66. Morrow C P, Townsend D E. Synopsis of gynecologic oncology, 3rd edn. New York: Churchill Livingstone, 1991: p 123.

67. FIGO Cancer Committee. Staging announcement. Gynecol Oncol 1989; 35: 125–127.

68. van Nagell J R, Greenwell N, Powell D F et al. Microinvasive carcinoma of the cervix. Am J Obstet Gynecol 1983; 145: 981.

69. Yajima A, Noda K. The results of treatment of microinvasive carcinoma of the cervix by means of simple and extended hysterectomy. Am J Obstet Gynecol 1979; 135: 685.

70. Kolstad P. Follow-up study of 232 patients with stage 1a1 and 411 patients with stage 1a2 squamous cell carcinoma of the cervix (microinvasive carcinoma). Gynecol Oncol 1989; 33: 265.

71. Greer B E, Figge D C, Tamini H et al. Stage 1A2 squamous carcinoma of the cervix: Difficult diagnosis and therapeutic dilemma. Am J Obstet Gynecol 1990; 162: 1406–1411.

72. Sedlis A, Sol S, Tsukada Y et al. Microinvasive carcinoma of the uterine cervix. A clinical-pathologic study. Am J Obstet Gynecol 1979; 133: 64.

73. Farnsworth A, Laverty C, Stoler, M H. Human papillomavirus messenger RNA expression in adenocarcinoma in situ of the uterine cervix. Int J Gynecol Pathol 1989; I: 321–330.

74. Neilsen A L. Human papillomavirus type 16/18 in uterine cervical adenocarcinoma in situ and adenocarcinoma. A study by in situ hybridization with biotinylated DNA probes. Cancer 1990; 65: 2588–2593.

75. Wilczynski S P, Bergen S, Walker J, Liao S, Pearlman L F. Human papillomavirus and cervical cancer. Human Pathol 1988; 19: 697–704.

76. Tase T, Okagaki T, Clark B A et al. Human papillomavirus types and localization in adenocarcinoma and adenosquamous carcinoma of the uterine cervix: A study by in-situ DNA hybridization. Cancer Res 1988; 48: 993–998.

77. Cullen A P, Reid R, Campin M, Lorincz A. Analysis of the physical state of different papillomarvirus DNA's in intraepithelial and invasive cervical neoplasms. J Virol 1991; 65:

78. Gilks C B, Young R H, Aquirre P et al. Adenoma malignum (minimal deviation adenocarcinoma) of the uterine cervix. Am J Surg Pathol 1989; 13: 717–729.

79. Young R H, Scully R E. Villoglandular papillary adenocarcinoma of the uterine cervix. Cancer 1989; 63: 1773–1779.

80. Stoler M H, Mills S E, Gersell D J, Walker A. Small-cell neuroendocrine carcinoma of the cervix: A human papillomavirus type 18-associated cancer. Am J Surg Pathol 1991; 15: 28–32.

3. Vulvar intraepithelial neoplasia

Catherine M. McLachlin   Christopher P. Crum

INTRODUCTION

Cancer of the vulva is an uncommon disease with an incidence of approximately 1.8 per 100 000,[1–3] or approximately one-eighth that of cervical carcinoma.[4,5] Risk factors for vulvar cancer include other genital carcinomas, chronic vulvar inflammatory disorders, smoking, prior history of genital warts and vulvar carcinoma-in-situ (vulvar intraepithelial neoplasms or VIN).[6,7] VIN has long been considered a precursor to some invasive carcinomas. Based upon both morphologic and clinical data, it appears that approximately 30% of vulvar carcinomas are associated with VIN. However, the incidence rate of VIN has nearly doubled in the last 20 years, while that of vulvar carcinoma has remained relatively stable.[8] This chapter will address these relationships, including the morphological definition of VIN, the role of papillomaviruses in its genesis, the manner in which these factors link VIN to invasive carcinomas, and how they may influence therapy of vulvar precursors.

TERMINOLOGY

Precancerous squamous lesions of the vulva have traditionally encompassed a variety of entities, including carcinoma *in situ*, Bowen's disease,[9] bowenoid papulosis,[10] erythroplasia of Queyrat, and a portion of the lesions previously termed carcinoma simplex[9] or vulvar atypia.[11] All of these vulvar lesions share epithelial atypia and a variable risk of progressing to invasive carcinoma.[9,10,12] In 1965 Kaufmann grouped precancers into three categories, corresponding to erythroplasia of Queyrat, bowenoid carcinoma in situ and carcinoma simplex.[13] Erythroplasia of Queyrat and bowenoid carcinoma in situ represented nearly identical lesions in the penile and vulvar mucosa, respectively.[14] They were distinguished by the presence of disordered epithelial growth which usually involved the entire thickness of the epithelium with loss of cellular polarity, enlarged and multinucleated cells, hyperchromatism and dyskeratosis. Carcinoma in situ simplex designated lesions in which nuclear atypia was most conspicuous in the lower portions of the epithelium while the surface layers maintained squamous maturation and only minor atypia.[9,13] This terminology was simplified in 1976 to carcinoma-in-situ and vulvar atypia.[11] 'Atypia' applied to those lesions in which only a portion of the epithelium was dysplastic.[11] Recently, this terminology has been refined further with the introduction of the term vulvar intraepithelial neoplasia, or VIN.[14] Under this classification, carcinoma-in-situ and most vulvar atypias would simply be termed VIN, and assigned a grade from 1 to 3 depending upon their degree of maturation. In contrast to similar grading systems of the cervix, there is essentially no data on the progression rates of various grades of VIN to invasive carcinoma.

HISTOPATHOLOGY

General concepts

Irrespective of how it is subclassified, the fundamental morphologic alteration in VIN is abnormal cell growth with nuclear atypia present in the mid or lower cell layers of the squamous epithelium. This parameter will serve to separate these lesions from conventional condylomata and has been correlated with the presence of aneuploid cell populations. Condylomata, which are diploid or polyploid, possess nuclear atypia which is confined to the surface epithelial cells.[12]

Grading of VIN is based upon the extent of cellular atypia and the degree of maturation of the neoplastic epithelium. It should be emphasized that, providing that the cytologic features of a VIN are present, there is no evidence to support a specific grading scheme, given the lack of information concerning its biologic meaning. However, as will be mentioned below, subsets of VIN may differ in pathogenesis and warrant subdivision for the purposes of gathering additional information about risk of progression to invasive carcinoma.

Morphology

The most consistent parameter for diagnosis of a VIN lesion is the presence of anisokaryosis and variations in staining of the cells in the lower third of the epithelium (parabasal). Nuclei will vary at least three-fold in size, and should be accompanied by differences in staining intensity and the presence of multinucleation. These features are relatively constant, and will serve to distin-guish these lesions from condylomata, podophyllin treated condylomata, seborrheic keratoses, and epithelial hyperplasia (Fig. 3.1). Condylomata exhibit nuclear atypia in the upper two-thirds of the epithelium and virtually never contain enlarged, hyperchromatic nuclei or multinucleated cells in the parabasal region.[12] The importance of comparing nuclear size in a given lesion is that this parameter is independent of variations in fixation which may produce the general appearance of nuclear enlargement. Other parameters, such as loss of polarity, hyperchromatism, dyskeratosis, and uneven maturation are frequently present and aid in the diagnosis of VIN.

The histologic parameters which correlate most consistently with aneuploidy are the presence of abnormal mitotic figures and the character of the cellular atypia in the constituent cells.[12,15–17] Abnormal mitotic figures include multipolar mitoses, 2 and 3 group metaphases, irregularly dispersed mitoses, and coarse clumping of the chromosomes on the mitotic spindle.[17]

Subsets of VIN

Although the VIN classification currently is justi-

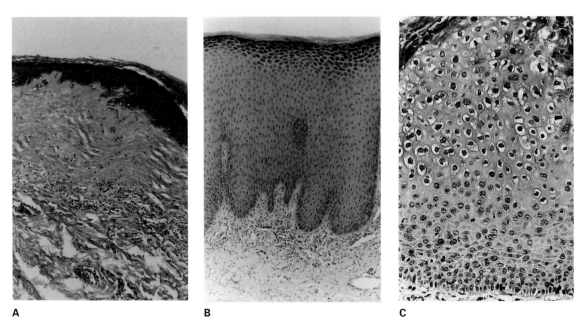

A   **B**   **C**

Fig. 3.1 Benign epithelial alterations distinguished from VIN: **A** lichen sclerosis, **B** epithelial hyperplasia, **C** condyloma accuminata.

fied for the purpose of simplifying terminology and therapy, certain distinct histologic patterns exist, and are worthy of note for reasons discussed later. They fall into three general categories which are separable using three parameters; the degree of differentiation of the neoplastic cells, the degree of maturation of the affected epithelium, and the distribution of the abnormal cells within the epithelium. Architectural alterations, including acanthosis, verruciform or 'warty' appearances, may be observed in all of the lesions in these categories.

The most common group includes those lesions in which the neoplastic cells are moderately differentiated, occur within an epithelium which is undergoing minimal surface maturation, and occupy the entire thickness of the squamous epithelium. Such lesions fall into the categories of Bowen's disease, bowenoid papulosis, and bowenoid dysplasia. Most VIN lesions exhibit one or more of the features described by a number of authors as Bowen's disease of the cutaneous epithelium.[9-14] These include multinucleation, dyskeratosis, individual cell keratinization, abnormal mitoses, and corps ronds (Fig. 3.2). These lesions

often contain koilocytotic atypia, but in contrast to condylomata, the koilocytes are confined to the most superficial areas of the epithelium, are few in number, and the delicate perinuclear halos are replaced by compact concentric clear spaces around obviously abnormal nuclei.

Despite attempts to group Bowen's disease and erythroplasia of Queyrat into one group (VIN 3/carcinoma-in-situ), an entity emerged which initially appeared to represent a distinct clinical–pathological subset. Bowenoid papulosis presents clinically as discrete papular, often pigmented lesions and which preserve the histological features of Bowen's disease.[10] These lesions appeared unique, since they were confined primarily to young individuals, were clinically innocuous, and a portion were reported to regress spontaneously after biopsy alone.[10,18-20] Another related subset, bowenoid dysplasia, was reported by Ulbright et al,[21] who described lesions with many clinical features of bowenoid papulosis except that the degree of nuclear atypia was less marked and pilosebaceous involvement was absent. However, these authors described enlarged nuclei and multinucleation in a portion of all bowenoid dysplasia,

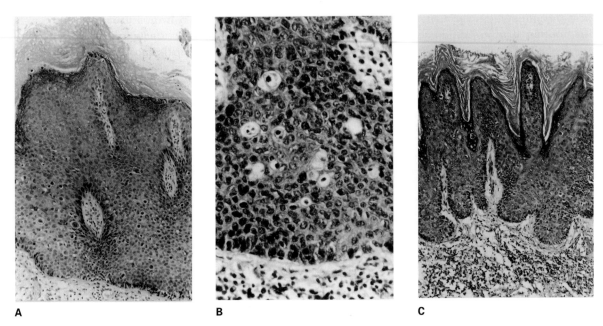

A   **B**   **C**

Fig. 3.2 Moderately differentiated VIN lesions in the general category of Bowenoid lesions: **A** lesion containing full thickness nuclear atypia and slight maturation; **B** a higher power view of a similar lesion illustrates nuclear atypia in the lower layers of the epithelium; **C** similar lesion with papillary architecture.

suggesting that they represent aneuploid lesions with less striking nuclear abnormalities. In this sense, the term dysplasia is more descriptive than indicative of a biological process which can be readily distinguished from VIN. The current classification of vulvar disease does not recognize these entities as distinct.[21] Although these lesions predominate in young patients, there is considerable overlap in the clinical appearance between these papules and classic VIN, which may be multifocal, pigmented, and also found in young women. Some authors have reported invasive cancer adjacent to lesions otherwise fulfilling the clinical criteria for bowenoid papulosis, suggesting further that bowenoid papulosis cannot be excluded from the spectrum of precancerous vulvar lesions.[22] Further similarities, specifically those associated with HPV, will be discussed subsequently.

The second group of vulvar lesions is substantially less common than the others and consists of undifferentiated neoplastic cells occurring in an epithelium which undergoes minimal to no differentiation, and which occupy the entire full thickness of the lesion. These are analogous to lesions designated as carcinoma-in-situ of the cervix (Fig. 3.3).

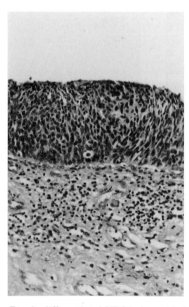

Fig. 3.3 Poorly differentiated VIN lesion with features of classic carcinoma-in-situ. Note the absence of maturation in the cells and diffuse distribution of nuclear atypia.

The third category of VIN includes lesions which are characterized by neoplastic cells of variable differentiation, occurring in an epithelium which is conspicuous for prominent maturation and keratinization, and which are frequently located exclusively in the lower or parabasal cell layers (Fig. 3.4). The term vulvar atypia was adopted in 1975 by the nomenclature committee to address those vulvar lesions which were often associated with hyperplastic or atrophic vulvar lesions, contained nuclear atypia, but which exhibited epithelial maturation.[19] At their worst, these lesions were identical to those described by Abell as carcinoma simplex, and were termed 'severe atypia', denoting an obvious precancerous neoplastic process.[9] In 1984 the nomenclature committee proposed combining the severe atypias with carcinomas-in-situ (including bowenoid lesions) under the term VIN.[14] This necessitated defining a strict cut-off between what would be termed nonspecific inflammatory lesions and precancerous neoplasia. If significant parabasal cell atypia and/or mitoses were present, the diagnosis of VIN should be made; if not, a narrative report (hyperplasia, inflammation, etc.) would convey the benign nature of the lesion. This distinction may be of importance, since vulvar dystrophies and vulvar atypia are frequently detected adjacent to invasive cancers.[23–25] The significance of this finding will be addressed at the end of this chapter.

EPIDEMIOLOGY AND PATHOGENESIS

General

The incidence of VIN has increased almost two-fold in the past 20 years, rising from 1.1 to 2.1 per 1 000 000 woman years.[8] This trend appears most significant for white woman under the age of 35, as the incidence rate in this group has nearly tripled. Presently, more than half of the women with VIN are less than 40 years of age.[12] Several factors, including most likely a change in sexual mores and a rapid increase in cigarette smoking in this group, may be responsible for this trend. Interestingly, the incidence of vulvar cancer has remained stable. Although the relative increase in VIN may be due to early diagnosis and treatment of the preinvasive disease or the

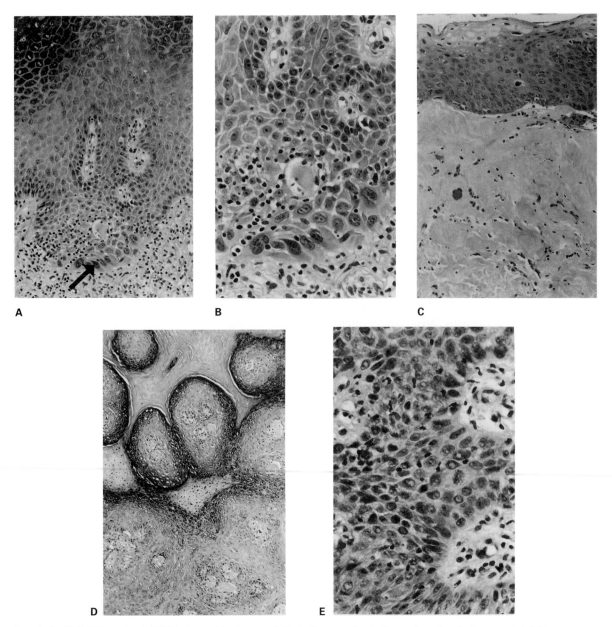

Fig. 3.4 Well differentiated VIN lesions with the morphologic features classically attributed to 'vulvar atypia:' **A** Low-power photomicrograph illustrates conspicuous maturation and similarity to vulvar hyperplasia (compare to Fig. 1B); note the small focus of atypical parabasal cells (arrow); **B** higher power view details nuclear enlargement and hyperchromasia in the parabasal cells; **C** Lichen sclerosis with coexisting nuclear atypia; **D** and **E** low- and high-power photomicrographs of a papillary lesion of the vulva with maturation and prominent keratohyaline changes **D**; however, the parabasal cells display conspicuous nuclear atypia **E**. These lesions are usually not associated with negative for HPV nucleic acids.

population at risk may not have had sufficient time to develop carcinoma.

The epidemiology of vulvar neoplasia shares several similarities with cervical neoplasia but differences do exist. Like cervical neoplasia, vulvar carcinoma is linked to a defined precursor lesion, vulvar intraepithelial neoplasia, which in turn is strongly linked to HPV 16.[26,27] In this respect, the scenario of HPV 16 infection, followed by VIN followed by cancer (after several years) is fulfilled.

However, as will be discussed subsequently, there are distinct differences between populations with vulvar intraepithelial and invasive neoplasms and these include cigarette smoking, presence of HPV nucleic acids, and most importantly age. These differences are summarized schematically in Fig. 3.5.

Relationship to papillomaviruses

The human papillomavirus has emerged as the major suspect in the genesis of intraepithelial and invasive neoplasms of the female genital tract. A number of studies have closely linked HPV and neoplasia at the clinical, histological and molecular levels. The close association of HPV with precancerous genital lesions was first appreciated morphologically when approximately 20–30% of cervical or vulvar intraepithelial neoplasms were observed in continuity with classic condylomata.[12] In addition, there exist lesions with features of both neoplasia and condyloma in the same epithelium and the coexistence of koilocytotic atypia with abnormal mitoses and nuclear atypia suggested a common etiology.[17,28]

The discovery, isolation, and subclassification of HPV types resolved many of the questions concerning the relationship of HPV to these different forms of precancers. HPV types 6 and 11, isolated from genital warts, were frequently detected in benign condylomata, particularly in the vulva, comprising from 60 to 80% of HPV found in these lesions.[29] In contrast, HPV 16 was found in up to 80% of koilocytotic CIN lesions, about 50% of classic CIN lesions, and 80% of VIN lesions.[30,31] Nearly 80% of invasive squamous cell cancers contain either HPV 16 or 18 DNA sequences.[32,33] HPVs have also been detected in endocervical adenocarcinomas and adenosquamous carcinomas, suggesting that HPV may not be limited to the squamous epithelium and derived tumors.

Certain HPV DNA types, such as types 16, 18, 31, 33, 35, and 51, have been associated with genital neoplasia,[34] and this subset of HPV types contains transforming 'genes' (E6 and E7) which have the capacity *in vitro* to bind regulatory cellular proteins encoded by such 'antioncogenes' such as P53 and the Rb (retinoblastoma) genes.[35] Other characteristics of oncogenic papillomaviruses include a capability to integrate into the host

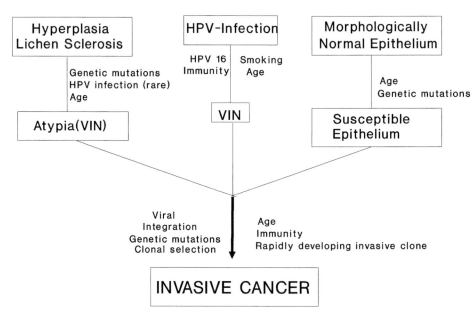

Fig. 3.5 Schematic diagram of potential pathogenetic mechanisms for the development of vulvar carcinoma. This pathway includes HPV associated (center) and unassociated (left) VIN lesions. A portion of cancers (right) may evolve without a precursor.

chromosomal DNA. In contrast, the distribution of HPV in condylomata and intraepithelial neoplasms is primarily extrachromosomal.[36] Whether chromosomal integration is required for invasion remains to be determined.

At present the possible cofactors in HPV-related neoplasia have not been clarified. Sun exposure, lesion site, and immune status are important to the genesis of some human tumors containing HPV.[37,38] Cigarette smoking is likely important in others, in particular verrucous tumors occurring in the larynx of heavy smokers.[39] The role of smoking in the genesis of genital tumors is unclear, although an association has been reported.[7] Oncogene amplification has been detected in some cervical tumors, specifically c-*myc* and h-*ras*, suggesting that host genes are also involved.[40] However, alterations in these genes have not been associated with vulvar neoplasia.[41]

Herpes simplex virus, which was intensively investigated in the 1970s, has no certain role. Despite a number of studies linking herpes simplex virus to cervical and vulvar neoplasms, they employed primarily seroepidemiological, histochemical and in-situ hybridization analyses.[42] Unlike HPV, HSV has not been consistently demonstrated in cancer precursors or invasive neoplasms using highly specific techniques such as Southern and Northern blot hybridization. Despite suggestions that it may cooperate with HPV to promote neoplastic transformation, there is little hard data identifying the role of HSV at present.[42] Moreover, Kreider et al,[43] in their preliminary studies with the nude mouse model, did not detect morphological changes in the cervical grafts which had been incubated with inactivated herpes.[43]

Relationship to vulvar carcinoma

Traditionally, vulvar squamous cancer has predominated in women in their seventh and eight decades, and rarely observed in women under age 30.[1-3] In a case-control study of vulvar carcinoma, Brinton et al identified preexisting genital warts as a significant risk factor, which with smoking increased the relative risk of vulvar cancer patients to 35 times that of controls. Smoking status was also an important risk factor in the group with VIN (current smoker: RR 4.65 vs 1.19). Up to a three-fold increase in risk was noted with five or more (in contrast to none to one) sexual partners.[7]

Papillomaviruses provide the strongest direct link between a sexually-transmitted disease and vulvar cancer. Being an infectious disease, it may explain both the multicentric nature of lower genital squamous neoplasia and the strong relationship between vulvar carcinoma and either genital warts or VIN. If HPV nucleic acids and sexual factors are associated with vulvar precancers, it would be expected that a proportion of invasive cancers would contain HPV DNA as well, given the association between the two.[7] It is of interest however, that some differences emerge as patients with VIN of different ages are evaluated, in particular with respect to the presence of HPV nucleic acids. For example, Twiggs et al[44] and Park et al[45] noted that older women had fewer HPV-16-positive lesions as compared to a younger cohort. In our experience, older women with typical forms of VIN (Bowen's disease/CIS) still have a frequency of HPV positives. However, so-called differentiated forms of VIN which are HPV negative predominate in the older group.[46] Brinton et al[7] identified number of sexual partners was a risk factor for VIN (RR up to 5.08 vs 3.32) but not for invasive cancer.[7] This would suggest that there may be two different groups of women with intraepithelial neoplasia, with the lesions in the older group occurring in the absence of HPV. An older study by Mabuchi et al[6] found little relationship between sexual factors and invasive vulvar carcinoma. In their study, which exclusively involved women with invasive cancer, over 80% of the study patients were 50 years of age or older, and 57% were over 60 years of age. Although they did not obtain data on number of sexual partners, they failed to associate early age of coitus, first marriage and multiple miscarriages, or venereal factors with vulvar cancer. They observed a relationship to prior history of vulvar inflammation and urogenital cancer, and the relationship to prior cervical cancer (6 cases out of 149) was of borderline significance.[6] This is similar to the findings of Brinton et al[7] who noted a RR of 1.5 for a previous cervical cancer. Additional studies suggest that, from an epidemiological perspective, vulvar cancer may encompass more than one distinct group.[47]

With use of a variety of techniques for analyzing HPV DNA in genital lesions it has become possible to explore by more direct means the relationship between HPV and vulvar neoplasia. It has become apparent that the detection rate of HPV in vulvar carcinoma is related to the age of the population under study, the associated precursor lesions, and the morphologic appearance of the invasive tumors. From 80 to 90% of VIN contain HPV 16 or related DNA types, but the association of HPV with cancer decreases as a function of age.[7,44] This is partially explained by the fact that cancers associated with VIN lesions — the group most strongly associated with HPV — are more likely to be younger in age than cancers in general.[48] Histological analysis of invasive vulvar carcinomas reveals that although only 20–30% of invasive vulvar carcinomas contain HPV, certain variants of vulvar cancer which bear a close similarity to genital warts ('warty carcinomas') are more frequently HPV positive.[48-50] This includes variants of HPV 6 nucleic acids in which genomic integration of the viral DNA has taken place.[51] In particular, vulvar carcinomas associated with VIN and vulvar carcinomas which exhibit a growth pattern resembling VIN (intraepithelial-like or basaloid patterns) are significantly more likely to be HPV+, with up to 66% positive (vs 13% for conventional carcinomas).[49,50] As one would expect, these same patients are more likely to be younger.[49,50]

The most interesting evidence that vulvar carcinomas may evolve from multiple precursor types comes from two morphological studies examining the epithelium adjacent to invasive vulvar cancers. Both Buscema et al[23] and Zaino et al[24] noted that in only approximately one-fourth of invasive cancers was there evidence of a classic vulvar intraepithelial neoplasm (carcinoma-in-situ) in the adjacent epithelium. In contrast, over one-half of cases were associated with epithelial hyperplasia or atrophy and inflammation, with or without cytological atypia (lichen sclerosis, squamous hyperplasia, atypia, etc.).[23-25] Whether these associations were merely fortuitous or actually signified that such inflammations place the patient at risk is not clear. However, they suggest that a significant proportion of vulvar carcinomas do not evolve from a long-standing precancerous lesion. Also, only a fraction of women with chronic inflammatory diseases of the vulva develop cancer. However, the strong topographical association between cancer and these changes supports the concerns by Mabuchi et al[6] that environmental factors may alter genital mucosa in some way to increase its susceptibility to cancer independent of HPV infection. In rare instances we have observed HPV positive VIN lesions in association with Lichen Sclerosis, suggesting further that several factors may coexist in the same patient.[46]

NATURAL HISTORY

There is relatively little information on the natural history of untreated vulvar precancers, but potential pathways are illustrated in Fig. 3.1. Although a portion of invasive cancers have been associated with VIN, the actual percentage of VIN which evolve into invasive cancer is unknown. Similar to condylomata, VIN has been observed more frequently in young women, often develop rapidly like genital warts, may coexist with genital warts, and may regress.[10,18-20]

The spontaneous regression rate for genital warts (including treatment via hypnosis) has ranged up to 80%.[52] VINs have been observed to regress spontaneously, particularly in younger women,[18-20] but there are no substantial long-term follow-up studies of untreated patients. Factors influencing regression are the age of the patient, the presenting clinical picture, and the duration of time required for resolution. Young women presenting with discrete papules (bowenoid papulosis) appear to comprise a distinct clinical group for which spontaneous regression is more likely, despite the fact that these lesions look similar to other precancerous lesions and often contain HPV-16 nucleic acids. In one review of 12 cases of bowenoid papulosis which regressed and in which the patients age was known, nine were under 30 years of age and three were under 20 years.[20] The time required for spontaneous resolution ranged from one to 22 months with most lesions resolving in less than 6 months. Thus it would appear that VIN lesions presenting as discrete papules in young women have a higher regression rate than those presenting as extensive disease in older age groups.

The greatest risk factor for progression to or association with invasive cancer appears to be age, with up to 19% of women in their late 50s with VIN harboring occult carcinoma.[53] A less commonly observed association is in younger patients with immune defects.[24] In one follow-up study of women with VIN, Jones and McClean observed five of five VIN lesions progress to invasion over follow-up, all in women in their late 40s or early 50s.[54] In women under the age of 40, progression to carcinoma appears to be uncommon. Studies have shown that up to 25% of patients treated for VIN III by local excision will develop recurrent disease[12] and an additional 10% may develop invasive squamous carcinoma. Their risk for vaginal or cervical dysplasia or carcinoma is also increased.[55]

Clinical correlations

The most important clinical issues concerning HPV are (1) the diagnosis and treatment of HPV-related neoplasia, (2) defining the morphological spectrum of HPV infection, (3) the mechanism(s) by which HPV related genital lesions recur, and (4) treatment of the male sexual partner.

The fact that a high proportion of VIN lesions in young women contain HPV 16 is intriguing since most of these lesions do not progress to invasive carcinoma over short-term follow-up.[12] The high prevalence of bowenoid papulosis or dysplasia in the young population would further reinforce the assumption that such VIN lesions are relatively innocuous and represent a variant of HPV 16 infection in cutaneous epithelium which may warrant a different therapeutic approach. However, it is difficult to delineate a subpopulation suitable for observation alone. Cases have been reported of young women with lesions containing all of the features of 'bowenoid papulosis' which were associated with invasive carcinoma.[22] Thus, with the exception of very young patients for whom ablation may be too traumatic, removal is warranted.

With respect to altering therapeutic approaches for lesions containing different HPV types, it is now possible to type lesions and determine if potentially oncogenic viral DNAs such as type 16 are present. However, the clinical value or feasibility of this approach is questionable at present. It is clear that although HPVs type 6 and 11 predominate in benign lesions, they may be found in some invasive cancers and verrucous carcinomas. Schinella et al[56] detected HPV sequences closely related to type 6 in anal carcinomas associated with condylomata in homosexual men. Others have detected either HPV 6 or a very closely related HPV in squamous cancers in women.[50] In our experience, this is an uncommon occurence. Others have found HPV 6 DNA sequences in 6% of vulva carcinomas (Beckman A, personal communication). Although this association requires further study, it would be imprudent to allow the HPV type to dictate the therapeutic approach to neoplasia. When multiple lesions are present in the genital tract, variability in lesion morphology (and multiplicity of HPV types) may be striking.[57] Therapy is usually dictated by the accessibility of the lesion, its configuration and size.

FUTURE CONSIDERATIONS

Several issues remain to be addressed which are germane to the concept of VIN as a cancer precursor. They include (1) the rising incidence of this disease and its potential relationship to behavioral (e.g., smoking) factors, (2) resolving the factors which promote the development of invasive carcinoma in a small subset of women with VIN, (3) the role of age in this process, and (4) the etiology and biology of those vulvar precursors and cancers which are not associated with papillomaviruses. With the exception of preliminary studies identifying p53 mutations in a minority of vulvar neoplasms, there is scant data linking HPV-negative tumors to a specific etiologic agent or molecular alteration.[41,58] Because many of these tumors arise in a background of vulvar hyperplasia or lichen sclerosis, resolving the etiology of these lesions may provide clues to the genesis of their related cancer precursors, irrespective of the relatively low prospective risk for cancer in patients with uncomplicated vulvar dystrophies. Because the genesis of many vulvar carcinomas may involve a normal to hyperplasia to atypia (VIN) to invasive cancer progression, understanding the factors which operate in the genesis of these HPV negative precursor lesions may be applicable to other systems, including cervix, where a series of molecular events must precede invasive carcinoma. Moreover, their resolution is particularly important to placing papillomaviruses in proper perspective as a causative agent in vulvar neoplasia.

REFERENCES

1. Silverberg E. Statistical and epidemiological information on gynecologic cancer. Atlanta: American Cancer Society, 1980: p 9.
2. Cramer D W, Cutler S J. Incidence and histopathology of malignancies of the female genital organs in the United States. Am J Obstet Gynecol 1974; 118: 443–460.
3. Krain L S. Carcinoma of the vulva in California 1942–1969. The California Tumor Registry experience. Oncology 1973; 28: 110–116.
4. Zaino R J. Carcinoma of the vulva, urethra, and bartholin's glands. In Wilkinson E J, ed. *Pathology of the vulva and vagina*. New York: Churchill Livingstone, 1987: pp 119–153.
5. Henson D, Tarone R. An epidemiologic study of cancer of the cervix, vagina, and vulva based upon the Third National Cancer Survey in the United States. Am J Obstet Gynecol 1977; 129: 525–532.
6. Mabuchi K, Bross D S, Kessler II. Epidemiology of cancer of the vulva. A case-control study. Cancer 1985; 55: 1843–1848.
7. Brinton L A, Nasca P C, Mallin K, Baptiste M S, Wilbanks G D, Richart R M. Case-control study of cancer of the vulva. Obstet Gynecol 1990; 75: 859.
8. Sturgeon S R, Brinton L A, Devesa S S, Kurman R J. In situ and invasive vulvar cancer incidence trends (1973 to 1987). Am J Obstet Gynecol 1992; 166: 1482–1485.
9. Abell M R, Gosling J R G. Intraepithelial and infiltrative carcinoma of the vulva: Bowen's type. Cancer 1961; 14: 318–329.
10. Wade T R, Kopf A W, Ackerman A B. Bowenoid papulosis of the genitalia. Arch Dermatol 1979; 115: 306.
11. International Society of Gynecologic Pathology: New nomenclature for vulvar disease I. Obstet Gynecol 1976; 47: 122.
12. Friedrich E G, Wilkinson E J, Fu Y S. Carcinoma in situ of the vulva: a continuing challenge. Am J Obstet Gynecol 1980; 136: 830.
13. Kaufman R H, Gardner H L. Intraepithelial carcinoma of the vulva. Clin Obstet Gynecol 1965; 8: 1035–1050.
14. Report of the committee on terminology of the International Society for the Study of Vulvar Disease. J Reprod Med 1990; 35: 483.
15. Crum C P, Egawa K, Fu Y S et al. Intraepithelial squamous lesions of the vulva: biologic and histologic criteria for the distinction of condyloma from vulvar intraepithelial neoplasia. Am J Obstet Gynecol 1982; 144: 77.
16. Fu Y S, Reagan J W, Richart R M. Definition of precursors. Gynecol Oncol 1981; 12: S220–S231.
17. Winkler B, Crum C P, Fujii T et al. Koilocytotic lesions of the cervix: the relationship of mitotic abnormalities to the presence of papillomavirus antigens and nuclear DNA content. Cancer 1984; 53: 1081.
18. Bhawan J. Multicentric pigmented Bowen's disease. A clinically benign sqamous cell carcinoma in situ. Gynecol Oncol 1980; 10: 201.
19. Skinner M S, Sternberg W H, Ichinose H et al. Spontaneous regression of Bowenoid atypia of the vulva. Obstet Gynecol 1973; 42: 40.
20. Halasz C, Silvers D, Crum C P. Bowenoid papulosis in a 3 year old girl. J Am Acad Dermatol 1986; 14: 326.
21. Ulbright T M, Stehman F B, Roth L M et al. Bowenoid dysplasia of the vulva. Cancer 1982; 50: 2910.
22. Bergeron C, Naghashfar Z, Canaan C, Shah K, Fu Y, Ferenczy A. Human papillomavirus type 16 in intraepithelial neoplasia (bowenoid papulosis) and coexistent invasive carcinoma of the vulva. Int J Gynecol Pathol 1987; 6(1): 1.
23. Buscema J et al. The significance of the histologic alterations adjacent to invasive vulvar carcinoma. Am J Obstet Gynecol 1980; 137: 902.
24. Zaino R J et al. Epithelial alterations in proximity to invasive squamous carcinoma of the vulva. Int J Gynecol Pathol 1982; 1: 173.
25. Neill S M, Lessana-Leibowitch M, Pelisse M, Moyal-Barracco M. Lichen sclerosis, invasive squamous cell carcinoma and human papillomavirus. Am J Obstet Gynecol 1990; 162: 1633–1634.
26. Gross G, Hagedorn M, Ikenberg H et al. Bowenoid papulosis: presence of human papillomavirus (HPV) structural antigens and of HPV 16-related DNA sequences. Arch Dermatol 1985; 121: 858.
27. Ikenberg H, Gissman L, Gross G et al. Human papillomavirus type-16-related DNA in genital Bowen's disease and bowenoid papulosis. Int J Cancer 1983; 32: 563.
28. Meisels A, Roy M, Fortin M et al. Human papillomavirus infections of the cervix: The atypical condyloma. Acta Cytol 1981; 25: 7–16.
29. Gissman L, Wolnick L, Ikenberg H et al. Human papillomavirus type 6 and 11 DNA sequences in genital and laryngeal papillomas and in some cervical cancers. Proc Nat Acad Sci USA 1983; 80: 560–563.
30. Crum C P, Ikenberg H, Richart R M, Gissman L. Human papillomavirus type 16 and early cervical neoplasia. New Engl J Med 1984; 310: 880–883.
31. Ikenberg H, Gissman L, Gross G, Grussendorf-Conen E-I, zur Hausen H. Human papillomavirus type-16-related DNA in genital Bowen's disease and Bowenoid papulosis. Int J Cancer 1983; 32: 563–565.

32. Durst M, Gissman L, Ikenberg H, zur Hausen H. A papillomavirus DNA from a cervical carcinoma and its prevalence in cancer biopsy samples from different geographic regions. Proc Nat Acad Sci USA 1983; 80: 3812–3815.

33. Boshart M, Gissman L, Ikenberg H et al. A new type of papillomavirus DNA, its presence in genital cancer biopsies and in cell lines derived from cervical cancer. EMBO J 1984; 3: 1151–1157.

34. zur Hausen H. Papillomaviruses as carcinomaviruses. In: Klein G, ed. *Advances in viral oncology*. New York: Raven Press, 1989: pp 1–27.

35. Werness B A, Levine A J, Howley P M. Association of human papillomavirus types 16 and 18 E6 proteins with p53. Science 1990; 248: 76–79.

36. Cullen A P, Reid R, Campion M, et al. Analysis of the physical state of different human papillomavirus DNAs in intraepithelial and invasive cervical neoplasia. J Virol 1991; 56: 606–612.

37. zur Hausen H. Human papillomaviruses and their possible role in squamous cell carcinomas. Curr Topics Microbiol Immunol 1977; 78: 1–29.

38. Schneider V, Kay S, Lee H M. Immunosuppression as a high risk factor in the development of condyloma accuminatum and squamous neoplasia of the cervix. Acta Cytol 1983; 27: 220.

39. Abramson A L, Brandsma J, Steinberg B, Winkler B. Verrucous carcinoma of the larynx. Arch Otolaryngol 1985; 111: 709.

40. Riou G, Sheng Z M, Zhou D, Lusinchi A, Le Doussal V, Barrois M. C-*myc* and c-Ha-*ras* proto-oncogenes in cervical cancer: prognostic value. Bull Cancer (Paris) 1990; 77: 341.

41. Tate J, Mutter G M, Prasad C J, Berkowitz R, Goodman H, Crum C P. Analysis of HPV positive and negative vulvar squamous cell carcinomas for alterations in the c-myc, Ha, Ki, and N ras genes (in preparation).

42. Crum C P. Vulvar intraepithelial neoplasia: the concept and its application. Human Pathol 1982; 13: 187–189.

43. Kreider J, Howett M K, Wolfe S A et al. Morphological transformation *in-vivo* of human uterine cervix with papillomavirus from condyloma acuminata. Nature 1985; 317: 639.

44. Twiggs L, Okagaki T, Clark B, Fukushima M, Ostrow R, Faras A. A clinical, histopathologic, and molecular biologic investigation of vulvar intraepithelial neoplasia. Int J Gynecol Pathol 1988; 7: 48.

45. Park J S, Jones R W, McLean M R, Currie J L, Woodruff J D, Shah K V, Kurman R J. Possible etiologic heterogeneity of vulvar intraepithelial neoplasia. Cancer 1991; 67: 1599–1607.

46. Haefner H A, Tate J E, McLachlin C M, Crum C P. Vulvar intraepithelial neoplasia: age, morphological phenotype, papillomavirus DNA, and coexisting invasive carcinoma. Human Pathol 1995; 26: 147–154.

47. Parazzini F, Vecchia C L, Garsia S, Negri E, Sideri M, Rognoni M T, Origoni M. Determinants of invasive vulvar cancer risk: an Italian case-control study. Gynecol Oncol 1993; 48: 50–55.

48. Bloss J D, Liao S Y, Wilczynski S P, Macri C, Walker J, Peake M, Berman M L. Clinical and histologic features of vulvar carcinomas analyzed for human papillomavirus status: Evidence that squamous cell carcinoma of the vulva has more than one etiology. Human Pathol 1991; 22: 711–718.

49. Andersen W A, Franquemont D W, Williams J, Taylor P T, Crum C P. Vulvar squamous cell carcinoma and papillomaviruses: two separate entities? Am J Obstet Gynecol 1991; 165: 329–336.

50. Toki T, Kurman R J, Park J S, Kessis T, Daniel R W, Shah K V. Probable nonpapillomavirus etiology of squamous cell carcinoma of the vulva in older women: a clinicopathologic study using in situ hybridization and polymerase chain reaction. Int J Gynecol Pathol 1991; 10: 107–125.

51. Kasher M S, Roman A. Characterization of human papillomavirus type 6b DNA isolated from an invasive squamous carcinoma of the vulva. Virology 1988; 165: 225–233.

52. Allington H V. Review of the psychotherapy of warts. Arch Dermatol Syphilol 1952; 66: 316–326.

53. Chafe W, Richards A, Morgan L et al. Unrecognized invasive carcinoma vulvar intraepithelial neoplasia (VIN). Gynecol Oncol 1980; 31: 154–162.

54. Jones R W, McClean M R. Carcinoma in situ of the vulva: a review of 31 treated and five untreated cases. Obstet Gynecol 1986; 68: 499–503.

55. Mitchell M F, Prasad C J, Silva E, Rutledge F, McArthur M C, Crum C P. Second primary squamous neoplasms in patients with vulvar carcinoma: viral (HPV) and histopathologic correlates. Obstet Gynecol 1993; 81: 13–18.

56. Schinella R A, Selvaggi S M, Morgan D M et al. Papillomavirus in anorectal condyloma acuminatum with malignant transformation detected by molecular hybridization and immunoperoxidase technique. Lab Invest 1985; 52: 59 (abstract).

57. McCance D J, Clarkson P K, Dyson J L et al. Human papillomavirus types 6 and 16 in multifocal intraepithelial neoplasias of the female lower genital tract. Br J Obstet Gynecol 1985; 92: 1093.

58. Pilotti S, Donghi R, D'Amato L et al. Papillomavirus, p53 alteration and primary carcinoma of the vulva. Eur J Cancer 1993; 29A: 924–925.

4. The epidemiology of cervical neoplasms

Melissa R. Krone   Nancy B. Kiviat   Laura A. Koutsky

INTRODUCTION

The role of sexual activity in the epidemiology of cervical neoplasia has been appreciated for decades. As early as 1842, Rigoni-Stern[1] reported that cancer of the uterus (site, unspecified) occurred less frequently among cloistered nuns than among married women. Since this initial report, several studies have confirmed the association between squamous cell neoplasms of the uterine cervix and various measures of sexual exposure including multiple sexual partners, and early age of first intercourse.[2] Recent investigations have persuasively demonstrated that the observed epidemiologic association between sexual behavior and cervical cancer is, in large measure, due to the underlying etiologic relationship between oncogenic types of sexually transmitted human papillomavirus (HPV) and cervical neoplasia.

Papanicolaou's observation (1943) that exfoliated cervical cells that pooled in the vaginal fornices could be used for early detection of even a small intraepithelial cervical lesion was a major breakthrough. This discovery permitted both the opportunity to investigate the natural history of cervical neoplasia and to develop effective cervical cancer control programs. Although the concept that premalignant intraepithelial lesions are stages in a continuum initially provided the basis for implementing population-based cytologic screening programs in the early 1950s, it was not until Richart and Barron[3] reported their observations on the natural history of mild dysplasia in 1969 that the progressive potential of early precancerous lesions became widely accepted.

The goal of this chapter is to provide an overview of epidemiologic trends in the incidence of cervical neoplasia. The focus is on data from the US, but, when available, information concerning international trends is presented. Squamous cell neoplasms of the vagina, vulva, penis and anus have also been linked with sexually transmitted papillomavirus infections. Comparisons between rates of cervical cancer and these other anogenital tract cancers are provided to illustrate unanswered questions concerning the relationship of epithelial site, type of infecting virus, and other factors in the pathogenesis of HPV-associated tumors. A discussion of the changing epidemiology of cervical neoplasia in the setting of human immunodeficiency virus (HIV) is included.

INVASIVE CERVICAL CANCER

International trends

Among women, carcinoma of the uterine cervix is the second most common cancer in the world, and the most common cancer in many developing countries of Africa, South and Central America, Asia, and the Pacific.[4] There were an estimated 465 600 new cases of cervical cancer detected worldwide in 1980, with a crude incidence rate ranging from four cases per 100 000 in Western Asia to 33 per 100 000 in the Eastern Asia regions of Hong Kong, Korea, and Mongolia. Among both sexes, cancer of the uterine cervix is the fifth most dominant cancer, following carcinomas of the stomach, lung, breast, and colon or rectum.

Unlike many carcinomas, cervical cancer is easily preventable because the uterine cervix is accessible to cytologic, colposcopic and histopathologic examination and because simple surgical excision or destruction of intraepithelial neoplastic or dysplastic lesions has proven to be highly effective in preventing progression to malignancy. However, because Papanicolaou (Pap) smear screening for cervical intraepithelial neoplasia (CIN) and referral for histologic confirmation and treatment is prohibitively expensive to implement and maintain in most developing countries, the global incidence of invasive cervical cancer is likely to remain high.

The estimated incidence of carcinoma of the cervix and penis in several countries with tumor registries in place between 1968–1971 and 1977–1982[5,6] is shown in Fig. 4.1. In all of the countries shown, the incidence of cervical cancer exceeds the incidence of penile cancer. Except for Recife, Brazil, the incidence of cervical cancer declined between the two time periods; in comparison, cancer of the penis underwent a slight increase in incidence in most areas. The relatively high incidence of of both cervical and penile cancer shown for Brazil may in part be due to incomplete denominator data.

Data from the SEER Program

The Surveillance, Epidemiology, and End Results (SEER) Program, based within the Surveillance Program at the National Cancer Institute, routinely collects cancer data from nine population-based cancer registries located throughout the US. The geographic regions that comprise the SEER Program database are adequately representative subsets of the USA, involving about 9.6% of the population. The SEER Program provides data on incidence, mortality, and survival rates for a broad spectrum of cancers over time; the National Center for Health Statistics provides cancer mortality data for the entire USA.

The monograph entitled 'SEER Statistics Review 1973–1990' contains the most current cancer data available from the SEER Program.[7] The data presented below come from this publication. Unless otherwise noted, incidence and mortality rates are calculated for women only and are age-adjusted to the 1970 USA standard million.

In 1990 there were an estimated 13 500 new cases and 4627 actual deaths from invasive cervical cancer in the USA. The US mortality rate (1986–1990) for cervical cancer was 3.0 per 100 000, and for women diagnosed between 1983 and 1989, the 5-year relative survival rate was 66.8%. With an incidence of 8.7 cases per 100 000

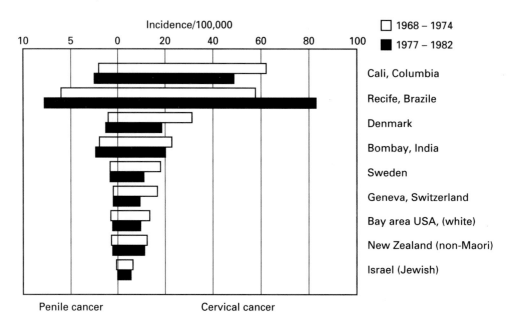

Fig. 4.1 Age-adjusted sex-specific incidence of invasive cancer of the cervix and penis in countries with established tumor registries during the years 1968–1974 and 1977–1982. (From Paavonen et al (1990);[12] reprinted with permission.)

during 1986–1990, cancer of the cervix uteri was the third most common female genital tract malignancy, following cancer of the corpus uteri (20.9 per 100 00) and ovary (14.3 per 100 000). In comparison, the incidence of breast cancer among women was considerably higher (108.4 per 100 000) as was the incidence for cancer of the testis in men (107.7 per 100 000). However, while the incidence for all of these malignancies except corpus uteri increased between 1973 and 1990, cervical cancer experienced a 34.8% decline (Fig. 4.2). Furthermore, during this same time interval mortality from cervical cancer decreased by 41.3%.

Trends over time

Since 1950, the change in incidence of cervical cancer has been dramatic, declining 75.1%, with an estimated annual percent change of −3.5. These data represent white women only, because prior to 1973 data for other racial groups were not complete. However, between 1973 and 1990, the estimated annual percent change in incidence of cervical cancer was −4.5 among black women compared to −2.6 among whites. In 1950 there were over 8000 deaths due to cervical cancer among American women,[8] and since then the mortality rate among all white women has decreased by 73.6%. From 1973 to 1990, mortality from cervical cancer declined by 41.1% among whites and 45.2% among blacks. The 5-year relative survival among white women has increased from 59% (1950–1954) to 69% (1983–1989); among black women it has increased from 47% (1960–1963) to 57% (1983–1989). The development and implementation of Pap smear screening for early detection of precancerous cervical lesions in the 1950s has generally been credited with the major portion of the decline in incidence and mortality over the past 30 years.[9]

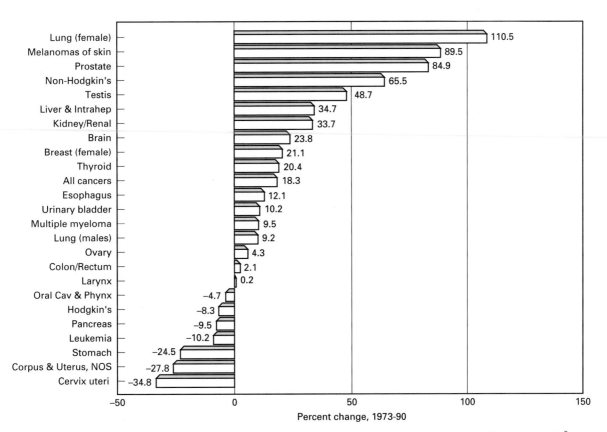

Fig. 4.2 Trends in incidence of primary cancer sites, SEER Program, USA, 1973–1990. (From Miller et al (1993);[7] reprinted with permission.)

Table 4.1 Age-adjusted genital and anal cancer incidence for 1969–1971, 1973–1977, 1981–1985, and 1986–1990, all races, SEER Programs, USA

	1969–1971 incidence per 100 000		1973–1977 incidence per 100 000		1981–1985 incidence per 100 000		1986–1990 incidence per 100 000	
	Females	Males	Females	Males	Females	Males	Females	Males
Cervix	16.7		12.4		8.0		8.7	
Vagina	0.6		0.7		0.7		0.6	
Vulva	1.8		1.6		1.5		1.7	
Penis		1.0		0.9		0.8		0.7
Anus	0.6	0.4	0.7	0.5	0.9	0.7	0.9	0.8

The change in incidence of cancer of the cervix, vagina, vulva, penis, and anus since 1969 is shown in Table 4.1.[7,10,11] while rates of cervical cancer have generally declined, the incidence of carcinomas at these other genital and anal sites remained relatively low and steady over the past two decades, at least five times lower than the rates of cervical cancer. Routine screening programs comparable to Pap smear screening for cervical neoplasia have never been implemented for early detection of premalignant lesions of the vulva, vagina, penis, and anus because rates of these tumors have remained so low over time.[12] One of the remaining questions relating to the epidemiology of HPV-associated cancers concerns the apparent paradoxical finding of a similarly high prevalence of oncogenic HPV infection of the penis, vulva, vagina, anus, and the cervix, but a relatively low occurrence of anogenital carcinomas exclusive of the cervix.

Whether the slight increase in invasive cervical cancer incidence noted for the most recent time interval (1986–1990) presented in Table 4.1 is an indication of a true change or of statistical fluctuation is not yet known. As discussed below, the change in incidence appears to be particularly striking for white women less than 50 years of age.

Age-specific rates

The incidence of invasive cervical cancer increases with age, rising sharply to 15 per 100 000 between the ages 20 and 35 years (premenopausal years), then fluctuating around 15–20 cases per 100 000 through the ninth decade of life (Fig. 4.3).[7] The age-specific incidence for other HPV-associated genital tract and anal cancers increases much more slowly and remains relatively low throughout life, except that of vulvar cancer, which increases sharply among women sixty years of age or older, up to about 20 cases per 100 000.

Ethnic comparisons

The incidence of carcinoma of the cervix is about two times higher for black women than for white women (Table 4.2).[7,10] Rates of vaginal, penile, and anal carcinoma are only slightly elevated among blacks compared with whites. Rates of vulvar cancer are higher among whites than blacks. Mortality rates for genital tract and anal cancers are also generally higher among blacks, with a cervical cancer mortality rate about 2.5 times higher among blacks compared with whites. Moreover, for all of these genital and anal cancers except vaginal, the 5-year relative survival is better for whites than for blacks. The median age of diagnosis for cervical cancer among all races is 47 years, which is at least 15 years younger than the median age of diagnosis of cancer of the vagina (70 years), vulva (71 years), penis (67) and anus (females, 67 years; males, 62 years). However, black women are diagnosed with cervical cancer at an older age (52 years) than white women (47 years) and at a more advanced stage (Table 4.3).[7] Fifty-one per cent of cervical tumors among whites were diagnosed at a localized stage, showing no regional or distant spread, compared with only 36% among blacks.

The fact that cervical cancer is diagnosed at an earlier age and growth stage in whites suggests

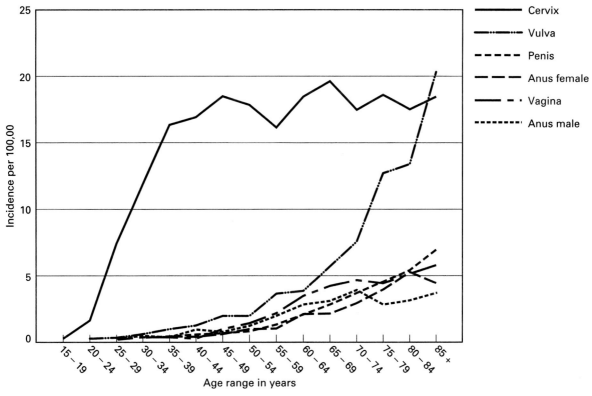

Fig. 4.3 Age- and sex-specific incidence of invasive cancers of the cervix, vulva, vagina, penis, and anus, SEER Program, USA, 1986–1990.

Table 4.2 Age-adjusted incidence, mortality, and 5-year relative survival rates for genital tract and anal cancer, SEER Programs, USA

	Incidence/100 000 (1986–1990)		Mortality/100 000 (1986–1990)		% Survival (1983–1989)		Median age of diagnosis in years (1986–1990)	
	Blacks	Whites	Blacks	Whites	Blacks	Whites	Blacks	Whites
Cervix	14.3	7.9	6.9	2.6	57.0	69.1	52	47
Vagina	1.1	0.6	0.4	0.2	50.3	41.3	66	71
Vulva	1.4	1.8	0.3	0.3	65.6	73.9	59	71
Anus								
Female	1.0	0.9	0.1	0.1	51.3	65.7	62	68
Male	1.1	0.8	0.2	0.1	31.9	60.7	59	62
Penis	0.9	0.7	0.3	0.1	71.0	70.6	65	67

Table 4.3 Tumor growth stage at diagnosis of invasive cervical cancer, SEER Programs, USA, 1986–1990

	Stage distribution (%)	
	Blacks	Whites
Localized	36	51
Regional	41	32
Distant	14	10
Unstaged	9	7

differences in the use and/or outcome of Pap screening programs. Women among lower socio-economic groups (lower income and education level), who until recently have had less access to Pap screening and gynecological services, have a higher risk of cervical cancer. This may explain some of the observed difference in incidence between blacks and whites.[8]

For white women under 50 years of age, the incidence of cervical cancer appears to be gradually increasing after a decline in the 1970s and early 1980s (Fig. 4.4).[7] While the rates for black women under the age of 50 years remain higher than those of whites up through the 1980s, the increase in incidence among whites and the continuing decrease among blacks over time have substantially reduced the disparity. Among women over the age of 50 years, the incidence of cervical cancer for black women continues to be at least two times higher than the incidence for whites (Fig. 4.5).[7] Mortality rates have remained considerably higher among black women of all ages since the early 1970s.

Ethnic comparisons of incidence, mortality, and stage of tumor at diagnosis are important because they provide clues as to the etiology of cervical carcinoma and to the level to which women have access to Pap screening, diagnostic, and therapeutic services. The observed increased incidence of cervical cancer among white women less than 50 years of age during a time interval when the incidence continued to decline among similarly aged black women may reflect both an increase in oncogenic HPV infection among younger white women initiating sexual activity at earlier ages[13] and to an increase in access to Pap screening services among black women.[9]

CERVICAL CARCINOMA-IN-SITU

There are few data concerning the incidence of cervical carcinoma-in-situ (CIS) among well-defined populations. The Washington State SEER Program has routinely collected information on histologically confirmed cases of cervical carcinoma since the mid-1970s. The incidence rates of CIS among women for the most populous county in Washington state, King County, are shown in Fig. 4.6 for the years 1979–1981 and 1989–1991. The two curves reflect the same trend of a dramatic increase up through 30 years of age, followed by a substantial decrease in incidence thereafter. Between 1989 and 1991, a statistically significant increase in incidence of CIS among young women 15 to 19 years of age was noted. Although changes in the classification of Pap smear findings took place during this time, particularly with the introduction of the Bethesda System in 1988, the data presented in Fig. 4.6 are based on evidence of histologically confirmed cervical CIS, a diagnosis that the Washington state SEER program has not revised since the

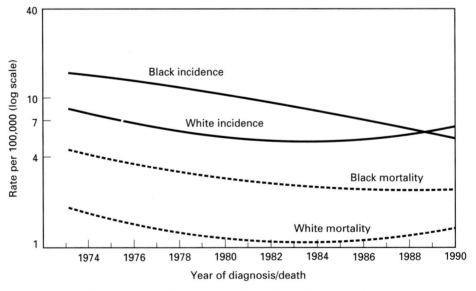

Fig. 4.4 Age-adjusted race-specific incidence and mortality of invasive cervical cancer among women under the age of 50, SEER Program, USA. (Adapted from Miller et al (1993);[7] reprinted with permission.)

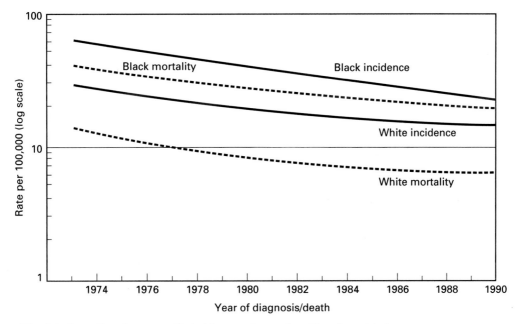

Fig. 4.5 Age-adjusted race-specific incidence and mortality of invasive cervical cancer among women over the age of 50, SEER Program, USA. (Adapted from Miller et al (1993);[7] reprinted with permission.)

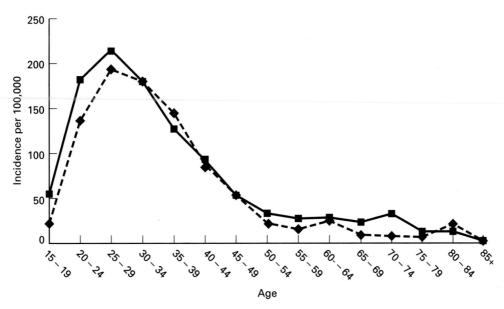

Fig. 4.6 Age-specific incidence of cervical carcinoma-in-situ, King County, Washington state. Solid line represents rates for 1989–1991; dashed line represents 1979–1981.

1970s. Nevertheless, changing cytologic criteria may explain part of the observed increase in incidence of CIS noted for the most recent time period.

The age-specific rates of CIS presented in Fig. 4.6 include in the denominator, women who, by virtue of never having had a Pap smear and/or of having had a hysterectomy could not be con-

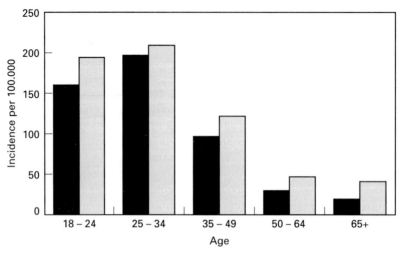

Fig. 4.7 Age-specific incidence of cervical carcinoma-in-situ, King County, Washington state, 1989–1991. Solid bars represent unadjusted rates; shaded bars represent rates adjusted for pap smear and hysterectomy rates.

sidered at risk of a diagnosis of cervical CIS. The CIS incidence rates for the 1989–1991 period were recalculated using data for Washington state from the Centers for Disease Control Behavioral Risk Factor Survey[14] to approximate the number of women in King County who had an intact cervix, and who reported having had at least one prior Pap smear during that time. As shown in Fig. 4.7, the adjusted incidence is considerably higher than the unadjusted incidence rate, particularly among the youngest and oldest age groups. This difference reflects the lower rate of Pap smear screening among younger women and substantially higher hysterectomy rates among older women. Importantly, for the years 1989 to 1991, the adjusted incidence rate for women 18–24 years of age (196 per 100 000) approximated the rate observed for women 25–34 years of age (212 per 100 000).

Overall, the incidence of cervical carcinoma-in-situ is much higher than the incidence of invasive cervical cancer through the fourth decade of life. Between 1987 and 1991 in the state of Washington, the age-adjusted rates of invasive cervical cancer and cervical carcinoma-in-situ were 7.9 and 62.4 per 100 000, respectively.[15] CIS has a younger age distribution, with incidence rates about thirty to over one hundred times

higher than rates for invasive cervical cancer among adolescent and young adult females. Current literature indicates that there has been an increase in sexual activity among young women in recent years.[16] As discussed above, two important risk factors for abnormal Pap smear results are early age of first intercourse and multiple sex partners. Current evidence suggests that adolescents are increasingly susceptible to developing cervical CIS.

Prevalence of cervical intraepithelial neoplasia (CIN)

The reported prevalence of cytologic changes consistent with CIN is quite variable, ranging from 0.43 to 24%, with the highest prevalence reported for a sexually transmitted disease (STD) clinic in Wales. In general, the prevalence of CIN varies with the type of clinic population screened, with clinics serving sexually active females between the ages 18 and 35 years reporting the highest prevalence estimates. Most gynecology clinic populations report annual prevalences for CIN of about 2%.[12]

Despite the fact that Pap smear screening has been widespread in industrialized countries including the USA for the last two decades, methods of obtaining exfoliated cells and interpreting and reporting microscopic findings have never been well standardized, making it nearly impossible to compare results from different laboratories and different time periods. For example, during the early to mid-1980s, the prevalence of cytologically diagnosed CIN in two similar STD clinics (Denver[17] and Seattle[18]) was 1.72% and 13.66%, respectively.

There are no good data on the prevalence of intraepithelial neoplasia or CIS of the vagina, vulva, anus or penis, but it is thought that the prevalence of these lesions is much lower than for cervical neoplasia. Vaginal intraepithelial neoplasia in the upper vagina usually represents a distal extension of CIN. Ferguson and MacLure[19] in 1963 published 27 cases of vaginal CIN or dysplasia that were found among 151 patients who had 'false positive' Pap smears. Timonen et al[20] identified 23 primary vaginal dysplasias among 12 000 patients screened during one year, giving a prevalence of 2 per 1000. Woodruff[21] in 1981 reported that less than 300 cases of CIS of the vagina had been recorded in the literature. Since vaginal cancer is so uncommon, screening for vaginal cancer has not received the same degree of emphasis as screening for cervical neoplasms.

HIV AND CERVICAL NEOPLASIA

The importance of immune system surveillance for prevention of HPV-associated neoplasia of the skin and genital tract has been well documented.[22–24] For example, patients with a rare condition, epidermodysplasia verruciformis, have been found to be particularly prone to develop multiple common skin warts, with up to one third of these individuals going on to develop skin cancers at the site of such lesions.[25] Interestingly, the HPV types associated with both warts and squamous cell cancers among patients with epidermodysplasia verruciformis differ from those found among the general population. A number of investigators have shown that renal transplant patients are also at increased risk for various manifestations of HPV infection including genital warts and cervical neoplasia.[24,26] Unlike patients with epidermodysplasia verruciformis, the types

of HPV detected among transplanted patients are usually similar to those seen in the general population. However, some investigators find that the relative distribution of HPV types differs among renal allograft recipients as compared to the general population, with an excess of the 'high-risk' HPV types being detected among transplanted patients.[27,28] Patients with either iatrogenic or congenital immunosuppression have been estimated to be from 14 to 100 times more likely than those with a normal immune system to develop carcinoma in situ, the lesion most likely to progress to invasive disease.[29] Several investigators have also suggested, although this has not been adequately substantiated, that squamous cell cancers of the cervix in immunosuppressed women differ from those in non-immunosuppressed women with respect to the types of HPV detected and to their natural history. For example, squamous cell cancers in immunosuppressed women compared with immunocompetent women are more often found with similar tumors at other genital sites and are more likely to occur in younger women.[29]

HIV and invasive cervical cancer

Despite the fact that invasive cervical cancer has been added to the list of AIDS defining illnesses, currently, there are no population-based data supporting an association between HIV and invasive cervical cancer. Up to the present time, studies have generally focused on the relationship between HIV, cervical HPV infection, and cervical intraepithelial neoplasia. Most of the studies primarily reported on women with CIN 1 and CIN 2 with a minority of women in these studies diagnosed with CIN 3/CIS. Current evidence suggests that, among immunocompetent women, only a minority of lesions classified as CIN 1 or CIN 2 would progress to invasive cancer if left untreated. It is well established that the majority of CIN 1 lesions spontaneously regress and represent self-limited infection with HPV.

Published data supporting an association between HIV and invasive cervical cancer is currently limited to isolated case reports and small case series.[30–34] Indirect evidence supporting an association between HIV and invasive cervical cancer comes from reports and studies of invasive anal cancer in homosexually active, HIV-positive men. Using a linkage between an AIDS database (Center for Disease Control HIV/AIDS Reporting System) and cancer registries from the same geographic locations, Melbye and colleagues[35] compared the number of expected cases of anal epidermoid cancer (based on general population rates) to the number of observed cases of epidermoid anal cancers, at and after the diagnosis of AIDS. By using this approach they were able to show a significant increased risk of anal cancer among patients with AIDS. However, when a similar approach was used to assess the association between cervical cancer and HIV infection there was only a small increase in the number of observed as compared to expected cases of invasive cervical cancer among women with AIDS. In addition, a study among 200 Kenyan women (mean age of 42 years) presenting with cervical cancer found an HIV seroprevalence of only 1.5%, an estimate that was comparable to the seroprevalence of 2% for the population from which the cases were detected.[36]

It is likely that HIV does increase the risk of cervical cancer and our current inability to demonstrate an increased risk may reflect the fact that HIV infected women are dying of other opportunistic diseases before the development or detection of cervical cancer. In the USA where HIV infection has been introduced into the female population only relatively recently, and where most women have access to Pap screening, and to diagnostic and treatment services, it is not surprising that an association between HIV and invasive cervical cancer has not yet been detected.

HIV and CIN

Women with HIV infection appear to be at increased risk for CIN. Odds ratios for the association between HIV and CIN have ranged from 1.0 to 14.7 (Table 4.4).[32,37-43] As with detection of HPV, the frequency of detecting CIN varies with level of immunosuppression.[43] Most studies reporting an association of HIV with CIN have involved relatively immunocompromised populations. In the one study that involved relatively immunocompetent women, no association between HIV and CIN was observed.[42]

SUMMARY

In developing countries where cervical cancer control programs are either nonexistent or inadequate, cervical cancer is the leading cause of cancer mortality among women. In the USA, as in other developed countries, significant reductions in the rates of, and mortality due to cervical cancer have been achieved though the widespread implementation of Pap screening programs. Important advances in the ability of minority populations to access these prevention programs in recent years is evident by data showing a shrinking disparity between rates of cervical cancer for white and black women in the USA. Although rates of cervical cancer for black women continue to show a decline, the trend for younger white women appears to be changing. With the most recent data (1986–1990), an increase in the rate of cervical cancer for white women less than 50 years of age was noted. Rates of cervical CIS also appear to be increasing among adolescent females. Whether these recent trends represent short-term

Table 4.4 Associations of HIV and cervical neoplasia in published studies

HIV positive	HIV negative	Odds ratio	(95% CI)	Reference
11/35 (31%)	1/23 (4%)	10.1	(1.2, 453)	38
14/35 (40%)	3/32 (9%)	6.4	(1.5, 38.3)	39
46/111 (41%)	7/76 (9%)	7.0	(2.8, 19.5)	33
2/10 (20%)	2/10 (20%)	1.0	(0.06, 17.1)	41
17/51 (33%)	6/45 (13%)	3.3	(1.1, 11.1)	40
11/42 (26%)	5/21 (24%)	1.1	(0.3, 4.9)	43
11/41 (27%)	1/41 (3%)	14.7	(1.8, 647)	42
15/43 (35%)	8/43 (19%)	2.3	(0.8, 7.1)	44

statistical fluctuations or a true reversal in the gains made in the prevention of cervical cancer is not yet clear. How the worldwide increase in HIV infection among heterosexual women will impact the rates of cervical cancer is largely unknown because of the difficulties encountered in studies of cervical neoplasia in individuals with declining immune function and poor survival.

REFERENCES

1. Rigoni-Stern D. Fatti statistici relativi alle malattie cancerose. Gior Serv Progr Pathol Terap 1842; 2: 507–517.
2. Cramer D W. Uterine cervix. In: Schottenfeld D, Fraumeni J F, eds. Cancer epidemiology and prevention. Philadelphia: Saunders, 1982; p 881–900.
3. Richart R M, Barron B A. A follow-up study of patients with cervical dysplasia. Am J Obstet Gynecol 1969; 105: 386–393.
4. Parkin D M, Laara E, Muir C S. Estimates of the worldwide frequency of sixteen major cancers in 1980. Int J Cancer 1988; 41: 184–197.
5. Muir C S et al. Cancer incidence in five continents, vol V. Lyon: International Agency for Research on Cancer, 1988.
6. Waterhouse J, Muir C, Correa P et al. Cancer incidence in five continents, vol III. Lyon: International Agency for Research on Cancer, 1976.
7. Miller B A, Ries L A G, Hankey B F et al (eds). SEER Cancer Statistics Review: 1973–1990, NIH Pub. No. 93-2789. Bethesda, NCI, 1993.
8. Devesa S S. Descriptive epidemiology of cancer of the uterine cervix. Obstet Gynecol 1984; 63: 605–612.
9. Harlan L C, Bernstein A B, Kessler L G. Cervical cancer screening: Who is not screened and why? Am J Public Health 1991; 81: 885–890.
10. National Cancer Institute: Division of Cancer Prevention and Control. 1987 Annual Cancer Statistics Review, NIH Publ 88-2789. US Department of Health and Human Services, 1988.
11. Young J L Jr et al (eds): Surveillance, Epidemiology and End Results: Incidence and Mortality Data: 1973–77, NIH Publ 81-2330. Bethesda: NCI, 1981.
12. Paavonen J, Koutsky L A, Kiviat N B. Cervical neoplasia and other STD-related genital and anal neoplasias. In: Holmes K K, Mardh P A, Sparling P F, Wiesner P J, eds. Sexually transmitted diseases. New York: McGraw-Hill, 1990, p 561–592.
13. Holmes K K. Human ecology and behavior and sexually transmitted bacterial infections. Proc Nat Acad Sci USA 1994; 91: 2448–2455.
14. CDC. Special focus: behavioral risk factor surveillance — United States, 1991. Morbidity and Mortality Weekly Report 1993; 42: 11–14.
15. Wiggins C L, Thomas D B, Potts, M S. Cancer in Western Washington state 1974–1991. Seattle: Cancer Surveillance System, Fred Hutchinson Cancer Research Center, 1993.
16. Roye C F. Abnormal cervical cytology in adolescents: A literature review. J Adolescent Health 1992; 13: 643–650.
17. Tavelli B G, Judson F N, Hetrick A E, Root C J. Cost-yield of routine Papanicolaou smear screening in a clinic for sexually transmitted diseases. Sex Trans Dis 1985; 12: 110–113.
18. Kiviat N B, Koutsky L A, Paavonen J et al. Prevalence of genital papillomavirus infection among women attending a college student health clinic or a sexually transmitted disease clinic. J Infect Dis 1989; 159: 293–302.
19. Ferguson J H, Maclure J G. Intraepithelial carcinoma, dysplasia, and exfoliation of cancer cells in the vaginal mucosa. Am J Obstet Gynecol 1963; 87: 326–336.
20. Timonen S, Numers C, Meyer B. Dysplasia of the vaginal epithelium. Gynaecologia 1966; 162: 125–138.
21. Woodruff J D. Carcinoma in situ of the vagina. Clin Obstet Gynecol 1981; 24: 485–501.
22. Penn I. Cancers of the anogenital region in renal transplant recipients. Cancer 1986; 58: 611–616.
23. Sillman F H, Sedlis A. Anogenital papillomavirus infection and neoplasia in immunodeficient women. Obstet Gynecol Clinics North Am 1987; 15: 537–538.
24. Halpert R, Fruchter R G, Sedlis A, Butt K, Boyce J, Sillman F H. Human papillomavirus and lower genital neoplasia in renal transplant patients. Obstet Gynecol 1986; 68: 251–258.
25. Orth G. Epidermodysplasia verruciformis. A model for understanding the oncogenicity of human papillomaviruses. Ciba Found Symp 1986; 120: 157–174.
26. Schneider V, Kay S, Lee H M. Immunosuppression as a high-risk factor in the development of condyloma accuminatum and squamous neoplasia of the cervix. Acta Cytol 1983; 27: 220–224.
27. Alloub M I, Barr B B B, McLaren K M, Smith I W, Bunney M H, Smart G E. Human papillomavirus infection and cervical intraepithelial neoplasia in women with renal allografts. Br Med J 1989; 298: 153–156.
28. Dyall-Smith D, Trowell H, Dyall-Smith M L. Benign human papillomavirus infection in renal transplant recepients. Int J Dermatol 1991; 30: 785–789.
29. Sillman F, Stanek A, Sedlis A et al. The relationship between human papillomavirus and lower genital intraepithelial neoplasia in immunosuppressed women. Am J Obstet Gynecol 1984; 150: 300–308.
30. Tirelli U, Vaccher E, Zagonel V et al. Malignant tumors other than lymphoma and Kaposi's sarcoma in association with HIV infection. Cancer Detect Prevent 1988; 12: 267–272.
31. Maiman M, Fruchter R, Serur E, Remy J C, Feuer G, Boyce J. Human immunodeficiency virus infection and cervical neoplasia. Gynecol Oncol 1990; 38: 377–382.
32. Schafer A, Friedmann W, Mielke M, Schwartlander B, Koch M A. The increased frequency of cervical dysplasia-neoplasia in women infected with the human immunodeficiency virus is related to the degree of immunosuppression. Am J Obstet Gynecol 1991; 164: 593–599.
33. Rellihan M A, Dooley D P, Burke T W, Berkland M E,

Longfield R N. Rapidly progressing cervical cancer in a patient with human immunodeficiency virus infection. Gynecol Oncol 1990; 36: 435–438.

34. Schwartz L B, Carcangiu M L, Bradham L, Schwartz P E. Rapidly progressive squamous cell carcinoma of the cervix coexisting with human immunodeficiency virus infection: Clinical opinion. Gynecol Oncol 1991; 41: 255–258.

35. Melbye M, Cote T R, Kessler L, Gail M, Bigger R J, and the AIDS/Cancer Working Group. High incidence of anal cancer among AIDS patients. Lancet 1994; 343: 636–639.

36. Rogo K O, Kavoo-Linge. Human immunodeficiency virus seroprevalence among cervical cancer patients. Gynecol Oncol 1990; 37: 87–92.

37. Schrager L K, Friedland G H, Maude D, et al. Cervical and vaginal squamous cell abnormalities in women infected with human immunodeficiency virus. J AIDS 1989; 2: 570–575.

38. Feingold A R, Vermund S H, Burk R D et al. Cervical cytologic abnormalities and papillomavirus in women infected with human immunodeficiency virus. J AIDS 1990; 3: 896–903.

39. Vermund, S H, Kelley K F, Klein R S et al. High risk of human papillomavirus infection and cervical squamous intraepithelial lesions among women with symptomatic human immunodeficiency virus infection. Am J Obstet Gynecol 1991; 165: 392–400.

40. Smith J R, Botcherby M, James M, Byrne M, Mason P, Forster S M. Influence of HIV on lower genital tract neoplasia. Antibiot Chemother 1991; 43: 150–155.

41. Laga M, Icenogle J P, Marsella R et al. Genital papillomavirus infection and cervical dysplasia — Opportunistic complications of HIV infection. Int J Cancer 1992; 50: 45–48.

42. Kreiss, J K, Kiviat N B, Plummer F A et al. Human immunodeficiency virus, human papillomavirus, and cervical intraepithelial neoplasia in Nairobi prostitutes. Sex Trans Dis 1992; 19: 54–59.

43. Smith J K, Kitchen V S, Botcherby M et al. Is HIV infection associated with an increase in cervical neoplasia? Br J Obstet Gynecol 1993; 100: 149–153.

5. Costs and benefits of cervical screening

S. Wilson   C. B. J. Woodman

INTRODUCTION

Screening — 'actively seeking to identify a disease or predisease condition in people who are presumed and presume themselves to be healthy' is an area of health care which has generated considerable debate and discussion.[1] Cervical screening, based on the premise that women with premalignant disease will progress to clinically invasive carcinoma unless detected and successfully treated, has stimulated more discussion than most.[2-7] The debate persists because of uncertainty relating to the scale of benefits attributable to the cervical screening programme and the paucity of information on what it costs. This review attempts to inform this debate by reporting what is and is not known about the balance between costs and benefits.

Cervical screening benefits women when screening succeeds in identifying disease at a point when the prevention, or cure of invasive disease is still possible. Benefits will also be accrued by those who would have been cured even at the time of symptomatic presentation but in whom earlier diagnosis following screening reduces morbidity. The act of screening for disease can move an individual from a 'healthy' to a 'diseased' state. Those women whose smear is reported as normal may be reassured. False negative results will promote false reassurance and may cause delays in presentation when symptoms are observed. False positive results cause anxiety and morbidity.[8]

THE BENEFITS OF SCREENING — EVIDENCE ADDUCED FROM TRENDS IN INCIDENCE AND MORTALITY

A randomized controlled trial is the preferred method of establishing the effectiveness of a screening program in reducing mortality. No randomized controlled trials demonstrating the effectiveness of cervical screening have been undertaken and evidence for the efficacy of cervical screening has largely been adduced from trends in incidence and mortality.

Trends in the incidence of, and mortality from cervical carcinoma in northern Europe have been extensively examined.[9-14] Iceland, Denmark, Finland and Sweden have achieved near complete coverage of their target populations since the mid-1960s and reductions in incidence and mortality were observed soon after this time. Norway, unlike the other Nordic countries, had no organized program in the 1960s and continued to report increased incidence rates into the late 1970s.[15] Within Denmark, the reduction in incidence was greatest in areas with well organized screening programs.[16] Similarly, in Aberdeen, where a 5-yearly screening program was introduced in 1960, the incidence rate fell steadily after that time; in 1960 incidence rates in Aberdeen were considerably higher than in the rest of Scotland but by 1981 the standardized rate was less than 50% of that in Scotland as a whole.[17]

The aim of the cervical screening program is to reduce mortality from carcinoma of the cervix.[18] A reduction in incidence may be an interim indicator of the beneficial effect of screening, but a reduction in mortality is required to prove effectiveness. Mortality is the only valid outcome measure as it is not subject to selection or diagnostic biases. These well-recognized sources of bias follow from the possibility that screening may preferentially detect tumors with a good prognosis.

Reductions in mortality which have been

attributed to the introduction of screening have been reported in the Nordic countries, areas of Canada and the USA.[9,10,13] It is difficult, however, to quantify the contribution that the cervical screening program has made towards reducing the mortality attributable to cervical cancer. Mortality rates have been declining gradually, for many years, in many parts of the world, even in countries with no organized screening program. In the UK, a reduction in mortality has been observed since the early 1960s, long before organized screening was introduced in 1988. This fall in mortality has occurred predominantly among women aged over 45 years.[19] In contrast, incidence rates have remained constant until recent years. It is difficult to reconcile this reduction in mortality with the constancy of incidence rates even when the survival of patients is taken into account.

There has been little change in the overall 5-year relative survival of patients with cervical cancer over the last two decades. However, it is difficult to interpret temporal trends in survival without access to stage-specific survival rates. These data are not routinely available on a national basis. A comprehensive review of cervical cancer in the West Midlands region of England did, however, compile a well-validated dataset covering a 25-year period and incorporating information on stage of disease.[20] The 5-year survival rates for invasive cancers of the uterine cervix increased from 43% during the period 1957–1961 to 55% in 1977–1981 ($t = 5.03$, $P < 0.001$). This improvement in survival can be attributed to the increased proportion of stage 1a disease, from 5% in the quinquennia 1962–1966 to 22% by 1977–1981. When these cases were removed from the series the incidence of clinically invasive disease is seen to decline but disappointingly survival rates appear to have remained constant in these patients over the 20 year period (Table 5.1).

Changes in clinical practice, for example the number and type of hysterectomy, may confound attempts to interpret temporal changes in both incidence and mortality rates. Stern et al reported on the increased use of total hysterectomies as opposed to subtotal hysterectomies.[21] The observed fall in mortality may be attributed to a reduction in the numbers of cervices at risk. Commonly, the computation of rates uses the age-specific female population as the denominator whereas, as Knox has suggested, the number of cervices at risk is a more appropriate measure.[22] An analysis of Canadian cervical cancer statistics for the period 1952–1976 suggested that the mortality rate for women aged 30–64 fell from 15 to 6 per 100 000 during this 25 year period but after correcting for the numbers of hysterectomies performed the respective rates were 16 and 9 per 100 000.[23] Thus the utilization of a more appropriate denominator suggested a 44% rather than 60% reduction in mortality during this period.

It has been suggested that an increase in the number of registered cases of CIN 3 provide a useful proxy measure for the effectiveness of the screening program. This is based on the premise that without screening many of these lesions would have progressed to invasive disease. The number of new cases of CIN 3 registered each year in the North West Region of England increased from 290 to 1640 between 1974 and 1992, from a rate of 14.5 per 100 000 to 75.8 (Centre for Cancer Epidemiology, unpublished data). The interpretation of this increase is confounded by changes in screening coverage and

Table 5.1 Temporal trends in survival for cervical cancer in the West Midlands Region (UK) 1957–1981*

	Number of cases	5-year survival rate (%)	Stage 1a		5-year survival rate (%) excluding Stage 1a
			n	%	
1957–1961	1819	44.9	3		44.0
1962–1966	2118	49.6	110	5.2	47.1
1967–1971	2130	51.8	233	10.9	46.2
1972–1976	1993	52.3	262	13.1	45.0
1977–1981	2155	55.9	472	21.9	43.8
	10 215	X^2 for trend $t = 5.03$ ($P < 0.001$)			$t = 0.7$ not significant

*Source: West Midlands Regional Cancer Registry.

clinical practice. CIN 3 is an asymptomatic condition, only diagnosed following the detection of cytological abnormality, and its prevalence will in part reflect the level of screening activity. The traditional approach to diagnosis and treatment is a two-stage process of colposcopically directed punch biopsy followed by laser ablation or loop diathermy excision of the CIN. There is evidence that punch biopsies are an unreliable method of diagnosis; small biopsies may miss areas of more severe dysplasia or microinvasive disease whereas large loop excision biopsies of the transformation zone allow a more thorough histological examination.[24] The increased use of loop diathermy and multiple biopsies may have contributed to the rise in the number of registrations for CIN 3 since the use of this technique allows a more precise histological characterization of the severity of the lesion.

Unfortunately, the interaction between changes in incidence which are themselves confused by birth cohort effects, which may be mediated by sexual behavior, the intensity of screening and changes in clinical practice confound attempts to interpret the individual impact of any of these factors on mortality rates.

EVIDENCE FROM CASE-CONTROL STUDIES

Case-control studies have been used to investigate the effectiveness of cervical screening. These studies have examined the screening history of cases (patients presenting with cervical carcinoma) and controls (age and residence matched women without evidence of disease). The results suggest that previous participation in the screening program is higher amongst controls and the relative risk of developing cervical cancer usually ranges from 0.25 to 0.37 in women who have been screened compared with those who have never been screened. The protective effect increased with the number of screening smears and declines with increasing time since the last smear.[25,26]

The use of case control studies to evaluate the benefits of screening presents a number of problems. These include difficulties in distinguishing between diagnostic and routine screening smears and deciding how cases of invasive disease diagnosed as part of the screening program should be treated in the analysis. The exclusion of cases of disease detected by screening may overestimate the benefits of screening, whereas the inclusion of such cases may underestimate the benefits as a lead time bias may be introduced.[27] The next problem relates to inadequate control over confounding factors. The uptake of screening may be associated with a low risk of developing cervical cancer and a negative correlation between the uptake of screening and the occurrence of cancer may be no more than a reflection of this association. There is a more fundamental problem; a negative smear in itself protects no-one. Protection follows from the intervention which succeeds a positive test. At a minimum those studies which aim to describe the protective efficacy of cervical screening should provide information on the frequency of positive tests and subsequent treatments.[28] The failure to provide this information and the methodological flaws inherent in this approach suggest that results derived from reported case control studies cannot be considered to provide sound estimates of procedural efficacy.

UNCERTAINTY SURROUNDING THE NATURAL HISTORY

Attempts to reduce mortality from cervical carcinoma by the introduction of well-organized screening programs are based on the presumption of progression from premalignant disease to invasive disease. Estimates of the rate and tempo of progression from dysplasia to invasive disease are not based on studies designed for this purpose and only small numbers of cases who have inadvertently progressed to invasive disease are available; consequently estimates of the rates of progression vary widely. Some estimates of the probability of transition through dysplasia and CIN 3 to invasive disease are illustrated in Table 5.2.

Most of the published studies are based on prevalent cases of cervical abnormality and are inevitably left censored as the abnormality has been present for an unknown period of time before diagnosis. They differ with respect to the disease entry criteria, endpoints, period of follow-up, and the age distribution of the study population. It is therefore difficult to derive robust estimates of progression.

Table 5.2 Selected studies aiming to describe the natural history

Reference	Study population	Follow-up	Endpoint	
Flannelly (1994)[29]	902 women with abnormal smears, age 18–62 (mean 31.1)			
			Reversion to normal	158 (30%)
	Mild dyskaryosis, n = 538		CIN 1	92 (17%)
		0–24 months	CIN 2	101 (19%)
			CIN 3	187 (35%)
	Moderate dyskaryosis, n = 255	0–24 months	Reversion to normal	54 (21%)
			CIN 1	28 (11%)
			CIN 2	38 (15%)
			CIN 3	135 (53%)
McIndoe (1986)[30]	Carcinoma-in-situ managed only by diagnostic biopsy and observation, age NK, n = 25	0–8 years	Invasive carcinoma	9 (36%)
Robertson (1988)[31]	1781 women with mild dyskaryosis 1347 with complete follow-up 434 lost to follow-up, age range NK	0–12 years	Reversion to normal	625 (46%)
			CIN 1–2	355 (26%)
			CIN 3	201 (15%)
			Invasive cancer	10 (0.6%)
Campion (1986)[32]	100 women with mild dyskaryosis, all age < 30 years	8–30 months	Reversion to normal	11 (11%)
			Reversion-no recurrence	7 (7%)
			CIN 3	26 (26%)
Kirby (1992)[33]	498 women with mild or moderate dyskaryosis, age NK	0–10 years	Reversion to normal	232 (46%)
			CIN 3	92 (18%)
			Invasive cancer (inc 1a)	5 (1%)
Hirschowitz (1992)[34]	437 women with borderline smears, age 15–72	13–106 months	CIN 2–3	77 (18%)
			Invasive cancer (inc 1a)	10 (2.3%)
Kinlen (1978)[35]	60 women with mild or moderate dysplasia who had not been biopsied or treated. Mean interval to clinical carcinoma 5.3 years, all regressions in women aged < 40	min 2 years	Reversion to normal	19 (32%)
			Invasive carcinoma (inc 1a)	13 (21.7)%

Our imperfect understanding of the natural history of the disease follows from the inability of light microscopy to confidently predict which cases will progress and which will regress. The identification of more certain prognostic factors is a necessary prerequisite to improving the efficiency of the screening program. In their absence it is inevitable that many women with lesions which may have spontaneously regressed will continue to be unnecessarily treated.

MATHEMATICAL MODELING AS A MEANS OF DESCRIBING THE NATURAL HISTORY AND ASSESSING THE BENEFITS OF SCREENING

There is no direct evidence available to measure the impact of the screening program on morbidity, mortality or life years gained. The lack of con-trolled experiments to assess the effectiveness of the cervical screening program, has led to the development of mathematical models which attempt to simulate the natural history of the disease, assess the merits of the different programs and hence optimize the schedule of screening visits.[22,36–42]

These models should aim to incorporate all those factors which are likely to influence the impact of a screening program. These include, the age distribution of the population, background age-specific incidence and mortality rates, the natural history of disease, the efficacy of different medical interventions, the performance of diagnostic tests and uptake of the screening program. A full-scale mathematical model attempts, thereby, to estimate the effects that are to be expected from a screening program when all factors and interactions are parameterized in the model.

Barron used a Markov chain model to predict

the natural history of cervical dysplasia and carcinoma-in-situ (CIS) and to derive estimates of the time for progression from dysplasia to CIS.[36] His assumptions included (i) CIS does not spontaneously regress, (ii) age-specific incidence rates of CIS are constant over time, (iii) progression rates of 85% for mild dysplasia, 90% for moderate and 95% for severe dysplasia to CIS, and (iv) a 10% false positive rate for routine cytological screening. Baron estimated the progression times to CIS to be 37.3, 29.4 and 11.5 months for mild, moderate and severe dysplasia respectively Coppleson & Brown produced a simpler model which, grouped all dysplastic lesions together and used a discrete-time Markov process to estimate transition probabilities.[37] This model assumed that (i) both dysplasia and CIS can regress, (ii) the risk of progression and time to progression from dysplasia and CIS were age dependent, the average transit time decreasing substantially with age, (iii) a 25% false negative rate for cytological examination, and (iv) a zero false positive rate. Albert used a probabilistic model which did not distinguish between normal and dysplastic smears and included only the categories; disease free, CIS, occult invasive and clinically invasive.[38] The assumptions of this model included (i) CIS could regress, (ii) the CIS category also included micro-invasive cancers, (iii) progression rates were not age or time dependent, and (iv) zero false negative rates for cervical screening. Progression rates were estimated as 3.7% per year from CIS to occult invasive and, 48% per year from occult to clinically invasive. Progression rates from disease free to CIS were only reported in terms of person years of observation and were 1.1/per 1000 person years per year. Knox also used models with a Markov structure but refined the model to include a life table of the population screened which incorporated the background mortality experience, annual transition frequencies between disease states by age and duration, and age at time of screening.[22] The optimal parameterization of the model suggested that one-third of CIS cases would not progress to invasive disease.

Parkin also used the model proposed by Knox which included transition states and allowed for changes in the age, marital status and parity of the study cohort.[43,44] His assumptions included (i)

survival for screen detected cancers was 100%, (ii) the prevalence rates of dysplasia, CIS, occult invasive cancer and clinically detectable cancer were age dependent, and (iii) dysplasia was a transient condition (75–80% of cases regress), 40% regressing within 2 years. His best-fitting model suggested a 14.8 year median duration for the preclinical detectable phase of invasive lesions.

All of the above models used some form of Markov process. This strategy however, limits the possibility for modelling interactions between important parameters and, therefore, Monte Carlo simulation models have been developed to circumvent these limitations.[45]

Habbema et al used a Monte Carlo simulation to model the natural history of preclinical lesions.[39] The assumptions used in the model included (i) progression and regression were independent of age, (ii) transition times were the same for lesions that progressed or regressed, and (iii) 50% spontaneous regression rates for preclinical invasive cancer. They concluded that the mean duration period for preclinical carcinoma (defined as severe dysplasia, carcinoma in situ and invasive cancer that is not clinically apparent) was 18 years. Gustafsson & Adami have attempted to model the natural history of the disease and estimate the effect of the screening program on the incidence of invasive carcinoma.[46] The proportion of cases progressing from CIS to invasive disease was assumed to be age dependent ranging from 16.7 to 22.1%, with a mean of 19.9% and a mean progression time to invasive carcinoma of 12.3 years. They concluded that, by 1981, screening in Sweden between 1958 and 1981 may have reduced the number of invasive cancers by 42–69%.

Other authors have also used computer simulation to attempt to quantify the benefits of screening. Using a series of assumptions based on Dutch health care practice, Ballegooijen predicted the outcome of three screening strategies (based on screening intervals of 2, 5 and 10 years).[47] For each million women invited per year and assuming a 65% attendance rate the simulation predicted that 20 deaths from cervical cancer will be avoided and 446 life years saved by implementation of 5-yearly screening. This invitation schedule would generate 78 700 smears per annum, 299 of which would show minor cytological abnormality, 113 cases of CIN 3, 6 microinvasive carcinomas and 43 invasive cancers; a further 92 women are likely to present each year with symptomatic disease.

Parkin assuming 80% attendance rates, 70% sensitivity and 99.5% specificity for the test and 5-yearly screening of women aged 35–65 estimated that for every 1000 women invited, 193 000 screening tests would be undertaken of which 1.7% would be positive.[43] It was estimated that this policy would prevent 62% of cancers and 54% of deaths over a 30-year period. This microsimulation study was extended to estimate the effectiveness of various screening policies in England.[44] It was concluded that over the 30-year period (1961–1990) 5-yearly screening of a notional 100 000 women would have saved 21 deaths and 1380 person years of life assuming 80% attendance.

In summary, these studies reveal little consistency in the definition of disease status, the assumptions made, or the data used for model fitting. Many conclusions derived from the models, for example, the estimated duration of CIS, are both model and data dependent. Several authors have used simplified models and unrealistic assumptions; such as the failure to distinguish between different grades of dysplasia or 100% sensitivity for the screening test. The Markov process assumes that the rate of transfer between states is independent of the duration of time spent in one state — this assumption may be unsound. The difficulty with all the models is in interpreting the appropriateness of the fitted parameter values. Some are well documented, for example, stage specific survival rates for treated patients or attendance for screening. Many, however, cannot be given a fixed value. Morbidity and mortality rates derived from simulation models are compared with available data and parameter values adjusted until the output matches reality. The large number of factors which can be included and range of parameter values results in an enormous number of feasible sets of values which generate output that approaches the observed data.

THE FINANCIAL COSTS OF SCREENING PROGRAMS

Establishing the cost of screening is problematic because the costs are distributed over several institutions and a considerable time period. Furthermore, these costs may vary both temporally and geographically. The costs of administering the screening program include the maintenance of population registers, sending out of invitations, the follow-up of nonresponders and notification of results. These costs will vary depending on the age distribution of the population, the frequency of screening, the rate of compliance and the prevalence of disease in the population.

The costs borne in the taking and processing of smears include professional costs incurred in taking and reading smears. Smears can be taken by a variety of staff (nurses, general practioners, other clinicians) on a wide range of salaries. The time required to take a smear will vary, as will the cost of the spatula or brush used. The total number of tests will be dependent on the percentage of inadequate smears that require repeating and the proportion of cases that are double read. The number of abnormal smears identified will depend on the prevalence of abnormality in the screened population and the opinion of cytoscreeners which may in turn reflect their experience. The action taken, either referral for colposcopy or repeat smear, is also dependent on local policy.

Treatment may take place at the first assessment visit (see and treat) or be delayed until histological confirmation of disease is obtained and can take place in either a inpatient or outpatient setting. The treatment of CIN is not uniform and the choice of cone biopsy, loop excision, laser, diathermy or hysterectomy depends in part on clinical preference and the availability of equipment as well as the extent of disease and the presence of comorbidity. There is also variability in the type, intensity and duration of post-treatment surveillance before the patient is returned to the screening program.

MODELING AS A MEANS OF ASSESSING THE COST-EFFECTIVENESS OF SCREENING

Cost-effectiveness studies address the technical efficiency of a health care program and assess the extent to which the costs of generating a given output (restoration of cytological normality, year of life gained, etc.) are minimized or output is maximized for a set cost.

Computer simulation models have been used to model the costs of screening, subsequent diagnosis and treatment and to measure cost-effectiveness in terms of the incremental costs per life year gained.

Ballegooijen estimated that, with a 5-yearly program, 3900 screening smears, 13 referrals and 6 minor treatment procedures are required to prevent one death.[47] A 2-yearly program would require 7300 smears, 22 referrals and 8 minor treatments for each death prevented. A deteriorating balance between beneficial and adverse effects is found as the frequency of screening increased due to the increased detection of women with minor abnormalities which were more likely to undergo spontaneous regression. The model predicted that the number of women with cytological abnormality who were likely to undergo regression would rise from 77 to 121 per million women per year if the screening interval was reduced from 5 years to 2. It was, therefore, concluded that screening women more frequently resulted in an increased risk of inappropriate referral and treatment.

The potential cost of a comprehensive screening program for the Dutch population was estimated by Ballegooijen and colleagues.[47] Assuming attendance rates of 65 and 75% and a screening interval of 3 years the total costs of the screening program were estimated as US$163 million and US$176 million, the costs per life year gained at US$12 400 and US$11 800 respectively. The model suggested that a 6-yearly program with the higher attendance rates was likely to be the most cost-effective option. Increasing attendance rather than shortening the screening interval was the optimal method of maximizing cost effectiveness because (i) the costs of screening are largely comprised of the costs of the organization of the program rather than those of the diagnosis and treatment of abnormality, and (ii) more high-risk women would be included in the program.

More recently the Dutch group have attempted to assess the savings on treatment and care of cervical cancer resulting from the screening program.[48] This costing study is based on only 35 cases, all with advanced disease, and the results from the earlier analyses which estimated the costs of the screening program. The authors concluded that the screening program resulted in a saving of DFl 37 million on the costs of treating advanced disease. Those potential savings were equivalent to only 10% of the cost of the national screening program and indicate that the cervical screening will not pay for itself.

OTHER COSTING STUDIES

Estimates of the cost of the screening program should include the follow-up of false positive smears and the costs of investigation and treatment of abnormal smears. The estimates of the monetary costs of investigating and treating women with abnormal cytology vary substantially. Our own estimate of the cost to the health service of investigating and treating women with cytological abnormality at 1986–1987 prices was £116. These estimates were based on a random sample of 365 women referred for colposcopic assessment.[49]

Roberts estimated the cost of the screening program based on the assumption that each 1000 smears read would generate 5 excision biopsies at a cost of £5 per smear and £500 per excision biopsy.[50] These costs relate only to inpatient treatment and have little relevance today when the majority of cases of CIN are treated in the out-patient department. Parkin and Day used a cost of £15 per smear but made no reference to the costs incurred in the investigation and treatment of women discovered to have abnormal cytology.[51] Lyce estimated the cost of an opportunistic Papanicolaou (Pap) smear to be between US$8 and US$30 and estimated the costs of screening, diagnosis and treatment to be US$340 per case.[52] Havelock estimated the cost of the screening program which included the investigation of abnormal smears (cytology, colposcopy and histology services) as between £27.40 and £30 per routine smear but failed to incorporate the costs of treatment for those cases identified as abnormal.[53]

The costs of the screening program are the activity costs. They cannot with any certainty be related to outcome. A pathological diagnosis is a process rather than an outcome measure. We cannot, at present, say how many cancers have been prevented or lives saved by cervical screening. Costs presented relate to the intervention necessary to restore a state of cytological normality to women identified as having abnormal smears. Whilst this outcome measure may be acceptable to patients and some clinicians, the measure by which the cervical screening program must be judged is deaths avoided or cancers prevented. To answer the question how much does it cost to prevent a death from cervical cancer or more pertinently what are the benefits which are likely to accrue from our investment in this program we require (i) the number of screening smears taken from women with invasive cancer (these may be considered a benefit or a cost depending on whether treatable or incurable disease is found), (ii) the cost of treatment or palliation of cancers of different stages using different therapeutic modalities and (iii) an estimate of the number of deaths from cancers prevented by the screening program. This work is in progress. Our best current estimate is derived from Ballegooijen's estimate of 3900 smears at £15 each and 13 referrals at £1465 (1986–1987 costs adjusted to 1990–1991 prices) which suggests £60 400 per death prevented.[47,48]

THE ESTIMATED COST OF THE SCREENING PROGRAMME IN ENGLAND 1991–1992

It is possible to tentatively estimate the costs of the screening program utilizing the information obtained from the Körner return (KC 53) for the financial year 1991–92.[54] The KC 53 collects information from the computerized call and recall system for Cervical Cancer Screening. Conclusions based on these statistics are circumscribed with caveats relating to the quality of the data returned, its completeness and the imputation methods necessary to overcome these deficiencies. In England, however, it would appear that 1 195 789 women were screened during that period.

If we estimate therefore that 1.2 million women were screened in England in 1991–1992 and the cost of taking a smear was £15, then the cost of these screening smears will be £18 million. The cost of taking a smear is critical to this calculation. Parkin and Day's estimate of £15 was made in

1985 and was a total rather than an itemized cost. We found the unit costs for two laboratories were £2.9 and £3.3 (Woodman et al, unpublished data). Further work is necessary to more precisely define the current professional and administrative costs of taking a smear in the screening situation.

In 1991–1992 4.2% of the screened population had an abnormal smear and 1% had a positive smear. These women will have been managed in one of two ways: (i) by immediate or delayed referral for hospital investigation and treatment, or (ii) continuing cytological surveillance until spontaneous regression of the abnormality occurs. Estimates of the proportion of the screened population referred for hospital investigation are also not yet widely available. If we assume that 3.73% will be referred (all of the positive smears and 65% of those with lesser abnormalities) and set the mean cost per case investigated at £146 (1986–1987 costs adjusted to 1990–1991 prices using a 5% rate of inflation) then the total costs arising from hospital investigation and treatment will be approximately £6.5 million. These costs were based on a sample of 100 women referred for investigation of cytological abnormality, with lesions considered suitable for outpatient laser vaporization.

The recent guidelines suggest that treated cases should have further smears before returning to the normal recall schedule.[55] There will be, therefore, an additional cost incurred in the follow-up of these patients after hospital discharge (£3.4 million). Calculation of the costs incurred in cytological surveillance is even more problematic because robust estimates of the rate and tempo with which untreated cytological abnormality undergo spontaneous regression are not available. If we estimate, however, that the remaining 1.47% of the screened population with an abnormal smear will have an additional 5 smears on average, before returning to the normal screening interval, then the costs arising from this part of the program will be approximately £1.3 million.

The costs ascribed to the screening program in 1991–1992 must be considered somewhat speculative given our uncertainties as to the current cost of taking a smear and the natural history of untreated cytological abnormalities. This estimate also, does not include the administrative costs.

This exercise indicates, however, that a substantial proportion of the total costs of £29.2 million (22%) arises from the referral of women with abnormal smears for investigation and treatment. The number of women referred is determined by the reported prevalence of different grades of cytological abnormality and the referral criteria employed, both of which vary geographically. Their normalization is a necessary prerequisite to controlling the cost of this screening program.

REFERENCES

1. Holland W W, Stewart S. Screening in health care: Benefit or bane? London: Nuffield Provincial Trust, 1990.
2. Cervical Cancer Screening. The Pap smear. Summary of an HIH consensus statement. Br Med J 1980; 281: 1264–1266.
3. Clarke E, Anderson T. Does screening by pap smears help prevent cervical cancer? Lancet 1979; ii: 1–4.
4. Richards T. Poor organisation and lack of will have caused the failure of cervical screening. Br Med J 1985; 291: 1135.
5. Wolfendale M R, King S, Usherwood M M. Abnormal cervical smears: are we in for an epidemic? Br Med J 1983; 287: 526–528.
6. Murphy M F G, Campbell M J, Goldblatt P. Twenty years of screening for cancer of the uterine cervix in Great Britain 1964–84: further evidence for its ineffectiveness. J Epidemiol Commun Health 1988; 42: 49–53.
7. Cook G A, Draper G J Trends in cervical cancer and carcinoma in situ in Great Britain. Br J Cancer 1984; 50: 367–375.
8. Wilkinson C, Jones J M, McBride J. Anxiety caused by abnormal result of cervical smear test: a controlled trial. Br Med J 1990; 300: 400.
9. Ashluwalia H S, Path M C, Doll R. Mortality from cancer of the cervix uteri in British Columbia and other parts of Canada. Br J Prev Soc Med 1968; 22: 161–164.
10. Cramer D W, The role of cervical cytology in the declining morbidity of cervical cancer. Cancer 1974; 34: 2018–2027.
11. Hakama M. Trends in the incidence of cervical cancer in Nordic countries. In: Magnus K, ed. Trends in cancer incidence, causes and practical implications. Washington D C: Hemisphere Publishing Corporation, 1982; pp 279–292.
12. Jonanneson G, Geirsson G, Day N, Tulinius H. Screening for cancer of the uterine cervix in Iceland 1965–78. Acta Obstet Scand 1982; 61: 199–203.
13. Läärä E, Day N E, Hakama M. Trends in mortality from cervical cancer in the Nordic countries: association with organised screening programmes. Lancet 1987; 1: 1247–1249.
14. Sigurdsson K. Effect of organised screening on the risk of cervical cancer. Evaluation of screening activity in Iceland 1964–199. Int J Cancer 1993; 54: 563–570.
15. Bjørge T, Steinar Ø, Thoresen G, Skare B. Incidence, survival and mortality in cervical cancer in Norway, 1956–90 Eur J Cancer 1993; 29A(16): 2291–2297.
16. Lynge E, Poll P. Risk of cervical cancer following negative smears in Maribo County, Denmark vol 7, no 3. Lyon: IARC Sci Publ Res Surveys, pp 379–401.
17. MacGregor J, Moss S, Parkin K, Day N. A case-control study of cervical cancer screening in NE Scotland. Br Med J 1985; 290: 1543–1546.
18. Department of Health, Health Service Management. Cervical cancer screening health circular (88). London, DoH.
19. Cancer Research Campaign. Cancer of the cervix uteri. Factscheet 12.2. London: Cancer Research Campaign, 1994.
20. Meanwell C A, Kelly K A, Wilson S et al. Young age as a prognostic factor in cervical cancer: analysis of population-based from 10 022 cases. Br Med J 1988; 296: 386–392.
21. Stein E. Misczznski M, Greenland B, Damust, Coulson A. 'Pap' Testing and Lysterectomy Prevalence: a survey of communities with high and low cervical cancer rates. Am J Epidemiol 1977; 106: 296–305.
22. Knox G, Woodman C. Prospects for the primary and secondary prevention of cervix cancer. Cancer Surveys 1988; 7: 379–401.
23. Miller A B. Evaluation of the impact of screening for cancer of the cervix. In: Hakama M, Miller A B, Dey N E eds. Screening for cancer of the uterine cervix. (IARC Scientific Publication no. 76). Lyon: IARC, 1986: pp 149–160.
24. Skehan M, Soutter W P, Lim K et al. Reliability of colposcopy and punch directed biopsy. Br J Obsetet Gynaecol 1990; 97: 811–816.
25. IARC Working Group on the Evaluation of the Cervical Cancer Screening Programme. Screening for squamous cervical cancer: duration of low risk after negative results on cervical cytology and its implications for screening policies. Br Med J 1986; 293: 659–664.
26. Geirsson G, Kristiansdottir R, Sigurdsson K. Cervical cancer screening in Ireland: a case control study in screening for cancer of the uterine cervix (Scientific Publication No 76). Lyon: IARC.
27. Moss S M, Case-control studies of screening. Int J Epidemiol 1991; 20: 1–6.
28. Knox G. Case-control studies of screening procedures. Public Health 1991; 105: 55–61.
29. Flannelly G, Anderson D, Kitchenere H C et al. Management of women with mild and moderate dyskaryosis. Br Med J 1994; 308: 1399–1403.
30. McIndoe W A, McLean M R, Jones R W, Mullins P. The invasive potential of carcinoma in situ of the cervix. J Am Coll Obstet Gynecol 1984; 64(4): 457–458.
31. Robertson J H, Woodend B E, Crozier E H, Hutchinson J. Risk of cervical cancer associated with mild dyskaryosis. Br Med J 1988; 297: 18–21.
32. Campion M J, McCance D J, Cuzick J, Singer A. Progressive potential of mild cervical atypia: prospective cytological colposcopic and virological study. Lancet 1986; i: 237–240.

33. Kirby A J, Spiegelhalter D J, Day N E et al. Conservative treatment of mild/moderate cervical dyskaryosis: long term outcome. Lancet 1992; 339: 828–831.

34. Hirschowitz L, Raffle A E, Mackenzie E F D, Hughes A O. Long term follow-up of women with borderline cervical smear test results: effects of age and viral infection on progression to high grade dyskaryosis. Br Med J 1992; 304: 1209–1212.

35. Kinlen L J, Spriggs A I. Women with positive cervical smears but without surgical intervention: A follow-up study. Lancet 1978; i: 463–465.

36. Barron B A, Cahill M C, Richart R M. A statistical mode of the natural history of cervical neoplasia disease: the duration of carcinoma in situ. Gynecol Oncol 1978; 6: 196–205.

37. Coppleson L W and Brown B. Observations on a model of the biology of carcinoma of the cervix: a poor fit between observation and theory. Am J Obstet Gynecol 1975; 127–136.

38. Albert A. Estimated cervical cancer disease state incidence and transition rates. J Nat Cancer Inst 1981; 571–576.

39. Habbema J D F, van Oortmarssen G J, Lubbe J T N, van der Maas P J. Model building on the basis of Dutch cervical screening data. Maturitas 1985; 7: 11–20.

40. Gustaffson L, Adami H O. Optimization of cervical cancer screening. Cancer Causes Control 1992; 3: 125–136.

41. Knox E G. Ages and frequencies for cervical cancer screening. Br J Cancer 1976; 34: 444–452.

42. Koopmanschap M A, van Oortmarssen G J, van Agt H M A et al. Cervical cancer screening. Attendance and cost-effectiveness. Int J Cancer 1990; 45: 410–415.

43. Parkin D M. A computer simulation model for the practical planning of cervical screening programmes Cancer 1985; 51: 551–568.

44. Parkin D M, Moss S M. An evaluation of screening policies for cervical cancer in England and Wales using a computer simulation model. J Epidemiol Commun Health 1986; 40: 143–153.

45. Oortmarssen G J van, Habbema J D F, Lubbe J T H N, Jong G A de, Mass P J van der. Predicting the effects of mass screening for disease — a simulation approach. Eur J Operat Res 1981; 6: 399–409.

46. Gustafsson L, Adami H O. Cytological screening for cancer of the uterine cervix in Sweden evaluated by identification and simulation. Br J Cancer 1990; 61: 903–908.

47. Ballegooijen M van, Koopmanschap M A, Oorthmarssen G J, van, Habbema J D F, Lubbe K T N, Agt H M A van. Diagnostic and treatment procedures induced by cervical cancer screening. Eur J Cancer 1990; 26(9): 941–945.

48. Ballegooijen M van, Koopmanschap M A, Subandono Tjokrowardojo A J, Oortmassen G J van. Care and costs for advanced cervical cancer. Eur J Cancer 1992; 28a, 10: 1703–1708.

49. Woodman C, Wilson S. A Compassion between the cost effectiveness of immediate intervention and surveillance in the management of cytological abnormality (submitted for publication 1994)

50. Roberts A. Cervical cytology in England & Wales: 1965–1980. Health Trends 1982; 14: 41–43.

51. Parkin D M, Day N E. Evaluating and planning screening programmes. (IARC Scientific Publication no. 66). Lyon: IARC, 1985: pp. 45–63.

52. Lyce R. Allocating costs and benefits in disease prevention programmes; an application to cervical cancer screening (Case study #7). Washington DC: Office of Technological Assessment.

53. Havelock C. The cost of the cervical screening programme an activity based approach. London: National Co-ordinating Network, NHS Cervical Screening Programme, 1994.

54. Department of Health. Cervical cytology 1991/92 Part one summary information form KC53 (SMI2B1). London: DoH.

55. Duncan I. Guidelines for clinical practice and programme management. National Health Service Cervical Cancer Screening Programme.

6. Immunology of the lower female genital tract with emphasis on genital infections

Per-Anders Mårdh   Marius Domeika

INTRODUCTION

Knowledge of the immunology of the lower female genital tract, i.e., of the vagina (vulva) and the cervix, and of the exchange between these sites and other immunocompetent organ systems is still surprisingly poor. This is, inter alia, a drawback for the development of vaccines for sexually transmitted diseases (STDs). Most immunological studies related to the genital tract have concerned reproductive aspects, such as the response or non-response to foreign proteins like those of spermatozoa, seminal fluid components and to the fetus. This communication will elaborate mainly on the nonreproductive aspects, as these have been scarcely highlighted as compared to the reproductive ones. Thus, studies on immunoglobulins and the presence of inflammatory immunocompetent cells in genital secretion, such as the complement factors and the cytokines, will be reported on. The co-occurrence and possible synergistic effects between immunogenic and nonimmunogenic anti-infectious principles are also reported on. The vaginal contents, and variations thereof caused by infections of the lower genital tract will be covered. Also discussed will be the immune response to selected sexually-transmitted agents, such as *Chlamydia trachomatis, Neisseria gonorrhoeae,* human papilloma virus (HPV), the human immunodeficiency viruses (HIV 1 and 2) and *Trichomonas vaginalis.* Genital candidiasis and bacterial vaginosis are also described, including the oncogenic potential of the bacterial flora occurring in the vagina in the latter condition.

ORIGIN, COMPOSITION AND THE ROLE OF GENITAL SECRETION COMPONENTS

The vaginal fluid contains components transmitted through the vaginal wall as a normal physiological process and from genital glands, like those of Skene and Bartholin. During sexual stimulation the secretion in the vagina increases and its composition changes. To the vaginal secretion is added fluid secreted from the cervical mucosa and to a lesser extent from the upper genital tract; a contribution which is maximal during menstruation, but does not occur during pregnancy. The vaginal fluid in sexually-active women is from time to time also exposed to ejaculate, which will increase the vaginal pH in healthy women and introduce foreign proteins and other potentially immunogenic components and cells. The fluid also contains constituents that can influence the efficiency of the immune system in the vagina (see below).

Mucus consists of glycoproteins, which in the female genital tract are produced by epithelial cells of the endocervix and the endometrium. It serves as a lubricator and selective barrier for these cells. Hormonal conditions during the menstrual cycle cause dramatic changes in the viscosity of the mucus.[1] Mucus creates a proper environment for phagocytic cells and cell-mediated immune actions. It also provides a target for bacterial attachment and thus a means for the body to discharge organisms as well as engaging in the immune mechanisms (see also below). Activation of the bactericidal capacity and of some bactericidal proteins by some redox-active agents may also occur.[2]

POLYMORPHONUCLEAR LEUKOCYTES AND MACROPHAGES

Both neutrophils and monocytes are involved in a variety of microbial defense processes in the lower female genital tract, i.e., in chemotaxis as well as in binding and digestion of offending microorganisms.

There is scanty information on polymorphonuclear (PMN) leukocytes in the female genital tract.

However, in the majority of lower genital tract infections an increased number of PMN leukocytes can be found which have the capacity to phagocytize causative agents of genital infections. Thus, interaction between *Neisseria gonorrhoeae*, *Chlamydia trachomatis*, *Treponema pallidum*, *Trichomonas vaginalis* and group B streptococci and the type of phagocytes have been demonstrated.[3] Some strains of STD pathogens are less susceptible to phagocytosis, e.g., gonococci not expressing OMP protein II,[4] which is believed to facilitate opsonin-independent ingestion of bacteria.[5]

A significant role of PMN leukocytes in the clearance of indigenous bacteria in the lower genital tract is, however, questionable as neutropenia is not associated with vaginitis and cervicitis.

Fibronectin can be found in connective tissue but also free in some body fluids, such as vaginal secretions. Some bacterial inhabitants of the vagina can adhere to fibronectin[6] and it is known that such a binding will promote phagocytosis, at least in experimental systems.

An inflammatory process causes an abundance of L-lactate secretion by phagocytes. Gonococci use this substrate to consume oxygen more aggressively than phagocytes.[7] Under these circumstances the phagocytes attacking gonococci cannot generate superoxide as shown in vitro studies. As the environment becomes anaerobic, gonococci use nitrite secreted by phagocytes as part of their microbicidal capacity, e.g., as a terminal electron acceptor.[8] Although oxygen-independent microbicidal proteins kill gonococci in vitro, survival of the organisms in vivo suggests, however, that this defense is not very effective.

Macrophages represent a target for infection with *C. trachomatis*.[9] Replication of the organism can be prevented by using a critical substrate, tryptophan, which is mediated through the action of the enzyme indoleamine-2,3-dioxygenase. The enzyme is activated by interferon. *C. trachomatis* can be taken up by macrophages where they may reproduce as shown in in vitro experiments.[10] The role of macrophages in producing cytokines and thereby a role in the regulation of the intracellular reproduction of chlamydiae in such cells remains to be established.

Macrophages (which occur in great numbers in the uterine epithelium) may be involved in eliminating microbial antibodies and immune complexes.

It is notable that there is a paucity of macrophages in the decidualized endometrium of *Listeria*-infected women, which is in contrast to other sites affected with this bacterium. This may contribute to the tissue tropism for *Listeria monocytogenes* in pregnant women.

IMMUNOGLOBULINS

Cervical and vaginal secretions contain immunoglobulins of several Ig classes. The fallopian tubes also contain Ig-producing cells which, as in the vagina and cervix, are located subepithelially. A great number of immunoglobulin-producing cells are seen in the tubes in cases of acute and chronic salpingitis.

A number of papers have been published concerning IgA produced in the lower female genital tract, while few publications have dealt with locally produced IgM and IgG at this site.

IgG makes up about one-third of the concentration of Ig in the cervicovaginal secretion. IgM makes up about 10%, while the rest of Ig consists of secretory IgA (sIgA) and IgA. No obvious differences are found between endo- and ectocervical secretion on one hand and the vaginal secretion on the other.[11]

IgG

Locally produced IgG antibodies to a variety of infectious agents have been demonstrated, e.g., to bacteria, chlamydiae, viruses, fungi and parasites.[12]

Of the immunoglobulin-producing cells in the

endo- and exocervix and in the vagina, 15%, 11% and 7% produce IgG, respectively.[11]

Although cells able to synthesize IgA predominate in the cervical mucosa, IgG-producing cells can also be demonstrated. IgG can block attachment of pathogens to vaginal mucosal cells and facilitate their elimination by fixation of complement. As a result susceptible pathogens can be killed by lysis. Another mechanism of IgG in the vagina is opsonization, facilitating phagocytosis.

The subepithelial cervical immunocytes capable of synthesizing IgG increase in number when progesterone is in excess, as in the luteal phase of the menstrual cycle. Their level declines during the follicular phase.

Antibody to sperm antigens belonging to IgG has been demonstrated.

Through the deposit of seminal fluid in the vagina an IgG-Fc-binding protein may contribute to the local microbial-resistence in the vagina.[13]

IgA

IgA circulates in serum as a monomeric structure. By the additition of a j-chain (formed by IgA committed plasma cells found adjacent to the mucosa) formation of an IgA dimer can take place. This occurs when IgA traverses the mucosal epithelium of the lower genital tract. The addition of the j-chain or the so-called secretory component increases the molecular weight of sIgA to 395 000, as compared with 160 000 for monomeric serum IgA.

The majority of IgA found in the vagina is derived from the uterus and transported through the cervical channel to the vagina or is produced in the endocervical mucosa. sIgA found in vaginal secretions can also be produced by immunocytes of the vaginal mucosa.

Seminal fluid deposited in the vagina may add IgA to the vaginal contents. It may have been produced locally in the prostate and the epididymis (sIgA), or transudated from serum into the seminal fluid of the male partner.[14]

In all mucosal secretions, including those of the cervical canal and the vagina, the concentration of sIgA exceeds those of IgG.

In the cervicovaginal secretion, sIgA is the predominant immunoglobulin with a concentration more than double that of monometric IgA. The latter constitutes roughly one-fifth of the total Ig concentration of that secretion.

sIgA$_1$ is the predominant antiprotein antibody, but when the antigens are lipopolysaccharides or lipoteichoic acid, it is IgA$_2$ that predominates. Carbohydrate antigens induce IgA$_1$ and IgA$_2$ antibodies in roughly the same concentrations, while IgA$_1$ may predominate in some instances when the antigen is a carbohydrate. This distribution is common for mucosal compartments, but the ratio of IgA$_1$ to IgA$_2$ may differ from that of serum.

The IgA found in the lower genital tract that comes from the uterine cavity in normal women is mostly derived from the circulation and the j-chain is added during passage through the uterine epithelium. A similar transudation seems to occur in the cervix.

Locally produced IgA antibodies occurring in female genital secretion are, inter alia, induced by N. gonorrhoeae, C. trachomatis, HIV, T. vaginalis and Candida albicans.

The role of IgA and sIgA seems to be to facilitate agglutination of organisms and thereby inhibit their attachment to the mucosal lining of the lower genital tract. IgA deficiency, which compared to many other immunodeficiences is comparatively common (1: 600 people), does not, however, seem to result in an increased susceptibility to genital tract infections. Another aspect of this phenomenon is that sIgA may hinder diagnosis of microorganisms in cases where cell culture techniques are used for their detection, e.g., of chlamydiae and viruses.

sIgA also has a role in activating the complement system by the alternative pathway.

The secretory form of IgA is obviously more resistent to proteolytic enzymes than the serum form. However, some microorganisms, i.e., N. gonorrhoeae, are able to destroy IgA by expressing IgA protease.[15] Such an enzyme can cleave IgA$_1$, but not IgA$_2$. We have found other organisms in the vagina which seem to be able to cleave IgA$_2$; organisms that can be found in women with vaginal flora changes such as bacterial vaginosis.

Antisperm antibodies of the IgA$_1$ isotype in cervical secretion are susceptible to bacterial IgA$_1$ protease.[16] Fragments of these antibodies, generated by proteolytic cleavage do not interfere, however, with sperm motility due to their mono-valency and consequent inability to cross-link antigens.

IgE (see also the 'Allergic reactions' section, below)

A role of locally produced IgE in allergic reactions of the lower female genital tract, e.g., to sperm proteins and to microbial antigens, has been proposed.

Seminal fluid containing IgE that has emerged from sensitization of the male partner to female vaginal secretion components may, when deposited in the vagina, cause allergic reactions in the female.

IgE antibodies to *C. albicans*, seminal fluid components, and to spermicides have been identified in vaginal fluid of women with recurrent vaginitis.[17,18] In many instances a vaginal IgE production is accompanied by the presence of prostaglandin E_2.[19] In such women, eosinophils can be demonstrated in vaginal secretions.[20] In sensitized women, there are mast cells in the basal layer of the vaginal epithelium, containing bound IgE of various specificities. Exposure to an allergen in the vagina is followed by transport of the allergen through interepithelial channels where it becomes bound to homologous IgE. This induces mast cell degranulation and release of histamine and other inflammatory mediators in the vaginal wall, causing symptoms of vaginitis.[21]

T-LYMPHOCYTES

Only a few lymphocytes are found in the genital tract of healthy women at any stage of the menstrual cycle. The few lymphocytes that occur are found in the subepithelial layers.[22] Other immunocompetent cells, like granulocytes and macrophages, occur in large numbers during menses, but are few during the proliferate phase.[23]

Natural killer (NK) cells also occur, although in low numbers, in the cervix of healthy women.

The majority of T-lymphocytes in the cervical epithelium belong to the T8-suppressor/cytotoxic subset, but there are also cells belonging to the T4-helper/inducer subset. The ratio by which they have been demonstrated differs considerably between different studies. The T-cells are found exclusively in the basal layers of the squamous epithelium. However, they may also occur in high numbers in the transformation zone of the ectocervix.

Approximately 95% of circulating T-lymphocytes have antigen receptors on their surface, that contain α- and β-chains. The rest of the cells contain such receptors composed of one γ- and one δ-chain. Unlike αβ-T-cells, most γδ-T-cells lack CD4$^+$ or CD8$^+$ surface molecules. Similar to αβ-T-cells, γδ-T-cells are CD3$^+$-positive. The function of the γδ-cells remains to be established, but there is some evidence suggesting that these cells may provide the first line of defense in mucosal infections. However, their function may be to recognize a small number of specific alterations in epithelial cell surfaces rather than a wide repertoire of bacterial, viral, fungal, and protozoan antigens.[24]

The γδ-T-cells in vaginal epithelium of healthy women increase in number after infection by several different organisms.[21] Like other T-cells most of the vaginal γδ-T-cells are associated with the basal layer of the vaginal epithelium.[25,26]

As CD4$^+$ lymphocytes carry receptors for HIV, their presence in genital secretion is of special interest owing to the risk of a person acquiring infection by this virus when having intercourse with an infected person. The transmission rate of HIV may be increased in infectious conditions of the lower genital tract when a high number of such cells may occur in the vaginal secretion.

Langerhan's cells are present in lamina propria.[22] This type of cell occurs in cervical squamous epithelium and stains positive for HLA-DR antigen and OK T6. Its concentration in the vagina is lower than in the epithelium of the cervix. Langerhan's cells express cell surface receptors for the Fc region of the IgG and for complement factor C3. Class II major histocompability antigens (HLA-DR) are also present on the surface of Langerhan's cells. This last property allows Langerhan's cells to present antigens to T-lymphocytes and thereby initiate a specific immune response in the lower genital tract.[27]

Sperms can induce an increased concentration of T-lymphocytes, macrophages, and poly-morphonuclear leukocytes in the cervix.[28] These lymphoid cells migrate into the vagina after coitus. Semen also contains CD4$^+$ and CD8$^+$ T-lymphocytes and $\gamma\delta$-T-cells.[29,30] Exposure to these allogeneic immune cells can probably activate the cell-mediated vaginal immune system and increases the local concentration of cytokines and vaginal lymphoid cells.

A cellular immune response occurs both in uncomplicated and complicated genital infections caused by at least some sexually transmitted agents, e.g., in cervicitis and salpingitis caused by *C. trachomatis*.[31] It may play an important role in tubal factor infertility occurring as a sequelae of chlamydial salpingitis.

Cell-mediated immunity to microbial pathogens seems to play a minor role in the protection of the host against infections of the lower genital tract as compared to infections caused by the same agent(s) at other sites. For example, cell-mediated immunity which is important in fungal infections (by *Candida*). In female HIV/AIDS patients *Candida* vaginitis is, however, not particularly common as compared to *Candida* infection at other sites.

A cell-mediated immune response to sperms can also be detected, at least in experimental animal models.[32]

COMPLEMENT

The concentration of complement is low in vaginal secretion, i.e., 15% of that of serum.

The complement system in the vagina can be activated both by the classical and alternative pathway in case of microbial challenge.

By complement fixation and IgG antibody binding, microbes can be eliminated from the lower female genital tract.

C3b fragments are recognised by gonococcal receptors on PMN cells. Antigonococcal IgM and IgG serum antibodies can activate complement.

CYTOKINES

Of the interleukins (IL), IL-5 selectively enhances IgA synthesis and this effect is synergized by IL-2. IL-5 also enhances IL-2 receptor expression on IgA-producing cells, thereby also the synthesis of this immunoglobulin. IL-6 is another cytokine

which contributes to clonal expression of cells synthesizing IgA.

Interferon can induce intracellular production of NO, which interferes with intracellular reproduction of *C. trachomatis*.[33]

The levels of interferon-γ in genital secretion is age-related, being higher in older than younger women. This interferon was found in higher levels (6.7 ± 2.8 U/ml) in endocervical secretion of 47 women infected by *C. trachomatis* as compared to 52 currently noninfected women (14 ± 0.4 U/ml) ($P \leq 0.002$).[34] The levels did not correlate with the presence of chlamydial organisms (as detected by culture studies), signs of inflammation or levels of interferon-γ in plasma.

ALLERGIC REACTIONS

Components of seminal plasma may, as mentioned, have an immunosuppressive effect.[35] On the other hand, allergy to semen deposited in the vagina ('allergic seminal vulvovaginitis')[36] has been reported, but most often only as separate case reports.[37] Usually it seems to be glycoproteins in the ejaculate to which the allergic woman reacts. Thus, delayed hypersensitivity, skin reactions and passive transfer (Prausnitz–Küstner) reactions have been demonstrated. Even anaphylaxis[38] to seminal fluid has been described in women.

Vaginal allergic reactions include urticaria, edema, pruritus and erythema. Affected women often have atopy, or have relatives with it. A history of surgery, pregnancy or insertion of an intrauterine device often precede allergic episodes; a fact which has been difficult to explain. Sensitization may occur over months or years. Potentially allergic substances ingested by a male sexual partner and present in his semen may induce immune-mediated vaginitis.[21]

Genital allergic reactions to *Candida* antigens have been demonstrated.[19,29] In *Candida* allergy vulvar vesicles and vaginal discharge may be seen. The condition may be mistaken for vulvovaginitis of unknown etiology rather than mere genital candidiasis (see below). However, allergy to *Candida* may occur concomitantly with clinical vaginal candidiasis. A local IgE antibody response in women with assumed allergy to *Candida* allergens has been demonstrated. Suppression of cellular immunity, induced by prostaglandin E_2 may also be seen. Histamine and viable *C. albicans* organisms can act synergistically to induce even higher levels of prostaglandin E_2 to be released from macrophages.[39] As mentioned, the prostaglandin E_2 production is accompanied by IgE production.[19]

Allergy to microbial antigens other than those of *C. albicans* of a protein or of a carbohydrate nature, particularly to antigens of anaerobic bacteria, is thought to occur. However, convincing data are lacking.

Medical drugs or possibly even certain foods may induce an allergic vaginitis in susceptible women. Rarely exogenic allergens introduced into the vagina by application of creams or other vehicles may cause hypersensitive reactions. Even seasonal allergic vulvovaginitis due to pollen has been described.[40]

While sexual abstinence or condom-use throughout coitus may eliminate allergic manifestations to semen, these would not do so if the causative organism is a part of the indigenous microbial flora.

INFLUENCE OF THE VAGINAL MILIEU ON THE EFFICIENCY OF IMMUNE REACTIONS

The pH of a given woman seems, to a large extent, to be genetically determined and may be either on the acid or alkaline side of the physiological range. The span of physiological vaginal pH-values changes somewhat during the reproductive period of the woman, that is, to the alkaline side with increasing age.

Menstruation will also change the pH to the alkaline side which, along with the disappearance of the cervical plug, may facilitate the establishment and ascending exogenic STDs. Thus gonococcal salpingitis is found more often in conjunction with menstruation than during other phases of the menstrual cycle. This may also be true for endogenous infections caused by organisms found in the vaginal flora, for example, of women with bacterial vaginosis (BV). The vaginal microorganisms in women with BV may represent a large number of facultatively and strictly anaerobic bacterial species.

Lactobacilli of a variety of species produce

proteases which may cleave IgA thereby making these antibodies noncompetent to opsonize bacteria. As mentioned such proteinases are produced by some STD agents, such as gonococci.

Proteinases of a male sexual partner, occurring in the seminal fluid, may be deposited in the vagina at intercourse.

Vaginal lavage fluid suppresses mitogen-induced proliferation in in vitro experiments. Neither menstruation nor seminal fluid deposit in the vagina seems to influence this suppressive capacity.

Seminal fluid contains zinc, spermin, spermidine, pregnancy-associated protein-A, transglutamine, 94 kDa Fc-receptor-binding protein, prostaglandins and prostasomes, all of which may have a immunosuppressive capacity.[41]

Spermicides, like nonoxynol-9, may be toxic to immunocompetent cells, e.g., protective lymphocytes and macrophages. This may be of potential concern when discussing the virocidal effect of nonoxynol-9 for HIV and other STD agents.

Hormones definitely influence the immunocapacity of the lower female genital tract. Estrogen therapy (2 mg estriol daily) of 20 postmenopausal women decreased the IgA level in vaginal secretion from 41.5 ± 5.7 mg/l to 20.8 ± 5.7 mg/l. In 20 fertile women the level was lower both before (20.8 ± 5.7 mg/l) and after (16.4 ± 3.7 mg/l) such therapy. In both groups the difference was significant both before and after the therapy.[42] It is notable, that estrogen can in one subject stimulate the production of IgA in the uterus but in the same subject decrease the production in the vagina.[43]

Sex hormones have also been found to influence the production of IgA in experimental animal models by increasing its production in the uterus and decreasing it in the vagina.[44]

Sex hormones affect the function of T- and B-lymphocytes. Also NK cells and macrophages are under the influence of such hormones. The way they have such an influence is not known.

Sex hormones can also influence the uptake of intracellular parasites, like *C. trachomatis,* in host cells. This has been shown in both in vitro studies[45] and animal models.[46] Sex hormones can also influence the spread of a chlamydial infection from the cervix to the Fallopian tubes.[47] In animal models, hormone treatment can also change the natural course of chlamydial infection, e.g., by the guinea pig inclusion conjunctivitis agent.

IMMUNE RESPONSE TO SOME INFECTIOUS AGENTS

Chlamydia trachomatis

Intrauterine infection of mice with *C. trachomatis*, serotype F, results in development of salpingitis. In some of the animals thus challenged, infertility due to tubal occlusion has been described. Parenteral immunization with purified, heterologous recombinant major outer membrane protein (MOMP) protected three-fourths of challenged animals from salpingitis. However, it did not prevent colonization of the lower genital tract. Interestingly, few chlamydiae challenged in the vagina were isolated from that site in mice immunized using Peyer's patches. In these latter animals, there was no protection from tubal damage after *C. trachomatis* infection. Presacral immunization caused high levels of humoral anti-MOMP IgG in vaginal secretion. Low levels of such IgA antibodies did not tend to reduce the severity of salpingitis and did not protect against tubal factor sterility in mice infected by chlamydiae by intravaginal challenge.[48]

Using a lymphogranuloma venereum serovar (L$_2$) of *C. trachomatis* to infect BALB/c mice by the oral route, an IgA response was detected. At subsequent intravaginal challenge a booster effect was obtained and significant protection to infection with the L$_2$ agent was seen. Passive immunization of the animals with serum IgG did not influence the vaginal shedding of the organism and did not protect against infection by L$_2$ after challenge.[49]

In chlamydial infections, lymphoid follicles are formed in the cervix; this is one of the hallmarks of such infections at any site of the body as, for example, can be seen by the naked eye in the eyelid mucosa at the earlier stages of trachoma. Lymphocytes otherwise occur only in low numbers in genital tract tissues.

In the uterine mucosa in cases of chlamydial endometritis, which occurs in up to 40% of all cases of female genital tract infections by chlamydiae, there is an intensive infiltration by plasma cells.[50] Plasma cell endometritis has also been reported

to occur in cases of gonorrhea. However, as these observations were made before the discovery of *C. trachomatis* and with the knowledge that double infections with gonococci and chlamydiae are very common, it remains to be established whether or not gonococci may really cause such a plasma cell infiltration.

Trichomonas vaginalis

Knowledge of the immunology of trichomoniasis is limited. Although immunologic factors are likely to be involved in the natural history of the disease, extensive studies have failed to show a protective effect or immune response.

Antibodies to *T. vaginalis* have been detected in serum and vaginal secretion of infected persons, but only in low titers. The formation of antibodies against intracellular structures of *T. vaginalis*[51] suggests that these antibodies are not only elicited by live parasites attached to the vaginal surface, but also by disintegrated organisms.

A local antibody response (IgA) to *T. vaginalis* can be demonstrated in cases of trichomoniasis.[52] IgG antibodies can be detected against a 230 kDa *T. vaginalis* surface antigen.[53] Antibody and complement, activated by the alternative pathway, can lyse the parasite.

T. vaginalis can cause vaginitis. An inflammatory response and a large number of PMN cells are recruited,[54] which can be seen in vaginal wet smears along with mobile trichomonades. The PMN cells are capable of phagocitizing the flagellate. *T. vaginalis* stimulates chemotaxis of polymorphonuclear cells, which may contribute to the development of symptoms.

T. vaginalis contains constituents that elicit proliferation of T-lymphocytes in infected persons.[55] A cell-mediated immune response can be demonstrated in up to one-fourth of cases of trichomoniasis.

Trichomonades may produce proteinases. Trichomonal antiproteinase antibodies were detected in the sera of 71% and in vaginal lavage in 86% of women with trichomoniasis.[56]

Candida albicans

In women with recurrent candida vaginitis, a

deficient lymphocyte proliferative response to *Candida* antigens can be demonstrated.[57]

Germination tube formation of *C. albicans* is related to the virulence of the invading fungus. In in vitro experiments, it reaches a maximum with sera obtained during the luteal phase. The hormonal status of women may thus alter the immune response in such a way that it may influence the resistance to invasion by *C. albicans*.[58] During the luteal phase the germination can be inhibited by products of activated peripheral blood mononuclear cells. Interferon-γ can inhibit germ tube formation in the presence of prostaglandin E_2.

Candida vaginitis occurs more often during pregnancy than otherwise and more often in the late luteal phase before menstruation than at other phases of the menstrual cycle. These and above-mentioned observations assume an important hormonal influence on the development of *Candida* vaginitis. Variations in the immune response to *C. albicans* is much less in women taking oral contraceptives; once more indicating a relationship between hormonal and immunological factors in the resistance to infections by *C. albicans* and certain other *Candida* species.

Antibody to *C. albicans* can be demonstrated in cervicovaginal secretion.[59] Such antibodies do not prevent *Candida* vulvovaginitis. Antibody to purified macrophages incubated with *C. albicans* and lymphocytes, can inhibit recognition by lymphocytes[60] and uptake of *Candida* antigens by macrophages.

The immune system of some women with recurrent candidal vaginitis responds to infection by *C. albicans* by producing prostaglandin E_2, which can be identified in vaginal secretion. An immune-mediated hypersensitivity to *C. albicans* results in the release of histamine, which in turn stimulates macrophages to release high levels of prostaglandin E_2.[20] Prostaglandin E_2 blocks the production of IL-2,[61] a T-lymphocyte-derived lympholeukin essential for lymphocyte proliferation.[57]

Cellular immunodeficiency, e.g., in HIV infection, increases the susceptibility to candidiasis, but it is not obvious that this accounts for genital candidiasis in women.

The presence of specific IgE antibodies in the vaginal fluid of women with genital candidasis suggests a localized vaginal hypersensitivity response.[19] Allergic reactions to *Candida* allergens were discussed earlier in this Chapter.

Neisseria gonorrhoeae

Gonorrhea is, apart from HIV/AIDS, probably the most extensively studied disease of the human STDs on a molecular level with regard to host–parasite interactions and pathogenic mechanisms.

PMN leukocytes, which can phagocytize gonococci, (a phenomenon which can be observed in stained smears and which still forms an important basis for the diagnosis of gonorrhea)[7] possess lectin-like receptors that recognize carbohydrate structures present in the cell wall of the gonococcus.[62] *N. gonorrhoeae* that do not express, an outer membrane protein II, can avoid phagocytosis by PMN cells. The protein is believed to facilitate opsonin-independent phagocytosis.[5] In vitro, phagocytosis of gonococci by PMN cells may be increased by gonococcal antipilus antibodies.

Phagocytes use L-lactate to increase their consumption of oxygen.[7] Under these circumstances phagocytes attacking gonococci cannot generate superoxide in vitro. When the environment becomes anaerobic, gonococci use nitrite (secreted by phagocytes) as a terminal electron acceptor.[8]

Gonococci that possess pili are less readily phagocytized than such bacteria lacking these structures. On the other hand, it has been shown that human monocytes are capable of phagocytizing nonpiliated gonococci.[63] In experimental studies in humans using nonpiliated gonococci the infection rate was only 40% of that when using a piliated strain to challenge the volunteers.

IgA antibodies to *N. gonorrhoeae* are produced by plasma cells localized in the lamina propria of the endocervix. IgA antibodies can inhibit attachment of *N. gonorrhoeae* to the mucosa of the cervix, although this effect is limited.

Gonococcal OMP antibodies can interfere with the attachment of gonococci.[64-66] IgG_1 and IgG_3 antigonococcal lipopolysaccharide (LPS) antibodies may lyze gonococci, but the protection of such antibodies is often limited.

Many species of the indigenous vaginal bacterial flora produce proteases that can cleave IgA. *N. gonorrhoeae* is well known to be a potent producer of IgA$_1$ protease which represents one of the virulence factors of this microorganism.[67]

Pili antigen protein II, a 23–33 kDa antigen, and presumably also LPS are predominant gonococcal antigens which can react with gonococcal serum IgG antibodies. IgA reacts also with gonococcal protein II and 46–48 kDa protein. In vaginal fluid, IgA antibodies are expressed against gonococcal pili proteins I and II, while such IgG antibodies are formed against the 46–48 kDa protein. Antigonococcal immunoglobulins in vaginal fluid showed more reactivity with protein I than corresponding serum immunoglobulins.[68]

Immunization of mice with a ribosomal fraction of *N. gonorrhoeae* protected against intravaginal challenge with the homologous strain of gonococci. The protection correlated with the presence of bactericidal antibody to the purified ribosomal fraction in serum as well as in vaginal secretion. Such antibodies may play a major role in the protection against gonococcal infection.[69]

To what extent the hormonal status of the individual, as for *C. trachomatis* and *C. albicans*, also influences the susceptibility of women to *N. gonorrhoeae* is poorly understood. Gonococcal PID, as mentioned, debut more often in conjunction with menstruation than elsewhere during the menstrual cycle. It is not known if this is due merely to the disappearance of the viscous cervical plug.

Human immunodeficiency virus (HIV)

The rate of sexual transmission of HIV appears to correlate to the level of lymphoid cells present during coitus in genital secretion.[70] Therefore, factors influencing the concentration of CD4$^+$ cells in the vagina carrying the receptor for the HIV virus are of importance for the transmission rate, e.g., many types of genital infections.

The predominant cell infected by HIV is the T-lymphocyte carrying CD4$^+$ receptors, but other cells including monocytes, macrophages, endothelial, epithelial and neural cells can become infected by the virus.[71] Some of these cell types express either CD4$^+$ mRNA or CD4$^+$ protein.[72]

If vaginal T-cells are chronically activated, a constant source of target cells for HIV would be generated. This might explain an increased susceptibility to HIV in women infected with sexually-transmitted agents, such as *Haemophilus ducreyi*. Comparing HIV-seropositive and -negative women, all of whom had leukorrhea from presumed infection(s), CD4$^+$ T-lymphocytes were identified in combined vaginal and exocervical secretions from all subjects studied.[73]

Infection of Langerhan's cells and cervical monocytes with HIV virus has been reported.[74,75] Infection of Langerhan's cells by HIV and simian immunodeficiency virus (SIV) might occur through the ability of HIV/SIV to bind to HLA-DR and/or by binding of IgG HIV antibody or complement receptors.[21]

In mice, exogenous proteins can be absorbed by interepithelial Langerhan's cells after vaginal administration.[76] This finding raises the possibility that Langerhan's cells might transport HIV antigen to regional lymph nodes and serve as antigen preserving cells in the vagina. Thus, migration of Langerhan's cells to regional lymph nodes provides one mechanism for the progress of HIV from a localised genital infection to a systemic infection.[21]

In monkeys infected by SIV, IgG antibodies to SIV can be demonstrated in vaginal secretion. IgA-containing plasma cells were absent from the vaginal and cervical basal lamina of infected animals.[77]

In naturally occurring HIV infection both IgG and IgA antibodies can be detected. Genital IgA is mainly directed against the HIV core proteins p18 and p25, the p68 reverse transcriptase, and the gp160 and gp41 glycoproteins. IgA antibodies against the glycoprotein gp120 can, rarely, be recovered.[78]

To conclude, the protective effect, if any, of the immune system of the lower female genital tract against HIV infection is poorly documented.

Human papilloma virus (HPV)

Generally speaking comparatively little is still known about host defence mechanisms to HPV. Some HPV types, e.g., 6, 11, 16 and 18 are related with cervicitis. Types 16 and 18, as well as certain other types, are associated with cervical carcinoma.[79] The human cervical mucosa seems to be the source of sIgA and IgG antibodies to HPV.[80] In the vaginal secretion of 29 patients with genital condylomas, IgA antibodies against synthetic peptides E_2 and E_7, could be demonstrated in 18 cases. Such antibodies in 28 control persons were found in 8 and 5 cases, respectively.[81]

HPV replicates poorly in the keratinized squamous epithelial cells which line the vagina. Junctional epithelium, as is found for example in the cervix, is especially prone to HPV infection. The profound nuclear and cytoplasmic changes induced by HPV infection lead to formation of koilocytes which are mainly found in the granular layer of the epithelium of the cervix and the vagina.[82]

Cervical immune response to HPV remains detectable for more than 30 days.[83]

Since there are no suitable target cells available for HPV in vitro, it has been difficult to investigate, for example, cell-mediated immune response to HPV. Technologies which rely upon the recognition of specific antigens by primed lymphocytes have recently been introduced. However, only a minor and transient response in patients with a long history of genital warts has been demonstrated.[84] Clinical HPV infection is associated with inhibition of cell-mediated immune reactions. Thus, an HPV infection may cause localized vaginal immunosuppression.

NK cells may play a role in the resistence to HPV infection. Such cells are found predominantly in the subepithelial stroma of the cervix. The frequency and pattern of distribution of these cells are similar in all stages of cervical intraepithelial neoplasia. The number of NK cells present in HPV infections is usually small, but the degree of infiltration by Leu-11 positive cells is pronounced.[85]

REFERENCES

1. Gibbons R A. Mucus of the mammalian genital tract. Br Med Bull 1978; 34: 34–38.
2. Root R K, Cohen M S. The microbicidal mechanisms of human neutrophils and eosinophils. Rev Infect Dis 1981; 3: 565–598.
3. Cohen M S, Weber R D, Mårdh P-A. Genitourinary mucosal defenses. In: Holmes K K, Mårdh P-A, Sparling P F, Wiesner P J, eds. Sexually transmitted diseases, 2nd edn. New York: McGraw-Hill, 1990: pp 117–127.
4. Hagman M, Danielsson D. Increased adherence to vaginal epithelial cells and phagocytic killing of gonococci and urogenital meningococci associated with heat modifiable proteins. APMIS 1989; 97: 839–844.
5. Britigan B E, Cohen M S, Sparling P F. Neisseria gonorrhoeae: A model of molecular pathogenesis. New Engl J Med 1985; 312: 1683–1694.
6. Nagy E, Fröman G, Mårdh P-A. Fibronectin binding of Lactobacillus species isolated from women with and without bacterial vaginosis. J Med Microbiol 1992; 37: 38–42.
7. Britigan B E, Klapper D, Svedsen T, Bean K, Cohen M S. Phagocyte derived lactate stimulates the metabolism of Neisseria gonorrhoeae: An unrecognised aspect of the O_2 metabolism on phagocytosis. J Clin Invest 1988; 81: 318–324.
8. Hassett D J, Cohen M S. The response of bacteria to oxidant stress. Implications for interaction with phagocytic cells and microbial pathogenesis. FASEB J 1989; 6: 214–218.
9. Byrne G I, Carline J M. Interferon-mediated induction of indoleamine 2,3-dioxygenase by human mononuclear phagocytes. In: Proceedings of 7th International Congress of Immunology. Berlin, 1989: p 212
10. Fröman G, Yxfeldt G, Wilén-Winter B, Grönvik K-O, Mårdh P-A. Large scale growth of Chlamydia trachomatis in macrophage suspension. In: Proceedings of the 2nd Meeting of the European Society for Chlamydia Research. P.-A. Mårdh, M. LaPlaca and M. Ward, eds. Stockholm, Uppsala University, Uppsala: Centre for STD Research, 1992: p 24
11. Kutteh W H, Hatch K D, Blackwell R E, Mestecky J. Secretory immune system of the female reproductive tract. I. Immunoglobulin and secretory component-containing cells. Obstet Gynecol 1988; 71: 56–60.
12. Kutteh W H, Edwards R P, Menge A C, Mestecky J. IgA immunity in female reproductive tract secretions. In: Griffin P D, Johnson P M, eds. Local immunity in reproductive tract tissues. Delhi: Oxford University Press, 1993: pp 229–244.
13. Witkin S S, Richards J M, Bangiovanni M, Zelikowski G. An IgG-Fc binding protein in seminal fluid. Am J Reprod Immunol 1983; 3: 23–27.
14. Brandtzaeg P, Christiansen A, Müller F, Purvis K. Humoral immune response patterns of human mucosae, including the reproductive tracts. In: Griffin P D, Johnson P M, eds. Local immunity in reproductive tract tissues. Delhi: Oxford University Press, 1993: pp 97–130.
15. Plaut A G, Gilbert J V, Artenstein M S. Neisseria gonorrhoeae and Neisseria meningitidis extracellular enzyme cleaves human immunoglobulin A. Science 1975; 190: 1103–1105.
16. Bronson R A, Cooper G W, Rosenfeld D L, Gilbert J V, Plaut A G. The effect of an IgA1 protease of immunoglobulins bound to the sperm surface and sperm cervical mucus penetrating ability. Fertil Steril 1987; 47: 985–991.
17. Witkin S S. Immunology of recurrent vaginitis. Am J Reproduc Immunol 1987; 15: 34–37.
18. Witkin S S. Immunologic factors influencing susceptibility to recurrent candidal vaginitis. Clin Obstet Gynecol 1991; 34: 662–668.

19. Witkin S S, Jeremias J, Ledger W J. A localized vaginal allergic response in women with recurrent vaginitis. J Allergy Clin Immunol 1988; 81: 412–416.

20. Witkin S S, Jeremias J, Ledger W J. Vaginal eosinophils and IgE antibodies to *Candida albicans* in women with recurrent vaginitis. J Med Vet Mycol 1989; 27: 57–58.

21. Witkin S S. Immunology of the vagina. Clin Obstet Gynecol 1993; 36: 122–128.

22. Edvards J N, Morris H B. Langerhan's cells and lymphocyte subsets in the female genital tract. Br J Obstet Gynaecol 1985; 92: 9774–9778.

23. Hill J A, Anderson D J. Human vaginal leukocytes and the effects of vaginal fluid on lymphocyte and macrophage defence functions. Am J Obstet Gynecol 1992; 166: 720–726.

24. Janeway C A J. Frontiers of the immune system. Nature 1988; 333: 804–806.

25. Itohara S, Farr A G, Lafaille J J. Homing of a (γ/δ) T-thymocyte subset with homogeneous T-cell receptors to mucosal epithelia. Nature 1990; 243: 754–757.

26. Deusch K, Luling F, Reich K, Classen M, Wagner H, Pfeffer K. A major fraction of human intraepithelial lymphocytes simultaneously expresses the (γ/δ) T-cell receptor, the CD8 accessory molecule and preferentially uses the V_c1 gene segment. Eur J Immunol 1991; 21: 1053–1059.

27. Boog C J P, Kast W M, Timmers M, Boes J, de Waal L P, Melief C J M. Abolition of specific immune response defect by immunization with dendritic cells. Nature 1985; 318: 59–62.

28. Thompson L A, Tomlinson M J, Barratt C L, Balton A E, Cooke I D. Positive immunoselection: a method of isolating leukocytes from leukocytic reacted human cervical mucus samples. Am J Reprod Immunol 1991; 25: 58–61.

29. Witkin S S, Goldstein M. Reduced level of T suppressor/cytotoxic lymphocytes in semen from vasectomised men: relationship to sperm autoantibodies. J Reprod Immunol 1988; 14: 283–290.

30. Munoz G, Posnett D N, Witkin S S. Enrichment of cd T lymphocytes in human semen: relation between βδ T cell concentration and antisperm antibody status. J Reprod Immun 1992; 22: 47–51.

31. Hallberg T, Wølner-Hansen P, Mårdh P-A. Pelvic inflammatory diseases in patients infected with *Chlamydia trachomatis*: in vitro cell-mediated immune response to chlamydial antigens. Genitourinary Med 1985; 61: 247–251.

32. Shelton J A, Goldberg E. Induction of cell-mediated cytotoxic immunity to sperm-specific lactate dehydrogenase-C4 in SJL/J female mice. Biol Reprod 1985; 32: 556–560.

33. Dutertre Y, Haglund O, Fröman G, Bioteau O, Mårdh P-A. Cycloheximide reduces nitric oxide production and increases infectivity of *Chlamydia trachomatis* in McCoy cells. In: Proceedings of the Tenth Meeting of the ISSTDR. Helsinki, 1993; p 239.

34. Arno J N, Ricker V A, Betteiger B E, Katz B P, Caine V A, Jones R B. Interferon gamma in endocervical secretions of women infected with *Chlamydia trachomatis*. J Infect Dis 1990; 162: 1385–1389.

35. Anderson D J, Tarter T H. Immunosuppressive effects of mouse seminal plasma components *in vitro* and *in vivo*. J Immunol 1982; 96: 577–581.

36. Ohman J L, Malkiel S, Lewis S, Lorusso J L. Allergy to human seminal fluid: characterisation of the allergen and experience with immunotherapy. J Allergy Clin Immunol 1990; 85: 103–107.

37. Jones W R. Adverse immune response in the female genital tract. In: Griffin P D, Johnson P M eds. Local immunity in reproductive tract tissues. Delhi: Oxford University Press, 1993: pp 399–408.

38. Friedman S A, Bernstein I L, Enrione M, Marcus Z H. Successful long-term immunotherapy for human seminal plasma anaphylaxis. J A M A 1984; 251: 2684–2687.

39. Witkin S S, Kalo-Klein A, Galland L, Teic M, Ledger W J. Effect of *Candida albicans* plus histamine on prostaglandin E_2 production by peripheral blood minonuclear cells from healthy women and women with recurrent candidal vaginitis. J Infect Dis 1991; 164: 396.

40. Berman B H. Seasonal allergic vulvovaginitis caused by pollen. Ann Allergy 1964; 22: 594–597.

41. Hargreave T B, James K, Kelly R, Skibinski G, Szymaniec S. Immunosuppressive factors in the male reproductive tract. In: Griffin P D, Johnson P M, eds. Local immunity in reproductive tract tissues. Delhi: Oxford University Press, 1993: pp 161–176.

42. Milsom I, Nilsson L A, Brandberg A, Ekelund P, Mellström D, Eriksson O. Immunoglobulin A (IgA) levels in post-menopausal women: influence of oestriol therapy. Maturitas 1991; 13: 129–135.

43. Sullivad D A, Wira C R. Morphological and immunohistochemical evidence suggesting human papilloma virus (HPV) involvement in the dysplastic lesions of the uterine cervix. Int J Gynaecol Obstet 1983; 21: 261–269.

44. Ahmed S A, Talai N. Sex hormones and the immune system. Part 2. Animal data. Baillière's Clin Rheumatol 1990; 4: 13–31.

45. Mårdh P-A. Some constituents of body fluids influencing the capability of *Chlamydia trachomatis* to multiply in McCoy cell cultures. In: Proceedings of the 4th Meeting of the ISSTDR. Heidelberg, 1981: p 14.

46. Rank R G, White H J, Hough A J, Pasley J N, Barron A L. Effect of oestradiol on chlamydial genital infection of female guinea pigs. Infect Immun 1990; 38: 699–705.

47. Möller B, Thorsen P, Mårdh P-A. Experimental inoculation of *Chlamydia trachomatis* in animal models. In: Mårdh D A, Saikku P, eds. Chlamydial infections of the genital and respiratory tracts and allied conditions. Uppsala: Uppsala University Centre for STD Research, 1991: pp 47–53.

48. Tuffrey M, Alexander F, Conlan W, Woods C, Ward M. Heterotypic protection of mice against chlamydial salpingitis and colonisation of the lower genital tract with a human serum F isolate of *Chlamydia trachomatis* by prior immunisation with recombinant serovar L_1 major outer membrane protein. J Gen Microbiol 1992; 138: 1707–1715.

49. LaScolea L, Cui Z-d, Kopti S, Fisher J, Ogra P L. Prevention of pulmonary and genital chlamydia infection by oral immunization. In: Meheus A, Spier R E, eds. Vaccines in sexually transmitted diseases. London: Butterworth, 1989: pp 86–91.

50. Mårdh P-A, Möller B R, Ingerslev H J, Nüssler E, Weström L, Wølner-Hansen P. Endometritis caused by *Chlamydia trachomatis*. Br J Ven Dis 1981; 57: 191–195.

51. Mathews H M, Moss D M, Callaway C S. Human serologic response to subcellular antigens of *Trichomonas vaginalis*. J Parasitol 1987; 73: 601–610.

52. Rein M F, Müller M. *Trichomonas vaginalis* and trichomoniasis. In: Holmes K K, Mårdh P-A, Sparling

F R. Sexually transmitted diseases. New York: McGraw Hill, 1990: pp 481–492.

53. Alderate J F, Newton E, Dennis C, Neale K A. The vagina of women infected with *Trichomonas vaginalis* has numerous proteases and antibody to trichomonad proteinases. Genitourinary Med 1991; 67: 469–474.

54. Mason P R, Forman L. Polymorphonuclear cell chemotaxis to secretion of pathogenic and nonpathogenic *Trichomonas vaginalis*. J Parasitol 1982; 6: 536–541.

55. Mason P R, Petterson B A. Proliferative response of human lymphocytes to secretory and cellular antigens of *Trichomonas vaginalis*. J Parasitol 1985; 71: 265–268.

56. Bozner P, Gombosova A, Valent M, Demes P, Alderete J F. Proteinases of *Trichomona vaginalis*: antibody response in patients with urogenital trichomoniasis. Parasitology 1992; 105: 89–91.

57. Witkin S S. Immunologic aspects of recurrent vaginitis. In: Horowitz B J, Mårdh P-A, eds. Vaginitis and vaginosis. New York: Wiley, 1991: 247–250.

58. Kalo-Klein A, Witkin S S. Regulation of the immune response to *Candida albicans* by monocytes and progesterone. Am J Obstet Gynecol 1991; 164: 1351–1354.

59. Waldman R H, Cruz J M, Rowe D S. Immunoglobulin levels and antibody to *Candida albicans* in human cervicovaginal secretions. Clin Exper Immunol 1971; 10: 427–434.

60. Witkin S S. Inhibition of candida-induced lymphocyte proliferation by antibody to *Candida albicans*. Obstet Gynecol 1986; 68: 696–699.

61. Chouaib S, Welte K, Mertelsmann R, Dupont B. Prostaglandin E2 acts at two distinct pathways of T-lymphocyte activation: Inhibition of interleukin-2 production and down regulation of transferrin receptor expression. J Immunol 1985; 135: 1172–1179.

62. Kinane D F, Weir D M, Blackwell C C, Winstanley F P. Binding of *Neisseria gonorrhoeae* by lectin-like receptors on human phagocytes. J Clin Lab Immunol 1984; 13: 107–110.

63. Mezzatesta J R, Rest R F. Phagocytic killing of *Neisseria gonorrhoeae* by human monocytes. Infect Immun 1983; 42: 99–105.

64. Rebello R, Green F H, Fox H. A study of the secretory immune system of the female genital tract. Br J Obstet Gynaecol 1975; 82: 812–816.

65. O'Reilly R J, Lee L, Welch B G. Secretory IgA response to *Neisseria gonorrhoeae* in the genital secretions in infected females. J Infect Dis 1976; 133: 113–125.

66. McMillan A, McNeillage G, Young H, Bain SSR. Secretory antibody response of the cervix to infection with *Neisseria gonorrhoeae*. Br J Ven Dis 1979; 55: 265–270.

67. Kilian M, Mastecky J, Russel M W. Defense mechanisms involving Fc-dependent functions of immunoglobulin A and their subversion by bacterial immunoglobulin A proteases. Microbiol Rev 1988; 52: 296–303.

68. Lammel C L, Sweet R L, Rice P A, Knapp J S, Schoolnik G K, Heilbron D C. Antibody-antigen specificity in the immune response to infection with *Neisseria gonorrhoeae*. J Infect Dis 1985; 152: 990–1001.

69. Kita E, Kashiba S. Analysis of immune responses in genital tracts of mice immunised with purified ribosomal fractions of *N. gonorrhoeae*. Br J Ven Dis 1984; 60: 219–225.

70. Bernstein G S. Presence of HIV in cervical and vaginal secretions. In: Alexander N J, Gabelnick H L, Spieler J M, eds. Heterosexual transmission of AIDS. New York: Wiley/Liss, 1990: pp 213–221.

71. Kozarsky P E, Blumberg H M, DuPuis M H. The acquired immunodeficiency syndrome. In: Morse S A, Moreland A A, Thompson S E, eds. Atlas of sexually transmitted diseases. Philadelphia: Lippincott, 1990: pp 8.2–8.42.

72. Koenig S, Fauci A S. Immunology of HIV infection. In: Holmes K K, Mårdh P-A, Sparling P F et al eds. Sexually transmitted diseases. New York: McGraw-Hill, 1990: pp 317–330.

73. Van de Perre P, DeClerq A, Cogniaux-Leclerc J, Nzaramba D, Butzler J P. Detection of HIV p17 antigen in lymphocytes but not epithelial cells from cervicovaginal secretions of women seropositive for HIV: implications for heterosexual transmission of the virus. Genitourinary Med 1988; 64: 30–33.

74. Pomerantz R J. Human immunodeficiency virus infection of the uterine cervix. Ann Int Med 1987; 108: 321–329.

75. Tschachler E. Epidermal Langerhan's cells — a target for HTLV III/LAV infection. J Invest Dermatol 1987; 88: 233–237.

76. Parr M B, Parr L E. Antigen recognition in the female reproductive tract: I. Uptake of intralaminal protein tracers in the mouse vagina. J Reprod Immunol 1990; 17: 101–114.

77. Miller C J, Kang D W, Marthas M. Genital secretory immune response to chronic simian immunodeficiency virus (SIV) infection: a comparison between intravenously and genitally inoculated *Rhesus macaques*. Clin Exper Immunol 1992; 88: 520–524.

78. Belec L, Georges A J, Steenman G, Martin P M. Antibodies to human immunodeficiency virus in vaginal secretions of heterosexual women. J Infect Dis 1989; 160: 385–391.

79. Meng X. Role of Langerhan's cells against cervical human papilloma virus infection and development of cervical carcinoma. Chung Hua I Hsueh Tsa Chih 1992; 72: 155–157.

80. Dillner L, Bekassy Z, Johnsson N, Moreno-Lopez J, Blomberg J. Detection of IgA antibodies against human papilloma virus in cervical secretions from patients with cervical intraepithelial neoplasia. Int J Cancer 1989; 43: 36–40.

81. Dillner L, Fredriksson A, Persson E, Forslund O, Hansson B G, Dillner J. Antibodies against papilloma virus antigens in cervical secretions from candyloma patients. J Clin Microbiol 1993; 31: 192–197.

82. Chardonnet Y, Bejui-Thivolet F, Viac J. Epitheliums malphigiens et infections papillomavirus. Arch Anat Cytol Pathol 1992; 40: 201–211.

83. Roche J K, Crum C P. Local immunity and the uterine cervix: implications for cancer associated viruses. Cancer Immunol Immunother 1991; 33: 203–209.

84. Shah K V. Biology of human genital tract papillomaviruses. In: Holmes K K, Mårdh P-A, Sparling P F et al eds. Sexually transmitted diseases. New York: McGraw-Hill, 1991: pp 433–441.

85. Tay S K, Jenkins D, Singer A. Natural killer cells in cervical intraepithelial neoplasia and human papilloma virus. Br J Obstet Gynaecol 1987; 94: 901–906.

7. Viral infections and lower genital tract neoplasia

H. Kitchener

INTRODUCTION

It is almost 40 years since viral infection of the lower genital tract was recognized, and more recently the principal interest in this area has centered on the link which has developed with cervical cancer. It was also in the 1950s that the first major epidemiological studies were carried out in cervical cancer. These early studies indicated a lack of disease in virgins,[1,2] indeed squamous cancer did not occur in such women. This indicated that sexual activity, and by implication transmission of an oncogenic agent, was necessary for cervical carcinogenesis. Such protection, in this case afforded by virginity, is very unusual in cancers and suggests that transmission of an oncogenic agent is essential in initiating oncogenesis in the cervix. Berenblum's classic model of carcinogenesis is of a multistage, multifactorial process,[3] and this remains generally accepted. This means that a process of malignant change initiated by a sexually-transmitted oncogen would require the continued action of other substances (promoters) to produce irreversible malignancy.

A current discussion of lower genital tract neoplasia is inevitably dominated by the cervix but its consideration collectively in this volume is highly relevant because etiological factors are very likely to be similar. One of the most striking aspects of the lower genital tract is the fact that it is lined almost entirely by squamous epithelium. This varies however. The cervix is covered by a native squamous epithelium which does not undergo significant change during life. By contrast, the columnar epithelium of the endocervix undergoes a process of metaplasia on the so-called transformation zone to produce new squamous epithe-

lium. The vagina is lined by a nonkeratinized squamous epithelium, which is inherently a stable epithelium. The vulva is covered by skin, a keratinized squamous epithelium with an epidermis and dermis and the associated appendages such as hair follicles and sweat glands.

All of these components of the lower genital tract undergo physiological changes in the course of a woman's life; this is principally a process of maturation during adolescence which is maintained during the reproductive years and then a process of atrophy postmenopausally. All three organs, the cervix, vagina and vulva are susceptible to malignant disease and in all three, there is a recognized preinvasive phase. The cervix is affected by neoplasia, far more commonly than the other two, presumably because of the rapid cell turnover at the squamocolumnar junction of the cervix. The vagina with its much more stable epithelium is affected much less commonly, and later in life than cervical cancer. Vulval cancer is somewhere in-between in terms of its incidence possibly because it is more susceptible to chronic trauma than the vagina.

Cervical carcinogenesis has become a major focus for medical science in recent years for three reasons. The first of these is that a great deal is understood of its natural history, the second is that there is a strong candidate oncogen and thirdly, the lower genital tract offers relatively non-invasive access for cytological and histological material for study.

The lower genital tract harbors many different microorganisms but whereas bacteria are frequently only commensals, it is viruses that are more frequently pathogenic. The two most common DNA viruses that are pathogenic in the lower genital tract are the human papillomavirus (HPV) and herpes simplex virus types 1 and 2 (HSV 1 and 2). Another herpes virus known to be shed from the cervix is the Epstein–Barr virus (EBV) but this does not lead to clinical infection in the lower genital tract. Papillomaviruses and herpes viruses are both oncogenic in nature and there is abundant in vitro evidence of their oncogenic potential, which has led to their proposal as candidate oncogens in cervical neoplasia. There is less interest now in HSV but a huge body of epidemiological and molecular evidence now links HPV with cervical cancer. Indeed, it is now difficult to accept that HPV does not play a role at least in the early stages of the disease. This therefore now dominates any general discussion of etiology of lower genital tract neoplasia and cervical neoplasia in particular, and though less evidence is available for carcinogenic events in the vagina and vulva, the cervix is very much the model for researching the other two sites.

HUMAN PAPILLOMAVIRUS

The human papillomavirus is a small nonenveloped virus with a double-stranded circular DNA genome of 8000 base pairs. This genome has coding regions called open reading frames (ORFs). These segments of DNA code for proteins involved in the regulation of viral functions as well as structural proteins required for viral assembly. There are eight early genes (E1–8) and two late genes (L1, L2). The early genes are responsible for transforming properties and the late genes code for the structural proteins. The functions of the HPV open reading frames are listed in Table 7.1.[4]

Table 7.1 Functions of HPV open reading frames

ORF	Function
E1	Episomal replication
E2	Regulation of transcription
E3	Not known; probably does not code for any protein
E4	Production of a late cytoplasmic protein
E5	Epithelial cell proliferation
E6	Transformation; binds with tumor suppressor p53
E7	Major transforming protein; binds with tumor suppressor RB
E8	Not known
L1	Production of major capsid protein
L2	Production of minor capsid protein

From Shaw (1992);[4] reprinted with permission.

Human papillomavirus infection

By far the commonest clinical viral lesions seen in the lower genital tract are anogenital warts, classically known as condylomata acuminata. These lesions first appeared in the West in the form of penile warts on American servicemen serving in the Korean War, but it was not realized until 1954 that these were caused by the papillomavirus.[5] They are sexually acquired and usually occur around the vulva, perineum and perineally. They vary from small isolated lesions to large fungating crops of warts. They may be symptomless but usually cause itch and discomfort, and their mere presence generally causes offence to the sufferer. Lesions are found less frequently inside the vagina and on the cervix but their occurrence on the vulva should prompt a careful inspection of the whole lower genital tract. The factors influencing their natural history are ill-understood and their behavior is unpredictable. They may resolve spontaneously within a short period of time or persist for many years. Male partners may also have clinical penile lesions but frequently do not. They are more frequently found in immunosuppressed women and may be exacerbated by pregnancy. Treatment is by podophyllin for small isolated warts; larger lesions are effectively treated by thermal destruction using local diathermy. Sometimes destruction of some of the warts will be followed by disappearance of the rest. Stimulating an immune response by inoculation with a crude wart homogenate has been tried in the past but yielded unreliable results.

The link between HPV and cervical neoplasia

Interest in infection by HPV was not really aroused until the late 1970s when koilocytosis, the cytopathic change produced by HPV was identified in smears of women who did not exhibit condyloma;[6] it was only colposcopically that these flat lesions or non condylomatous wart virus infection could be seen on the cervix. Histology of these lesions showed koilocytosis and the proof of HPV infection was demonstrated by immunoperoxinase staining using HPV antibody to identify the viral antigen in the tissue.[7] It was this discovery of subclinical HPV infection of the cervix that led to the subsequent evidence linking HPV and cervical neoplasia. Following the identification of cytological features attributable to HPV, these were then identified admixed with those of cervical intraepithelial neoplasia (CIN).[8] These lesions were usually noncondylomatous and could not be distinguished colposcopically from CIN of a similar grade without the viral changes. These were termed by some, atypical condylomas, which was confusing but meant atypical warty lesions.

Human papillomaviruses exist as many different types, which are differentiated by nonhomology with one another. The advent of DNA–DNA hybridization enabled typing of HPV, such that a virus with less than 50% homology with any other type is reported as distinct and given a type number. There are currently around 60 HPV types of which about eight are associated with infection of the cervix (Table 7.2).[9] Certain HPV

Table 7.2 Human papillomavirus types and clinical associations

HPV Type	Location	Clinical Associations
1–4	Cutaneous	Verruca plantaris, plana, vulgaris
5	Cutaneous	Epidermodysplasia verruciformis (EV)
6	Genital mucosa	Condyloma acuminatum; cervical intraepithelial neoplasia (CIN) Laryngeal papillomas Buschke–Löwenstein's tumors
7	Cutaneous	Butcher's wart
8, 9	Cutaneous	EV
10	Cutaneous	Verruca plana
11	Genital mucosa	Condyloma acuminatum; CIN Laryngeal papillomas
12	Cutaneous	EV
13	Oral mucosa	Focal epithelial hyperplasia (FEH)
14, 15	Cutaneous	EV
16	Genital mucosa	CIN; cervical carcinoma
17	Cutaneous	EV
18	Genital mucosa	CIN; cervical carcinoma
19–25	Cutaneous	EV
26–29	Cutaneous	Verruca vulgaris, plana
30	Genital, oral mucosa	CIN
31	Genital mucosa	CIN; cervical carcinoma
32	Oral mucosa	FEH
33	Genital mucosa	CIN; cervical carcinoma
34	Genital mucosa	CIN
35	Genital mucosa	CIN; cervical carcinoma
36	Cutaneous	EV
37	Cutaneous	Keratoacanthoma
38	Cutaneous	Malignant melanoma
39	Genital mucosa	CIN; cervical carcinoma
40	Genital mucosa	CIN
41	Cutaneous	Squamous cell carcinoma
42–44	Genital mucosa	CIN
45	Genital mucosa	CIN; cervical carcinoma
46, 47	Cutaneous	EV
48	Cutaneous	Squamous cell carcinoma
49	Cutaneous	Verruca plana
50	Cutaneous	EV
51, 52	Genital mucosa	CIN; cervical carcinoma
53	Genital mucosa	Normal mucosa
54	Genital mucosa	Condyloma acuminatum
55	Genital mucosa	Bowenoid papulosis
56	Genital mucosa	CIN; cervical carcinoma
57	Genital oral mucosa	CIN
58	Genital mucosa	CIN
59	Genital mucosa	Vulvar intraepithelial neoplasia
60	Cutaneous	Epidermoid cyst

From Werness et al (1991);[9] reprinted with permission.

types produce certain lesions, e.g., the common cutaneous warts or plantar warts or anogenital warts. Using DNA–DNA hybridization, the HPV responsible for anogenital warts was designated HPV-6.[10]

In 1983 a new HPV type was identified, HPV-16, which was identified in invasive cervical cancers from various geographical regions.[11] This was a very significant discovery because not only had HPV genomes been discovered in cervical cancer, but given the specificity of HPV types for different lesions, this became a strong candidate for a cervical carcinogen. A further important development at this time was the realization that high- and low-grade cervical precancerous lesions when probed using Southern blot hybridization, were associated with different HPV types. What was found, was that high-grade lesions (CIN 3) contained HPV 16 genomes whereas in the low-grade lesions, mainly HPV 6 was identified.[12] In other words, lesions of negligible malignant potential contained the viral type normally found in anogenital warts, but high grade lesions, regarded as cervical cancer precursors, were linked with HPV-16 already identified in cervical cancers. These data provided very persuasive evidence of a strong link between HPV, particularly HPV 6, and cervical cancer. This evidence, however, was circumstantial, and it remained to be proven that there was a causal link. The subsequent identification of HPV 16 DNA in cervical cancers has been a remarkably consistent finding in many subsequent reports from different populations.[13,14]

Once this link between HPV-16 and cervical cancer had been established, research reports took a greater interest in control subjects and in internally controlled biopsies from unaffected regions of a diseased cervix. Using Southern blot analysis, the initial findings were of an unexpectedly high prevalence of HPV DNA sequences in cervical biopsies from cytologically normal women[15] as well as in internal normal control biopsies from women with abnormal cytology.[16] These findings raised the obvious question: could HPV be a harmless or passive agent which was able to multiply in cervical cells rather than acting as a pathogen?

NATURAL HISTORY OF HPV INFECTION

Research up to this point had been concerned with essentially cross-sectional studies, with little information about the natural history of HPV infection. If HPV infection were to be considered of etiological important in cervical carcinogenesis, it would be far more convincing if it could be shown that HPV-infected cells were associated with the subsequent development of high-grade CIN, which can be regarded as a cancer precursor. Two such studies provided some supportive evidence of this. An Australian case control study reported on the relative risk of women, known to have cytological changes of HPV in otherwise normal smears, developing CIN 3 six years later.[17] Women who were 25 years or younger at the time of the original smear, had a relative risk of 30 compared with cytologically normal controls. This very significant association showed that if not actually etiological, at the very least, the presence of HPV is a powerful marker for the subsequent development of CIN 3. A second approach to the same question came from Finland where women with cytological and colposcopic evidence of HPV infection were placed under continuing surveillance until the smear showed significant dyskaryosis.[18] Twelve percent of these women developed CIN 3, though 50% of this latter group had in fact HPV 6 and 11 normally associated with low-grade lesions, and 50% had HPV 16 and 18 the so-called oncogenic types. Because it is now unethical to observe cervical lesions beyond the point where CIN 3 is suspected, CIN 3 must be used as the surrogate in this context for the eventual development of cervical cancer.

Accurate evaluation of the natural history of HPV infection is methodologically difficult to pursue. The cytological changes seen in HPV infection are also associated with underlying high-grade CIN in up to 20%. Establishing the diagnosis with certainty would therefore involve a biopsy which would undoubtedly affect the natural history of HPV changes in the cervix. Another parameter for studying the natural history of HPV infection is not at the clinicopathological level but at the molecular level. In one such study,[59] women who had HPV changes in the cervix confirmed by means of colposcopy and biopsy had serial biopsies at 6-month intervals. These biopsies were probed for HPV DNA sequences by DNA–DNA hybridization. This study showed that both histological evidence of HPV infection and HPV genome detection fluctuated within the same individual with time. The factors which might influence this fluctuation remain to be elucidated; however if the virus is truly oncogenic then its persistence is probably necessary in the early stages of carcinogenesis. The converse of this would be that any factors which could interrupt HPV replication might interrupt in time any oncogenic process being driven by the virus.

This was the situation by the late 1980s. HPV, particularly HPV 16 had been found in almost all cervical cancers probed and in high-grade precancers, but to a far lesser extent in low-grade CIN lesions. However, HPV 16 had also been detected in cytologically normal women. Natural history studies were conflicting but there appeared to be a consensus that the women with evidence of HPV infection were at significant risk of developing CIN 3 several years later.

POLYMERASE CHAIN REACTION AND HPV INFECTION

A very significant advance came in the late 1980s with the development of the polymerase chain reaction (PCR), by which means DNA could be amplified greatly, thus rendering the detection of specific DNA sequences at a far greater level of sensitivity than had been possible hitherto.[19] This method is described in greater detail elsewhere but one of the problems posed by the method was contamination because of the extremely small amounts of DNA which can be detected. One of the advantages of PCR is that exfoliated cells rather than biopsies can be used as a source of DNA. This, in turn, avoids the need for a more invasive biopsy, which not only may affect natural history but also usually includes a large amount of stroma in the material for DNA extraction, which will dilute the epithelial DNA. Another advantage of PCR is that it is far less labor intensive than was Southern blotting. DNA can

be more simply extracted and up to 60 samples of DNA can be processed by the PCR machine at the same time. This means that far larger scale studies can be undertaken than hitherto. This has enabled larger populations to be analysed in order to assess for example, the relative risk of HPV infection for the development of cervical cancer in case control studies.

Recent PCR studies

Early studies of HPV-16 sequences in exfoliated cervical cells using PCR reported very high prevalence rates not only in women affected by cervical neoplasia but also in control subjects. One response to these data was, that if HPV infection was so common, it must therefore be of little significance when so many individuals were positive compared with the relatively small number who developed CIN 3 or cervical cancer. However, with the realization of the need for the very highest quality control, recent results show much smaller HPV 16 positive results in control groups of women. A recent large Dutch study[20] revealed that of 1300 symptomless women being screened only 1.5% were positive for an oncogenic HPV type (16, 18 or 31). Of interest was the fact that of 593 women with gynecological symptoms, 7% were oncogenic HPV positive: of these, 78% had a history of abnormal cytology. These data together with very high detection rates of HPV in cervical neoplasia tell us that there is a very close association of HPV with cervical cancer. Not only that, but the risk factors for cervical carcinoma are strongly associated with HPV genital infection. This was convincingly demonstrated in a study of 467 female college students in California[21] which showed that the risk of HPV infection was independently strongly associated with increasing numbers of sexual contacts, use of oral contraceptives and younger age. This type of study suggests that it is HPV that is the etiological agent conferring the increased risk of cervical cancer related to sexual activity.

Another approach in correlating HPV-16 infection with cervical neoplasia has been to look at viral load by employing a semiquantitative method of PCR.[22,23] The method of semiquantitative

PCR involves running several known standards of various concentrations of the DNA being probed for. The viral DNA signal in the material being probed is compared with that of the known standards on the autoradiograph. These studies have shown that mildly abnormal smears which contain higher quantities of HPV are more likely to be associated with the underlying high-grade CIN than if the smear contained only low amounts. This again demonstrates the degree of the association between infection by HPV 16 and significant cervical neoplasia.

HPV ONCOGENESIS

Although the above data provide a convincing epidemiological case for HPV having a direct etiological role in cervical neoplasia, the evidence until recently was still regarded by many as being of an essentially circumstantial nature. However, in the last 2 or 3 years, possible molecular pathways have been elucidated which involve interaction between oncogenic HPV proteins and tumor suppressor genes as a potential scenario for explaining how HPV 16 may initiate cellular transformation.

Designing experimental models to investigate possible mechanisms for an oncogenic effect of HPV in the human cervix has proven difficult for several reasons. Cervical cancer does not occur in nonhuman species making in vivo study impossible, although the bovine papillomavirus model offers some insight. Furthermore HPV will not replicate in in vitro systems which makes it difficult to study its effect on cells in culture. A nude mouse system has been described[24] where cervical tissue grafted under the renal capsule can be subjected to cell-free extracts of genital warts, with dysplasia of cervical cells being observed. Although this is not necessarily a good model for the cervix it does demonstrate that HPV can produce abnormal cellular changes in vivo.

Cell culture of the cervical epithelium is notoriously difficult although the use of serum-free growth media has improved results. Using such a culture system, the HPV 16 and HPV 18 protein coded by the E7 open reading frame has been shown capable of producing immortalization of cultured cells.[25] Furthermore, these immortalized cells can be morphologically transformed by the addition of the ras oncogene protein.[26] It has also been shown that such immortalisation can be achieved by transfecting HPV 16 and HPV 18 DNA into the cells, but not if HPV 6 is employed.[27] Maintenance of this transformed state in vitro requires continued expression of the HPV 16 E7 oncoprotein.[28] This two-stage process of transformation of cells using an HPV 16 oncoprotein and oncogene product lends insight into the possible role of virus and oncogene combining to produce cervical cellular changes in vivo.

A further observation which has been made in vitro is that the tumor promoter, phorbol ester, can stimulate HPV 18 expression.[29] This suggests that continued HPV expression which is required to maintain the transformed state of cultivated cells maybe encouraged by promoters. A plausible model therefore is of initiation of oncogenic change brought about by HPV 16 or HPV 18, and other agents promote further malignant change in the cell driving it towards uncontrolled growth associated with tumor invasion. All of these data point clearly to the tumorigenic potential of HPV 16 and HPV 18. Recently, possible mechanisms for this viral oncogenicity have been elucidated which have advanced progress in this field.

HPV AND TUMOR SUPPRESSOR GENES

In the previous section reference was made to oncogenes whose coded products or oncoproteins are thought to result in loss of control over cellular growth. These oncogenes which may be growth factors or kinases act at different points of cellular control. Recently, there has been increasing interest in relation to HPV 16 and the tumor suppressor genes, p53 and the retinoblastoma gene Rb-1. It is now widely believed that retinoblastoma occurs when both Rb-1 alleles are defective. If one defective Rb-1 is inherited, then a somatic point mutation which renders the other one defective will result in the development of retinoblastoma.[31] If both alleles are inherited in a defective form the retinoblastoma will be congenital. Thus, the intact retinoblastoma gene protects against tumor development. In vitro support for this concept is demonstrated when Rb-1 defective cell lines can be made non tumorigenic by introducing an Rb gene.[32] In HPV 16 it is the protein expressed by the E6 and E7 open reading frames, i.e., the E6 and E7 oncoproteins which confer immortalization on transfected cell lines. Significantly, therefore, the Rb-1 gene product will complex with oncoproteins such as those of the transforming virus adeno-5.[33] Furthermore, the binding domain on these vital proteins for the Rb-1 protein shares homology with a sequence on the HPV 16 E7 protein. This suggests that Rb-1 can complex and thereby be inactivated by the HPV 16 oncoprotein. This in turn could result in deregulated cellular growth in infected cervical cells.

p53 and cervical cancer

It is now recognized that mutations of the p53 gene are amongst the commonest genetic alterations seen in human cancer.[30] p53 was originally found in extracts of SV40 transformed cells and complexes with the SV40 oncoprotein, large T antigen.[34] The originally found p53 was in fact a mutated form and true p53 is now regarded as an antioncogene which will suppress cell transformation in vitro.[35] In a similar way to the Rb-1 gene, it has been demonstrated that the HPV 16 E6 oncoprotein will bind p53 but this capability is apparently limited to the oncogenic HPV types.[36] Inactivation of p53 in cervical cells by HPV 16 may confer oncogenic potential.

Not all cervical cancers are HPV positive; indeed HPV negative tumors, in one report, had a worse prognosis.[37] In one study of 28 cervical cancers, 25 were found to be HPV positive and 3 negative. In the HPV positive cancers, the p53 was wild type or normal, but in the HPV negative cancers the p53 demonstrated a point mutation.[38] The hypothesis therefore is that in HPV positive lesions the p53 is inactivated by HPV oncoproteins, and in HPV negative lesions, somatic mutation accounts for the inactivation of p53.

It can be appreciated from the foregoing data that there is an abundance of evidence to suggest that HPV 16 confers a greatly increased risk of subsequent high-grade cancer precursor lesions in the cervix, that HPV 16 is an oncogenic virus and that it interacts in a crucial way with genes which regulate cellular control. It is now difficult to doubt that this virus exerts a causative effect in the development, at least, of cervical intraepithelial neoplasia.

SMOKING AND CERVICAL CANCER

Accepted tumor models support the concept that single agents are not solely responsible for tumor development; that this occurs in a multistage multifactorial fashion. There is every reason to believe this is the case with cervical neoplasia. While HPV 16 is the likeliest initiator of carcinogenesis and its continued expression may be necessary, other agents are necessary to act as promoters. The likeliest candidate example in women who smoke is cigarette carcinogen.

The evidence that smoking is related to cervical neoplasia is based mainly on extensive epidemiological work and more recently there has been some experimental evidence of smoking-related products being identified in the cervix. One of the earliest reports of the increased risk conferred by cigarette smoking was a case control study from Oxford[39] which showed a very significant independent relative risk, although this study did not control for the other major risk factor in cervical neoplasia which is the number of sexual partners. This issue was addressed however by an American study which after adjusting for age, oral contraceptive use and socioeconomic status as well as number of sexual partners, demonstrated a dose–response relationship between number of cigarettes smoked and risk of cervical cancer.[40] Since these studies in the early 1980s other epidemiological studies have tended to confirm not only the positive association between cigarette smoking and cervical neoplasia, but several other studies have confirmed this to be a dose–response relationship. The dose–response effect observed epidemiologically fits well with the idea that smoking is a promoter of neoplastic change in cells in which HPV infection has switched on abnormal cell growth.

From a biological point of view the basis for

cigarette smoke being related is the transmission to the cervix of blood-borne products of tobacco smoke which have been absorbed in the lungs. Cotinine and nicotine, for example, can be detected in cervical mucus, indeed at higher concentrations than in serum.[41] Chemical carcinogens exert their biological effect by means of covalently modifying DNA to form adducts. In the bronchial tree, biopsies from smokers show an increased level of DNA adducts compared with non-smokers.[60] Because smoking is unequivocally a cause of lung cancer, it is therefore significant that an increased level of DNA adducts can be identified in cervical biopsies of smokers compared with nonsmokers.[43] Another approach associating cigarette smoking with CIN has been to examine Langerhan's cells, which are thought to play a role in local immunocompetence. Langerhan's cells have been reported to be reduced in number in cervical biopsies of smokers compared with nonsmokers.[44] Such reduced immunocompetence could enhance any effects exerted by HPV infection of the cervix. Langerhan's cells are reduced in the presence of CIN and HPV induced change in cervical epithelium[42] but whether this is the result of external agents such as smoking or related to the HPV infection itself is not clear.

The strength of data implicating cigarette smoking as a causal agent in cervical neoplasia was analyzed in a recent thorough review which concluded that cervical cancer should be added to the list of smoking-related diseases, and that policies to control cervical cancer should take account of the role of cigarette smoking.[45]

HERPESVIRUSES AND CERVICAL NEOPLASIA

Although HPV now dominates discussion of virus-induced neoplasia in the cervix, two members of the herpesvirus family have been linked with this disease. Herpes simplex virus (HSV) type 2 emerged in the 1960s as the original viral candidate for a cervical oncogen. More recently another herpes virus, the Epstein–Barr virus (EBV), has generated some interest in this context.

Herpes simplex virus and cervical neoplasia

HSV exists as 2 types, types 1 and 2. HSV 1 typically is responsible for oral lesions and HSV 2 for genital lesions, though orogenital contact means that either type can be associated with lesions at either site. Following a primary infection, painful blisters form typically on the vulva although lesions may occur on the cervix and vagina, which contain enormous numbers of viral particles. Cell death occurs during this lytic phase following which crusting and healing occur. This process typically lasts about a week, after which the virus becomes latent in neural ganglia. Recurrent attacks typically occur, although not always, these subsequent attacks being triggered by mechanisms which are not yet elucidated. Because HSV infection produces cell lysis and death, a persistent infection must be by virus which has been mutated. Under such circumstances HSV 2 may achieve morphological transformation of mammalian cells. However, in life, although HSV 2 may be shed from the cervix for several months after an acute genital attack, persistent infection does not occur in the way it does with HPV.

During the 1960s it was observed that women who had cytological changes of HSV infection had an increased risk of CIN.[46] Similarly, women who were seropositive for HSV 2 had an increased relative risk of having cervical neoplasia.[47] With the advent of in situ hybridization in the 1970s, initial studies reported HSV-2 transcripts in cervical neoplasms.[48,49] However, these results were not generally substantiated by detection of HSV DNA sequences in cervical biopsies using Southern blotting, apart from one or two isolated reports.[50] With this failure to find HSV genomes in a high proportion of cervical neoplasia, and the concomitant identification of HPV genomes in most cervical cancers, interest in HSV as a cervical oncogen waned. More recent data continues to indicate a possible etiological role for HSV 2, with the demonstration that HPV 16 transformed cells can be rendered tumorigenic in nude mice by transfecting with HSV 2 DNA.[51] While mutant HSV 2 is undoubtably oncogenic in vitro, the relevance of wild-type infection to cervical carcinogenesis in vivo remains uncertain. One recent seroepidemiological study reported that HPV 16/18 positivity gave a relative risk of 4.3 for invasive cervical cancer which increased to 8.8 if positive for HSV 2 antibodies also.[52] The authors suggested this could point to a possible interaction between HPV and HSV. However, another case control study found that although HSV 1 and 2 antibodies were associated with cervical cancer, when HPV seropositive cases and controls were compared this association was weaker. The authors suggest that past infection with sexually-transmitted agents other than HPV may be simply surrogate markers of exposure to HPV and not of independent etiological significance.[53] It could also simply reflect increased sexual exposure. Further convincing evidence will be required to strengthen the case for HSV 2 being involved in cervical carcinogenesis.

EBV and cervical neoplasia

The other herpes virus to attract interest in the search for candidate oncogenic agents in cervical neoplasia is EBV. It is closely associated with another squamous neoplasm, nasopharyngeal carcinoma, in which the viral nuclear antigen or EBNA is frequently identified. This virus is generally regarded as lymphotrophic and is associated with three lymphoproliferative B-cell disorders; acute infectious mononucleosis, Burkett's lymphoma and lymphoma occurring in immunocompromised individuals.

EBV is a ubiquitous agent probably infecting 90% of the world's population, generally harmlessly, although if a primary infection is delayed until the teenage years, infectious mononucleosis or 'glandular fever' may occur. Primary infection is followed by persistent infection with individuals remaining seropositive and low levels of virus being detectable in saliva. The virus although primarily lymphotrophic can replicate in epithelial cells in vivo as demonstrated by the detection of replicating EBV in exfoliated nasopharyngeal cells[54] as well as in epithelial cells infected in vitro.[55] It is thought that only terminally differentiated cells are permissive for viral replication. The nuclear antigen, EBNA, is the only expressed gene in the basal epithelial cells and as differentiation occurs, early antigen and virus production can be seen.

Studying EBV expression is hampered by the lack of a robust culture system, however, transfection of human epithelial cells in culture, with the latent membrane protein gene of EBV has been shown to inhibit cell differentiation.[56] This gene is expressed in nasopharyngeal carcinoma. EBV therefore represents a potentially oncogenic virus known to be shed by the cervix,[57] and as such is a potential candidate virus in cervical carcinogenesis. A recent study from Greenland where both EBV-associated nasopharyngeal and salivary gland cancers are endemic, addressed the question of EBV and cervical cancer.[58] The use of PCR failed to detect EBV DNA in cervical tumors whereas 50% of the specimens tested did contain HPV 16 DNA. Further studies are required to elucidate the presence of EBV in cervical pathology in particular in normal and premalignant epithelial cells of the cervix.

CONCLUSION

A clearer picture is now beginning to form as to the role of HPV in cervical carcinogenesis. The epidemiological evidence for HPV involvement has become compelling and this is supported by in vitro work demonstrating the transforming potential of HPV oncoproteins. The exciting research into tumor suppressor genes is providing a possible explanation as to how HPV may be affecting cellular control mechanisms. If HPV is an important initiator we need to identify possible promotor agents, though in smokers it appears that tobacco products are probably of considerable importance (Fig. 7.1). During the last few years considerable effort has been devoted to the development of an HPV vaccine and very careful thought will require to be given as to how such a vaccine may be exploited.

Progress in this field has been fascinating and will certainly continue to preoccupy researchers for some years to come.

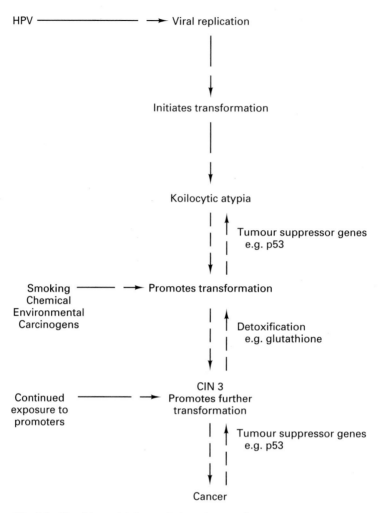

Fig. 7.1 Possible model for cervical carcinogenesis.

REFERENCES

1. Wynder E L, Cornfield J, Schroff P D, Doraiswami K R. A study of environmental factors in carcinoma of the cervix. Am J Obstet Gynecol 1954; 68: 1016–1052.
2. Gagnon F. Contribution to the study of the aetiology and prevention of cancer of the cervix of the uterus. Am J Obstet Gynecol 1950; 60: 516–527.
3. Berenblum I. The mechanism of carcinogenesis. A study of the significance of co-carcinogenic action and related phenomena. Cancer Res 1941; 1: 807–814.
4. Shah K V. Biology of the genital tract papillomavirus. Urologic Clinics North Am 1992; 19: 63–69.
5. Barrett T J, Silbar J D, McGinley J P. Genital warts — a venereal disease. JAMA 1954; 154: 333–334.
6. Meisels A, Fortin R, Roy M. Condylomatous lesions of the cervix. A cytologic, colposcopic and histologic study.

Acta Cytol 1977; 21: 379–390.
7. Morin C, Braun L, Casas Cordero M, Shah K, Roy M, Fortier M, Meisels a. Confirmation of the papillomavirus etiology of condylomatous cervix lesions by the peroxidase anti-peroxidase technique. J Nat Cancer Inst 1981; 66: 831–835.
8. Kurman R J, Jenson A B, Lancaster W D. Papillomavirus infection of the cervix II. Relationship to intraepithelial neoplasia based on the presence of specific viral structural proteins. Am J Surg Pathol 1983; 7: 39–40.
9. Werness B A et al. Role of the human papillomavirus oncoproteins in transformation and carcinogenic progression. Imp. Adv Oncol 1991; 3: 18.
10. Gissmann L, Villiers E M, zur Hausen H. Analysis of

human genital warts (condyloma acuminata) and other genital tumours for human papillomavirus type 6 DNA. Int J Cancer 1980; 29: 143–146.

11. Durst M, Gissmann L, Ikenberg H, and Zurhausen H. A papillomavirus DNA from a cervical carcinoma and its prevalence in cervical biopsy samples from different geographic regions. Proc Nat Acad Sci USA 1983; 80: 3812–3815.

12. Crum C P, Ikenberg H, Richart R M, Gissmann L. Human papillomavirus type 16 and early cervical neoplasia. New Engl J Med 1984; 310: 880–883.

13. McCancer D J, Campion M J, Clarkson P K, Chesters P M, Jenkins D, Singer A. Prevalence of human papillomavirus type 16 DNA in cervical intraepithelial neoplasia and invasive carcinoma of the cervix. Br J Obstet Gynaecol 1985; 92: 1101–1105.

14. Das B C, Sharma J K, Gopalkrishna D K, Das D K, Singh V, Gissmann L, ZurHausen H, Luthra U K. A high frequency of human papillomavirus DNA sequences in cervical carcinomas of Indian women as revealed by Southern blot hybridization and polymerase chain reaction. J Med Virol 1992; 36: 239–245.

15. Meanwell C A, Blackledge G, Cox M F, and Maitland N J. HPV 16 DNA in normal and malignant cervical epithelium: implications for the aetiology and behaviour of cervical neoplasia. Lancet 1987; 703–707

16. Murdoch J B, Cordiner J W, Macnab J C M. Histological and cytological evidence of viral infection and human papillomavirus type 16 DNA sequences in cervical intraepithelial neoplasia and normal tissue in the West of Scotland: evaluation of treatment policy. Br Med J 1988; 296: 381–386.

17. Mitchell H, Drake M, Medley G. Prospective evaluation of risk of cervical cancer after cytological evidence of human papillomavirus infection. Lancet 1986; 1: 573–576.

18. Syrjanen K, Mantyjarvi R, Saarikoski S, Vayrynen M, Syrjanen S, Parkkinen S, Yliskoski M, Saastamoinen J, Castren O. Factors associated with progression of cervical papillomavirus (HPV) infections into carcinoma in-situ during a long term prospective follow-up. Br J Obstet Gynaecol 1988; 95: 1096–1102.

19. Saiki R K, Gelfandi D H, Stoffels S et al. Primer directed enzymatic amplification of DNA with a thermostable DNA polymerase. Science 1988; 239: 487–491.

20. Van den Brule A J C, Walboomers J M M, Maine M D, Keemans P, Meijer J L M. Difference in prevalence of human papillomavirus in cytomorphologically normal cervical smears is associated with a history of cervical intraepithelial neoplasia. Int J Cancer 1991; 48: 404–408.

21. Ley C, Bauer H M, Reingold A et al. Determinants of genital human papillomavirus infection in young women. J Nat Cancer Inst 1991; 83: 997–1003.

22. Cuzick J, Terry G, Ho L, Hollingworth T, Anderson M. Human papillomavirus type 16 DNA in cervical smears as predictor of high grade cervical cancer. Lancet 1992; 339: 959–960.

23. Bavin P J, Giles J A, Deery A, Crow S, Griffiths P D, Emery V C, Walker P G. The use of semiquantitative PCR for human papillomavirus DNA type 16 to identify women with high grade cervical disease in a population presenting with a mildly dyskaryotic smear report. Br J Cancer 1993; 67: 602–605.

24. Kreider J W, Howett M K, Wolfe S A et al. Morphological transformation in-vivo of human uterine cervix with papillomavirus from condylomata acuminata. Nature 1988; 317: 639–641.

25. Gissmann L, Durst M, Oltersdorf T, Von Knebel Doeberitz M. Human papillomaviruses and cervical cancer. In: Steinberg B M, Brandsma T L, Taichman L B, eds. Cancer cells, vol V, The papilloma viruses. New York: Cold Spring Harbor Laboratory, 1987: p 275.

26. Matlashewski G, Schneider J, Banks L, Jones N, Murray A, Crawford L. Human papillomavirus type 16 DNA cooperates with activated ras in transforming primary cells. EMBO J 1987; 6: 1741–1746.

27. Pecoraro G, Morgan D, Defendi V. Differential effects of human papillomavirus type 6, 16 and 18 DNA's on immortalization and transformation of human cervical cells. Proc Nat Acad Sci 1989; 86: 563–567.

28. Crook T, Morgenstern J P, Crawford I, Banks L. Continued expression of HPV 16 E7 protein is required for maintenance of the transformed phenotype of cells co-transformed by HPV 16 plus EJ ras. EMBO J 1989; 8: 513–519.

29. Gius D, Laimins L A. Activation of human papillomavirus type 18 gene expression by herpes simplex type 1 viral transactivator and a phorbol ester. J Virol 1989; 63: 555–563.

30. Levine A J, Momand J, Finlay C A. The p53 tumour suppressor gene. Nature 1991; 351: 453–455.

31. Horowitz J M, Yandell D W, Park S H et al. Point mutational inactivation of the retinoblastoma anti-oncogene. Science 1989; 243: 937–940.

32. Bookstein R, Shew J Y, Chen P L, Scully P, Lee W H. Suppression of tumourigenicity of human prostate carcinoma cells by replacing a mutated RB gene. Science 1990; 247: 712–715.

33. Harlow E, Whyte P, Franza B R, Schley C. Association of adenovirus early region 1A proteins with cellular polypeptides. Molec Cell Biol 1986; 6: 1579–1589.

34. Lane D P, Crawford L V. T antigen is bound to a host protein in SV40 transformed cells. Nature 1979; 278: 261–263.

35. Baker S J, Markowitz S, Fearon E R, Willson J K V, Vogelstein B. Suppression of human colo-rectal carcinoma cell growth by wild type p53. Science 1990; 249: 912–915.

36. Werness P, Levine A J, Howley P M. Association of human papillomavirus types 16 and 18 E6 proteins with p53. Science 1990; 248: 76–79.

37. Riou G, Favre M, Jeannel D, Bourhis J, Le Doussal V, Orth G. Association between poor prognosis in early stage invasive cervical carcinomas and non-detection of HPV DNA. Lancet 1990; 335: 1171–1174.

38. Crook T, Wrede D, Tidy J A, Mason W P, Evans D J, Vousden K H. Clonal p53 mutation in primary cervical cancer: association with human papillomavirus negative tumours. Lancet 1992; 339: 1070–1073.

39. Harris R W C, Brinton L A, Cowdell R H et al. Characteristics of women with carcinoma in-situ of the cervix uteri. Br J Cancer 1980; 42: 359–369.

40. Trevathan E P, Layde L A, Webster D W et al. Cigarette smoking and dysplasia and carcinoma *in-situ* of the uterine cervix. JAMA 1983; 250: 499–505.

41. Hellberg D, Nilsson S, Haley N J et al. Smoking and cervical intraepithelial neoplasia: nicotine and cotinine in serum and cervical mucus in smokers and non smokers. Am J Obstet Gynecol 1988; 158: 910–913.

42. McArdle J P, Muller H K. Quantitative assessment of

Langerhan's in human cervical intraepithelial neoplasia and wart virus infection. Am J Obstet Gynecol 1986; 154: 509–515.

43. Simons A M, Phillips D H, Coleman D V. Damage to DNA in cervical epithelium related to smoking tobacco. Br Med J 1993; 306: 1444–1448.

44. Barton S E, Jenkins D, Luzick J et al. Effect of cigarette smoking on cervical epithelial immunity: a mechanism for neoplastic change? Lancet 1988; 2: 652–654.

45. Winklestein W. Smoking and cervical cancer — current status: a review. Am J Epidemiol 1990; 131: 945–957.

46. Naib Z M, Mahmias A J, Josey W E. Cytology and histopathology of cervical herpes simplex infection. Cancer 1966; 19: 1025–1029.

47. Rawls W E, Tomkins W A F, Figueriva M E, Melnick J L. Herpes virus type 2 association with carcinoma of the cervix. Science 1968; 161: 1255.

48. McDougall J K, Grum C P, Fenoglis C M, Goldstein L C, Galloway D A. Herpes virus specific RNA and protein in carcinoma of the uterine cervix. Proc Nat Acad Sci USA 1982.

49. Eglin R P, Sharp F, Maclean A B, Macnab J C M, Clements J B, Wilkie N M. The detection of RNA complementary to herpes simplex virus DNA in human cervical squamous neoplasms. Cancer Res 1981; 41: 3597.

50. Park M, Kitchener H C, Macnab J C M. Detection of herpes simplex virus type 2 DNA restriction fragments in human cervical carcinoma tissue. EMBO J 1983; 2: 417.

51. Di Paola J A, Woodworth C D, Porescu N C, Kovel D L, Lopez J V, Doniger J. HSV-2 induced tumorigenicity in HPV-16 immortalized human genital keratinocytes. Virology 1990; 177: 777–779.

52. Hildesheim A, Mann V, Brinton L A, Szklo M, Reeves W C, Rawls W E. Herpes simplex virus type 2: a possible interaction with human papillomavirus types 16/18 in the development of invasive cervical cancer. Int J Cancer 1991; 49: 335–340.

53. Prabhat K S, Beral V, Peto J et al. Antibodies to human papillomavirus and to other genital infections agents and invasive cervical cancer. Lancet 1993; 1: 1116–1118.

54. Sixbey J W, Nedrud J G, Raab-Traub N, Hanes R A, Pagano J S. Epstein Barr virus replication in nasopharyngeal epithelial cells. New Engl J Med 1984; 310: 1225–1230.

55. Sixbey J W, Vesterinen E H, Nedrud J G, Raab-Traub N, Walton L A, Pagano J S. Replication of Esptein–Barr virus in human epithelial cells infected in-vitro. Nature 1983; 306: 480–483.

56. Dawson C W, Rickinson A B, Young L S. Epstein-Barr virus latent membrane protein inhibits human epithelial cell differentiation. Nature 1990; 344: 777–780.

57. Sixbey J W, Lemon S M, Pagano J S. A second site for Epstein–Barr virus shedding: the uterine cervix. Lancet 1986; 2: 1122–1124.

58. Hording V, Daugaard S, Bock J E. Human papillomavirus, Epstein–Barr virus and cervical cancer in Greenland. Int J Gynecol Cancer 1992; 2: 314–317.

59. Kitchener H C, Neilson L, Burnett R A, Young L, Macnab J C M. Prospective serial study of viral change in the cervix and correlation with human papillomavirus status. Br J Obstet Gynaecol 1991; 98: 1042–1048.

60. Phillips D H, Schoker B, Hewer A, Bailey E, Kostic E, Vinze I. Influence of cigarette smoking on the levels of DNA adducts in human bronchial epithelium and white blood cells. Int J Cancer 1990; 46: 569–575.

8. The application of molecular biology to the detection of HPV infection

J. R. M. Ellis   L. S. Young

INTRODUCTION

Reliable techniques for identifying human papillomavirus (HPV) infection are a prerequisite for investigating the possible etiological role of the virus in the development of cervical neoplasia. As HPVs can not be propagated in vitro and suitable specific antibodies are not available, detection systems have used molecular biological analysis to identify viral DNA in pathological specimens.[1] Extracted DNA can be analysed by Southern, dot blot or 'filter in situ' hybridization while HPV-infected cells can be directly visualized in tissue sections by in situ hybridization. However, differences in the sensitivity of these methods (Table 8.1) and difficulties in the interpretation of the resulting data, combined with practical problems in the application of these complex techniques to large-scale epidemiological studies, has produced a wide variation of estimates of HPV prevalence in different populations of women. Thus, when data from 20 different laboratories in various parts of the world were compared the prevalence of HPV 16 was found to vary from 18 to 92% in cervical cancer biopsy specimens and from 0 to 38% in normal cervical epithelium.[2]

The advent of the polymerase chain reaction (PCR) has provided an opportunity to overcome these difficulties with a highly sensitive technique that can be applied to crudely extracted cervical smear cell DNA as well as paraffin-embedded material. Since its introduction in 1985 the PCR has lead to a veritable revolution in molecular biology and given its remarkable simplicity and tremendous range of applications, it is no surprise that this technique has had an huge impact on scientific research. PCR has been referred to as 'the molecular biologists photocopying machine' as it allows millions of copies of any specific DNA sequence to be generated within a few hours. The amplified DNA can then be visualized as a distinct band after standard agarose gel electrophoresis and the specificity of detection can be increased by subsequent hybridization with specific oligonucleotide probes.

The extreme sensitivity of PCR means that a single-copy gene (i.e., β-globin) can be readily detected from extremely small amounts of tissue and microorganisms present at low levels (i.e., virus infection of one in a million cells) can also be identified. Successful PCR does not require the DNA sample to be pure or of high quality and thus allows analysis of extracts where the majority of the DNA molecules are damaged and/or degraded to such an extent that examination by other molecular biological techniques is impossible.

PCR was originally used in the prenatal diagnosis of gene defects,[3] but has now become a valuable tool in the armory of the molecular biologist and can be used in a variety of research contexts including DNA sequencing, analysis of RNA transcription, mutagenesis, development of probes for genetic studies and screening of cDNA libraries.

In this chapter we will discuss the use of PCR for the detection of HPV infection and consider

Table 8.1 Detection of viral DNA: sensitivity of available techniques

Technique	Sensitivity
Dot blot	10 gene copies per diploid cell
Southern blot	0.1 gene copies per diploid cell
In situ hybridization	1–10 gene copies per diploid cell
Polymerase chain reaction	1 gene copy in 10^5–10^6 diploid cells

the impact of this technique on epidemiological studies.

HPV BIOLOGY

The papillomaviruses are a family of double-stranded DNA viruses infecting both humans and a variety of other animals.[1] Upon infection the viruses cause a range of benign and malignant lesions in such diverse species as rabbits, cattle and humans. Of the human papillomaviruses (HPVs) over 60 different genotypes have been identified on the basis of DNA homology, the individual viruses preferentially infecting mucosal or cutaneous epithelium.[4] Around 24 of these different HPVs are associated with infections of the anogenital tract, types 6 and 11 being most commonly isolated from benign warts (condylomata acuminata) and low-grade cervical intraepithelial neoplasia (CIN) and types 16 and 18 being consistently associated with more severe grades of CIN and the majority of invasive cervical carcinomas (HPV types 31, 33 and 35 are less frequently found in cervical tumors).[5]

The viral genome consists of a double-stranded circle of DNA of around 7.9 kb and, by analogy with bovine papillomavirus, is divided into two functional regions (Fig. 8.1). The 'early' region contains a number of open reading frames coding proteins involved in viral maintenance and replication while the 'late' region products form the viral capsid and are termed structural proteins.[4] The early region represents about 70% of the genome

and is sufficient to transform rodent cells. Transfection of this early region, and particularly the E6 and E7 open reading frames, into human keratinocytes will immortalize these cells and in cooperation with other factors such as the activated ras oncogene can bring about malignant transformation.[6] The regular expression of E6 and E7 in cervical carcinomas and derived tumor cell lines and the maintenance of these regions even after integration of the viral genome into host DNA emphasises the importance of these proteins.[7] As a result the possible functions of the E6 and E7 proteins has attracted much attention. Recent work has shown that the E6 and E7 proteins of the oncogenic HPV types interact with tumor suppressor gene products, E6 with p53 and E7 with the RB1 gene product.[8,9]

ESTIMATING HPV INFECTION BY DNA HYBRIDIZATION

The inability to culture HPVs has prevented the development of in vitro assays for detecting infectious virus and has hindered the generation of simple serological tests for HPV infection. Thus, HPV assays have relied upon techniques for detecting viral DNA in infected cells and tissues using the individually cloned HPV types as specific probes. A brief review of these techniques is set out below.

Southern blot

The Southern blot technique[10] was regarded as

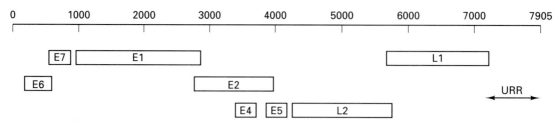

Fig. 8.1 The genomic organization of human papillomavirus type 16. The boxes represent open reading frames encoding 'early' (E) or 'late' (L) viral proteins. The 'early' proteins are involved in viral replication, control of viral transcription and cell transformation whereas the two 'late' proteins form the structural component of the HPV virion. The URR (or upstream regulatory region) contains enhancer elements that are responsive to cellular and viral transcriptional regulators. The majority of PCR studies have used primers to the E6 or E7 region as these encode the proteins responsible for cell transformation. Consensus PCR primers target the regions of the viral genome conserved amongst many different HPV types such as L1 and E1.

the 'gold standard' for identifying HPV infection in cell or tissue samples. Cellular DNA is first extracted from cells or biopsy material by proteinase K/sodium dodecyl sulfate digestion followed by purification with phenol–chloroform. The sample DNA is then digested with various restriction enzymes and the resulting fragments separated on the basis of size by electrophoresis on an agarose gel. The DNA in the gel is then denatured and transferred onto a nitrocellulose hybridization membrane (filter) before being probed with cloned HPV DNAs. These clones from various HPV genotypes are labeled (usually with radioactivity) and hybridize to their relevant target sequence on the nitrocellulose filter enabling identification of particular HPV types.

Often low stringency conditions (low temperature hybridization and washing) are used to identify infection with any HPV type, while higher temperatures (around 65°C) are used to impose high stringency conditions for the identification of specific HPV types. The filters can be stripped of probe and reprobed so that screening for infection with different HPV types can be performed on a single sample. If radiolabeled probes have been employed the data is read from an autoradiogram. Where the original sample was digested with the Pst1 restriction enzyme, HPV positivity can be identified as a specific pattern of different sized bands generated from the genome. The digestion of samples with specific restriction enzymes can be applied to identify integration of viral DNA into the host genome.[11]

Southern blotting can detect 0.01–0.1 copies of viral DNA per cell and has been widely applied for the investigation of HPV prevalence in various populations. Meanwell et al[11] demonstrated that 35% of cervical biopsies from normal women were HPV 16 positive while elsewhere only 1% of cervical smears from normal controls were found to be infected with types 16, 18, 31 or 33.[12] The low yield of DNA extracted from smear samples coupled with the sensitivity of Southern blotting prevents reliable detection of HPV in cytological material. Thus, variations in viral prevalence are common in HPV studies and probably reflect differences in the origin of the sample (biopsy versus smear) as well as differences in defining

'normal' populations and the varying conditions of stringency used to determine the type specificity of HPV positive individuals.

Dot blot

The dot blot technique uses the same DNA extraction protocol applied for Southern blot hybridization, but once extracted the DNA is not digested but is denatured and spotted directly onto a filter.[13,14] The sensitivity of dot blot is lower than that of Southern blotting but larger numbers of samples can be analyzed more rapidly. High stringency hybridization conditions are required to prevent the possibility of false-positives due to cross-reactivity with cellular DNA sequences present in the undigested sample. The filters can be stripped and reprobed with individual HPV types or mixtures of probes can be used, i.e., to identify either low-risk (HPV 6/11) or high-risk (HPV 16/18) types. Estimates of viral prevalence by the dot blot technique show less variation than other protocols, with two reports from Britain and Norway suggesting HPV 16 is present in 4% of women attending a family planning clinic and 8% of women attending their GP for a routine gynecological check-up.[15,16] However, the reduced sensitivity of this type of analysis must mean that some HPV positive individuals will be misdiagnosed as being negative, particularly in a largely normal population where the amount of virus present is low.

Filter in situ hybridization

Cells are filtered directly onto a membrane where they are lysed and denatured in alkaline buffer.[17] The DNA is then neutralized and the membrane baked at 80°C for about 4 h. Hybridization with cloned HPV specific probes is then performed under high stringency conditions to ensure specific recognition between probe and target. The membrane is then washed and processed for autoradiography.[18,19] As with dot blot this technique allows rapid screening of multiple samples but the sensitivity of filter in situ is lower and only high level HPV infection such as that found in biopsies of CIN or cervical carcinoma can be reliably detected. Detection of infected cells containing a low copy number of HPV DNA is problematic as backgound activity may reduce the clarity of the resulting autoradiogram.

In situ hybridization

The in situ hybridization technique enables direct visualization of HPV DNA or RNA in cytological preparations or tissue sections from frozen or fixed samples. The main advantage of in situ analysis is its application to paraffin-embedded material, enabling detection and typing of HPV infection in archival samples previously unavailable for HPV studies by Southern or dot blot. In addition, since the architectural detail of the tissue section is not disrupted the distribution of viral infection within the sample can be analyzed and morphological features associated with HPV infection can be identified.

Paraffin-embedded sections mounted on glass slides are first dewaxed and rehydrated before being treated with proteinase K. The exposed DNA (or RNA) is then denatured before being hybridized with labeled DNA or RNA probes. The slides are washed under varying conditions of stringency depending on the degree of specificity required for the probe being used and processed for autoradiography.[20] However, this assay is technically demanding and of varying sensitivity depending on the particular detection system employed. Using a radioactively labeled probe 10 copies of viral genome per cell can be detected but with biotin-labeled DNA the sensitivity is dramatically reduced requiring up to 800 copies of HPV DNA for a positive reaction.[21]

Schneider et al[22] were able to demonstrate striking differences in distribution of HPV 16 in various cervical lesions using in situ hybridization analysis. Viral DNA was restricted to areas of differentiated epithelium in CIN 2 but was more uniformily distributed in CIN 3 and invasive carcinomas. This data together with other in situ studies confirms the relationship between HPV replication and epithelial cell differentiation. More recently in situ hybridisation has been used to study the expression of HPV mRNAs.

Overall these hybridization techniques suffer from problems of specificity and sensitivity and in situ hybridization in particular is technically demanding precluding its use for large-scale analysis of samples for epidemiological studies. In addition, the differing relative sensitivities of these protocols has led to varying estimates of the level of HPV infection in normal and abnormal populations, thus hampering the interpretation of prevalence studies. The advent of PCR held out great hope that a simple, sensitive and specific technique was now available which could be used for analysis of both extracted DNA and archival material and stimulated great optimism that this technology would revolutionize epidemiological studies.

STANDARD PCR METHOD

PCR involves the enzymatic synthesis by DNA polymerase of millions of copies of a segment of target DNA. A pair of short DNA fragments referred to as oligonucleotide primers are synthesized to be complementary to sequences on opposite strands of the DNA flanking the fragment to be amplified (Fig. 8.2). Denaturation of the DNA sample is used to separate the double strands, enabling the primers to anneal to each of the resulting single strands. The annealed primers are then extended toward each other from their 3′ hydroxyl ends by a DNA polymerase in the presence of a mixture of deoxynucleotide triphosphates (dATP, dCTP, dGTP, dTTP), using the target sequence as a template. This initial extension produces fragments suitable for subsequent primer binding and template synthesis so that by repeated cycles of denaturation, primer binding and DNA synthesis large quantities of a specific product are accumulated.

Each successive PCR cycle doubles the amount of DNA synthesized in the previous round. This chain reaction results in the exponential accumulation of the specific DNA target fragment at approximately 2^n, where n is the number of cycles. The size of the amplified DNA fragment is determined by the boundaries of the two primers so that if the chosen region is 200 base pairs (bp) in length, as defined by the 5′ ends of the PCR primers, then the amplified product generated during the PCR will be 200 bp (Fig. 8.2). The amplified product of the predicted size can then

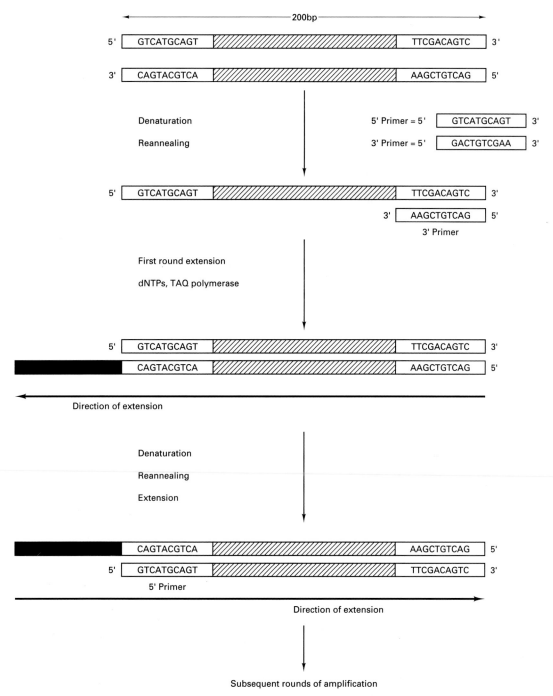

Fig. 8.2 Diagrammatic represenation of the PCR. For simplicity the oligonucleotide primers used to amplify the 200 bp fragment are represented as 10mers and the annealing/extension of only one strand is shown. The primers are synthesized to be complementary to DNA sequences on opposite strands of the DNA flanking the fragment to be amplified and thus after denaturation hybridize to their complementary sequences. First round extension in the presence of deoxynucleotide triphosphates (dNTPs) and Taq polymerase generates newly synthesized DNA strands of indeterminate length as represented by the solid lines. Subsequent cycles of denaturation, annealing and extension generates fragments whose length is now determined by the boundaries of the primers. Amplification products from previous cycles are used as substrates for subsequent cycles and thus amplified products of a fixed size (i.e., 200 bp) are exponentially produced.

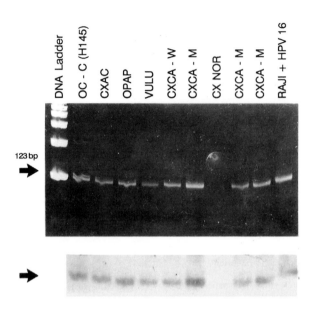

Fig. 8.3 PCR amplification of DNA isolated from a variety of human tissue biopsies and cell cultures using type-specific primers directed to the E6 region of the HPV 16 genome. The primers produced an amplified fragment of 120 bp, which can be seen as a distinct band after polyacrylamide gel electrophoresis and ethidium bromide staining (top panel). These DNA bands can then be transferred to a nitrocellulose membrane by the Southern blot technique and hybridised with an oligonucleotide probe end labeled with ^{32}P. Binding of this probe can be visualised by autoradiography to confirm specificity for HPV 16 (bottom panel). M — DNA size markers; OC-C (H145) — oral carcinoma culture; CXAC — human acanthoma; OPAP — oral papilloma; VULU — vulval leukoplakia; CXCA — W — well-differentiated cervical carcinoma; CXCA-M — moderately differentiated cervical carcinoma; CX NOR — normal cervix; Raji+HPV16 — positive control with one copy per cell of cloned human papillomavirus type 16 DNA added to DNA from Burkitt's lymphoma cell line negative for HPV 16; bp — base pair. (Reproduced from Ref. 24, by permission.)

be detected by electrophoresis on an agarose or polyacrylamide gel followed by direct visualization with ethidium bromide, which lights up the DNA when illuminated with ultraviolet light (Fig. 8.3). The specificity and sensitivity of the PCR can be further increased by subsequent Southern blotting and hybridization with an oligonucleotide probe internal to the amplified product.

In addition certain other conditions must be controlled to ensure reaction specificity, but with the ever-increasing variety of applications in which PCR is being used individual parameters may vary considerably. However, PCR is generally performed in a 100 µl volume of buffer containing 50 mM KCl, 10 mM TrisHCl (pH 8.4), 1.5 mM $MgCl_2$, 100 µg/ml gelatin, 0.25 µm of each primer, 200 µm of each deoxynucleotide triphosphate (dATP, dCTP, dGTP and dDTP) and 2.5 units of Taq polymerase. The influence of these individual components is not always entirely clear but variation in concentrations can markedly affect the accumulation of specific product. Thus, at high $MgCl_2$ concentrations the sensitivity and specificity of the PCR reaction are reduced as more mismatches between primer and target are tolerated enabling amplification of various non-specific fragments. With too little $MgCl_2$ the yield of amplified product is reduced. As secondary structure of target DNA can be a problem, addition of dimethyl sulfoxide (DMSO) to the PCR buffer has been used to improve primer annealing. However, DMSO may inhibit Taq polymerase activity and so reduce the yield of amplified product.

The DNA extension step is initiated by raising the temperature to 72°C which stimulates Taq polymerase, a heat-resistant DNA polymerase isolated from the thermophilic bacterium *Thermus aquaticus,* to copy the DNA template.[23] This extension step is stopped by denaturation and the cycle starts over again. The use of Taq polymerase has simplified the PCR procedure obviating the need to add DNA polymerase every time the newly synthesized DNA strands are denatured and has thus made the PCR more amenable to automation. Furthermore, the higher temperatures at which Taq polymerase catalyses the extension step increases the stringency of the PCR facilitating the amplification of large DNA fragments (over 1 kb) which are easily visible on ethidium bromide-stained gels. The concentration of Taq polymerase added to the PCR reaction will affect PCR specificity and may need to be adapted for particular assay requirements.

Each phase of the PCR cycle is performed at a discrete temperature to improve the efficiency and specificity of the reaction. Denaturation usually occurring at 90–98°C, primer binding at 37–65°C and template extension at 72°C. The wide range of primer binding temperatures reflects the varying composition of the primers used, the optimum binding temperature for each oligonucleotide being dependent upon its length and nucleotide content (i.e., GC content). A simple rule of thumb is that the higher the GC content of a primer the higher the required annealing (and extension) temperature. Successful PCR is usually achieved with 20 bp long primers comprising a GC content of 50% in a reaction buffer containing 1.5 mM magnesium chloride.

SAMPLE PREPARATION FOR PCR

The specificity of the PCR means that DNA can be amplified from relatively crude extracts and from samples where the DNA may be degraded or damaged. Whilst the technique was pioneered on purified DNA samples, the use of Taq polymerase has obviated the need for DNA prepared using the long-winded phenol–chloroform extraction procedure. Thus, cytological specimens in the form of cervical smears or cells isolated from cerebral spinal fluid, urine, pleural or peritoneal effusions can be directly analyzed by PCR.[24] Simply boiling the cells in distilled water or PCR buffer is often sufficient[25] but DNA is more efficiently extracted from small numbers of cells by proteinase K digestion followed by boiling. This latter approach can also be used to extract DNA from small tissue specimens or from cryostat sections. In addition, PCR can be used to analyze DNA extracted from fixed, paraffin-embedded tissue.[26] This ability is particularly powerful as it raises the possibility of retrospective analysis to determine the clinical usefulness of HPV typing, the changes in HPV prevalences over time and, ultimately, the role of HPV in oncogenesis.[26,27] Similarly, PCR can also be applied to archival Papanicolaou smears.[28]

Variable numbers of 5–10 μM paraffin-embedded sections, depending on the cross-sectional area of the tissue, can be used to extract amplifiable DNA by dewaxing followed by proteinase K digestion. Paraffin-embedded sections mounted on slides can be treated in the same way. However, meticulous attention to detail is required in all aspects of sample handling, and swabbing of the microtome blade with ethanol between the cutting of different paraffin blocks is a sensible precaution to reduce the risk of sample cross-contamination. In addition some workers have experienced problems with PCR on DNA extracted from fixed tissue possibly due to the variable fixation procedures used. Thus, the time taken to process a tissue block and the fixative used (i.e., Bouin's versus formal saline) may influence the overall sensitivity of the PCR. False negatives can also be a problem in PCR studies particularly when analyzing DNA extracted from paraffin-embedded tissue. In this situation checking that amplifiable DNA has been extracted using primers directed to a single copy cellular gene such as β-globin is a useful test

PCR ANALYSIS OF HPV INFECTION

A number of studies were initiated to compare the sensitivity and specifity of PCR with other techniques previously used for the detection of HPV DNA. Such studies demonstrated that PCR could detect the equivalent of a single copy of the HPV 16 genome in a million cells.[24] This level of detection was clearly a significant improvement on previous hybridization assays and explains the increased sensitivity of this technique compared to dot blot DNA hybridization.[15,16,29] This difference is particularly pronounced when a comparison of cytologically normal smear samples is analyzed resulting in a 5–10 fold increase in HPV detection.[15,29]

Similarly, PCR analysis identified HPV 16 DNA in 15 cervical biopsies originally declared to be negative by Southern blot hybridization, and indicated a higher prevalence of multiple virus infection than previously determined.[30] The sensitivity of PCR also compares favorably with that of in situ hybridization where HPV detection was increased from 72 to 96% of condyloma specimens[31] and from 50 to 85% of invasive anal neoplasias.[32] In the latter example previous studies of invasive anal disease had stated that the low prevalence of HPV 16 in such samples excluded its role as an etiological agent in the development of disease. The increased viral prevalence identified by PCR challenged that view and clearly showed the high incidence of viral infection in anal carcinomas.

PCR was shown to be more sensitive than immunochemical detection of viral antigens using antibodies specific for HPV 16 E4.[33] In this case, however, the level of antigen expression may change as abnormalities develop within the cervical tissue and during the infective cycle of the virus, and a negative result may reflect a loss of antigen expression rather than lower sensitivity.

Overall the use of primers targeting specific areas of DNA and generating amplified products of known size which can then hybridize with type-specific probes accounts for the superior specificity of PCR compared to these other techniques, and this superiority is further enhanced by the ability of the consensus PCR (see later) to detect previously unidentified HPV genotypes.[31,34,35]

As would be expected therefore early reports of PCR-based estimates of HPV 16 prevalence suggested that the level of infection in both cytologically normal and abnormal smear samples was much greater than previously reported. In one instance 70% of normal and 95% of abnormal smears were found to be HPV 16 positive[23] and in a second larger study 117 of 140 normal individuals were infected with HPV 16, while 100% of cervical neoplasia's had evidence of viral DNA.[36] These results were controversial as they raised the possibility that HPV infection was much more widespread in the normal population than previously assumed, questioning the putative role of HPV 16 as the sexually-transmitted agent responsible for the development of cervical carcinoma.[37] However, the high prevalence of HPV 16 infection in these studies could also result from accidental sample cross-contamination or more commonly from PCR product carryover of previous amplifications of the same DNA target. The high sensitivity of PCR and its ability to produce millions of copies of a sequence from minute quantities of DNA can easily lead to such contamination problems. Stringent laboratory procedures[38,39] are required to prevent DNA carryover, particularly when handling PCR products, and the physical separation of PCR preparation from the handling of amplified products is imperative.[38] In addition, strong positive controls should be avoided and the use of negative controls such as reactions containing no target DNA or, where appropriate, DNA negative for the sequence of interest are required in every assay.

As if to illustrate this point Beyer-Finkler et al[40] published a report comparing HPV16 detection using standard primers targeting the E6 open reading frame and newly developed anticontamination primers targeting the L1 region of the genome. These anticontamination primers were developed in an attempt to prevent false positives resulting following contamination of PCR specimens with cloned HPV plasmids, and were designed to anneal to the L1 open reading frame so that they flanked the BamHl cloning site (Fig. 8.1).[42,43] During the initial cloning procedure the HPV genome is enzymatically cut at this point before being inserted into the appropriate plasmid vector. The 'anticontamination' primers anneal to the HPV target DNA on either side of the plasmid, so that where recombinant plasmid DNA has contaminated a sample, amplification must occur across the plasmid potentially producing a fragment of around 3000 bp. Amplification of such a large target would be extremely inefficient but, if bona fide collinear HPV DNA is present the amplified fragment is only 152 bp and is easily amplifiable under normal PCR conditions.

Beyer-Finkler et al[40] showed that the standard E6 primers identified 23 out of 53 samples to be HPV 16 positive, but only 13 of these were also positive with the anticontamination PCR indicating a high level of plasmid contamination. Elsewhere the application of these primers produced lower estimates of viral prevalence than quoted previously, particularly within normal samples where only 6–12% of individuals were found to be HPV 16 positive.[41,42]

In order to extend the application of PCR other studies made use of general or consensus primers directed to highly conserved regions of the HPV genome that were able to amplify all genital HPV types including those of novel viruses.[43–48] These primers were either used under lower stringency conditions which allow DNA annealing with a number of base pair mismatches between primer and target, or the primers were 'degenerate' meaning that during their synthesis one of a number of nucleotides was inserted at certain variable positions. The resulting primers actually consisted of a mixture of oligonucleotides which could specifically recognize a variety of HPV types. The amplified PCR products could then be processed for Southern blot hybridization and probed using internal generic probes identifying conserved regions common to all HPVs, or using specific probes complementary to a range of previously sequenced viral types.

In HPV studies general primers yielded higher detection rates when compared to type-specific primers suggesting that infection with unsequenced

HPVs may be relatively common.[6,7] Similarly, analysis of cervical smear samples from a group of 467 female university students with the consensus PCR found that 13% were infected with novel, unidentified HPV types.[29] However, consensus primers can underestimate the real prevalence of infection with any one HPV type. For instance, if a sample has more than 10 000 copies of HPV 11 but only a single copy of HPV 16 this may affect the sensitivity of the consensus PCR with regard to HPV 16 detection. Furthermore, as the consensus PCR can amplify a variety of target sequences some workers feel unhappy about the specificity of this technique, arguing for the theoretical possibility that cross-reactive recognition may lead to nonspecific amplification of host cell DNA.

Despite these problems we have used consensus primers described by Manos et al[44] to examine the influence of HPV 16 and 18 infection on the subsequent progression of cervical neoplasia in a population of women with known cervical abnormalities. Women with histological evidence of viral infection alone or in association with CIN 1 and 2 were entered into the study and left untreated. These patients were kept under regular review for evidence of disease progression or spontaneous regression and biopsies were taken for determination of their HPV 16/18 status at the time of their referral. The application of the consensus primers in this study enabled simultaneous identification of HPV 16 and 18 infection from the same PCR amplification by the use of type specific internal probes. Analysis of the progression/regression follow-up data indicated a significant association of HPV 16/18 infection with those individuals whose abnormality progressed to a higher disease state (unpublished data). It should also be noted that some of the HPV 16/18 negative individuals also progressed, indicating that HPV infection is not the only cause of progressive cervical disease.

More recently the same primers have been applied in a large population based case-control study[49] designed to evaluate the association between HPV infection and cervical cancer. The results indicated a strong link between the presence of the oncogenic HPV viruses and the incidence of cervical cancer, and suggested that this association was indeed causal. However, PCR analysis did not detect some HPV positive controls identified by other DNA hybridization assays, and some 50% of cases originally determined to be negative by PCR analysis of smear cells were subsequently found to be positive when DNA was extracted from tissue biopsies. The lack of correlation between PCR and less sensitive hybridization assays in this case differs from all previous comparisons of assay sensitivity and suggests some problem either with the PCR protocol used in this study or with the sampling, handling or processing of biological specimens by the different laboratories involved. Such problems of inter-laboratory variation are common in HPV studies and must be addressed to ensure the reliability of PCR predictions of viral prevalence.

Further studies aimed at the development of a more reliable and rapid HPV screening method have combined the general PCR protocol with the anticontamination regimen. Cervical scrapes are prescreened using the general primers for the presence of a wide range of HPV types, the anticontamination type specific primers are then used to identify sequenced HPV types in the positive samples.[50] Using this strategy Melkert et al[51] identified an age-related association with HPV infection, with women of 35 years or more having lower viral prevalence. The level of HPV 16/18 infection in this study was below 4% for all ages, and comparable with earlier studies using the anticontamination protocol alone,[46–48] but significantly lower than quoted elsewhere using degenerate consensus primers[52] where 19% of cytologically normal smears contained HPV DNA.

Such reported differences in viral prevalence have made an assessment of the role of HPV in cervical disease problematic. Several explanations may account for these variable results:

(1) sample contamination and/or variation in sample processing are potential problems particularly when large sample numbers are being handled;
(2) geographical variations in the incidence of different HPV genotypes may influence level of infection reported in different countries;
(3) difficulties in defining what constitutes a

normal population with controls being taken from various populations of women;
(4) disparities in HPV infection rates could also be attributable to the use of different primers targeting various regions of the viral genome whose specificity and sensitivity may vary.

This last aspect is particularly relevant as shown in Table 8.2, where a range of estimates for HPV 16 prevalence among normal women is illustrated. The rate of infection varies considerably from 0 to 84%, and even where primers targeting the early E6 open reading frame are used by different laboratories estimations of viral prevalence still vary considerably. However, from our own work of comparative PCR analysis of HPV 16 infection in normal and abnormal cervical smears using different primers to various regions of the HPV genome, we have noticed varying detection rates which can not be explained on the basis of differences in the relative sensitivities and efficiencies of amplification of the primer sets alone.[52] In particular, variations in the estimation of HPV prevalence in cytologically normal cervical smears between primers targeting the early and late regions of the viral genome were apparent (Table 8.3). While the consensus and type-specific primers directed to the L1 open reading frame both identified 19% of this population to be HPV 16 positive, early region primers only detected 9%. Comparison of the efficiency of detection of these

Table 8.2 Prevalence of cervical HPV 16 infection by PCR in different studies of cytologically normal women

Country	HPV 16 prevalence (%)	Position of PCR primers
England[24]	70	E6
England[37]	84	E6 and URR
Netherlands[47]	8	GP-E1/GP-L1*
USA[45]	11, 0, 22	Con L1* and URR
USA[28]	73	E6
USA[30]	9	Con L1
Norway[16]	8	E7
England[15]	39	E6

*GP-E1/GP-L1 are consensus primers specific for either the E1 or L1 region of the HPV genome. Con L1 refers to a set of consensus primers specific to the L1 region but different to the GP-L1 primer set.
It should be noted that the HPV 16 E6 primers used in 7 out of the 11 studies referenced above differ between the individual laboratories.

Table 8.3 Prevalence of HPV 16 infection in normal and abnormal cervical smears

Primer	Normal	Abnormal
L1 consensus	11 (19%)	22 (38%)
L1 specific	11 (19%)	22 (38%)
URR	4 (7%)	23 (40%)
E6	5 (9%)	25 (43%)
E7	1 (2%)	22 (38%)

Table 8.5 Contribution of different primers to the detection of HPV 16 in cervical smears

Primer	Number positive ($n = 52$)
L1 consensus (L1 con)	33 (64%)
L1 con + L1 specific (L1 spec)	43 (83%)
L1 con + L1 spec + E6	47 (90%)
L1 con + L1 spec + E6 + E7	50 (96%)
L1 con + L1 spec + E6 + E7 + URR	52 (100%)

primers with dilutions of CaSki DNA, a cervical carcinoma cell line containing around 500 copies of the HPV16 genome per cell, demonstrated a 10-fold difference in sensitivity between the consensus and type specific L1 late region primers (Table 8.4). The L1 consensus and early E6 and E7 primers showed similar levels of sensitivity even though the E6 and E7 primers appear to underestimate the prevalence of HPV 16 infection in the cytologically normal population.

In this case it would be tempting to speculate that HPV 16 DNA sequence diversity over the early region is responsible for the differences in viral prevalence. As the various primers identified similar numbers of HPV 16 positive individuals among those with cytologically abnormal smears, it may be that subtypes of HPV16 exist with variable sequences over the early region and that these viruses are more common in the normal population. Alternatively, the physical state of the HPV genome (circular in normal infection and integrated in progressive disease) may influence the ability of the early region primers to efficiently anneal with their complementary sequences. However, it is more likely than a combination of factors are responsible for the differing estimates of viral prevalence, particularly when analyzing crudely extracted DNA where subtle differences in primer annealing and amplification may become more apparent. Despite this caution we are at present investigating the possibility of sequence

variation within the early region but have as yet not identified any specific deletions within the E6 and E7 open reading frames. For our HPV prevalence studies we have adopted the consensus primers as a standard technique. These primers alone identified 63% of the HPV 16 positive individuals in our primer study (Table 8.5), while type specific primers to L1 and the early E6, E7 and URR regions only detected an additional 19, 7, 6, and 4%, respectively. But the possibility of false negatives must be remembered as this study shows that no primer set is able to identify all those individuals infected with viral DNA.

In order to further investigate the influence of different primer sets on the reported prevalence of HPV 16, comparative sample swap studies have been initiated between ourselves and other PCR laboratories. Preliminary results from these analyses suggest that differences in primer concentrations used by various workers have a significant effect on viral detection, particularly in normal samples where the level of viral infection may be low. Completion of these determinations will help to establish standard PCR protocols for each laboratory and define the variation in HPV infection reported to date. In addition, such collaboration between HPV investigators will help to establish laboratory reference centres, an essential step before meaningful epidemiological studies of the natural history of HPV infection can be undertaken.

Table 8.4 Detection sensitivities of primers for CaSki DNA

Primer	Lowest amount detected (fg)
LI consensus	50
L1 specific	500
E6	50
E7	50

VARIATIONS OF THE PCR AND FUTURE APPLICATIONS

The PCR technique can be easily modified to amplify RNA so that gene expression can be analyzed in small amounts of tissue. In this situation extracted RNA is copied into double-stranded cDNA using the retroviral enzyme, reverse transcriptase and the PCR is then performed on the cDNA copies. By this method Johnson et al[53] identified quantitative differences in the level of early region transcription in cytologically normal and abnormal cervical samples. The suggestion from this work was that the level of E6 and E7 transcription could contribute to the malignant phenotype, but other factors must be important in the development of cervical neoplasia.

Investigation of HPV infection is not restricted to cervical tissue. PCR technology has also been applied to estimations of viral prevalence in lesions at various other sites including vulvar and penile warts and carcinomas, anal intraepithelial neoplasia and carcinoma, tumors of the upper respiratory tract and conjunctival and oral tumors.[32,54–60] Furthermore, the PCR has permitted detection of subclinical HPV infections in penile lesions histologically negative for condylomata,[61–63] and has been used to exclude a role for HPV in the development of ovarian carcinomas. New modifications of the PCR are continually being published. An example of this is the possibility of using PCR to analyze small numbers of cells that have been histologically identified under the microscope. In this technique specific cell subsets, identified in tissue sections by morphological criteria or by prior immunohistological staining for a particular marker, are protected from ultraviolet inactivation by an 'umbrella' in the form of a dot (made with a marker pen) placed physically over the cells of interest.[64] Direct ultraviolet radiation of the section will cross-link the DNA in all but the protected cells and thus subsequent PCR analysis for virus infection or genetic mutations can be directed to the specific cell subset originally identified.

The possibility of combining the sensitivity of PCR with the cellular localization afforded by in situ hybridization has recently been suggested and would be of value in both the clinical and biological analysis of HPV infection.[65,66] This technique is still very much in its infancy, but encouraging results have been obtained using multiple primers to generate DNA fragments with overlapping cohesive ends in an attempt to increase the retention of PCR products within specific cells in a tissue section. However, there are still a number of theoretical and practical problems with this technique. The kinetics of the entry of primers and of Taq polymerase into cells, the efficiency and specificity of in cell PCR amplification and the prevention of amplified product diffusion have yet to be thoroughly assessed. Attempts to validate PCR in situ as applied to tissue sections suggest that it is an extremely inefficient process (only 10–100 times amplification versus the 10^6-fold amplification achieved in solution) with significant cell-to-cell variation. Thus, whilst the theoretical potential of PCR in situ is vast, its practical application will have to await the development of more robust and carefully validated technologies.

A quantitative means of analyzing HPV infection may help differentiate between low-grade latent infections as may be present in cytologically normal individuals and replicative infections as observed in CIN. However, as described above variability in the amplification efficiencies of different samples even when using the same primers precludes the use of simple strategies for quantitation such as measuring the intensity of the amplified product band. As PCR amplification is an exponential process any small differences in any of the variables that affect the reaction rate (i.e., constituents of the PCR buffer, primer sequences, purity of the DNA sample) will significantly affect the yield of PCR product.

By far the best quantitative approach to date is the strategy involving coamplification of a competitive template that uses the same PCR primers as those of the target DNA.[67] Primers targeting the early E6 region of HPV have been used which coamplify sample DNA in the presence of increasing known concentrations of competitor DNA. The cloned fragment of the E6*I mRNA used as a competitor in these amplifications is recognized by the E6 primers but generates a smaller sized product (158 bp) compared to the wild type HPV16 genome (340 bp). Target DNA is coamplified with a dilution series of the competitor DNA of known concentration and the relative amounts of the two products are determined by direct scanning of the ethidium bromide-stained gel or by incorporation of radiolabeled dNTPs. Because the starting concentration of the competitive template is known, the initial concentration of the target DNA can be determined. This approach is promising although little is known about its reproducibility and suitability for large-scale epidemiological analysis.[67] In addition, multiple PCRs are required for each individual sample which is sometimes precluded by the lack of sufficient material.

Elsewhere quantitative analysis of HPV infection is now being developed for commercial assays using antibody immunoassay type analyses. Preliminary results with such assays suggest that detection levels compare favorably with standard methods such as Southern blot and that inter-assay agreement is at least 95%.

The sensitivity and specificity of PCR can be further increased by the use of 'nested PCR' where the PCR product obtained with one set of primers is reamplified with another set of primers. The second set of primers are complimentary to sequences within the amplified product from the first PCR and referred to as 'nested primers.' However, this procedure is notoriously prone to contamination, a common problem discussed earlier.

SUMMARY

Previously reported PCR estimates of HPV 16 infection among normal women from various laboratories range from 0 to 84%. This confusion has hindered a proper assessment of the virus's role in the development of cervical carcinoma, but recent attempts to standardize the detection methods used, together with improved laboratory practices have helped to reduce these inconsistencies. Certain HPV types are now associated with the development of cervical neoplasia, types 31, 33, 35 and particularly 16 and 18 being considered high-risk oncogenic strains. In some cases the increased sensitivity of PCR has enabled the identification of latent HPV infection in asymptomatic subjects. The clinical significance of such information is difficult to assess, but has certainly demonstrated that more individuals are infected with HPV16 than originally indicated. Accurately determining the prevalence of HPV in normal and abnormal populations awaits the widespread application of more standardized PCR procedures.

ACKNOWLEDGEMENTS

The authors' own work referred to in this chapter was supported by grants from the Cancer Research Campaign.

REFERENCES

1. Shah K V, Howley P M. Papillomaviruses. In: Fields B N, Knipe D M, eds. Fields virology. New York: Raven Press, 1990: p 1651.
2. Munoz N, Bosch X, Kaldor J M. Does human papillomavirus cause cervical cancer? The state of the epidemiological evidence. Br J Cancer 1988; 57: 1–5.
3. Saiki R, Scharf S, Faloona F et al. Enzymatic amplification of β-globin genomic sequences and restriction site analysis for diagnosis of sickle cell anemia. Science 1985; 230: 1350–1354.
4. Howley P M. Papillomaviruses and their replication. In: Fields B N, Knipe D M, eds. Fields virology. New York: Raven Press, 1990: p 1625.
5. Munger K, Phelps W C, Bubb V, Howley P M, Schlegel R. The E6 and E7 genes of the human papillomavirus type 16 together are necessary and sufficient for transformation of primary human keratinocytes. J Virol 1989; 63: 4417–4421.
6. Chesters P M, McCance D J. Human papillomavirus types 6 and 16 in cooperation with Ha-ras transform secondary rat embryo fibroblasts. J Gen Virol 1989; 70: 353–365.
7. Wilczynski S P, Pearlman L, Walker J. Identification of HPV16 early genes retained in cervical carcinomas. Virology 1988; 166: 624–627.
8. Werness B A, Levine A J, Howley P M. Association of human papillomavirus types 16 and 18 E6 proteins with p53. Science 1990; 248: 76–79.
9. Dyson N, Howley P M, Munger K, Harlow E. The human papillomavirus-16 E7 oncoprotein is able to bind to the retinoblatoma gene product. Science 1989; 243: 934–937.
10. Southern E M. Detection of specific sequences among DNA fragments separated by gel electrophoresis. J Molec Biol 1975; 98: 503–517.
11. Meanwell C A, Cox M F, Blackledge G, Maitland N J. HPV16 DNA in normal and malignant cervical epithelium: Implications for the aetiology and behaviour of cervical neoplasia. Lancet 1987; i: 703–707.
12. Schiffman M H, Bauer H M, Lorincz A T et al. Comparison of Southern blot hybridisation and polymerase chain reaction methods for the detection of human papillomavirus DNA. J Clin Microbiol 1991; 29: 573–577.
13. Kafatos F C, Jones C W, Estradtiadis A. Determination

of nucleic acid sequence homologies and relative concentration by a dot blot hybridisation procedure. Nucleic Acids Res 1979; 7: 1541–1552.

14. Denhardt D T. A membrane-filter technique for the detection of complementary DNA. 1966; 23: 641–645.

15. Hallam N, Green J, Gibson P, Powis J, Bibby J. Prevalence of HPV cervical infection in a family planning clinic determined by polymerase chain reaction and dot blot hybridisation. 1991; 34: 154–158.

16. Gjoen K, Siebke J C, Flikke M et al. Genital human papilloma virus infection in Oslo studied by dot blot DNA hybridisation and the polymerase chain reaction. 1991; 34: 159–164.

17. Wagner D, Ikenberg H, Boehm N, Gissman L. Identification of human papillomavirus in cervical swabs by deoxyribonucleic acid in situ hybridisation. Obstet Gynecol 1984; 64: 767–772.

18. Schneider A, Kraus H, Schuhmann R, Gissman L. Papillomavirus infection of the lower genital tract: detection of viral DNA in gynecological swabs. Int J Cancer 1985; 35: 443–448.

19. Schneider A, Sawada E, Gissman L, Shah K. Human papillomaviruses in women with a history of abnormal PAP smears and their male partners. Obstet Gynecol 1987; 69: 554–562.

20. Gall J G, Pardue M L. Nucleic acid hybridisation in cytological preparations. Methods Enzymol 1971; 38: 470–480.

21. Morin C, Bouchard C, Fortier M, Levesque R, Meisels A. A colposcopical lesion of the uterine cervix frequently associated with papillomavirus type 16 as detected by in situ and Southern blot hybridisation: a cytohistological correlation study. Int J Cancer 1988; 41: 531–536.

22. Schneider A, Oltersdorf T, Schneider V, Gissmann L. Distribution pattern of human papillomavirus 16 genome in cervical neoplasia by molecular in situ hybridisation of tissue sections. Int J Cancer 1987; 39: 717–721.

23. Saiki R K, Gelfand D H, Stoffel S et al. Primer-directed enzymatic amplification of DNA with a thermostable DNA polymerase. Science 1988; 239: 487–491.

24. Young L S, Bevan I S, Johnson M A et al. The polymerase chain reaction: a new epidemiological tool for investigating cervical human papillomavirus infection. Br Med J 1989; 298: 14–18.

25. Cuzick J, Terry G, Ho L, Hollingsworth T, Anderson M. HPV in cervical smears. Lancet 1992; 340: 112–113.

26. Shibata D K, Arnheim N, Martin W J. Detection of human papilloma virus in paraffin-embedded tissue using the polymerase chain reaction. J Exper Med 1988; 167: 225–230.

27. Resnick R M, Cornelissen M T E, Wright D K et al. Detection and typing of human papillomavirus in archival cervical cancer specimens by DNA amplification with consensus primers. J Nat Cancer Inst 1990; 82: 1477–1484.

28. Rakoczy P, Sterrett G, Kulski J et al. Time trends in the prevalence of human papillomavirus infections in archival Papanicolaou smears: analysis by cytology, DNA hybridisation and polymerase chain reaction. J Med Virol 1990; 32: 10–17.

29. Bauer H M, Greer C E, Chambers J C et al. Genital human papillomavirus infection in female university students as determined by a PCR-based method. J AMA 1991; 265: 472–477.

30. Tham K M, Chow V T K, Singh P et al. Diagnostic sensitivity of polymerase chain reaction and Southern blot hybridisation for the detection of human papillomavirus DNA in biopsy specimens from cervical lesions. 1991; 95: 638–646.

31. Skyldberg B, Kalantari M, Karki M, Johansson B, Hagmar B, Walaas L. Detection of human papillomavirus infection in tissue blocks by in situ hybridisation as compared with a polymerase chain reaction procedure. Human Pathol 1991; 22: 578–582.

32. Palefsky J M, Holly E A, Gonzales J, Berline J, Ahn D K, Grenspan J S. Detection of human papillomavirus DNA in anal intraepithelial neoplasia and anal cancer. Cancer Res 1991; 51: 1014–1019.

33. Palefsky J M, Winkler B, Rabanus J P et al. Characterisation of in vivo expression of the human papillomavirus type 16 E4 protein in cervical biopsy tissues. J Clin Invest 1991; 87: 2132–2141.

34. Snijders P J F, van den Brule A J C, Schrijnemakers H F J, Snow G, Meijer C J L M, Walboomers J M M. The use of general primers in the polymerase chain reaction permits the detection of a broad spectrum of human papillomavirus genotypes. J Gen Virol 1990; 71: 173–181.

35. Snijders P J F, Meijer C J L M, Walboomers J M M. Degenerate primers based on highly conserved regions of amino acid sequence in papillomaviruses can be used in a generalized polymerase chain reaction to detect productive human papillomavirus infections. J Gen Virol 1991; 72: 2781–2786.

36. Tidy J A, Parry G C N, Ward P et al. High rate of human papillomavirus type 16 infection in cytologically normal cervices. Lancet 1989; i: 434.

37. Editorial. Human papillomaviruses and the polymerase chain reaction. Lancet 1989; i: 1051.

38. Kwok S, Higuchi R. Avoiding false positives with PCR. Nature 1989; 339: 237–238.

39. Kwok S. Procedures to minimize PCR-related carry-over. In: Innis M A, Gelfand D H, Sninsky J J et al eds. Polymerase chain reaction protocols: a guide to methods and applications. San Diego: Academic Press, 1990: 142–145.

40. Beyer-Finkler E, Pfister H, Girardi F. Anti-contamination primers to improve specificity of polymerase chain reaction in human papillomavirus screening. Lancet 1990; i: 1289–1290.

41. Cornelissen M T E, Van den Tweel J G, Struyk A P H B et al. Localisation of human papillomavirus type 16 DNA using the polymerase chain reaction in the cervix uteri of women with cervical intraepithelial neoplasia. J Gen Virol 1989; 70: 2555–2562.

42. Van den Brule A J C, Claas E C J, du Maine M et al. Use of anticontamination primers in the polymerase chain reaction for the detection of human papilloma virus genotypes in cervical scrapes and biopsies. J Med Virol 1989; 29: 20–27.

43. Gregoire L, Arella M, Campoine-Piccardo J, Lancaster W D. Amplification of human papillomavirus DNA sequences by using conserved primers. J Clin Microbiol 1989; 27: 2660–2665.

44. Manos M M, Lee K, Greer C et al. Looking for human papillomavirus type 16 by PCR. Lancet 1990; i: 734.

45. Resnick R M, Cornelissen M T E, Wright D K et al. Detection and typing of human papillomavirus in archival cervical cancer specimens by DNA

amplification with consensus primers. J Nat Cancer Inst 1990; 82: 1477–1484.

46. Van den Brule A J C, Snijders P J F, Gordijin R L J, Bleker O P, Meijer C J L M, Walboomers J M M. General primer-mediated polymerase chain reaction permits the detection of sequenced and still unsequenced human papillomavirus genotypes in cervical scrapes and carcinomas. Int J Cancer 1990; 45: 644–649.

47. Snijders P J F, van den Brule A J C, Schrijnemakers H F J, Snow G, Meijer C J L M, Walboomers J M M. The use of general primers in the polymerase chain reaction permits the detection of a broad spectrum of human papillomavirus genotypes. J Gen Virol 1990; 71: 173–181.

48. Snijders P J F, Meijer C J L M, Walboomers J M M. Degenerate primers based on highly conserved regions of amino acid sequence in papillomaviruses can be used in a generalized polymerase chain reaction to detect productive human papillomavirus infections. J Gen Virol 1991; 72: 2781–2786.

49. Munoz N, Bosch F X, de Sanjose S et al. The causal link between human papillomavirus and invasive cervical cancer: A population-based case-control study in Colombia and Spain. Int J Cancer 1992; 5: 743–749.

50. Walboomers J M M, Melkert P W J, Van den Brule A J C, Snijders P J F, Meijer J L M. The polymerase chain reaction for human papillomavirus screening in diagnostic cytopathology of the cervix. In: Herrington C S, McGee J O D, eds. Diagnostic molecular pathology: A practical approach. Oxford: IRL Press, 1992: pp 153.

51. Melkert P W J, Hopman E, Van den Brule A J C. Prevalence of HPV in cytomorphologically normal cervical smears, as determined by the polymerase chain reaction, is age dependent. Int J Cancer 1993; 53: 919–923.

52. Tierney R J, Ellis J R M, Winter H et al. P C R for the detection of cervical HPV16 infection: the need for standardisation. Int J Cancer 1993; 54: 700–701.

53. Johnson M A, Blomfield P I, Bevan I S, Woodman C B J, Young L S. Analysis of human papillomavirus type 16 E6–E7 transcription in cervical carcinomas and normal cervical epithelium using the polymerase chain reaction. J Gen Virol 1990; 71: 1473–1479.

54. Bloss J D, Liao S-Y, Wilczynski S P et al. Clinical and histologic features of vulvar carcinomas analysed for human papillomavirus status. Human Pathol 1991; 22: 711–718.

55. Varma V A, Sanchez-Lanier M, Unger E R et al. Association of human papillomavirus with penile carcinoma. Human Pathol 1991; 22: 908–913.

56. Bryan R L, Bevan I S, Crocker J, Young L S. Detection of HPV 6 and 11 in tumours of the upper respiratory tract using the polymerase chain reaction. Clin Otolaryngol 1990; 15: 177–180.

57. Odrich M G, Jakobiec F A, Lancaster W D et al. A spectrum of bilateral squamous conjunctival tumors associated with human papillomavirus type 16. Ophthalmology 1991; 98: 628–635.

58. Maitland N J, Bromidge T, Cox M F, Crane I J, Prime S S, Scully C. Detection of human papillomavirus genes in human oral tissue biopsies and cultures by polymerase chain reaction. Br J Cancer 1989; 59: 698–703.

59. Shroyer K R, Greer R J. Detection of human papillomavirus DNA by in situ hybridisation and polymerase chain reaction in premalignant and malignant oral lesions. Oral Surg Oral Med Oral Pathol 1991; 71: 708–713.

60. Yeudall W A, Campo M S. Human papillomavirus DNA in biopsies of oral tissues. J Gen Virol 1991; 72: 173–176.

61. Nuovo G J, Hochman H A, Eliezri Y D, Lastarria D, Comite S L, Silvers D N. Detection of human papillomavirus DNA in penile lesions histologically negative for condylomata. Analysis by in situ hybridisation and the polymerase chain reaction. Am J Surg Pathol 1990; 14: 829–836.

62. Chow V T, Tay S K, Tham K M, Lim T S, Bernard H U. Subclinical human papillomavirus infection of the male lower genital tract: colposcopy, histology and DNA analysis. Int J STD AIDS 1991; 2: 41–45.

63. Kataoka A, Claesson U, Hansson B G, Eriksson M, Lindh E. Human papillomavirus infection of the male diagnosed by Southern blot hybridisation and polymerase chain reaction. J Med Virol 1991; 33: 159–164.

64. Shibata D, Hawes D, Li Z H, Hernandez A M, Spruck C H, Nichols P W. Specific genetic analysis of microscopic tissue after selective ultraviolet radiation fractionation and the polymerase chain reaction. Am J Pathol 1992; 141: 539–543.

65. Nuovo G J, MacConnell P, Forde A, Delvenne P. Detection of human papillomavirus DNA in formalin-fixed tissues by in situ hybridisation after amplification by polymerase chain reaction. Am J Pathol 1991; 139: 847–854.

66. Nuovo G J, Gallery F, MacConnell P, Becker J, Bloch W. An improved technique for the in situ detection of DNA after polymerase chain reaction amplification. Am J Pathol 1991; 139: 1239–1244.

67. Gilliland G, Perrin S, Blanchard K, Bunn H F. Analysis of cytokine mRNA and DNA: Detection and quantitation by competitive polymerase chain reaction. Proc Nat Acad Sci USA 1990; 87: 2725–2729.

9. The etiology and natural history of vulvar dysplasia

Vicki V. Baker

THE ETIOLOGY AND NATURAL HISTORY OF VULVAR DYSPLASIA

The etiology and natural history of vulvar dysplasia are poorly understood. Although the English language literature is replete with small series and case reports, there are relatively few studies which include large numbers of cases of vulvar dysplasia that focus upon these issues. Parallels concerning the etiology and natural history of squamous intraepithelial dysplasia of the vulva and cervix are occasionally suggested but such extrapolations are often inaccurate or unproved. Although there are certain similarities, there are also some striking differences between dysplasia of the vulva and cervix (Table 9.1).

Vulvar keratinocytes, adnexal glandular cells and melanocytes may each exhibit dysplastic growth and maturation (Table 9.2). Although the nomenclature for Paget's disease of the vulva and melanocytic dysplasia is straightforward, considerable confusion has resulted from the myriad of diagnostic terms used in the past for epithelial dysplasia of the vulva. The terminology for vulvar dysplasia has recently been standardized in an effort to obviate the confusion that has surrounded earlier descriptions.[1-3] The International Society for the Study of Vulvar Disease (ISSVD) has recommended that the term vulvar intraepithelial neoplasia (VIN) or vulvar squamous intraepithelial neoplasia be used in reference to keratinocyte dysplasia. Use of terms such as squamous cell carcinoma in situ, erythroplasia of Queyrat, bowenoid atypia, bowenoid dysplasia, bowenoid papulosis, and Bowen's disease is discouraged.

Table 9.1 Differences between vulvar dysplasia and cervical dysplasia

	Vulva	Cervix
Percent cases exhibiting dysplasia adjacent to invasive disease	~ 25%	80–100%
Invasive potential of dysplasia	Low	Significant
Time to progression from dysplasia to invasive disease	20–30 years	10–15 years
Embryologic derivation of kertinocytes	Ectoderm	Mesoderm
Microenvironment	Moist	Exposure to cervical mucus
Cellular turnover	Low to moderate	High

Table 9.2 Cellular components of the vulva that may exhibit dysplasia

Cell type	Dysplasia	Abandoned terminology
Keratinocytes	Vulvar intraepithelial neoplasia (VIN)	
	VIN 1	Bowenoid atypia
	VIN 2	Bowen's disease
	VIN 3	Bowenoid papulosis, simplex carcinoma in situ
		Queyrat's erythroplasia, squamous cell carcinoma in situ
Adnexal glandular cells	Paget's disease of the vulva	
Melanocytes	Melanocytic dysplasia	
	Melanoma in situ	

CLINICOPATHOLOGIC CHARACTERISTICS

The anatomic structures of the vulva include the clitoris, the prepuce of the clitoris, the labia majora, the labia minora, the external urethral meatus and the perineal body. Dysplastic lesions of the vulva may involve any of these structures (Fig. 9.1).

Dysplastic lesions of the vulva may be white, pigmented, or erythematous papular lesions with an irregular margin and surface contour. Typically, the central vulvar structures and the posterior vulva are the areas most commonly affected.[4,5] Extension with involvement of the anal mucosa may occur in 14–35% of cases of multifocal VIN that involve the posterior vulva.[6–9] VIN lesions of the posterior vulva are also more likely to exhibit foci of early invasive disease.[9]

The gross appearance of a vulvar lesion does not reliably establish the diagnosis. A punch biopsy should always be performed to differentiate VIN, condyloma, nevi, basal cell carcinoma, seborrheic keratoses, and postinflammatory hyperpigmentation, all of which may appear similar. In addition, the appearance of dysplastic lesions of the vulva is not necessarily predictive of the presence or absence of invasive disease. Schlaerth et al described six cases of VIN with foci of microinvasive carcinoma involving the perianal area which was clinically unsuspected in five.[9] Similar observations have been reported by Chafe et al[10] and Bergeron et al.[11]

Histologically, VIN is characterized by loss of cellular polarity, an altered nuclear/cytoplasmic ratio, and cellular pleomorphism. Based upon the severity of these changes and the level of epithelial involvement, vulvar dysplasia is classified as mild, moderate, or severe.[12] Ultrastructurally, dysplastic squamous epithelial cells of the vulva exhibit loss of desmosomes, disorganized tonofibrils, interchromatic and perichromatin granules, and increased free ribosomes and mitochondria.[13]

Three distinct histologic patterns of VIN have been described: keratinizing, warty and basaloid. Keratinizing VIN is characterized by marked nuclear pleomorphism, cellular enlargement, atypia and multinucleation with keratin production. Warty VIN also demonstrates marked nuclear pleomorphism, cellular enlargement, atypia and multinucleation in conjunction with cytoplasmic changes resembling koilocytotic atypia but keratin production is absent. Basaloid VIN is characterized by a uniform population of small cells with a high nuclear–cytoplasmic ratio. Not infrequently, warty and basaloid patterns may coexist and classification of the lesion is based upon the predominant pattern.

The average thickness of the vulvar epithelium is 0.52 ± 0.23 mm. The average thickness of VIN lesions ranges from 0.10 to 1.90 mm.[4] Typically, VIN lesions measure less than 0.77 mm in hair bearing vulvar areas and less than 0.69 mm in nonhairbearing areas on the vulva.[14] Sebaceous gland and hair follicle involvement by VIN occur in 21% and 32% of cases, respectively.

Although VIN is commonly found in the setting of normal skin, it may also be found amidst hyperplastic dystrophy, lichen sclerosis, or condyloma. Whether this reflects a causal or casual association has not been resolved.[15]

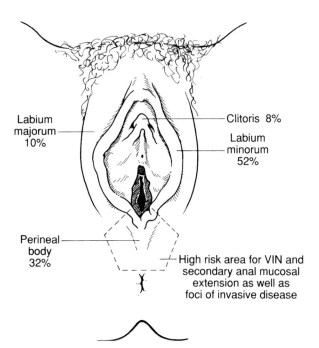

Labium majorum 10%
Clitoris 8%
Labium minorum 52%
Perineal body 32%
High risk area for VIN and secondary anal mucosal extension as well as foci of invasive disease

Fig. 9.1 The relative incidence of vulvar dysplasia by anatomic site.[45,54]

Paget's disease of the vulva, which is a dysplasia of the adnexal sweat gland cells, consists of large cells with pale cytoplasm and nuclei with a fine, vesicular pattern. Ultrastructurally, Paget's disease of the vulva is characterized by cells with pseudopod-like interdigitations among epidermal cells, irregularly distributed glycogen granules in the cytoplasm, and absent tonofibrils.[13]

Melanocytic dysplasia is characterized by atypical melanocytes that are generally restricted to the basal cell layer. The hypothesis has been advanced that this represents a precursor lesion for melanoma.[16] Ultrastructurally, melanoma in situ is characterized by cells with a loss of cohesion, prominent nucleoli, and compound melanosomes.[13]

ETIOLOGY OF VULVAR DYSPLASIA

Historically, vulvar intraepithelial neoplasia has been considered a disease of older women. However, a trend of increasing numbers of cases in younger women as well as an overall increase in the total number of cases has been documented.[8,17,18] Woodruff et al appear to be some of the earliest investigators to comment upon the increasing incidence of VIN, particularly in younger women.[8] Hilliard et al subsequently commented upon not only the increasing incidence of VIN in young women, but its multifocal distribution in this age group as well.[17]

The disproportionate increase in the number of younger women affected as well as the increase in total number of cases appears to mirror the increase in human papillomavirus (HPV)-related lesions of the cervix. Consistent with these observations is the recognition that the patient with vulvar dysplasia is at risk for concurrent, past, or future dysplasia at another site, most commonly the cervix. Caglar et al reported a series of 50 patients with VIN 3. Twelve of these patients, or 24%, had other preinvasive or invasive genital or extragenital neoplasms.[19] DiPaolo et al found that 28.5% of the patients in his group of 28 women diagnosed with VIN 3 had preexisting cervical dysplasia or invasive disease.[20] Ragnarsson et al reported a series of 74 patients with VIN 3 who were followed over a 10-year period.

Twenty-three percent of these patients had a history of cervical dysplasia.[5] Bernstein et al studied 65 women with VIN diagnosed between 1970 and 1979 and found that 65% had multifocal disease.[21] The mean age of this group was 38 years and 48% were younger than 41. Bornstein et al reported that 16 of 46 patients with VIN 3 had an additional site of dysplasia, usually the cervix.[22] In this study, the frequency of multicentric lesions decreased from 59% in women age 20–34 to 10% in women over the age of 50.

HPV has emerged as a risk factor for VIN although the true incidence of HPV associated VIN is difficult to ascertain. Referral bias, the diligence with which the diagnosis is sought, reports of relatively small numbers of cases, and the use of different viral detection techniques contribute to the wide range of values reported in the literature. Light microscopy diagnostic criteria of viral infection and immunohistochemical detection of viral capsid antigen are relatively insensitive methods that underestimate the incidence of HPV infection. Methods of detection utilizing amplification of HPV DNA by the polymerase chain reaction (PCR) are much more sensitive and may permit a more accurate estimation of the true incidence of infection. However, PCR-based methods are extremely sensitive and precautions must be taken to avoid contamination of the amplification reaction that would result in overestimates of the incidence of HPV infection.

Crum et al analyzed 41 VIN lesions using light microscopy that were diagnosed between 1966 and 1982.[18] VIN lesions exhibited pleomorphism and abnormal mitoses of the lower half of the lesion. Patients younger than age 45 more often exhibited associated condyloma and koilocytosis as compared to older patients. Based upon this series of patients, the authors concluded that the epidemiology of the disease had changed from one found predominantly in older women to one found in younger women (e.g., less than age 45) that was also associated with histologic changes suggestive of HPV infection.

Hording et al detected HPV 16 DNA sequences in 15 of 19 (79%) VIN lesions using PCR amplification of DNA from biopsies obtained from a group of women with a median age of 37 (range

22–55).[23] Jones et al, employing PCR and in situ hybridization, detected HPV 16 DNA in 15 of 29 VIN 3 lesions.[24] The mean age of the patients in this study was 48 and koilocytosis was a common histologic finding.

Similar results have been reported by Park.[25] Using in situ hybridization and PCR amplification, the presence of HPV 16 DNA in 16 of 30 VIN 3 lesions was reported. HPV 16 DNA positive lesions occurred in younger women (mean age 49 years) and the lesions more often demonstrated koilocytosis (94%) as compared to older women (60 years and 43%, respectively).

Buscema et al reported that HPV 16 DNA was present in 84% of VIN 3 lesions obtained from a group of 22 patients with a mean age of 38.[26] HPV 18 DNA and HPV 31 DNA were infrequently found. Pilotti et al studied 10 cases of VIN 3 in patients aged 31–68 and found that 90% of the lesions were HPV 16 DNA positive.[27] Interestingly, 3 of 10 lesions also contained DNA homologous to herpes simplex virus type 2 (HSV 2) DNA. Bornstein et al found HPV DNA in roughly 80% of patients with VIN 3.[22] In contradistinction to other studies, there were no differences between younger and older patients who had multifocal versus unifocal disease with respect to the presence or absence of HPV antigen, HSV 2 antigen, or antibodies to HSV 2.[22]

Collectively, these data indicate that VIN is often an HPV-associated condition. Based upon data from studies of the cervix, it is tempting to speculate that HPV, particularly type 16, plays a role in the etiology of vulvar dysplasia. It is also plausible that specific HPV types influence the biologic behavior of the dysplastic lesion. Toki et al[28] studied 30 cases of invasive vulvar disease and the adjacent epithelium for the presence of HPV DNA using PCR amplification and in situ hybridization. Eleven of 13 invasive lesions that were HPV DNA positive also exhibited adjacent areas of VIN whereas only three of 17 HPV DNA negative cancers had adjacent areas of VIN. Of the 13 HPV DNA positive invasive lesions, HPV 16 DNA was detected in nine, HPV 18 DNA in two, and both HPV DNA types in two. HPV 6 DNA and HPV 11 DNA were not detected. The mechanism by which HPV disrupts normal control of cell growth and proliferation appears to involve interactions of the E7 viral protein with the gene product of the p53 tumor suppressor gene.[29]

In addition to altered p53 gene activity, other molecular genetic alterations have been found in dysplastic lesions of the vulva. As an example, the histopathologic changes diagnostic of vulvar dysplasia are associated with alterations in the amount and distribution of keratin expression. Esquius et al have reported that the AE1 antibody, which recognizes 40–56.5 kDa keratins, and the CAM 5.2 antibody, which recognizes 39–50 kDa keratins, can be used to differentiate non-neoplastic epithelial disorders from VIN based upon differential staining patterns.[30] Normal vulvar squamous epithelium is stained by the AE1 antibody whereas VIN 1–2 lesions are not. Interestingly, AE1 stains VIN 3 lesions although the uptake is quite heterogeneous. VIN 1–2 lesions are not stained by the CAM 5.2 antibody whereas VIN 3 lesions are focally positive. Alterations of keratin gene expression have not been correlated with the presence or absence of HPV DNA. Like keratinocytes, Paget's cells also exhibit aberrant expression of low-molecular-weight keratins. Helm et al reported that Paget's cells expressed 40 kDa, 45 kDa, and 52.2 kDa low-molecular-weight keratins based upon detection with the CAM 5.2 monoclonal antibody.[31,32] In this regard, Paget's cells and squamous dysplasia cells are similar. Unlike squamous dysplastic cells, Paget's cells also express carcinoembryonic antigen (CEA), the epithelial membrane antigen (EMA) and antigross cystic diseases fluid protein (GCDFP). These cells also stain positive for B72.3, a tumor-associated antigen developed from human mammary tumor cells.[33]

Knowledge concerning the antigen reactivity of dysplastic cells is particularly useful in those cases in which the distinction between Paget's disease and amelanotic melanoma is unclear. Melanoma cells do not exhibit abnormal low-molecular-weight keratin expression and can be differentiated from Paget's cells on this basis.[34] In addition, melanoma cells are positive for the s100 protein, unlike Paget's cells. The alterations at the molecular level that are responsible for the abnormal expression of keratins and tumor associated antigens have not been defined.

Abnormalities of ploidy are common in dysplastic lesions of the vulva. Aneuploid cell populations are present in most cases of VIN 1 and VIN 2[7,35–37] as well as VIN 3 lesions. Crum et al analyzed the ploidy of 41 VIN 3 lesions and found that all were aneuploid.[35] Unlike cervix dysplasia in which aneuploid lesions are associated with higher grade lesions and a greater risk for progression, correlations between abnormalities of ploidy and the severity of the dysplastic lesion or its biologic behavior have not been reported.

Natural history of vulvar dysplasia

In contradistinction to cervical dysplasia, the risk of progression of VIN to invasive disease has not been well defined. Published estimates of the risk of progression to invasive disease are less than 5%.[7,38] With few exceptions, published series are small. In addition, review of published reports is hampered by the changing criteria for the histologic diagnosis of VIN during the past two decades and the frequent absence of information concerning the status of the margins of resection and the unifocal versus multifocal distribution of the disease. Table 9.3 presents a representative survey of the English languange literature to demonstrate the incidence of regression, persistence, and progression of VIN. These reports have been analyzed with respect to treated versus untreated lesions.

The general clinical impression is that older patients, who typically have unifocal, unicentric lesions, are at greater risk of progression to invasive vulvar cancer as compared to younger patients.[18,39–41] As an example, Barbero et al reported a case of VIN 1 in a 69 year old woman that progressed to invasive disease during a 24 month interval of time.[15] However, it is important to recognize that invasive carcinoma can and does occur in young women. Chafe et al reported a series of 69 patients with presumed VIN who were treated by wide local excision of the vulva.[10] Unsuspected invasive carcinoma was identified in 12 patients, the youngest of whom was 35.

Clues concerning the natural history of vulvar dysplasia may be found in observations concerning the relationship between various histologic patterns of squamous cell carcinoma of the vulva and adjacent areas of dysplasia. Buscema et al and Zaino et al have reported that roughly 25% of invasive vulvar carcinomas have areas of VIN 3 in adjacent epithelium.[42,43] Leibowitch et al found VIN 3 in 50% of 78 invasive squamous cell carcinomas of the vulva.[39] VIN was found in 31% and HPV DNA was detected in 6 of the 11 VIN lesions. The likelihood of finding dysplasia adjacent to invasive carcinoma is influenced by the histologic pattern of the carcinoma. Both warty and basaloid carcinomas exhibit adjacent VIN in over 75% of cases.[44] In contradistinction, keratinizing squamous cell carcinoma of the vulva

Table 9.3 Published examples of regression, persistence, and progression published in the English languange literature

Reference	N	Duration of follow-up	Recurrence or persistence	Progression	Regression
Patients treated for VIN					
38	102			3/102	
19	50		6/41	2/41*	
18	41	2–7 years		5/14	
20	28		1/28		
23	19	3–18 years		4/19	
55	32			1/32	
5	74		21/74	3/74	
56	18	1–5 years	3/18		2/18**
Patients followed for VIN					
11	2	6–40 years		2/2	
39	102	>5 years			2/102
55	4	2–8 years		4/4	

* These patients were diagnosed with invasive cancer 3 and 4 months after laser therapy and 5FU therapy, respectively. One suspects that these patients had invasive disease that was not diagnosed at the time of initial presentation.
** Regression of residual lesions noted at 4.8 and 5.2 years of follow-up after incomplete resection.

generally exhibits adjacent areas of hyperplastic dystrophy.[28] The age distribution also differs among these histologic types of cancer in that keratinizing carcinoma is typically diagnosed in older women (e.g., age greater than 60) whereas basaloid and warty carcinoma is diagnosed in younger women (e.g., age less than 60). In addition, keratinizing carcinoma is most commonly HPV negative and basaloid and warty carcinomas are typically HPV positive. Collectively, these observations provide indirect evidence that keratinizing versus warty/basaloid cancers are two biologically distinct diseases.

Because many cases of VIN are HPV DNA positive, it has been suggested that this virus may not only play a role in the etiology of VIN but in its natural history as well. In order to markedly disrupt the control mechanisms of cell growth and maturation, HPV DNA must be integrated into the genome of the host cell. Based upon in vitro models, incorporation of HPV DNA into the host genome may result in insertional mutagenesis and disruption of normal gene function. Integration of HPV DNA into the host genome has been found in VIN 3 lesions as well as invasive lesions of the vulva.[11,23,27] Bergeron et al reported two cases of multifocal VIN, one in a 30 year old and one in an 86 year old. In both cases, the aneuploid VIN lesions exhibited integrated HPV 16 DNA and were associated with loci of invasive disease.[11] However, there are no data from large series that have correlated the biologic behavior of VIN with respect to episomal or integrated HPV DNA.

The presence of HPV may predict the patient at increased risk of recurrent dysplasia following treatment. Hording et al found that patients with HPV 16 DNA positive lesions had a greater likelihood of recurrent dysplasia but there was no association between the presence of HPV 16 DNA and the occurrence of multicentric disease or the risk of malignant progression.[23] These patients were followed for a median of 5 years (range 2–16 years).

It has been postulated that the immune system influences the natural history of VIN lesions. Indirect evidence to support this hypothesis may be found in the high incidence of neoplasms and HPV-induced lesions in immunocompromised women.[45,46] Caglar et al reported a series of 50 cases of CIS of the vulva, five of which occurred in patients who were immunocompromised.[19] Sillman et al reported the outcome of 20 immunosuppressed women who had VIN.[47] Immunosuppression was the result of treatment administered for sarcoidosis, lupus, or renal transplantation. An altered CD4/CD8 ratio or a deficient response to mitogen stimulation were the criteria used to define immunosuppression. Evidence of HPV infection was based upon immunohistochemical detection of capsid antigen or electron microscopic visualization of viral particles. Twelve of the 20 women had persistent or recurrent VIN and one patient developed invasive disease.[47] Anecdotal case reports by Becagli and Cadore of three patients with Sjogren's syndrome, two of whom developed invasive vulvar cancer and one with VIN also suggest a possible relationship between altered immunologic function and vulvar neoplasia.[48] Buscema et al followed 106 patients with VIN 3 for 1–15 years and observed four cases of progression to invasive disease.[42] Of these four cases, two occurred in postmenopausal women and two occurred in immunosuppressed patients. Buscema and Woodruff also reported five cases of invasive cancer in women previously treated for VIN 3.[41] Based upon these and other reports in the literature, chronic immunosuppression has emerged as a risk factor for progression although the relative risk has not been defined.[11,41,49–51]

VIN that develops during periods of reversible immunosuppression may exhibit spontaneous regression when normal immune function is restored. As an example, VIN lesions diagnosed during pregnancy commonly regress during the postpartum period. Friedrich et al followed five pregnant patients prospectively and reported spontaneous regression in four.[7]

Spontaneous regression is also reported to occur in patients who are not immunologically compromised. Bernstein et al followed 13 untreated cases of VIN 3 and five underwent spontaneous regression within 6 months.[21] The ages of these women ranged from 23 to 55 and all were in good health. Spontaneous regression appears most likely to occur in younger patients with multifocal VIN.[52,53]

Paget's disease is characterized by frequent recurrence, largely attributable to incomplete surgical resection. Paget's disease may rarely exhibit minimally invasive loci but this is not commonly reported. Paget's disease is more notable for its association with adenocarcinoma of contiguous and noncontiguous structures.

Melanocytic dysplasia tends to mature into benign intradermal melanonaevus in the vast majority of cases.[16] However, melanocytic dysplasia progresses to melanoma in a small percentage of cases although the factors which influence this have not been defined.

SUMMARY

The number of new cases of vulvar dysplasia is increasing and younger women are disproportionately represented. Based upon epidemiological, clinical, and virology studies, it appears that vulvar dysplasia is a diagnostic term which encompasses at least two distinct subgroups based upon age (Table 9.4).

Table 9.4 Subgroups of vulvar dysplasia categorized by the age of the patient into younger (less than 45) and older (greater than 50)

	Younger patient	Older patient
Multicentric	Often	Uncommon
Multifocal	Often	Uncommon
HPV 16 DNA positive	Often	Less common
Likelihood of progression to invasive disease	Rare	Less common
Likelihood of spontaneous regression of VIN	Not considered unusual	Uncommon
Aneuploid lesion (s)	Common	Common
Unifocal	Rare	Common
Unicentric	Rare	Common
Histologic pattern	Basaloid or warty	Keratinizing

The human papillomavirus appears to play a role in the etiology of vulvar intraepithelial neoplasia although its role in the natural history is poorly defined at this time. The risk of progression from vulvar dysplasia to invasive disease appears to be small and when it occurs, it is usually seen in elderly or immunocompromised patients although exceptions to this generalization are well-documented in the literature.

REFERENCES

1. Ridley C M, Frankman O, Jones I S C et al. New nomenclature for vulvar disease: International Society for the Study of Vulvar Disease. Human Pathol 1989; 20: 495–496.
2. Wilkinson E J, Kneale B, Lynch P J. Report of the ISSVD Terminology Committee. J Reprod Med 1986; 31: 973–974.
3. Kiryu H, Ackerman A B. A critique of current classifications of vulvar disease. Am J Dermatopathol 1990; 12: 377–392.
4. Benedet J L, Wilson P S, Matisic J. Epidermal thickness and skin appendage involvement in vulvar intraepithelial neoplasia. J Reprod Med 1991; 36: 608–612.
5. Ragnarsson B, Raabe N, Willems J, Pettersson F. Carcinoma in situ of the vulva: longterm prognosis. Acta Oncologica 1987; 26: 277–280
6. Disaia P J, Rich W M. Surgical approach to multifocal carcinoma in situ of the vulva. Am J Obstet Gynecol 1981; 140: 136–142.
7. Friedrich E G, Wilkinson E J, Fu Y S. Carcinoma in situ of the vulva: a continuing challenge. Am J Obstet Gynecol 1980; 136: 830–883.
8. Woodruff J D, Julian C G, Puray T, Mermut S, Kayayama P. The contemporary challenge of carcinoma in situ of the vulva. Am J Obstet Gynecol 1973; 115: 677–684.
9. Schlaerth J B, Morrow C P, Nalick R H, Gaddis O. Anal involvement by carcinoma in situ of the perineum in women. Obstet Gynecol 1984; 64: 406–411.
10. Chafe W C, Richards A, Morgan L, Wilkinson E. Unrecognized invasive carcinoma in vulvar intraepithelial neoplasia (VIN). Gynecol Oncol 1988; 31: 154–162.
11. Bergeron C, Naghashfar Z, Canaan C, Shah K, Fu Y, Ferenczy A. Human papillomavirus type 16 in intraepithelial neoplasia (Bowenoid papulosis) and coexistent invasive carcinoma of the vulva. Int J Gynecol Pathol 1987; 6: 1–11.
12. Buckley C H, Butler E B, Fox H. Vulvar intraepithelial neoplasia and microinvasvie carcinoma of the vulva. J Clin Pathol 1984; 37: 1201–1211.
13. Stegner H-E. Ultrastructure of preneoplastic lesions of the vulva. J Reprod Med 1986; 31: 815–820.
14. Schatz P, Bergeron C, Wilkinson E J, Arseneau J, Ferenczy A. Vulvar intraepithelial neoplasia and skin appendage involvement. Obstet Gynecol 1989; 74: 769–775.
15. Barbero M, Micheletti L, Preti M et al. Vulvar intraepithelial neoplasia: a clinicopathologic study of 60 cases. J Reprod Med 1990; 35: 1023–1028.
16. Cook M G, Robertson I. Melanocytic dysplasia and melanoma. Histopathology 1985; 9: 647–658.
17. Hilliard G D, Massey F M, O'Toole R V. Vulvar neoplasia in the young. Am J Obstet Gynecol 1979; 135: 185–188.
18. Crum C P, Liskow A, Petras P, Keng W C, Frick H C. Vulvar intraepithelial neoplasia (severe atypia and carcinoma in situ): a clinicopathologic analysis of 41 cases. Cancer 1984; 54: 1429–1434.
19. Caglar H, Tamer S, Hreshchyshyn M M. Vulvar

intraepithelial neoplasia. Obstet Gynecol 1982; 60: 346–349.

20. DiPaolo G R, Rueda-Leverone G, Belardi M G, Vighi S. Vulvar carcinoma in situ: a report of 28 cases. Gynecol Oncol 1982; 14: 236–242.

21. Bernstein S G, Kovacs B R, Townsend D E, Morrow C P. Vulvar carcinoma in situ. Obstet Gynecol 1983; 61: 304–307.

22. Bornstein J, Kaufman R H, Adam E, Adler-Storthz K. Multicentric intraepithelial neoplasia involving the vulva: clinical features and association with human papillomavirus and herpes simplex virus. Cancer 1988; 62: 1601–1604.

23. Hording U, Daugaard S, Iversen A K et al. Human papillomavirus type 16 in vulvar carcinoma, vulvar intraepithelial neoplasia, and associated cervical neoplasia. Gynecol Oncol 1991; 42: 22–26.

24. Jones R W, Park J S, McLean M R, Shah K V. Human papillomavirus in women with vulvar intraepithelial neoplasia III. J Reprod Med 1990; 35: 1124–1126.

25. Park J S, Jones R W, McLean M R, Currie J L, Woodruff J D, Shah K. Possible etiologic heterogeneity of vulvar intraepithelial neoplasia: a correlation of pathologic characteristics with human papillomavirus detection by in situ hybridization and polymerase chain reaction. Cancer 1991; 67: 1599–1607.

26. Buscema J, Naghashfar Z, Sawada E, Daniel R, Woodruff J D, Shah K. The predominance of human papillomavirus type 16 in vulvar neoplasia. Obstet Gynecol 1988; 71: 601–606.

27. Pilotti S, Rotola A, D'Amato L et al. Vulvar carcinomas: search for sequences homologous to human papillomavirus and herpes simplex virus DNA. Modern Pathol 1990; 3: 442–448.

28. Toki T, Kurman R J, Park J S, Kessis T, Daniel R W, Shah K. Probable nonpapillomavirus etiology of squamous cell carcinoma of the vulva in older women: a clinicopathologic study using in situ hybridization and polymerase chain reaction. Int J Gynecol Path 1991; 10: 107–125.

29. Wemess B A, Levine A J, Howley P M. The E6 proteins encoded by human papillomavirus types 16 and 18 can complex p53 in vitro. Science 1990; 248: 76–79.

30. Esquius J, Brisigotti M, Matias-Guiu X, Prat J. Keratin expression in normal vulva, non-neoplastic epithelial disorders, vulvar intraepithelial neoplasia, and invasive squamous cell carcinoma. Int J Gynecol Path 1991; 10: 341–335.

31. Helm K F, Goellner J R, Peters M S. Immunohistochemical stains in extramammary Paget's disease. Am J Dermatopathol 1992; 14: 402–407.

32. Ganjei P, Giraldo K A, Lampe B, Nadji M. Vulvar Paget's disease. Is immunocytochemistry helpful in assessing the surgical margins? J Reprod Med 1990; 35: 1002–1004.

33. Olson D J, Fujimura M, Swanson P, Okagaki T. Immunohistochemical features of Paget's disease of the vulva with and without adenocarcinoma. Int J Gynecol Pathol 1991; 10: 285–295.

34. Bacchi C E, Goldfogel G A, Greer B E, Gown A M. Paget's disease and melanoma of the vulva: Use of a panel of monoclonal antibodies to identify cell type and to microscopically define adequacy of surgical margins. Gynecol Oncol 1992; 46: 216–221.

35. Crum C P, Fu Y S, Levine R U, Richart R M,

36. Townsend D E, Fenoglio C M. Intraepithelial lesions of the vulva: biologic and histologic criteria for the distinction of condyloma from vulvar intraepithelial neoplasia. Am J Obstet Gynecol 1982; 144: 77–83.

36. Fu Y S, Reagan J W, Townsend D E et al. Nuclear DNA study of vulvar intraepithelial neoplasia and invasive squamous neoplasms. Obstet Gynecol 1981; 57: 643–652.

37. Wilkinson E J, Friedrich E G J R, Fu Y S. Multicentric nature of vulvar carcinoma in situ. Obstet Gynecol 1981; 58: 69–74.

38. Buscema J, Woodruff J D, Parmley T H, Genady R. Carcinoma in situ of the vulva. Obstet Gynecol 1980; 55: 225–230.

39. Leibowitch M, Neill S, Pelisse M, Moyal-Baracco M. The epithelial changes associated with squamous cell carcinoma of the vulva: a review of the clinical, histological, and viral findings in 78 women. Br J Obstet Gynecol 1990; 97: 1135–1139.

40. Abell M R and Gosling J R. Intraepithelial and infiltrative carcinoma of the vulva: Bowen's type. Cancer 1961; 14: 31–35.

41. Buscema J, Woodruff J D. Progressive histolgic alterations in the development of vulvar cancer. Report of 5 cases. Am J Obstet Gynecol 1980; 138: 146–50.

42. Buscema J, Stern J, Woodruff J D. The significance of the histologic alterations adjacent to invasive vulvar carcinoma. Am J Obstet Gynecol 1980; 137: 902–907.

43. Zaino R J, Husseinzadeh N, Nahhas W et al. Epithelial alterations in proximity to invasive squamous carcinoma of the vulva. Int J Gynecol Pathol 1982; 1: 173–177.

44. Kurman R J, Toki T, Schiffman H. Basaloid and warty carcinoma of the vulva. Distinctive types of squamous cell carcinoma of the vulva frequently associated with human papillomavirus. Am J Surg Pathol 1993; 17: 133–145.

45. Koranda F C, Dehmel E M, Kahn G, Penn I. Cutaneous complications in immunosuppressed renal homograph recipients. JAMA 1974; 229: 419–424.

46. Marshburn P B, Trofatter K F. Recurrent condyloma acuminatum in women over age 40: association with immunosuppression and malignant disease. Am J Obstet Gynecol 1988; 159: 429–433.

47. Sillman F, Stanek A, Sedlis A et al. The relationship between human papillomavirus and lower genital intraepithelial neoplasia in immunosuppressed women. Am J Obstet Gynecol 1984; 150: 300–308.

48. Becagli L, Cadore L. Sjogren's syndrome and vulvar cancer. Clin Exper Obstet Gynecol 1987; 14: 69–71.

49. Rasthkar G, Okagaki T, Twiggs L B, Clark B A. Early invasive and in situ carcinoma of the vulva: clinical, histologic, and electron microscopic study with particular reference to viral association. Am J Obstet Gynecol 1982; 143: 814–820.

50. Wilkinson E J, Rico M J, Pierson K K. Microinvasive carcinoma of the vulva. Int J Gynecol Pathol 1982; 1: 29–34.

51. Pilotti S, Della Torre G, Rilke F et al. Immunohistochemical and ultrastructural evidence of papilloma virus infection associated with in situ and microinvasive squamous cell carcinoma of the vulva. Am J Surg Pathol 1984; 8: 751–757.

52. Skinner M S, Sternberg W H, Ichirose H, Collins J. Spontaneous regression of bowenoid atypia of the vulva. Obstet Gynecol 1973; 42: 40–46.

53. Kimura S, Hirai A, Harada R, Nagashima M. So-called multicentric pigmented Bowen's disease: report of a case and a possible etiologic role of human papillomavirus. Dermatologica 1978; 57: 229–237.

54. Andreasson B, Bock J E. Intraepithelial neoplasia in the vulvar region. Gynecol Oncol 1985; 21: 300–305.

55. Jones R W, McLean M R. Carcinoma in situ of the vulva: A review of 31 treated and 5 untreated cases. Obstet Gynecol 1986; 68: 499–504.

56. Ulbright T M, Stehman F B, Roth L M, Ehrlich C E, Ransburg R C. Bowenoid dysplasia of the vulva. Cancer 1982; 50: 2910–2919.

10. Vulvar and multifocal intraepithelial neoplasia

Rashna Chenoy   David Luesley

VULVAR INTRAEPITHELIAL NEOPLASIA

INTRODUCTION

As a clinical entity vulvar intraepithelial neoplasia (VIN) is of interest to practitioners of various medical disciplines including gynecology, dermatology, pathology and oncology. Numerous descriptive terms have been used to characterize this disorder in the past, resulting in complex and confusing terminology. Current nomenclature describes VIN as premalignant changes occurring within, and confined to, the squamous epithelium of the vulva.[1] Nonsquamous intraepithelial lesions such as Paget's disease and in situ melanomas are not included under VIN. The term VIN has now replaced previously used names such as 'mild, moderate or severe atypia', 'carcinoma-in-situ', 'Bowen's disease' and 'erythroplasia of Queyrat.'[2]

EPIDEMIOLOGY

Shifts in the epidemiological pattern of VIN have been noted over the past 30 years,[3,4] although it still remains an uncommon condition. Higher rates of detection in clinical practice may simply reflect an increased awareness of the condition and greater familiarity with its colposcopic appearances or referral bias. Others have suggested a true increase in incidence.[5-7] Data collected from the SEER programme[8] provide the best evidence to date that there has been a real increase in the incidence of VIN. This population-based study noted that the incidence has almost doubled between two examined cohorts (1973–1976 and 1985–1987). This group also noted that the inci-

dence of invasive vulvar cancer had remained stable over the same two cohorts.

VIN is now reported more frequently in women below the age of 40.[9-12] In young patients the disease is usually multifocal with frequent spontaneous regressions, and very rarely if ever, is progression to invasion seen in those who are not immunocompromised.[6,10] This contrasts with reports of VIN 30 years ago, when the disease was usually diagnosed in women over the age of 40 years, was unifocal in distribution and had a small but distinct malignant potential.[13] These changing trends have been attributed to greater exposure of the vulvar skin to sexually transmitted viral infections such as human papillomavirus 16 and 18 and herpes simplex virus 2.[14] The viruses implicated are believed to act synergistically with cofactors such as smoking and immunosuppressants, in the initiation of multicentric VIN lesions in young women.[15,16]

Although VIN is being diagnosed more frequently and at younger ages (28–35 years), the incidence of invasive vulvar cancer and its average age of occurrence (62–63 years) has remained unchanged for the last three or four decades.[3] This prolonged interval for transition to invasive disease implies that the preinvasive VIN lesions noted previously were biologically different from the nonprogressive intraepithelial changes being diagnosed at present. The two may well represent separate disease entities, of dissimilar pathogenesis and natural history.

HISTOLOGY

The main histopathological features of VIN are

abnormal cell maturation and *disordered stratification* of the vulvar squamous epithelium. The former is characterized by an increased nuclear to cytoplasmic ratio, cellular and nuclear pleomorphism, hyperchromasia, irregular chromatin clumping and bizarre mitotic figures. The latter is denoted by the presence of abnormal basal and parabasal cells in the more superficial layers of the epithelium usually associated with parakeratosis and hyperkeratosis. VIN is graded as 1,2, or 3 depending upon the degree of maturation or differentiation of the epithelial lesion.

The current classification of VIN was recommended for general use at the 8th World Congress of the International Society for the Study of Vulvar Disease (ISSVD) in 1986. When the epithelial abnormalities described above are confined to the lower third of the squamous epithelium of the vulva the condition is referred to as VIN 1 (mild atypia/dysplasia). Involvement of the lower two-thirds of the epithelium by these abnormalities is called VIN 2 (moderate atypia/dysplasia), and when the changes extend to the upper third the lesion is classed as VIN 3 (severe atypia/dysplasia; carcinoma-in-situ). Although the term VIN 3 has replaced 'severe atypia' and 'carcinoma-in-situ', the ISSVD classification has recommended the continuing usage of 'carcinoma-in-situ' terminology for lesions involving the full thickness of the squamous epithelium.

The changes of VIN may affect the pilosebaceous units as well as the surface epithelium and the depth of involvement can vary according to whether hairbearing or non-hairbearing skin is evaluated. This has an obvious effect on the way that treatment is planned. Several groups have commented on pilosebaceous unit involvement. Shatz et al[17] found that VIN involved sebaceous glands and hair follicles in 21 and 32%, respectively (62 cases). The mean depth of sebaceous gland involvement was 0.77 mm in hairy skin and 0.5 mm in non-hairbearing skin. The mean depth of hair follicle involvement was 1.04 mm and 99.5% of all hair follicles were involved to a depth of less than 2.55 mm. Mene et al[18] reported 56% involvement of skin appendages with the maximum depth of involvement reaching 4.6 mm.

Two distinct histological subtypes of VIN 3 have been described.[1,19] In addition to the usual features of VIN 3, the *bowenoid* type is characterized by premature cellular differentiation, individual cell keratinization and multinucleate giant cell formation in the deeper layers of the epidermis. In the *basaloid* type, atypical parabasal cells extend throughout the thickness of the nonstratified dysmature epithelium which is covered by a superficial layer of parakeratotic cells. This subclassification appears to have no practical clinical use and is therefore no longer specifically reported when diagnosing VIN 3.

Adoption of the VIN terminology is attractive to many clinicians because it draws an analogy with intraepithelial neoplasia in other parts of the female genital tract. This concept of a continuum of disease has, however, been challenged recently. In practice, many more cases of VIN 3 are diagnosed than the milder grades, which would not be expected if the lesions developed through a continuum of worsening pathological changes. The concept of a spectrum, implying separate entities without progression of milder forms to the more severe may seem more appropriate. A further explanation for this could be our inability to detect early changes of VIN which are often asymptomatic and can resemble nonneoplastic disorders of the vulva.

Difficulty is also experienced in distinguishing between the histological features of VIN and vulvar condyloma acuminata.[2,20] Human papillomavirus (HPV) antigens have been found in VIN lesions[21,22] and 'koilocytosis,' a virally induced cytoplasmic vacuolation of superficial epithelial cells is frequently found in both conditions. The differentiating histological feature between condylomas and VIN is the presence of abnormal mitosis and enlarged pleomorphic basal and parabasal nuclei found only in the latter. In condylomas, some nuclear enlargement may occur in the superficial and intermediate cells but no mitotic changes are seen and basal and parabasal pleomorphism is minimal. The ISSVD classification does not consider the presence of HPV infection while grading VIN.

ETIOLOGY

Since intraepithelial neoplasia of the vulva was first described by Bowen in 1912, there have been no large epidemiological studies to provide information regarding the etiology, pathogenesis or natural history of this disorder. Several small studies have investigated the role of various etiological agents in the development of VIN, but the exact mechanisms remain unclear. Consensus opinion now points to three main factors: a 'field change' affecting the vulvar skin, viral infections of the vulva and an impaired host immune response.

Field changes affecting the vulvar skin

The frequent association of intraepithelial neoplasia of the vulva and other sites in the anogenital tract has led to the concept of a 'field change' involving all the squamous epithelium in this region. The affected epithelium is susceptible to the carcinogenic effects of agents such as viruses which may be sexually transmitted. Multicentric disease in other areas of the genital tract have been found in up to 30% of women with VIN 3.[23,24]

Viral infections of the vulva

VIN is seen with increasing frequency in young sexually active women, and reports of its association with sexually transmitted diseases abound.[6,25,26] The viral agents most frequently implicated are HPV and herpes simplex virus 2 (HSV 2), both of which have shown correspondingly high rates of infection in women with VIN.

HPV is strongly linked with the genesis of VIN. Histological stigmata of HPV infection have been reported in upto 59% of patients with VIN.[11] Up to 40% of women with VIN give a history of vulvar warts, and the disease has been known to develop in typical condyloma acuminata associated with the 'benign' HPV types 6 and 11.[10,27] More frequently however, the capsid antigens and nucleic acids (DNA) of 'high-risk' HPV types 16 and 18 are found in VIN lesions, particularly in recurrent ones and in those which progress to invasion.[21,28–30]

The model of VIN as an infection with milder forms being frequently associated with spontaneous regression, and even some more high-grade lesions resolving is elegantly described by Crum.[2] Furthermore, the background information available on HPV-and HSV-related oncogenesis also fits this model.

Genital HSV 2 infection is not a prime initiator of neoplastic change, but is believed to act synergistically with HPV in the development of VIN. Kaufman et al[14] detected HSV 2 antigens in 50%, and HPV-DNA in over 80% of the cases of VIN 3 they studied.

Immunosuppression

Local or generalized immunosuppressive conditions can increase the burden of HPV and HSV infections in the genital tract, enhance the development of intraepithelial neoplasias and increase the rate of progression to invasive cancer.

Local immunosuppression may result from the effects of smoking, radiation or repeated exposure to seminal plasma. A generalized reduction in immunocompetence may be due to conditions such as lymphomas, HIV infection and immunosuppressant therapy for problems such as severe asthma, systemic lupus erythematosis and organ transplants.[15,16,31]

NATURAL HISTORY

Despite the accessibility of the vulva for various investigations, VIN remains a confusing condition, with very little known about its natural history. It is clear however, that the natural history of VIN is not comparable to that of CIN, being more indolent than the latter.

Spontaneous regression of VIN is well documented, particularly for the milder forms. For VIN 3 spontaneous regression rates as high as 38% have been reported.[10] Multifocal lesions in young women are most likely to regress untreated as are lesions detected during pregnancy.[6] Woodruff et al[32] have suggested that VIN in young women may simply be a proliferative response to viral infection and not a preinvasive disorder, so accounting for the high rates of regression.

The risk of progression to invasive disease is reported to be low, varying between 2 and 4%.[32,33] Lesions most likely to progress have aneuploid patterns[34] which do not revert to normal diploidy as in the case of regressive disease. Malignant transformation usually occurs in unifocal VIN lesions, in women over the age of 45 years, and in those who are immunosuppressed.[6,35-37] Invasion has also been reported more frequently in patients with multiple intraepithelial neoplasia of the anogenital tract.[23,33,38] The depth of invasion in the majority of these lesions has been reported as less than 5 mm (microinvasion/'early' squamous carcinoma of the vulva).[39,40]

CLINICAL PRESENTATION OF VIN

VIN may present in many guises, affecting women over a wide age range from as young as 15 years[3] to some in their 80s.[5,11] The majority of recent reports indicate that the age at presentation has dropped to the third or early fourth decade of life.

There is a dearth of information on the association between VIN and the race and parity of affected individuals. What literature there is pertaining to this, suggests that the disease is more common in white women and is not significantly related to parity.[5,41]

Presenting symptoms

The most frequent presenting symptom is *vulvar pruritus*. It is complained of by over 40% of patients and maybe severe and intractable. Other symptoms commonly reported include vulvar burning and/or soreness, superficial dyspareunia, warts or other lesions noticed by the patient. Less frequently patients complain of abnormal vaginal discharge or bleeding, sensation of vulvar swelling and discoloration of the skin.[5,11,41-43] A review of the literature shows that the duration of symptoms may vary from as little as a few weeks to several years. The average duration of symptoms prior to medical consultation is about 2 years in about half the cases seen.

A substantial number of women are asymptomatic, VIN being detected during the course of routine gynecological examination or while investigating abnormal cervical cytology and screening for sexually-transmitted diseases. In two recent series over 50% of the patients were asymptomatic and had a past or concurrent history of multifocal lower genital tract neoplasia.[4,44]

Physical signs

The clinical appearance of VIN may vary from flat papules to raised warty lesions. They may vary in their number, size and distribution. Multifocal pigmented lesions are commonly seen in young patients and often coalesce to form confluent patches of disease.[9,10,45] The lesions may have a white, gray, brown or red colour. Lesions on the lateral cutaneous surface of the vulva are normally white hyperkeratotic plaques — leukoplakia, whereas lesions on the medial surface of the labia minora are pink or red macules. 'Pigment incontinence' is found in approximately one third of all cases of VIN, and refers to the diffuse distribution of melanin throughout the epithelium instead of its normal confinement in the basal keratinocytes. Lesions of varying appearance and coloration may be seen occurring together in the same patient. Discrete unifocal lesions are usually seen in older women.

Other presenting features seen less commonly include fissuring, ulceration and generalized erythema. In some patients the only abnormality may be colposcopically detectable acetowhitening of the vulvar epithelium. One study has reported detection rates with an accuracy as high as 84% when epidermal thickening and discoloration were present together.[46]

VIN changes can occur in both the hair-bearing and the non-hairbearing areas, with a slight predilection for the latter. Extension into skin appendages such as the sweat glands and pilose-baceous units has been described.[18,47] Although some authors have suggested that the posterior vulvar skin — perineum, fourchette and perianal areas — has the highest rate of involvement,[41] lesions may involve any part of the vulva. Contiguous extension to the anus and vagina has been reported in less than 20% of cases. Reports of clitoral involvement range from 6 to 70% in different series.[19,41,48]

VIN is known to coexist with other genital tract neoplasias. Between 20 and 40% of women with VIN 3 have associated CIN and, 25–38% had associated CIN and vaginal intraepithelial neoplasia (VAIN).[11,41,43,49]

DIAGNOSIS OF VIN

The entire vulva is examined using the colposcope set initially at low or medium magnifications. The application of normal saline or a clear lubricant prior to the use of acetic acid, often aids the visualization of abnormal vascular patterns.

The vulva and perianal areas are colposcoped again after prolonged application of 5% acetic acid. It may take up to 5 min for the full development of acetowhite changes in the epithelium. The obscuring effects of keratin, hyperkeratosis and lichenification from chronic scratching make visualization of abnormal vascular patterns of mosaicism, punctation or atypical branching, very difficult. The medial surface of the labia minora and the periurethral area have nonkeratinized epithelium which allows better visualization of vascular changes. Features of subclinical or overt HPV infection may also interfere with the colposcopic diagnosis of VIN and invasive disease. The final diagnosis therefore, is invariably a histological one and requires full thickness skin biopsies from suspicious areas identified colposcopically.

Vulvar biopsies are easily performed under local anesthetic using the 3–4 mm diameter Keyes punch. Depending on the distribution of the lesions and their clinical appearance multiple biopsies may be necessary. Lesions with features of invasion — rapid increase in size, ulceration and abnormal vascular proliferation — should be widely excised under general anesthetic in preference to punch biopsies.

In view of the frequent association of multicentric lesions the whole lower genital tract and anal canal must be assessed colposcopically and abnormal areas biopsied.

The Collins Toluidine Blue test is also occasionally valuable although the results obtained can be misleading. Toluidine Blue (1%), a nuclear dye was previously used to identify areas of parakeratosis and abnormal maturation with nuclear atypia in the superficial epithelial cells. False-positive staining can occur in normal excoriated skin, while abnormal hyperkeratotic areas may stain poorly despite their malignant nature. Similarly, exfoliative cytology which yields little useful information, has also been abandoned.

A permanent record of lesion morphology may be obtained by simple colpophotographic documentation or by using more sophisticated digital imaging techniques. This not only provides a record for follow-up after treatment but also allows natural history studies on VIN of which there is a great dearth.

MANAGEMENT OF VIN

Factors to be considered in planning the management of patients with VIN include:

1. age of the patient and her general medical condition;
2. symptoms;
3. distribution and focality of the lesions;
4. involvement of skin appendages;
5. malignant potential of the lesions;
6. preservation of the structure and function of the vulvoperineal unit;
7. psychological issues; and
8. recurrence rates.

Various treatment options have been suggested and employed in the management of VIN, but as yet no definitive cure has emerged for the condition. Existing treatment modalities have yet to be evaluated in a prospective randomized manner. High rates of recurrence have been reported irrespective of the method used.[1,35] The importance of individualizing management cannot be overemphasized. Table 10.1 shows the broad categories of management.

Conservative management

Observation

The increasing occurrence of VIN lesions of low malignant potential in young women, demands the adoption of a conservative therapeutic approach which avoids both physical disfiguration and psychological damage to the patient. An expectant policy is justified in these patients

Table 10.1 Broad categories of management

Conservative	Radical
Observation	Skinning vulvectomy + grafts
Wide local excision	Simple vulvectomy
Laser vaporization	
Cryocautery	
5′-Fluorouracil	
Dichloronitrobenzene	
Interferons	

particularly as high rates of spontaneous regression have been reported,[5,6] progression to invasion being extremely rare below the age of 40. Similarly, asymptomatic indolent lesions and lesions first detected in pregnancy may also be managed expectantly.

Patients must be informed of the need for long-term follow-up involving colposcopy and interval biopsies to exclude malignant transformation. Accurate documentation of lesions is essential at each visit, and is best recorded photographically or by digital image capture techniques.

Surgical

The treatment of VIN is basically surgical. Surgical removal of lesions allows accurate histological diagnosis to be reached. Therapeutic intervention in young women is indicated only when distressing symptoms develop, lesions enlarge or ulcerate and bleed. Occasionally the patient may request removal of disfiguring lesions. Malignant transformation may occur in women who are immunosuppressed or have a history of neoplasia elsewhere in the genital tract. Older women, over the age of 45 years, are at a low but slightly increased risk of developing cancer.[5,50] In order to avoid anatomical deformity and to preserve the function of the vulvoperineal unit it is important to limit the amount of tissue that is surgically excised.

Wide local excision

Either a knife or laser on cutting supermode, may be used to widely excise unifocal or discrete multifocal lesions, the optimum margin of excision being 0.8–1 cm. The epidermis and dermis are undercut until the whole lesion has been removed. The wound is then closed with fine absorbable sutures. Primary closure of defects is achieved easily due to the laxity of tissues in this area, and postoperative deformity is minimal. Recurrence rates as high as 32% have been reported following wide excision treatment of VIN lesions.[5,25] Although margin involvement correlates closely with high recurrence rates, lesions may reappear even where the margins are free of disease.

Laser vaporization

Carbon dioxide laser vaporization of VIN lesions is usually performed under general anesthetic and is the treatment modality of choice when extensive multifocal disease affects young women. Small lesions may be ablated under local anesthesia. Early reports of laser surgery for VIN recommended a uniform depth of vaporization to 3 mm for all areas of the vulva.[51] More recently this policy has been described as unnecessarily hazardous in areas like the labia minora and clitoris where the skin thickness is less than 3 mm.[52] Lesions occurring in hairbearing areas are best removed by wide local excision as the VIN changes may involve skin appendages down to a depth of 4 mm.[18] Uniform laser ablation to a depth of 3 mm as suggested earlier would therefore fail to eradicate the disease in hairbearing areas of the vulva. On the other hand, deeper ablation would result in greater tissue destruction and slow cicatrization. Attempts have been made to measure the thickness of VIN epithelium and to tailor the depth of laser vaporization accordingly.[17,47] These studies suggest that laser vaporization to a depth of 2.5 mm will eradicate over 98% of VIN in hairbearing areas without totally destroying the pilosebaceous unit. Deeper ablations may result in superficial dyspareunia due to lack of lubrication from the destroyed sebaceous glands.

Laser ablation treatment produces considerable postoperative pain and edema but is acceptable to patients as the end result is cosmetically and functionally excellent. Recurrence rates of between 5 and 40% have been reported.[52-55] The main worry with this method of treatment is the possibility of inappropriately treating early invasion, missed at prior colposcopic assessment.

Cryocautery

This method is now no longer used as the depth of tissue destruction is inadequate for elimination of the disease, requiring repeated treatments and resulting in cosmetic deformity of the vulva.[6]

Medical

Topical 'chemoimmunotherapy' has been tried

in women who refuse surgery or have recurrent multifocal disease. The therapeutic effects of these agents on the vulva may be limited by their reduced absorption through the layers of keratin. Results of treatment have been disappointing, with few responses and high complication and recurrence rates.

5-Fluorouracil

5-Fluorouracil exerts its anticancer action by inhibiting DNA synthesis in the 'S' phase of cell division. In addition, it may be incorporated into the neoplastic cell and acts as a cell marker for the immune system to recognise and destroy.[56]

In the treatment of VIN, failure rates of greater than 75% have been reported[26] with many patients abandoning treatment due to severe vulvar pain and pruritus.

Dinitrochlorobenzene

This agent reverses vulvar atypia by inducing a type of delayed hypersensitivity reaction on topical application.[56,57] Patients often discontinue therapy due to side-effects.

Interferons

Topical gels and intralesional injections of α-interferon have been used to some benefit in the treatment of VIN.[58] Complete response rates of about 60% have been reported and side-effects are mild flu-like symptoms. Interferons act by reducing viral (HPV) multiplication and inhibiting cell proliferation.

Radical treatment of VIN

There is now a definite trend away from the radical surgical management of VIN as the outcome of such procedures is unsatisfactory, often leaving the vulva grossly disfigured and the patient psychologically scarred.[59,62] Sexual function may be significantly disrupted and patients may find psychosexual adjustment after radical vulvar surgery very difficult. However, such extensive surgery may be the only effective treatment open to women with widespread symptomatic disease with a distinct risk of invasion.

Skinning vulvectomy with skin grafting

This procedure was first described by Rutledge and Sinclair in 1968.[60] It is indicated in young women with multifocal disease affecting the hairbearing areas where laser treatment would be inappropriate because the depth of ablation required would result in gross deformity. It can also be used to treat unifocal lesions too large to treat by wide excision and primary closure.

Skinning vulvectomy involves the wide excision of vulvar lesions, cutting through the relatively avascular tissue immediately deep to the dermis. The subcutaneous tissue is vascular and forms a good graft bed. Every attempt is made to preserve the clitoris and any clitoral lesion is either shaved off it using a scalpel blade or superficially ablated with laser.

A split-thickness skin graft from the thigh is used to cover the vulvar defect. Alternatively, local flap or pedicle grafts maybe used resulting in less contractures and hence better preservation of vulvar anatomy.

Recurrence rates of 12–30% have been documented following this procedure,[7,39,41] with recurrences occurring in grafted and ungrafted skin.[61] In one series of patients who underwent this procedure graft rejection was noted in less than 15% and patients were able to resume sexual relations within 6–8 weeks, with no complaints of dyspareunia.[41]

Simple vulvectomy

This operation has little to recommend it in the treatment of VIN. It is a mutilating procedure associated with an understandably high incidence of psychosexual sequelae. Recurrences occur with the same frequency as in other treatments. Repeated local wide excisions are preferable to a simple vulvectomy in young women. The only place for this operation appears to be for the symptomatic relief of elderly patients with extensive VIN 3, in whom it is important to rule out occult cancer.

CONCLUSION

VIN though increasingly encountered in clinical practice remains a poorly understood condition. Little is known about its development, its presentation is variable, its diagnosis difficult and its treatment suboptimal. In the presence of so much uncertainty it is unjustified to subject patients with the disease to radical treatments of doubtful benefit. Until such time as more is known about the condition, treatment should be conservative and individualized. Patients should be closely monitored to detect any suspicious changes and to further our knowledge of the natural history of the disorder.

MULTIFOCAL DISEASE (MIN)

Whether MIN is a separate entity or a natural progression of some types of VIN or CIN is unknown and probably academic. For the purposes of definition MIN can be described as intraepithelial change in squamous epithelium occurring either simultaneously or at intervals in the lower genital tract. The lesions should be separated by normal squamous epithelium. This statement underlies the fact that the malignant process is occurring multicentrically and lesions do not involve adjacent sites by direct extension. The sites involved are:

— Cervix
— Vagina
— Vulva
— Perineum
— Anal canal
— Natal cleft

Any combination or all of these sites may be affected, either simultaneously, or in succession. Although it is still a relatively rare disorder clinical experience suggests a recent increase in the incidence of the condition but whether this reflects a true increase in disease or merely a greater awareness and detection of lesions, is not clear. There is little mention of MIN in medical literature and very few centers have any experience in its management.

Intraepithelial neoplasia affecting individual discrete sites such as the cervix, vagina and vulva have been extensively investigated in recent times, but the exact etiology, pathogenesis and natural history of this condition remains obscure. Even less is understood about MIN.

ETIOLOGY

It is well established that women with a history of CIN or invasive carcinoma are at increased risk of developing similar lesions in other parts of the lower genital tract, specifically the vagina and vulva, 25% of women with vulvar carcinoma have had cervical neoplasia at some time in their life. This has led to the concept of a 'field effect' involving the squamous epithelium of the anogenital tract.

Field change has already been suggested as a possible cause for observation of multicentric disease. The precise mechanism of such change is not understood. Recent observation of the interaction between viral oncoproteins and recognized tumor suppresser genes, particularly in CIN do support the concept of multistage, multicentric malignant transformation in the squamous epithelium of the lower genital tract. Our own clinical observation on certain subgroups of patients with MIN suggest that apart from lower genital tract malignancies, distant malignancies are more common. This would support a role for suppresser gene inactivation and or mutation in this disease. Furthermore there is a greater incidence of immunosuppression in patients with MIN.

Viral infections have been suggested as possible etiological factors in the development of multifocal squamous neoplasia of the female genital tract. The most commonly implicated agents are HPV, HSV and Epstein – Barr virus. Of the three, HPV most frequently affects the anogenital epithelium. Although HPV occurs as frequently in the vagina and vulva as on the cervix, the incidence of VAIN and VIN is much less than CIN. This is attributed to the absence of metaplastic squamous activity in the epithelium of the vulva and vagina which is believed to be important for the neoplastic activity of the virus. Women with a history of intrauterine diethylstilbestrol exposure who show metaplastic epithelial changes in the vagina are susceptible to viral oncogenic effects in this site. However, viral carcinogenesis alone is unlikely to be responsible for the development of MIN and several reports have indicated that local tissue immunosuppression resulting from the effects of cigarette smoking, or repeated exposure to seminal plasma, or previous radiation, could play a role in the development of this disorder. Immunocompromised patients have long been recognized as being at significantly increased risk of developing high-grade intraepithelial neoplasia and invasive disease in multiple sites. It is therefore most likely that all three factors — field change, viral infections and immunosuppression — are involved to varying degrees in the development of MIN.

PRESENTATION

MIN may be detected during the assessment of patients with abnormal smears, particularly those with recurrent cytological abnormalities following treatment. Colposcopically identifiable intraepithelial lesions may be seen involving the vulva, vagina and perineum.

A significant number of women present with long-standing vulvar symptoms, investigation of which may lead to the diagnosis of vulvar intraepithelial neoplasia and associated squamous lesions in other areas.

Regular and more intensive screening of high-risk patients, i.e. those on long-term immunosuppressive treatment for conditions such as organ transplants, autoimmune disorders, allergic conditions and cancer, or those with HIV-related problems may bring to light the presence of intraepithelial neoplasia in multiple sites.

NATURAL HISTORY OF MIN

The natural history of anogenital preinvasive disease is not well defined. The condition may arise independently, or be part of a generalized immunological disorder. In the case of cervical intraepithelial neoplasia, which has been extensively investigated, it is often assumed that progression to cancer occurs gradually from milder through more severe degrees of dysplasia to invasion. Although epidemiological studies would appear to support such a progression, there is however, no definite evidence for this incremental pattern of neoplastic change.

The natural history patterns of intraepithelial neoplasia occurring at multiple sites in the anogenital tract are not comparable. Very diverse disease incidence and rates of progression have been reported for the various lesions. For example, the rate of progression of VIN 3 to cancer is much lower than that of CIN 3, being reported as 2–4% over 10–15 years for the former, as compared to 36% for the latter.

The incidence of VAIN is approximately 0.2/100 000 women (CIN = 36.4/100 000) with over 70% of cases being associated with CIN. Approximately 25% of cases occur simultaneously with cervical lesions while others may develop anytime between 6 months to 16 years after the treatment of CIN.

It is possible that MIN represents abnormal clones of cells in the lower genital and anal tracts with each clone possessing its own degree of abnormality. Hence severely abnormal cells may develop at a particular site without necessarily being preceded by the minor changes. Varying degrees of abnormality may be found occurring either concurrently or successively in different parts of the anogenital tract. Likewise rates of progression and regression may vary from clone to clone.

The natural history of intraepithelial lesions is altered by diagnostic interventions and spontaneous regression too may occur from any level of abnormality.

MANAGEMENT

The clinical management of MIN poses a problem in that the measures required to treat the multiple disease sites may present as much or more of a risk to the well-being of the patient, as the disease itself.

Investigations for this condition are often as numerous as the sites involved. They include:

— Multiple biopsies;
— Full hematological and biochemical screening
— Viral subtyping
— HIV testing
— T-cell count and function

The biopsy should be colposcopically directed and be large enough to exclude invasion. The aim is to define disease extent and to identify the predisposing factors.

The management aims are chiefly to eradicate disease, alleviate symptoms and to preserve anatomical structure and function.

Cervical lesions are best managed separately, using an excisional technique. The upper vaginal lesions may be treated using laser ablation after excluding invasive disease, or by hysterectomy with removal of a vaginal cuff. The lower vagina, perineum, anus and natal cleft are managed as a unit because preservation of function takes priority in the treatment of disease at these sites.

Repeated local ablation is an option for symptom control but suspicious areas must be excised. Skin grafting is usually required if extensive multifocal disease is removed. Wide skinning excision with full-thickness skin grafts are often used in combination with laser ablation of anal canal lesions. Two-stage procedures involving initial colostomy followed by excision of disease have also been attempted successfully where the anal canal and perineal skin has been affected.

The psychological and physical distress caused to these women is considerable. Treatment should only be undertaken after the patient and her partner have been fully counselled and understand the implications of such therapeutic procedures.

Newer approaches such as interferons and retinoids are being evaluated.

CONCLUSION

Although when present MIN often produces distressing symptoms, it fortunately remains an uncommon condition. It challenges medical skills, requiring a global approach to its management, additional colposcopic expertise for its diagnosis, and varied expert clinical and surgical approaches for its eradication.

The efficacy of treatment in terms of preventing cancer remains unproven and in addition there is a high risk of malignant change occurring in other parts of the body. The current emphasis therefore is to do the least required.

REFERENCES

1. Buckley C H, Butler E B, Fox H. Vulvar intraepithelial neoplasia and microinvasive carcinoma of the vulva. J Clin Pathol 1984; 37: 1201–1211.
2. Crum C P. Vulvar intraepithelial neoplasia: The concept and its application. Human Pathol 1982; 13.3: 187–189.
3. Woodruff J D. Carcinoma in situ of the vulva. Clin Obstet Gynecol 1985; 28: 230.
4. Hussienzadeh N, Newman N J, Wesseler T A. Vulva intraepithelial neoplaxia. A clinicopathological study of carcinoma in situ of the vulva. Gynecol Oncol 1989; 33: 157–163.
5. Buscema J, Woodruff J D, Parmley T H, Genandry R. Carcinoma in situ of the vulva. Obstet Gynecol 1980; 55: 225–230.
6. Freidrich E G, Wilkinson E J, Fu Y S. Carcinoma in situ of the vulva. A continuing challenge. Am J Obstet Gynecol 1980; 136: 830–838.
7. Caglar H, Delgado G, Hreshchyshyn M M. Partial and total skinning vulvectomy in treatment of carcinoma in situ of the vulva. Obstet Gynecol 1986; 68: 504–507.
8. Sturgeon S R, Brinton L A, Devesa S S, Kurman R J. In situ and invasive vulvar cancer incidence trends (1973–1987). Am J Obstet Gynecol 1992; 166: 1482–1485.
9. Hilliard G D, Massey F M, O'Toole R V. Vulvar neoplasia in the young. Am J Obstet Gynecol 1979; 135: 185–188.
10. Bernstein S G, Kovacs B R, Townsend D E, Morrow C P. Vulva carcinoma in situ. Obstet Gynecol 1983; 61: 304–337.
11. Shafi M I, Luesley D M, Byrne P, Samra J S, Redman C W, Jordan J A, Rollason T P. Vulvar intraepithelial neoplasia — management and outcome. Br J Obstet Gynecol 1989; 96: 1339–1344.
12. Henson D, Tarone R. An epidemiological study of cancer of the cervix, vagina and vulva based upon the Third National Cancer Survey in the United States. Am J Obstet Gynecol 1977; 129: 525–532.
13. Japaze H, Garcia-Bunuel R, Woodruff J D. Primary vulvar neoplasia: a review of in situ and invasive carcinoma, 1935–1972. Obstet Gynecol 1977; 49: 404.
14. Kaufmann R H, Bornstein J, Adam E et al. Human papillomavirus and herpes simplex virus in vulvar squamous cell carcinoma in situ. Am J Obstet Gynecol 1988; 158: 862–871.
15. Shokri-Tabibzadeh S, Koss L G, Molnar J, Romney S. Association of human papillomavirus with neoplastic processes in the genital tract of four women with impaired immunity. Gynecol Oncol 1981; 12: S129–S138.
16. Sillman F, Stanck A, Sedlis A et al. The relationship between human papillomavirus and genital intraepithelial neoplasia in immunosuppressed women. Am J Obstet Gynecol 1984; 150: 300–308.
17. Shatz P, Bergeron C, Wilkinson E J, Arseneau J,

Ferenczy A. Vulva intraepithelial neoplasia and skin appendage involvement. Obstet Gynecol 1989; 74: 769–774.

18. Mene A, Buckley C H. Involvement of the vulvar skin appendages by intraepithelial neoplasia. Br J Obstet Gynecol 1985; 92: 634–638.

19. Powell L C, Dinh T V, Rajaraman S et al. Carcinoma in situ of the vulva. A clinicopathologic study of 50 cases. J Reprod Med 1986; 31: 808.

20. Purola E, Savia E. Cytology of gynaecologic condyloma acuminatum. Acta Cytol 1977; 21: 26–31.

21. Pillotti S, Rilke F, Shah K V, Torre G D, De Palo G. Immunohistochemical and ultrastructural evidence of papillomavirus infection associated with in situ and microinvasive squamous cell carcinoma of the vulva. Am J Surg Pathol 1984; 8: 751–761.

22. Rastkar G, Okagaki T, Twiggs L B, Clark B A. Early invasive and in situ warty carcinoma of the vulva: Clinical, histologic and electron microscopic study with particular reference to viral association. Am J Obstet Gynecol 143, 814–820.

23. Hansen L H, Collins C G. Multicentric squamous cell carcinomas of the lower female genital tract. Am J Obstet Gynecol 1967; 98: 982–986.

24. Marcus S L. Multiple squamous cell carcinomas involving the cervix, vagina, and vulva: the theory of multicentric origin. Am J Obstet Gynecol 1960; 80: 802–812.

25. Andreasson B, Bock J E. Intraepithelial neoplasia in the vulvar region. Gynecol Oncol 1985; 21: 300–305.

26. Forney J P, Morrow C P, Townsend D E, DiSaia P J. Management of carcinoma in situ of the vulva. Am J Obstet Gynecol 1977; 127: 801–806.

27. Gissman L, de Villiers E M, zur Hausen H. Analysis of human genital warts (condylomata acuminata) and other genital tumours for human papillomavirus type 6 DNA. Int J Cancer 1982; 29: 143–146.

28. Ferenczy A. Intraepithelial neoplasia of the vulva. In: Coppleson M, ed. Gynaecologic oncology, vol 1. Edinburgh: Churchill Livingstone, 1990: pp 443–456.

29. Teiggs L B, Okagaki T, Clark B, Fukushima M, Ostrow R, Faras A. A clinical, histopathologic and molecular biologic investigation of vulvar intraepithelial neoplasia. Int J Gynecol Path 1988; 7: 48–55.

30. Zachow K R, Ostrow R, Bender M, Watts S, Okagaki T, Pass F, Faras A. Detection of human papillomavirus DNA in anogenital neoplasia. Nature 1982; 300: 771–773.

31. Penn I. Cancers of the anogenital region in renal transplant recipients. Cancer 1986; 58: 611.

32. Woodruff J D, Julian C G, Puray T et al. The contemporary challenge of carcinoma in situ of the vulva. Am J Obstet Gynecol 1973; 115: 667–686.

33. Jones R W, McLean M R. Carcinoma in situ of the vulva: a review of 31 treated and 5 untreated cases. Obstet Gynecol 1986; 68: 499–503.

34. Fu Y, Reagan J W, Townsend D E, Kaufman R H, Richart R M, Wentz W B. Nuclear DNA study of vulvar intraepithelial and invasive squamous neoplasms. Obstet Gynecol 1981; 57: 643–651.

35. Hording V, Danguard S, Iversen A K N, Knudsen J, Bock J E, Norrild B. Human papillomavirus Type 16 in vulvar carcinoma, vulvar intraepithelial neoplasia, and associated cervical neoplasia. Gynecol Oncol 1991; 42: 22–26.

36. Barbero M, Micheletti L, Preti M et al. Vulva intraepithelial neoplasia. A clinicopathologic study of 60 cases. J Reprod Med 1990; 35: 1023–1028.

37. Crum C P, Liskow A, Petras P, Keng W C, Frick H C. Vulvar intraepithelial neoplasia (severe atypia and carcinoma in situ). Cancer 1984; 54: 1429–1434.

38. Jimerson G K, Merrill J A. Multicentric squamous malignancy involving both cervix and vulva. Cancer 1970; 26: 150–153.

39. Rettenmaier M A, Verman M L, DiSaia P J. Skinning vulvectomy for the treatment of multifocal vulvar intraepithelial neoplasia. Obstet Gynecol 1987; 69: 247–250.

40. Collins C G, Roman-Lopez J J, Lee F Y L. Intraepithelial carcinoma of the vulva. Am J Obstet Gynecol 1970; 108: 1187–1191.

41. DiSaia P J, Rich W M. Surgical approach to multifocal carcinoma in situ of the vulva. Am J Obstet Gynecol 1981; 140: 136–145.

42. Boutselis J G. Intraepithelial carcinoma of the vulva. Am J Obstet Gynecol 1972; 113: 733–738.

43. Benedet J L, Murphy K J. Squamous carcinoma in situ of the vulva. Gynecol Oncol 1982; 14: 213–219.

44. Wolcott H D, Gallup D G. Wide local excision in the treatment of vulvar carcinoma in situ: A reappraisal. Am J Obstet Gynecol 1984; 150: 695–698.

45. Townsend D E, Levine R U, Richart R M, Crum C P, Pettrilli E S. Management of vulvar intraepithelial neoplasia by carbon dioxide laser. Obstet Gynecol 1982; 60: 49–52.

46. Singer A, Mitchell H. The treatment of vulvar premalignancy. In: Clinical practice of gynecology. New York: Elsevier, 1990.

47. Baggish M, Sze E, Adelson M et al. Quantitative evaluation of the skin and accessory appendages in vulvar carcinoma in situ. Obstet Gynecol 1989; 74: 169–173.

48. Benedet J L, Wilson P S, Matisic J. Epidermal thickness and skin appendage involvement in vulvar intraepithelial neoplasia. J Reprod Med 1991; 36(8): 608–612.

49. Sherman K J, Daling J R, Chu J et al. Multiple primary tumours in women with vulvar neoplasms: a case control study. Br J Cancer 1988; 57: 423–427.

50. Rusk D, Sutton G P, Look K Y, Roman A. Analysis of invasive squamous cell carcinoma of the vulva and vulvar intraepithelial neoplasia for the presence of human papillomavirus DNA. 1991; 77: 918–922.

51. Baggish M S, Dorsey J H. CO_2 laser for the treatment of vulvar carcinoma in situ. Obstet Gynecol 1981; 57: 371–375.

52. Wright V C, Davies E. Laser surgery for vulvar intraepithelial neoplasia; principles and results. Am J Obstet Gynecol 1987; 156: 374–378.

53. Levani H, Ziv E, Segal J, Tadir Y, Ovadia J. Carbon dioxide laser therapy for vulvar intraepithelial neoplasia. Colposcopy Gynecol Laser Surg 1988; 4(2): 95–99.

54. Ferenczy A. Using the laser to treat vulvar condylomata acuminata and intradermal neoplasia. Can Med Assoc J 1983; 128: 135–137.

55. Leuchter R S, Townsend D E Hacker N F, Pretorius R G, Lagasse L D, Wade M E. Treatment of vulvar carcinoma in situ with the CO_2 laser. Gynecol Oncol 1984; 29: 314.

56. Mansell P W, Litwin M S, Ichinose H et al. Delayed hypersensitivity to 5-fluorouracil following topical chemotherapy of cutaneous cancers. Cancer Res 1975; 35: 1288–1294.

57. Foster D C, Woodruff J D. The use of dinitrochlorobenzene in the treatment of vulvar carcinoma in situ. Gynecol Oncol 1981; 11: 330–339.

58. Spirtos N M, Smith L H, Teng N N H. Prospective randomised trial of topical alfa-interferon (alfa-interferon gels) for the treatment of vulvar intraepithelial neoplasia III. Gynecol Oncol 1990; 37: 34–38.

59. Anderson B L, Hacken N F. Psychosexual adjustment after vulvar surgery. Obstet Gynecol 1983; 62.4: 457–462.

60. Rutledge F, Sinclair M. Treatment of intraepithelial carcinoma of the vulva by skin excision and graft. Am J Obstet Gynecol 1968; 102: 806–818.

61. Cox S M, Kaufman R H, Kaplan A. Recurrent carcinoma in situ of the vulva in a skin graft. Am J Obstet Gynecol 1986; 155: 177–179.

62. Andersen B L, Turnquist D, LaPolla J, Turner D. Sexual functioning after treatment of in situ vulva cancer: preliminary report. Obstet Gynecol 1988; 71: 15–19.

11. Vulvar warts: clinical and subclinical

Alex Ferenczy

DEFINING LESIONS

Lesions that result from human papillomavirus (HPV) infections of the vulvar epithelium can be divided into two categories: clinically visible and clinically poorly to nonvisible, subclinical macules.[1]

Clinical vulvar lesions are usually referred to as condylomata acuminata or genital warts and can be further subdivided into *hyperplastic,* cauliflower type lesions, *sessile based* and *hyperkeratotic* lesions resembling verruca vulgaris or cutaneous warts. The hyperplastic variants are soft, pink to flesh-colored with a micropapillary surface and double loop central (feeding) capillaries. They typically are found on the moist surface of the nonhairy skin of the vulva, namely the inner surface of the labia minora, the vestibular epithelium, hymen and the urethral meatus (Fig. 11.1). Sessile condylomatous papules and the hyperkeratotic lesions tend to occur on the hairy skin on the vulva and the outer surface of the labia minora. These lesions are firm and vary in size. The surface of sessile and hyperkeratotic variants is micropapillary and macropapillary, respectively (Figs 11.2 and 11.3). Subclinical lesions by definition are *slightly elevated,* often confluent macules and are appreciated with the colposcope after the application of 5% acetic acid solution. They are most often located on the nonhairy skin of the vulva, particularly along the areas that are susceptible to trauma such as the labia minora, introitus and the posterior fourchette (Fig. 11.4). However, the hairy skin may also be involved with subclinical macules, often together with acuminate, hyperkeratotic condylomata (Table 11.1). For example, in a series of 100 consecutive patients referred for anogenital HPV infections, we ob-

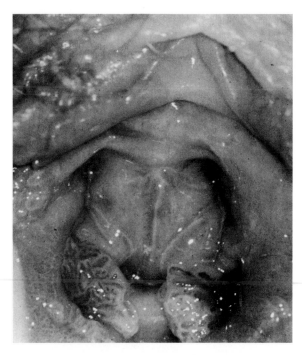

Fig. 11.1 Hyperplastic condylomata: Soft, papillary lesions in the vestibule arising from Bartholin's duct ostia. Note double looped capillaries in papillae.

served 38 of 55 (69%) subclinical, acetowhite macular lesions in association with acuminate condylomata.

THE CONDYLOMA MIMICS

These are presented in Table 11.2. Molluscum contagiosum, intradermal nevi and micropapillomatosis labialis (MPL) are the conditions most often confused with condylomata acuminata, whereas in the acetowhite subclinical lesion

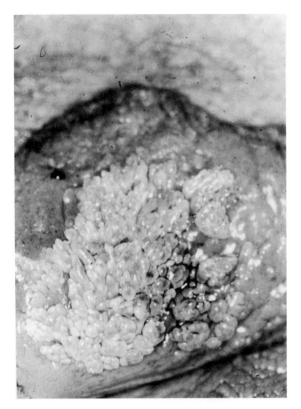

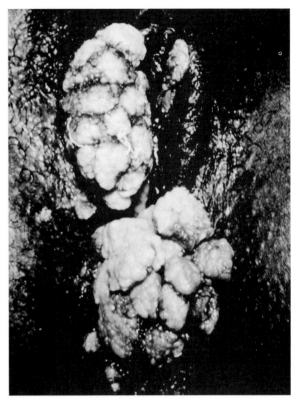

Fig. 11.2   Sessile-based lesions with micropapillary surface on labia minora.

Fig. 11.3   Hyperkeratotic condylomata on exterior surface of labia minora with macropapillary surface pattern.

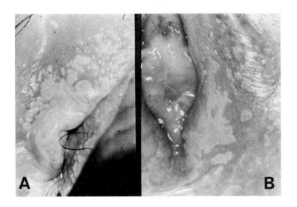

Fig. 11.4   Subclinical acetowhite macules on labia minora. **A** Note slightly elevated epithelium. **B** Acetowhite, confluent epithelium on the inner surface of vestibular skin. The patient had candidiasis and negative HPV test.

Table 11.1   Distribution of vulvar HPV infection by clinical and colposcopic presentation*

	Clinical Number	%	Subclinical Number	%
Nonhairy skin				
Labia minora, vestibule, hymen, urethra	20	44	31	56
Hairy skin				
Labia majora	8	18	7	13
Both	17	38	17	31
Total	45	100	55	100

* 100 consecutive referral patients.

category are candidiasis, contact dermatitis and folliculitis.

Molluscum contagiosum presents as scattered and occasionally clustered papules which, on high magnification inspection contain an umbilicated center and a smooth, rather than a papillary surface. They are most often located on the hairy skin of the vulva with great predilection for the pubic area. In our experience, about 10% of patients with condylomata acuminata also have molluscum contagiosum of the external genitals.[1] Occasionally, molluscum contagiosum may grow

Table 11.2   Condyloma mimics of the vulva

Molluscum contagiosum
Micropapillomatosis labialis (MPL)
Intradermal nevus
VIN (bowenoid papulosis)
Hypertrophic sebaceous glands
Lichen nitidus
Seborrheic keratosis
Folliculitis
Vulvar dermatoses:
   Candidiasis
   Contact dermatitis
   Lichen simplex chronicus
   Lichen planus
   Psoriasis, etc.

to pea size and the surface may be slightly papillary without central umbilication. If a biopsy is obtained, histology is diagnostic.

Intradermal nevus presents as either a pigmented or nonpigmented elevated lesion. Its surface may be slightly papillary and it is usually located on the hairy skin of the vulva and perineal/perianal area. In the nonpigmented cases, histology is diagnostic.

MPL consists of clinically visible, finger-like papillary projections located on the inner labial, vestibular and hymenal epithelium (Figs 11.5A and 11.5B). Typically, the condition is bilateral, symmetrical, and unlike acuminate condylomata in which multiple papillary projections converge to a single base, in MPL each finger-like papilla has its own base (Figs 11.1–11.3). The vast majority of patients with MPL are fair-skinned, young women aged less than 40 years, and a significant proportion have had recurrent urogenital infections particularly candidiasis.[2] Vulvar pain (vulvodynia) in the form of pruritus and burning before or after the menstrual periods (cyclic vulvitis) and dyspareunia *after* intercourse are the most significant clinical manifestations of MPL. Earlier morphologic and immunohistochemical studies suggested that MPL is HPV-related because HPV antigen was found in some patients with MPL by immunoperoxidase technique.[3] However, more recently, two independent correlative studies using molecular hybridization technology failed to demonstrate HPV DNA rates higher than those found in the control population, namely 6% and 8% in the Bergeron et al[2] and the Moyal-Barracco et al[4] study, respectively. The currently available data do not support the HPV-relatedness of most cases of MPL. Rather it represents a nonspecific, 'hypertrophic', epithelial–stromal reaction to chronic, recurrent vulvovaginal candidiasis and/or other urogenital infections.

Patients with symptomatic MPL are best managed by long-term topical and/or oral medications according to the infectious agents or irritants identified or suspected. For example, MPL patients with candidiasis respond well to oral fluconazole (Diflucan, Pfizer), 100 mg 2/week for 3–6 months. The use of nondrying vaginal lubricating gels during intercourse helps to relieve further local irritation due to friction. In nonresponding patients with longstanding dyspareunia and vaginismus, psychosexual dysfunction may be a contributing factor, and if confirmed, the patient should be managed accordingly.

It is important for the vulvoscopist to distinguish between acetowhite macules and acetowhite epithelium (Figs 11.4A and 11.5). Acetowhitening is *not pathognomonic* of HPV infection, although in both instances a positive staining reaction occurs with 5% acetic acid solution. Subclinical, aceto-white macules are slightly elevated, often contain punctate vessels and are likely to be HPV-induced (Fig. 11.6A). Acetowhite epithelium is not elevated, is devoid of vascular structures and is unlikely to be related to HPV infection (Fig. 11.6B). Contact dermatitis and vulvar candidiasis are frequently associated with acetowhite epithelium.

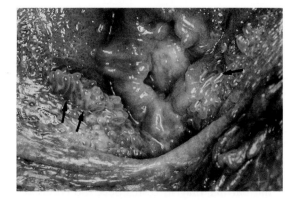

Fig. 11.5   Micropapillomatosis labialis. Both the labial and vestibular epithelium contain numerous finger-like projections. The involvement is symmetrical. Each finger-like projection has its own base (arrows) compared to the branching pattern of acuminate condylomata (Fig. 11.2).

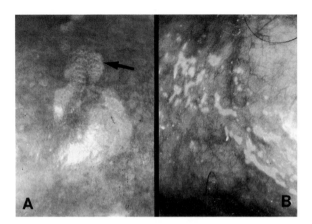

Fig. 11.6 Subclinical lesions. **Left** Slightly elevated acetowhite papules with punctate vessels (arrow) typical of subclinical HPV infection. **Right** Acetowhite epithelium presenting as 'flakes'. Such findings are not specific of HPV infection. The patient had chronic candidiasis.

When in doubt, it may be appropriate to obtain tissue specimens for histology. Acetowhite subclinical macules contain acanthosis (hence their elevated nature) and surface parakeratosis. Koilocytosis, the morphologic hallmark of HPV infection may be inconspicuous. In such cases, molecular demonstration of HPV DNA by in situ hybridization may help to establish the diagnosis. Biopsies obtained from acetowhite epithelium uniformly lack koilocytosis (which by definition contains nuclear atypia) and often have morphologic alterations including inflammatory exudate and epithelial cell degeneration chiefly located at the epithelial–dermal interface. In cases of candidiasis, hyphae are seen with the PAS stain in the upper epithelial strata.

EPIDEMIOLOGY

Despite a wealth of clinical, morphologic and molecular data on genital HPV infections, information on the precise prevalence and incidence of anogenital condylomata in nonselected populations are fragmentary at best. Nevertheless, in young adults attending health clinics or sexually-transmitted disease (STD) clinics, a steady increase in the prevalence of overt condylomata acuminata of the external anogenital skin has been reported in Europe and North America as well as, in Australia from the early 1980s to the late 1980s.[5] In general, the prevalence has doubled to tripled in Western countries with a rate of 9% and 13% of female and male patients, respectively, at risk of STDs.[5] In another epidemiologic survey, 1% of sexually active females and males aged 15–49 years were estimated to carry clinically overt condylomata of the anogenital skin.[5] Ever-smoking women and those on long-term (5 or more years) use of oral contraceptives have, respectively, a 3.7 and 9.8 times relative risk for developing genital warts.[6] Data on the prevalence or incidence of subclinical vulvar macular lesions are not available; however, on the basis of personal experience, they seem to be more frequent than overt clinical lesions (Table 11.1).

CLINICAL SIGNIFICANCE

The vast majority (95%) of vulvar condylomata acuminata contain low oncogenic-risk HPV types, namely types 6 or 11, and neoplastic transformation of overt warts is an extremely rare event.[5-7] The so-called giant condyloma of Buschke–Löwenstein is in fact a very well differentiated squamous cell carcinoma which is believed to develop de novo from an HPV 6 infected genital tract squamous epithelium (Fig. 11.7). Although both clinical and subclinical HPV-related lesions are frequent, invasive carcinoma of the vulva is a rare disease and has not increased in incidence for the past 30–40 years.[8] It appears that from a clinical point of view, histologically benign HPV infections of the vulvar skin in the nonimmunodepressed patient lack significant cancer risk potential. However, overt lesions are cosmetically and many times psychologically unacceptable to informed patients, and both clinical and subclinical macules may be a source of sexually-transmittable viruses. About 5% of acuminate and 50% of subclinical acetowhite lesions contain high to intermediate oncogenic risk HPV types by molecular hybridization and PCR technology.[9] These viruses, when contracted by the male sexual partner may in turn infect the cervix of a new sexual partner perpetuating HPV infections, and in the susceptible individuals, contribute to the development of cervical cancer and its precursors.

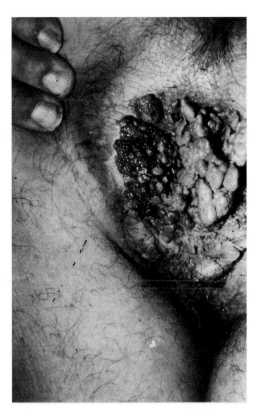

Fig. 11.7 Verrucous carcinoma of anus. The entire anal orifice is replaced by vegetative papillary lesions which histologically contained voluminous rete pegs extending deep into the dermis.

MECHANISMS OF TRANSMISSION

Most clinical and subclinical lesions are considered to be sexually transmitted by developing direct lesion-to-genital-skin contact between an infected and uninfected person.[10–12] In general, recently developed (less than 4 months) clinically visible condylomata have high viral load, and at least in one study viral type and copy number together with duration and frequency of exposure were related to increased potential for transmission.[13] In this study, HPV 6 was the most frequent viral type (73%) in the warts of both of the heterosexual partners, and the mean copy numbers of HPV 6 was much higher in couples with both partners infected (20 000/cell) than in those with only one partner infected (5000/cell). Also, couples in which both partners had warts had sexual relationships of longer duration (mean 22 months) than did the couples in which only one partner

was infected (mean 17 months). Oriel[10] found that men whose sexual contacts developed condylomata had had their lesions for an average of 3.5 months prior to sexual intercourse, whereas men whose female sexual contacts remained disease-free had had their lesions for an average of 1 year. These observations seem to correlate with molecular studies in which viral replication was noted to be at its maximum during the first 4 months of lesional tissue development.[14]

While the mechanism of HPV infection is largely venereal, it is not necessarily so in every case of genital warts. Autoinoculation of HPV from one anatomic site to another (vulva first, perianal skin after and vice versa) is a relatively common phenomenon; heteroinoculation is another way to acquire HPV infection. About two-thirds of intraanal condylomata are a result of anodigital insertion in patients with perianal condylomata.[15] Lesbians have external anogenital condylomata (without prior sexual intercourse with HPV-infected men); oral lesions contain genital type HPVs[16] and can develop in susceptible individuals as a result of frequent oral sex.[17] Subungual squamous cell carcinomas contain genital type oncogenic HPV 16 or 18.[18] Children and infants born from mothers with anogenital warts may very rarely become infected during delivery and develop recurrent (formerly juvenile) laryngeal papillomatosis (RLP) or warts in the anogenital area.[12] In the latter case, the lesions typically develop at a distance from the introitus or the anal orifice and appear in infants less than nine months of age.[19] HPVs are highly site specific, but occasionally warts in the genital area contain nongenital type HPVs.[20] In a recent study[21] 7 of 34 children with anogenital warts tested positive for HPV type 2, two of them had a similar virus type in their subungual warts and the parents of three children had HPV type 2 positive common hand warts.

The degree of exposure to the lesion(s) and cell-mediated immunity or the host's defence against HPV infection are suspected to be important factors for contracting or not contracting HPV, although hard data on the HPV-immune state 'connection' are not on hand. Similarly, information on periods of HPV incubation are limited. In fact, there is only one prospective study that specifically addressed this issue by following 88 persons who had sexual intercourse with those known to have external genital condylomata at the time.[10] After 9 months, 60% of them had developed genital warts, with an average incubation time of 2.8 months (range 3 weeks to 8 months). In another retrospective study of children, the incubation period ranged from one month to 20 months.[22]

Non-sexual transmission via fomites may occur although scientific evidence in support of this concept is lacking. Indeed, HPV does not grow in cell cultures and thus the issue remains unanswered. Nevertheless, HPV DNA has been identified on various instruments used in patients with genital HPV infections including speculum,[23] gloves, biopsy punches, cryoprobe tips, CO_2 laser- and electrosurgery-generated plume of smoke,[24-26] and the underwear of patients with external anogenital warts.[27] HPV DNA was found by Southern blot hybridization in 65, 45 and 10% of warts exposed for 5 min to liquid nitrogen ($-196°C$), podofilotoxin and 5% trichloroacetic acid, respectively.[28] Unfortunately, none of these studies was able to demonstrate whether the HPV DNA identified was in the form of virion with the potential for infection or if the HPV DNA was devoid of its protein coat. In the latter situation, HPV is not considered to be infectious. It may be pertinent to note, however, that bovine papillomaviruses isolated in the plume of smoke generated by the CO_2 laser or electrosurgical generator remained infectious in a tissue culture bioassay.[29] From a clinical point of view, the most appropriate means to avoid using 'contaminated' instruments is to clean them in formaldehyde containing solutions or expose them to heat in an autoclave or by steaming at over 100°C for at least 10 min.

EVALUATING THE PATIENT WITH VULVAR WARTS

HPV infection of the vulvar skin is almost always multifocal and may be associated with HPV infections in other sites of the female lower genital tract (multisite disease), particularly the cervix (Fig. 11.8A–11.8C). In several studies of patients with external anogenital condylomata, the cervix

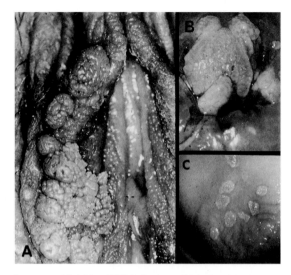

Fig. 11.8 Multisite HPV infections. **Left** Condylomata acuminata of vulva. **Upper right** Same patient with acetowhite lesion with granular surface of cervix. **Lower right** Multifocal punched out lesions in the vagina with similar color tone and surface pattern to that of the cervical lesion. Histologically, both lesions were of the low grade squamous intraepithelial neoplasia type.

was found to be involved by HPV infection in from 25 to 100% of the cases.[1,30,31] It may thus be appropriate to examine with the colposcope the perianal skin, the vagina and the cervix in patients with vulvar disease. In practices in which colposcopy is not available, the cervix, vagina and anus should be examined thoroughly with the naked eyes, and if clinically visible lesions are not seen, an exoendocervical Papanicolaou (Pap) test be taken.

In the experience of the author, HPV infection of the urethra is relatively infrequent (Table 11.1), but when present it is almost always associated with lesions of the vulva and perianal skin. Meatal lesions are of the soft, hyperplastic type, and in the vast majority of the cases they are confined to the posterior meatus. The distal end (fossa navicularis) of the urethra may be examined with the colposcope at 7× or 15× magnification by gently dilating the orifice using either an endocervical speculum or a nasal speculum. In the rare cases of extensive intraurethral condylomatosis, in which the inner limit of the lesional tissue cannot be visualized with the colposcope, a urethrocystoscopy should be requested from a urologist colleague.

It is debatable whether typical vulvar warts must be biopsied prior to therapy. The advantage of obtaining a histologic diagnosis is to verify the clinical impression. In legal cases, it serves as evidence of disease for which the treatment was delivered. All other lesions that may resemble condyloma but clinically are not typical of condylomata acuminata or are suspicious of cancer must be investigated by histology (Table 11.2). Such lesions include confluent verrucous lesions (Fig. 11.7) pigmented, papular disease (Fig. 11.9), red, raised, infected bleeding growths (Fig. 11.10), and treatment-resistant lesions.

The application of 5% acetic acid solution to the external anogenital skin using either a vinegar-soaked 4" × 4" sponge or spraying the skin with vinegar is of value only in cases in which the Pap test is positive but neither the cervix nor the vagina contain obvious lesions. Indeed, in such instances, HPV-related subclinical macular lesions may be demonstrated on the inner surface of the labial epithelium and/or posterior fourchette and be the source of the abnormal Pap test (Fig. 11.4). Another frequent cause of abnormal Pap tests without cervical-vaginal lesions is micropapillomatosis labialis (MPL) with acetowhite surface parakeratosis (Fig. 11.5A and 11.5B) (Table 11.2). In these instances, parakeratotic cells desquamate, are 'retrotransported' to the vaginal fornices and recovered in the cervicovaginal samples when taking a Pap test. In cytology laboratories in which parakeratosis is considered suggestive of HPV infections, overcalls are often made. Hence, once cervical disease, including that in the canal, has been ruled out and the benign nature of the asymptomatic vulvar condition is verified, the

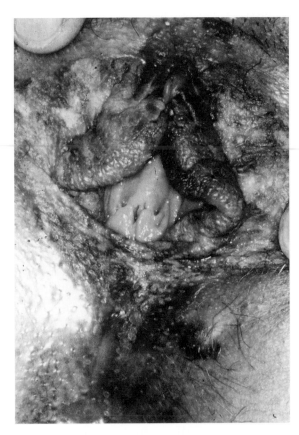

Fig. 11.9 Vulvar intraepithelial neoplasia. Pigmented to whitish, multifocal papules of the vulva consistent with 'bowenoid papulosis'.

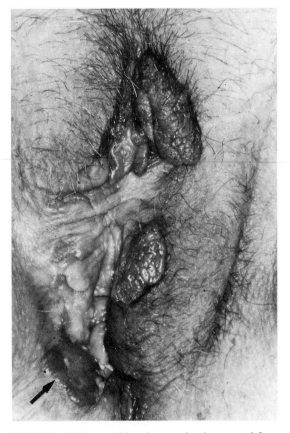

Fig. 11.10 A 58-year-old patient previously operated for condylomata acuminata. Now presents with recurrent warts and a slightly elevated ulcer (arrow) which on wide excision proved to be invasive squamous cell carcinoma.

patient may be followed on an annual basis and a cone biopsy thus avoided.

The clinical pertinence of demonstrating subclinical macular lesions that may coexist with acuminate condylomata is subject to debate. Some investigators reported better cure rates (87%) of clinical warts when coexistent subclinical macules were included in the treatment-field using the so-called extended CO_2 laser surgery technique.[32] Curiously, in a later study, the same investigators reported only 40% cure rates with extended CO_2 laser ablation of genital warts.[33] These rates are similar to those which have been reported by others after laser surgery without removal of coexisting subclinical macules.[34–36]

In cases in which the histological diagnosis is uncertain as to the HPV-relatedness of the lesional tissue, consultation with a pathologist with expertise in gynecologic dermatopathology may be appropriate. As suggested earlier, an alternative approach is to process the formalin-fixed paraffin-embedded biopsy specimen for in situ hybridization with one of the commercially available HPV DNA detection kits or the polymerase chain reaction technique.

There are also other clinical situations in which viral testing may help to make the appropriate management decisions. These include immunosuppressed patients whose condylomatous lesions are refractory to standard therapy, those with extensive, asymptomatic subclinical macules and patients who practice polygamous sexual relationships but do not wish to be treated. If they test positive for high oncogenic-risk HPVs, they should be followed at regular 6–12 month intervals. Although data with respect to risk of progression to invasive disease in the two latter types of patients are not available, immunocompromised patients may be at higher risk of developing malignancy than their immunocompetent counterparts.[37] In one recent study, 14 of 39 cases of condylomata acuminata were positive for both low and high oncogenic risk HPVs, particularly in immunosuppressed individuals.[38] Patients with low oncogenic risk HPV positive lesions are not at risk for cancer, however, those who are polygamous, should be encouraged to use condoms in an effort to control HPV transmission. In pediatric patients with external anogenital warts

and without clinical evidence of sexual abuse, HPV typing may 'exonerate' a suspected molester.

THE IMMUNOSUPPRESSED PATIENT

A number of clinical observations made over the past 20 years indicate that the response to therapy for genital HPV infections is comparatively less favorable in patients with cell-mediated immunodepression than in their nonimmunocompromised counterparts.[38] For example, in most patients with lymphoproliferative diseases, Crohn's disease, sarcoidosis, renal transplants, AIDS, etc., despite multiple attempts at therapy, cure of disease more often than not is fruitless. Also, these patients tend to have more extensive disease than those with an intact immune system.

Kidney transplant patients have been shown to be at increased risk for HPV-related cervical neoplasia, cutaneous warts and cancer,[38] as well as genital warts and probably external anogenital tract neoplasia. In one study of 107 transplant recipients, a 17-fold increase in the rate of low-grade and nine-fold increase in the rate of high-grade squamous intraepithelial lesions was observed when compared to an immunocompetent cohort.[39] The rates of anogenital condylomata in renal transplantees range from 10 to 45%.[39] The rate of anogenital cancer in renal transplant recipients and other immunocompromised patients is not known and information on this issue is mainly anecdotal. In one study of 120 kidney transplantees, six (15%) patients had anogenital squamous cell carcinomas two of which were HPV 16 positive.[39] All of the six patients with cancer also had warts. In another report, invasive carcinoma developed from vulvar condylomata in four immunosuppressed patients.[40] The same trend seems to occur in patients with primary immunodeficiency diseases, including lymphoproliferative disease, Hodgkin's disease and AIDS.[37] Since all these conditions have some degree of cell-mediated immune (CMI) deficiency and since myeloma patients with humoral immune deficiency have no more HPV infections than controls, CMI seems to be important in both the prevention and response to treatment of HPV infections. The clinical implication of HPV infection in patients who are candidates for organ transplants is that attempts have to be made to treat all clinically visible anogenital warts prior to transplantation. Once immuno-suppressed, warts can achieve giant sizes and cover the entire external anogenital skin. These are difficult to remove and require general anesthesia.

A relative depression of cell-mediated immunity in pregnancy[41] may provide 'permissiveness' for HPV infection. Estrogens and progesterone during pregnancy stimulate viral replication,[42] and accumulation of large amounts of interstitial glycosaminoglycans together with vascular en-gorgement may be additional contributing factors for the extensive and voluminous nature of exter-nal genital warts during periods of gestation.

BIOPSY TECHNIQUE

Specimens for histologic examination are obtained according to the clinical appearance, size and location of the vulvar lesions. For example, condy-lomata acuminata may be biopsied under local anesthesia using a small biopsy punch (Fig. 11.11) or a small 1.0 cm × 0.4 cm loop electrode (Fig. 11.12A) or scissors. When both the diagno-sis and treatment of noncondylomatous lesions are the aim, excisional biopsies are performed using either a scalpel or a microneedle electrode (Fig. 11.12B) and the tissue defect is closed with a 3/0 catgut. For dermatosis type lesions, a Keyes' punch used by dermatologists is the preferred

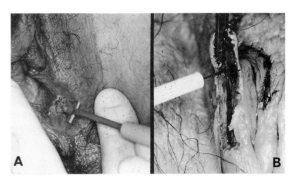

Fig. 11.12 **A** Loop electrode used both for diagnosis and therapy for vulvar condylomata acuminata. **B** Microneedle electrode for excising clinically suspicious areas.

tool. Lesions located on the clitoris or subclinical, acetowhite macules are 'elevated' above the adja-cent epithelium by infiltrating the subepithelial connective tissue with local anesthetic solution (Fig. 11.13). This will 'separate' the lesion from the underlying papillary dermis. Then by grasping

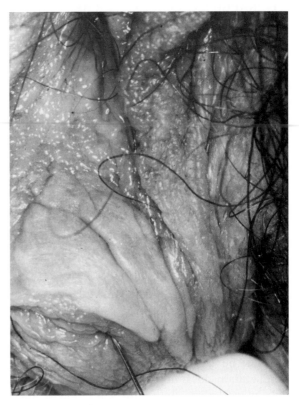

Fig. 11.13 Well-circumscribed papular lesion elevated by infiltrating the anesthetic solution just beneath the lesional tissue into the papillary dermis.

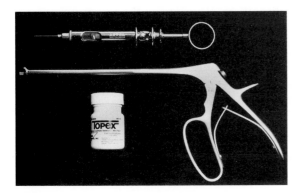

Fig. 11.11 Biopsy punch (middle), local (upper) and topical (lower) 20% benzocaine anesthetic gel. The relatively small jaw of the punch prevents deep penetration into the dermis and bleeding and scarring.

the apex of the lesion with the first half of the biopsy forceps jaw, the lesional tissue is excised. In this way, deep penetration into the underlying tissue is prevented as is bleeding and scarring. Biopsy sites may be treated with Monsel's paste or gel to insure hemostasis. However, it is important to remove the excess Monsel's paste/gel from the wound to prevent scarring. Topical antibiotic therapy is not necessary.

Accurate histological interpretation is greatly enhanced by well-oriented histologic sections. These are obtained when larger specimens are placed in plastic pathology laboratory cassettes or, if not available, on a cardboard or paraffin plate and pinned down while being fixed in 10% neutral-buffered formalin. Smaller punch biopsy specimens are placed on lens paper with the dermis facing the paper (on 'end' orientation). Tissue adherence is enhanced by placing a drop of lubricating gel on the lens paper.

THERAPEUTIC CONTROVERSIES

There are several situations in which the removal of lesions is indicated, whereas in other situations, therapy may not only be redundant but also cost-ineffective. The majority of patients who have been informed about the sexually transmittable viral nature of their clinically visible condylomata acuminata seek therapy. In others, the lesions are cosmetically unacceptable and, feel physically and psychologically unclean, a situation which may lead to psychosexual dysfunction. Some patients have associated symptoms such as pruritus and less frequently, bleeding, pain and infections. The latter symptoms are more common in women and men with large introital or anal disease, respectively.

Managing subclinical macular lesions

Whether the male sexual partner of a patient with overt clinical vulvar warts should be evaluated for subclinical acetowhite HPV macules and, if present, be treated are issues for debate.[37,43,44] The author does not recommend therapy for subclinical lesions unless the condition is associated with symptoms (burning, pruritus) that are not relieved by conservative, topical agents, and/or

the condition is simply unacceptable to the patient. In the male patient who is polygamous or is engaged in short term, serial, monogamous unions, the consistent use of condoms is stressed. It is not necessary to treat the male partner with subclinical lesions who is engaged in long-term monogamy for their removal does not seem to improve the treatment results of the clinically visible warts in his female partner.[43,44] In an ongoing prospective study, we have specifically addressed the issue of the role of the male sexual partner in influencing treatment results of the external genital condylomata in his female partner. In this cohort study of 160 women with anogenital warts, 108 (68%) of their 'steady' (6 months or longer) male sexual partners had either clinical and/or subclinical acetowhite macules on the penis. The men were then randomized for either continuous wave CO_2 laser therapy and thereafter condom use (55 patients) or no therapy and no condom use (53 patients). The entire cohort has been, so far, followed for a minimum of 6 weeks, maximum 24 weeks, mean 12 weeks. Table 11.3 clearly shows that treatment results in the women are similar irrespective of whether their current male sexual partners were treated. Our preliminary results reinforce the concept that 'post-therapy recurrences (within 3 months after therapy) are due to the later activation of latent HPV DNA rather than to reinfection from the current sexual partner'.[45]

It has been suggested that removal of the 'viral reservoir' by CO_2 laser vaporizing coexistent subclinical HPV-related lesions contributes significantly to (1) reducing the recurrence rates of external anogenital condylomata[32] and (2) the number of repeat laser ablative procedures.[32,33] However, in a large prospective, multicenter,

Table 11.3 Role of the male sexual partner in treatment results of vulvar/anal condylomata

Male partners*	Recurrence**	
	Number	%
CO_2 laser + condom (n = 55)	92	58
No therapy/no condom (n = 53)	98	62
Total: 108	160	100

* After single CO_2 laser therapy.
** With clinical/subclinical lesions.

double-blind, placebo-controlled study using CO_2 laser vaporization followed by subcutaneous injections of interferon-α2a 3 times per week for 4 weeks, recurrence and complete response rates in patients with coexistent subclinical lesions were similar.[35] In view of these findings and the potential risk of severe postoperative discomfort, and later dyspareunia, attempts at compulsive removal of subclinical macular lesions that are associated with overt clinical warts are not cost-effective at best and may lead to gynecologic cripples at worst (Fig. 11.4). This is particularly true when depth of vaporization is extended deeper than the first surgical plane or papillary dermis.

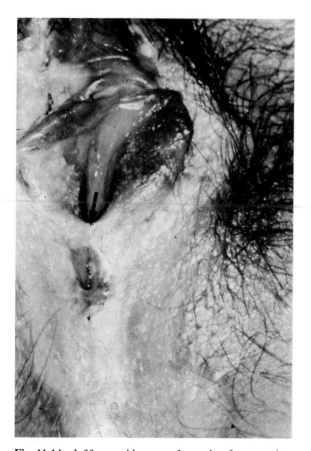

Fig. 11.14 A 23-year-old woman 3 months after extensive CO_2 laser photovaporization for subclinical, macular lesions. There is coaptation of labia minus (arrow), scarring and loss of substance. Even after repair, the patient complained of severe dyspareunia due to poor lubrification secondary to destruction of vestibular and sebaceous glands.

MANAGING THE PREGNANT PATIENT

The management of pregnant patients with clinically visible acuminate condylomata is also controversial,[46] except when the lesional tissues obstruct vaginal delivery. In such cases, caesarean-section may be indicated; however, this situation occurs very rarely. The controversial issue revolves around the competitive risk of transmitting HPV to the fetus during delivery which may lead to the development of recurrent laryngeal papillomatosis (RLP) and the cost and side-effects of therapy. The school that favors therapy argues that untreated genital warts may represent a 'substantial' risk for the infant to develop RLP and that RLP imposes a tremendous physical and psychological burden on the affected child and family.[47] The school which proposes no therapy suggests that the risk for developing RLP is exceedingly low and is significantly smaller than are complications related to either caesarean-section or ablative therapies, particularly when the lesions are extensive but none obstructive to vaginal delivery.[48] The risk of RLP has been crudely estimated in the USA at 1 in 360 pregnancies with genital warts.[49] Although in two studies, 75% of women with affected infants had condylomata during pregnancy,[12,50] the very small number of cases observed in the general population (1:100 000) and the fact that none of the 44 000 children examined clinically from birth to 7 years was found with RLP, suggest that this disease represents a very small complication of HPV infection during pregnancy. According to the recommendations of the Centers for Disease Control, caesarean section should not be performed solely to prevent transmission of HPV infection to the newborn.[51]

If the informed pregnant patient wishes to have therapy for her genital warts, treatment modalities may include topical application of a 50% trichloroacetic acid solution once a week starting therapy 8 weeks prior to delivery or, if the lesional tissue is extensive, laser ablation or electroexcision/fulguration. Treatment results are generally excellent (Table 11.4) when carried out between the 27th and 30th weeks of gestation.[46] It may not be necessary to remove all of the lesions but to aim at 'debulking'. This in turn decreases

Table 11.4 Treatment results with 50% TCA and CO_2 laser vaporization in pregnant patients with anogenital warts

Gestational age (weeks)	Recurrence (%)	
	TCA	Laser
< 24	53	26
> 25	13	0

viral load and at least theoretically, further decreases the already minimal risk of HPV transmission to the neonate. It may also be appropriate to suction thoroughly the oral cavity and clean the eyes and anogenital regions of the newborns to reduce or eliminate HPV infection to these sites.

Another infrequent complication of genital HPV infections during pregnancy is the development of external anogenital[46] and conjunctival condylomata[52] in the offspring. From 1940 to 1989, 50 cases of anogenital condylomata in infants and children have been reported;[46] however, it is suspected that there are many more cases, particularly in recent years.[53] Of the reported cases, about one in three developed after contact with anogenital condylomata during delivery. The younger the child (less than 9 months) with anogenital warts, the greater the likelihood of 'innocent' contact with the mother's warts. In elder children, however, sexual abuse or auto- or heteroinoculation of HPV from cutaneous verruca vulgaris of the extremities should be investigated. Lesions that should be suspected to be a reflection of sexual abuse are located near the anal orifice or introitus, in the anal canal or behind the hymen and occur in children between the ages of 1 and 12 years. When genital warts are associated with vaginal trauma (posterior hymenal cleft, tears, fissures, fibrous ridges, etc.) or concomitant venereal infections they are clinical evidence of sexual abuse. Approximately 50% of pediatric cases of genital warts in North America are documented to be a result of sexual abuse.[54]

TREATMENT MODALITIES

General considerations

These can be classified into four categories: (1) cytolytic/chemical agents; (2) cytodestructive

physical means; (3) immunomodulation, on an experimental basis; and (4) antiviral agents and vaccines. Regardless of mode(s) of therapy, recurrence rates of condylomata are high, of the order of 50%, and most recurrences develop within six weeks after initial treatment.[45] Conversely, up to 30% of condylomata acuminata regress with placebo therapy with either subcutaneous injections or topical applications of inert substances.[55,56] In the experience of most investigators, treatment results appear to be influenced negatively but not necessarily statistically by the volume of clinical disease, the age of the patient (over 20 years old), the age of the lesional tissue (< 4 months) and immunosuppressed states.

Cytolytic/chemical agents

Podophyllin

These are applied topically, and the most widely used agent has been 20% podophyllin solution applied at weekly intervals for up to 3 months. The cumulative therapeutic effect of podophyllin, however, is poor ranging between 22 and 58% (Table 11.5).[55,57,58] Podophyllin is a crude and nonstandardized extract from the roots of either podophyllum peltatum or emodi, potentially very toxic, and its content of quercetin may be mutagenic. The latter is also found in bracken fern which has been associated with carcinogenic transformation of bovine papillomavirus-related warts in the upper digestive tract of cattle.[59] Podophyllin is highly unstable, and the therapeutically effective agents are rapidly degraded into inactive isomers. Because of the risk of local and systemic toxicity including respiratory failure and coma and because of its enhanced absorption in young children and pregnant women, podophyllin should not be used in these situations, nor should

Table 11.5 Treatment results with topical agents*

Agents	Cure rates (%)
20% podophyllin	22–58
0.5% podofilox	48–82
50–80% TCA	55–73
5% 5-FU (Efudex)	90**

* Based on personal experience and literature review.
** Meatal warts.

the adult, nonpregnant patient apply the solution herself. These problems put a heavy burden on the medical staff, and make this form of therapy cost-ineffective.

Podofilox

Topical podophyllotoxin or podofilox (Condyline™, Europe and Canada and Condylox™, in the USA) (Fig. 11.15) is a variant of podophyllin. Podofilox is the most potent cytotoxic agent (lignan) in podophyllin and interferes with DNA synthesis and mitosis of squamous epithelial cells by 'paralyzing' the sliding of the mitotic (microfilamentous) spindle. Unlike podophyllin in which the concentration of podofilox may range between 3 and 10%, in Condyline/Condylox, it is only 0.5%. It contains, furthermore, no other potential toxic or systemic ingredients and its vehicle is 70% ethanol. To date, no systemic reactions have been reported with 0.5% podofilox, and it is approved for home use for external anogenital warts. Warts located on mucus membranes (vagina, anus) are not to be treated, however, for podofilox may be absorbed into the systemic circulation through mucus membranes, particularly if fissures are present. The area treated should not be washed for at least four hours after use. Side effects are limited to local skin irritation, burning and erosion. In most patients the symptoms are mild and transient. In the experience of most investigators, treatment-results were superior to podophyllin[55,60,61] and placebo (Table 11.5) but relapse of warts can be expected in between 34%[62] and 38%[55] of the cases.

In the experience of the author, topical podofilox solution is effective as initial monotherapy for soft, nonkeratinized warts or for 'rescuing' warts that recur soon after cytodestructive therapy with CO_2 laser or electrosurgery. To make therapy with podofilox more convenient for women, the agent is being investigated in the form of a cream preparation. The preliminary results of a double-blind, placebo-controlled study with 0.5% podophyllotoxin cream indicated a 91% complete response rate compared with 8.3% with placebo after 3 weeks of therapy.[61] Relapse of disease within 3 months after completion of three treatment cycles was 14% in the active agent group, resulting in an overall cure rate of 38 of 44 (77%) of women. Further studies with long-term follow-up are needed to verify the preliminary findings and determine the lowest possible concentration of podofilox in the form of gel that is associated with the lowest rate of local skin irritation.

The therapeutic effects of podofilox solution are comparable to either 50% or 80% trichloro- (TCA) or bichloroacetic acid solutions (Table 11.5). These are applied also with cotton-tipped applicators once a week on soft warts and two to three times a week on keratinized warts for a maximum of 8 weeks. TCA, in a concentration of 80% seems to be more effective for smaller, hyperkeratotic lesions than podofilox. However, TCA is associated with comparatively more frequent and severe side-effects including pain and deep ulcerations than is 0.5% podofilox (Fig. 11.16) and it has not been approved for home use. Application of local anesthetic gel such as 2% xylocaine (Astra Pharmaceutical Products, Inc.) or 20% benzocaine (Freulich, Inc.) reduces temporary pain. TCA is not absorbed into the vascular system and is the therapy of choice for warts during pregnancy.[63]

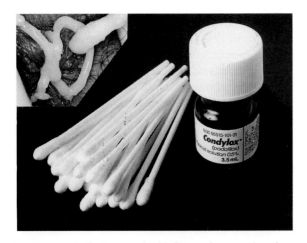

Fig. 11.15 A Topical 0.5% podofilox and cotton-tipped applicator for home treating extended anogenital warts. Insert: to prevent exposure of normal skin to podofilox, the lesions are separated from the adjacent skin by petroleum jelly.

5% 5-Fluorouracil (Efudex)

This agent is an antimetabolite, a pyrimidine

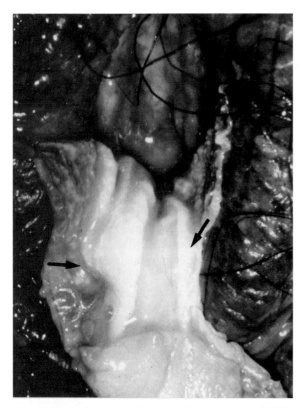

Fig. 11.16 Patient exposed to excessive use of topical TCA solution resulting in complete epithelial desquamation (arrows) of the labiovestibular epithelium.

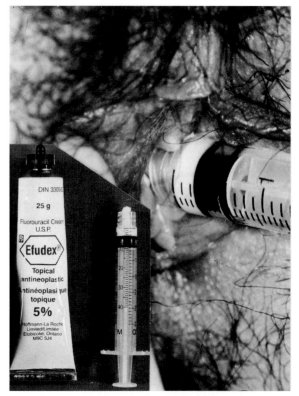

Fig. 11.17 Five percent 5-FU cream (Efudex) delivered into meatus by syringe. Insert: Efudex cream and 3 cm^3 plastic syringe.

analog, that competes with thymidilate synthetase and substitutes for uracil. It interferes with DNA and RNA synthesis in epithelial cells. In current practice, many have abandoned its use as primary therapy[32] other than for meatal warts.[43,64,65] In the latter case, intrameatal application of the cream nightly for 7–14 days results in over 90% cure rates (Table 11.5). The author instructs the patient or her partner to deliver 0.3 cm^3 of cream into the meatus with a 3 cm^3 plastic or tuberculin syringe subsequent to voiding, three times per week for 3 weeks (Fig. 11.17). The patient is hydrated with two glasses of water per hour, starting 2 h before therapy. In this way, the cream is voided off about 3–5 h after the intrameatal application of cream. Although dysuria, coaptation of the distal urethral epithelium and urinary retention may be rare complications of meatal Efudex therapy, the author has not encountered a single instance

of clinically significant side effects in a series of 84 women treated with Efudex over the past 15 years. 5-Fluorouracil (5-FU) cream is available also in 1% concentration (Fuluroplax™) but its therapeutic effectiveness has not been extensively investigated. Efudex should not be used in women in whom absolute contraception cannot be established for its absorption into the general circulation during pregnancy may lead, at least theoretically, to fetal toxicity and birth defects.[66] Also, fair-skinned women are hypersensitive to Efudex and often develop extensive denudation of the vulvar skin and dyspareunia (Fig. 11.18).

When treating external anogenital warts, relatively good results are obtained only if the cream is applied in an occlusive form overnight for 5–10 days on the genital warts.[67] This in turn may produce extensive sloughing of the epidermis, denudation, chemical dermatitis (Fig. 11.17) and

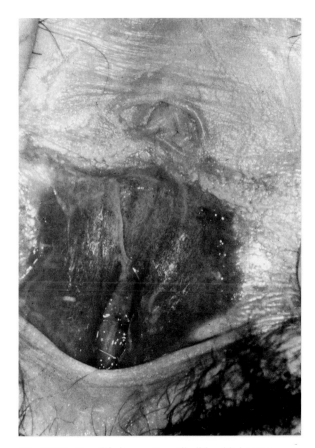

Fig. 11.18 Post-Efudex acute vestibulitis with intense erythema and epithelial erosion.

folliculitis if the hairbearing skin is also included in the treatment field.

In recent years, some have used topical 5% 5-FU cream given once or twice weekly as an adjuvant therapy subsequent to CO_2 laser ablation in an effort to reduce recurrence rates.[32,33,68] The results in one study have been encouraging,[68] particularly in immunosuppressed patients,[69] whereas others failed to demonstrate its superior therapeutic efficacy over extended CO_2 laser ablation alone.[32] The scientific rationale for this form of 'rescue' therapy has not been clearly established, nor are there data generated by multicenter, double-blind, placebo-controlled studies. Also, using 5-FU for 6 months results in relatively high rates of drop-out and the long-term effects of Efudex therapy in organ transplant patients has not been fully documented. Moreover, 5-FU

is unlikely to penetrate the thick, highly keratinized surface of vulvar condylomata.[70]

Cytodestructive techniques

These include cryotherapy,[71,72] scissor excisions,[73] electrodesiccation, electroexcision and fulguration[36,71] and CO_2 laser vaporization.[32–34,74,75] All of these modalities are appropriate for removing bulky lesions or those which failed to respond to conservative topical therapy. Using one over another technique depends on the availability of the equipment, technical skills of the operator and the number and location of condylomata. With few exceptions,[32] treatment results of the order of 75–85% are obtained only with multiple repeat treatments or by combining surgical removal with subsequent rescue therapy with podofilox, 50–85% TCA or interferons.[32,76]

Cryotherapy is probably the cytodestructive technique most often used by dermatologists and venerologists to treat external anogenital warts[63,72] but is less frequently used by gynecologists.[77] The most commonly employed refrigerants are liquid nitrogen and nitrous oxide, both of which may be delivered as drops or sprays or by using a cryogun with cryoprobe tips (Fig. 11.19). The treatment does not require local anesthesia, and the average number of cryotherapy sessions to achieve cure is six. Prospective studies on large patient samples showed comparable cure rates

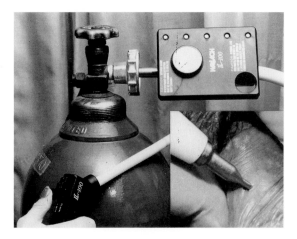

Fig. 11.19 Cryo-gun with nitrous oxide refrigerant. Insert: Needle-shaped cryotip on lesional tissue.

Table 11.6 Treatment results of cytodestructive methods*

Therapy	Cure rates (%)	
	Single therapy	Repeat therapy
Cryosurgery	42	74
Electrosurgery	50	75
CO_2 laser	50	87

* As per available literature review.

with cryotherapy, electrosurgery and podophyllin[63,72,77] (Tables 11.5 and 11.6).

In patients with only a few condylomata, scissors or a biopsy punch (Fig. 11.11) may be used under local anesthesia to excise larger lesions.

During the past decade, CO_2 laser vaporization has gained popularity for surgical treatment of genital warts.[32–34,74,75] The advantages of laser therapy in expert hands are rapid removal of lesions, rapid healing, particularly when the heat containing ultrapulsed chopped/laser energy is used,[32] and excellent cosmetic results (Fig. 11.20A–11.20C). The main disadvantage of laser surgery is the high cost of the equipment precluding many physicians from having access to its use. In a controlled, randomized study on patients with recurrent anogenital condylomata, excision and/or electrocauterization was as effective as continuous wave CO_2 laser treatment, and in this study, there was no difference in the incidence of postoperative pain, healing time or scarring between CO_2 laser and conventional surgical methods.[75]

The authors and his colleagues treated 180 patients with external anogenital condylomata measuring at least 2 cm^2 in area.[36] To avoid selection bias, in each patient half of the lesions were treated with loop electrosurgical excision/ball electrofulguration and the other half with CO_2 laser excision/vaporization using continuous wave form (Figs 11.21A and 11.21B). As in the Duus et al study,[75] we were unable to demonstrate statistically significant differences in the duration of operative time, healing time, degree of postoperative discomfort and the rate of complications between the electrosurgical and laser-treated areas. Complete clearance of warts after a single (51%) and multiple (75%) treatments were similar in areas treated with electrosurgery and CO_2 laser (Table 11.6).

Immunomodulators

Theoretically, interferons (IFNs) have a unique

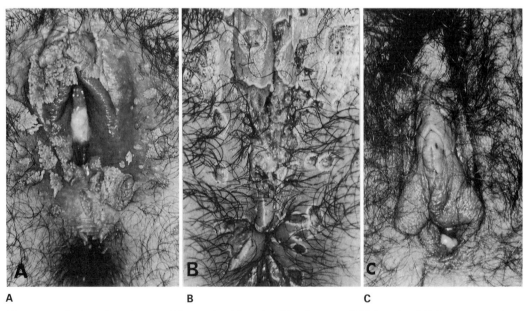

A   B   C

Fig. 11.20 **A** Extensive vulvar condylomatosis with perianal involvement. **B** Vulva after CO_2 laser vaporization of genital warts. **C** Vulva 3 months after CO_2 laser vaporization with excellent cosmetic results.

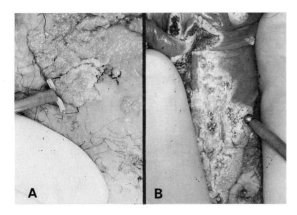

Fig. 11.21 Electrosurgery for vulvar warts.
A Electroexcision of lesions with loop electrode.
B Electrofulguration of all lesions with ball-shaped electrode.

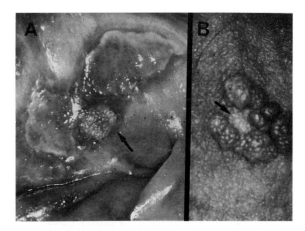

Fig. 11.22 The Koebner phenomenon. **Left** New lesion developed at laser margin (arrow) three weeks after photovaporization. **Right** 'Ring recurrence': multiple new lesions surrounding previous treatment site (arrow).

application to the treatment of genital warts for they have antiviral, antiproliferative and immuno-modulatory activities. Also, IFNs may act not only on mature virions found in lesional tissues, but also on latent HPV DNA which may be present in about 45% of patients with external anogenital warts.[45] Latent HPV DNA may be activated and produce fully formed virions soon after therapy and produce new lesional tissue (Koebner's phenomenon) (Fig. 11.22).

Although several reports in the literature have documented the efficacy of various IFN preparations for the treatment of genital warts, others failed to confirm favorable responses to the same type of IFNs (Table 11.7), and for all purposes, it is impossible to assess the practical role of IFNs in the treatment of external anogenital condylomata.[33,35,56,76,78–83] Indeed, the preparations used in clinical trials vary from recombinant to

natural IFNs, some use IFNα, others IFNβ, and still others IFNγ. The dosage and administration range from intramuscular[80] and subcutaneous[35,79] to intralesional.[56,81–83] The major pitfall in many studies, however, is lack of using a placebo to control for spontaneous regressions (Table 11.7). An example to illustrate this problem is the Reid et al study[33] vs the experience of the Collaborative International Condyloma Study Group (CICSG).[35] In both studies, the same IFNα2a (Roferon, Roche Laboratories) was used to prevent recurrences after CO_2 laser ablation of genital warts. The Reid study was not placebo-controlled, whereas the CICSG was, and in both studies IFN was administered subcutaneously at variable distances from the treatment fields 3 times per week for 4 weeks in the CICSG study[35] and 10 weeks in the Reid et al study.[33] The outcome was

Table 11.7 Placebo-controlled IFN therapy for anogenital condylomata

IFN*	Dose(U)	Route/schedule	Complete response (%)		Reference
			IFN	Placebo	
β	2×10^6	i.m. q.d. × 10 days	82	18	80
α/R	$1 \times 10^{5-6}$	Intralesional 3/week × 3 weeks	53	14	81
α2b	1×10^6	Intralesional 3/week × 3 weeks	36	17	82
αN	1.2×10^6	Intralesional 2/week × 8 weeks	62	21	56
αN αN/R	1×10^6	Intralesional 3/week × 4 weeks	16.5	9.5	83
α2a	$1–9 \times 10^6$	Subcutaneous 3/week × 4 weeks	22	25	79
α2a	3×10^6	Subcutaneous 3/week × 10 weeks	32	39	35
α2b	3/w	Subcutaneous 3/week × 10 weeks	54	23	76

* N — natural; R — recombinant.

82 vs 32% in the Reid study and the CICSG study, respectively. Cure rates in the CICSG study were similar to those observed with placebo (39%). Better response rates in the Reid study were attributed to the longer (10 weeks) administration of IFNα2a, and the complete removal of coexistent acetowhite subclinical macular lesions as opposed to the 4 weeks duration and failure of treating subclinical lesions in the CICSG study.[35] Our unpublished, placebo-controlled, double-blind multicenter experience with a 10 week long subcutaneous administration of Roferon produced similar rates of complete response as the placebo, and as mentioned earlier, in the two CICSG studies, patients with coexistent subclinical HPV reservoirs have as many recurrences as cures.[35,79]

In reviewing the literature on the subject and based on personal experience, it is clear that IFN therapy is indicated for patients with recalcitrant warts, only as an adjunct to other treatment modalities rather than primary therapy. Dosages, the most appropriate number of injections and mode of IFN administration have yet to be clearly defined to maximize cure rates and minimize side-effects, mostly flu-like syndrome, fatigue and headache.

COMBINATION ('RESCUE') THERAPY FOR RECALCITRANT CONDYLOMATA ACUMINATA

In recent years, it has become increasingly evident that patients with recalcitrant lesions are best managed by 'wart debulking' using cyto-destructive means followed by the application of an adjunct which is believed to be effective either in preventing activation of latent HPV DNA or removing newly formed lesions. Although the precise immune deficit, if any, in otherwise healthy persons who have repeatedly recurrent and/or recalcitrant condylomata is not known, one factor that may be useful to obtain better treatment results is activation of natural killer cell activity. This in turn may keep in check latent HPV DNA from being activated leading to recurrences.[45] The logical choice in such cases is one of the commercially available interferons. In one study, a better response to intralesional

Table 11.8 Rescue therapy for recalcitrant anogenital warts with adjuvant IFNs

IFN	Cure rates (%)		Reference
	Laser + IFN	Laser alone	
α2a	82 vs	52	33
α2b	54 vs	23	76

IFNα2b was observed in patients with a greater increase in natural killer cell activity than in those without a significant increase.[78] In two prospective studies, one uncontrolled[33] and one controlled by placebo,[76] administration of IFNα2a and IFNα2b prior to[76] and after CO_2 laser vaporization,[33] respectively, was associated with significantly better treatment-results than either laser alone[33] or placebo[76] (Table 11.8).

When using IFNs after ablative therapy, the preparations are injected subepithelially at the edge of or close to the treatment field(s), twice per week for 8 weeks (Fig. 11.23). Intron-A (IFNα2b) has been approved by the FDA in the USA and the Health Protective Branch in Canada for the treatment of anogenital warts. The recommended maximum dosage is 5×10^6 (U) or 0.5 cm^3 per treatment session. The maximum duration of therapy should not exceed 8 weeks. Response to IFN therapy may be delayed two to three months after completion of IFN injections.

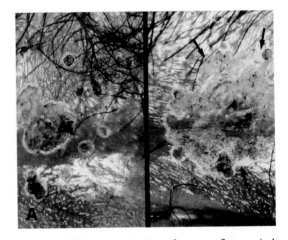

Fig. 11.23 **A** Laser vaporization of warts to first surgical plane (papillary dermis). **B** Normal epithelium adjacent to lesional tissue has been laser brushed to remove latent HPV DNA. Arrows indicate injection sites with α-interferons.

Table 11.9 Effect of 'rescue' therapy with adjuvent topical agents on repeat surgery for recalcitrant anogenital warts*

	Cure rates Number	%	Number of repeat CO_2 Laser or LEEP**
Laser/LEEP alone	160	76	2–7 (mean 4.0)
Laser/LEEP + 0.5% Podofilox	40	73	1–4 (mean 2.0)
Laser/LEEP + 50% TCA	33	77	1–3 (mean 2.0)

* Minimum follow-up 6 weeks; maximum 9 months; mean 4.5 months.
** LEEP — loop electrosurgical excision procedure.

Another adjunct to surgical debulking is the topical antimitotic 0.5% podofilox or 50% TCA solution. Table 11.9 contains our experience with 73 women who were treated at random with podofilox or TCA after electroexcision and fulguration of recalcitrant, external anogenital warts. In this study, the patients were instructed to apply the respective topical preparations on newly developing lesions as described earlier in this chapter. Although the overall cure rates are not additive, thus not different from other treatment modalities, using chemical 'rescuing' of recurrent lesions results in fewer repeat and relatively expensive cytodestructive, excisional/ablative procedures. None of these results have been controlled by placebo and, thus, generalization from our experience cannot be made. Prospective multicenter, placebo-controlled clinical trials should be conducted to assess the role of IFNs as an adjunct to 'prevent' recurrent warts after debulking therapy.

Experimental treatment modalities

Vitamin-A derivative retinoids are another theoretically attractive modality for the treatment of HPV-related diseases. They enhance both humoral and cell-mediated immunity,[84] are well known to promote cell differentiation and are potent inhibitors of malignant transformation. While several reports suggested beneficial results with systemic retinoids in patients with various immunologically impaired conditions and cutaneous warts, similar studies have not appeared in patients with anogenital warts.

Crude autogenous vaccines made of the patient's own warts were used in the early 1970s.[85]

However, a placebo-controlled study failed to demonstrate the therapeutic effectiveness of autogenous vaccines over placebo.[57] Also, the use of inactivated but not destroyed oncogenic viral DNA prevents commercial distribution of crude vaccines made of wart extracts. HPV vaccine research is in its infancy and is currently centered on identifying HPV-related proteins which may stimulate both the humoral and cell-mediated immune response against the many types of genital HPVs.

CONCLUSIONS

The natural history of vulvar HPV infections is fairly well documented; the acetowhite, subclinical, macular lesions are more frequent than the clinical acuminate condylomata acuminata, and both conditions should be distinguished from their mimics that range from a variety of dermatoses to carcinoma. The use of modern viral hybridization techniques may help in selected cases to reach appropriate diagnostic and therapeutic decisions. Therapy is indicated for clinically visible disease but patients with asymptomatic, subclinical lesions living in a long-term monogamous sexual union may be followed rather than subjected to costly and repeated therapies. Patients engaged in polygamous sexual relationships with asymptomatic subclinical lesions should be encouraged to use condoms consistently, whereas those with symptoms and psychological distress benefit from therapy. Attempts at removing extensive genital warts during pregnancy are not cost-effective for preventing the exceedingly rare RLP and anogenital warts in the newborn.

Among the most cost-effective topical therapeutic agents are 0.5% podofilox and 50–80% trichloroacetic acid. Topical 5% 5-FU (Efudex) is the treatment of choice for meatal condylomata. Voluminous, hyperkeratotic lesions are best excised with scissors, biopsy forceps, loop electrodes or ablated with cryosurgery, electrofulguration or photovaporized with the CO_2 laser beam. Patients with problematic recurrent/recalcitrant anogenital warts may benefit from combining electro- or CO_2 laser surgery with adjuvant agents. These include injections of IFNs in a subepithelial position near the operative field (to prevent activation of latent HPV DNA) or the application of topical agents (to destroy newly formed lesions) after surgical debulking of genital warts. The role of extended CO_2 laser vaporization aimed at removing subclinical HPV reservoirs from the external anogenital skin for obtaining superior therapeutic results of acuminate condylomata remains to be verified by multicenter, prospective studies on a large number of patients. Also, extensive prospective, placebo-controlled clinical trials with various

IFNs and topical agents combined with cyto-destructive methods are needed to gain insight into the most cost-effective therapeutic means of treating patients with anogenital condylomata, particularly those with recalcitrant disease. Future studies should also focus on preventing HPV infections and reinfections using vaccines and considerable attention should be given to public education, promoting long-term monogamous sexual relationships.

REFERENCES

1. Bergeron C, Ferenczy A. Clinical spectrum of genital HPV infection in the female. II. Vulva, perineum and anus. In: Winkler B, Richart R M, eds. Clinical practice of gynecology, vol 2. New York, NY: Elsevier Science Publishing, 1989: pp 59–72.
2. Bergeron C, Ferenczy A, Richart R M, Guralnick M. Micropapillomatosis labialis appears unrelated to human papillomavirus. Obstet Gynecol 1990; 76: 281–286.
3. Growdon W A, Fu Y S, Lebherz T B et al. Pruritic vulvar squamous papillomatosis: evidence for human papillomavirus etiology. Obstet Gynecol 1985; 66: 564–568.
4. Moyal-Barracco M, Leibowitch M, Orth G. Vestibular papillae of the vulva. Arch Dermatol 1990; 126: 1594–1598.
5. Koutsky L A, Galloway D A, Holmes K K. Epidemiology of genital human papillomavirus infection. Epidemiol Rev 1988; 10: 122–163.
6. Daling J R, Sherman K J, Weiss N S. Risk factors for condyloma acuminatum in women. Sex Trans Dis 1986; 13: 16–18.
7. Schmauz R, Owor R. Epidemiology of malignant degeneration of condyloma acuminata in Uganda. Pathol Res 1980; 170: 91.
8. Biometry Branch, Division of Cancer Prevention and Control, National Cancer Institute. Cancer incidence and mortality in the United States. Seer Program, 1973–81. (NIH publication no. 85–1837) (US Department of Health and Human Services, PHS, NIH). Bethesda, MD: National Cancer Institute, 1984: pp 53–158.
9. Aziz D C, Ferre F, Robitaille J, Ferenczy A. Human papillomavirus testing in the clinical laboratory. Part II: Vaginal, vulvar, perineal and penile squamous lesions. J Gynecol Surg 1993; 9: 9–15.
10. Oriel J D. Natural history of genital warts. Br J Ven Dis 1971; 47: 1–13.
11. Gross G, Ikenberg H, de Villiers E-M et al. Bowenoid papulosis: a venereally transmissible disease as reservoir for HPV 16. In: Peto R, zur Hausen H, eds. Viral etiology of cervical cancer. Cold Spring Harbor, NY: Cold Spring Harbor Laboratory, 1986: pp 149–165.
12. Quick C A, Watts S L, Krzyzek R A et al. Relationship between condylomata and laryngeal papillomata. Ann Otol Rhinol Laryngol 1980; 89: 467–471.
13. Wickenden C, Hanna N, Taylor-Robinson D et al. Sexual transmission of human papillomaviruses in

heterosexual and male homosexual couples, studied by DNA hybridisation. Genitourinary Med 1988; 64: 34–38.
14. Grussendorf-Conen E I, Gissman L, Holters J. Correlation between content of viral DNA and evidence of mature virus particles in HPV-1, HPV-4 and HPV-6 induced virus acanthomata. J Invest Dermatol 1983; 81: 511–513.
15. Sonnex C, Scholefield J H, Kocjan G et al. Anal human papillomavirus infection in heterosexuals with genital warts: Prevalence and relation with sexual behavior. Br J Med 1991; 303: 1243.
16. Chang F, Syrjanen S, Kellokoski J, Syrjanen K. Human papillomavirus (HPV) infections and their associations with oral disease. J Oral Pathol Med 1991; 20: 305–317.
17. Muretto P, Ferenczy A. Association of human papillomavirus type 16 with intraepithelial neoplasia of the vulva and oral cavity in a married couple. Cervix 1992; 10: 55–56.
18. Ashinoff R, Li J J, Jacobson M, Friedman-Kien A, Geronemus R G. Detection of human papillomavirus DNA in squamous cell carcinoma of the nail bed and finger determined by polymerase chain reaction. Arch Dermatol 1991; 127: 1813–1818.
19. Rock B, Naghashfar Z, Barnett N et al. Genital tract papillomavirus infection in children. Arch Dermatol 1986; 122: 1129–1132.
20. Fleming K A, Venning V, Evans M. DNA typing of genital warts and diagnosis of sexual abuse of children [Letter]. Lancet 1987; 2: 454.
21. Obalek S, Jablonska S, Favre M, Walczak L, Orth G. Condylomata acuminata in children: Frequent association with human papillomaviruses responsible for cutaneous warts. J Am Acad Dermatol 1990; 23: 205–213.
22. DeJong A R, Weiss J C, Brent R L. Condyloma acuminata in children. Am J Dis Children 1982; 136: 704–706.
23. McCance D J, Campion M J, Baram A, Singer A. Risk for transmission of human papillomavirus by vaginal specula. Lancet 1986; 2: 816–817.
24. Ferenczy A, Bergeron C, Richart R M. Human papillomavirus DNA in fomites on objects used for the management of patients with genital human papillomavirus infections. Obstet Gynecol 1989; 74: 950–954.
25. Ferenczy A, Bergeron C, Richart R M. Human papillomavirus DNA in CO_2 laser-generated plume of

smoke and its consequences to the surgeon. Obstet Gynecol 1990; 75: 114–118.

26. Andre P, Orth G, Evenou P, Guillaume J C, Avril M F. Risk of papillomavirus infection in carbon dioxide laser treatment of genital lesions. J Am Acad Dermatol 1990; 22: 131–132.

27. Bergeron C, Ferenczy A, Richart R M. Underwear: Contamination by human papillomaviruses. Am J Obstet Gynecol 1990; 162: 25–29.

28. Zhu W Y, Blauvelt A, Goldstein B A, Leonardi C, Penneys N S. Detection with polymerase chain reaction of human papillomavirus DNA in condylomata acuminata treated in vitro with liquid nitrogen, trichloroacetic acid and podophyllin. J Am Acad Dermatol 1992; 26: 710–714.

29. Dvoretzky I, Shober R, Chattopadhyay S K, Lowy D R. A quantitative in vitro focus assay for bovine papillomavirus. Virology 1980; 103: 369–375.

30. Walker P G, Colley N Y, Grubb C et al. Abnormalities of the uterine cervix in women with vulvar warts. Br J Ven Dis 1983; 59: 120–123.

31. Schneider A, Sawada E, Gissmann L et al. Human papillomaviruses in women with a history of abnormal Pap smears and in male partners. Obstet Gynecol 1987; 69: 554.

32. Reid R, Greenberg M D, Lorincz A T et al. Superficial laser vulvectomy. IV. Extended laser vaporization and adjuvant 5-fluorouracil therapy of human papillomavirus associated vulvar disease. Obstet Gynecol 1990; 76: 439–448.

33. Reid R, Greenberg M D, Pizzuti D J, Omoto K H, Rutledge L H, Soo W. Superficial laser vulvectomy. V. Surgical debulking is enhanced by adjuvant systemic interferon. Am J Obstet Gynecol 1992; 166: 815–820.

34. Ferenczy A. Laser treatment of patients with condylomata and squamous carcinoma precursors of the lower female genital tract. Can–Am Cancer J Clinicians 1987; 37: 334–347.

35. Condylomata International Collaborative Study Croup. Randomized placebo-controlled double-blind combined therapy with laser surgery and systemic interferon-α2a in the treatment of anogenital condylomata acuminatum. J Infect Dis 1993; 167: 824–829.

36. Wright T C, Richart R M, Ferenczy A. Electrosurgery for HPV-related diseases of the lower genital tract: A practical handbook for diagnosis and treatment by electroexcision and fulguration procedures. Montreal: BioVision, Inc. and New York: Arthur Vision, Inc., 1992.

37. Cobb M W. Human papillomavirus infection. J Am Acad Dermatol 1990; 22: 547–566.

38. Rudlinger R, Buchmann P, Grob R, Colla F, Steiner R, Meandzija M. Genitoanal HPV infections in immunodeficient individuals. In: Gross G, Jablonska S, Pfister H, Stegner H E, eds. Genital papillomavirus infections. Modern diagnosis and treatment. Berlin: Springer-Verlag 1990: pp 249–260.

39. Halpert R, Fruchter R G, Sedlis A et al. Human papillomavirus and lower genital neoplasms in renal transplant patients. Obstet Gynecol 1986; 68: 251–258.

40. Shokri-Tabibzadeh S, Koss L G, Molinar J, Romney M D. Association of human papillomavirus with neoplastic processes in the genital tract of four women with impaired immunity. Gynecol Oncol 1981; 12: 5129–5140.

41. Weinberg E D. Pregnancy-associated depression of cell-mediated immunity. Rev Infect Dis 1984; 6: 814–831.

42. Pater M M, Pater A. RU486 inhibits glucorticoid hormone-dependent oncogenesis by human papillomavirus type 16 DNA. Virology 1991; 183: 799–802.

43. Ferenczy A. Laser treatment of genital human papillomavirus infections in the male patient. In: Dorsey J H, ed. Obstetrics and gynecology clinics of North America: Lasers in gynecology. Philadelphia: WB Saunders, 1991: pp 515–535.

44. Krebs H B, Helmkamp B F. Treatment failure of genital condylomata acuminata in women: role of the male sexual partner. Am J Obstet Gynecol 1991; 165: 337–340.

45. Ferenczy A, Mitao M, Nagai N, Silverstein S J, Crum C P. Latent papillomavirus and recurring genital warts. New Engl J Med 1985; 313: 784–788.

46. Ferenczy A. HPV-associated lesions in pregnancy and their clinical implications. Clin Obstet Gynecol 1989; 32: 191–199.

47. Shah K V. Do genital warts untreated during pregnancy present a substantial risk for an infant developing laryngeal papillomas? J Gynecol Surg 1990; 6: 139–141.

48. Ferenczy A. Do genital warts untreated during pregnancy present a substantial risk for an infant developing laryngeal papillomas? J Gynecol Surg 1990; 6: 143–144.

49. Shah K, Kashima H K, Polk F et al. Rarity of cesarean delivery in cases of juvenile respiratory papillomatosis. Obstet Gynecol 1986; 68: 795.

50. Cook T A, Brunschwig J P, Butel J S et al. Laryngeal papilloma: etiologic and therapeutic considerations. Ann Otol Rhinol Laryngol 1973; 82: 649–655.

51. US Department of Health and Human Services, Centers for Disease Control and Prevention (CDC). 1993 sexually transmitted diseases treatment guidelines. Morbidity and Mortality Weekly Report 1993; 42: 87.

52. McDonnell P J, McDonnell J M, Kessis T et al. Detection of human papillomavirus type 6/11 DNA in conjunctival papillomas by in situ hybridization with radioactive probes. Human Pathol 1987; 18: 1115–1119.

53. Stumpf P G. Increasing occurrence of condylomata acuminata in premenarchal children. Obstet Gynecol 1980; 56: 262–264.

54. Renshaw D C. Treatment of sexual exploitation. Rape and incest. Psychiatric Clinics North Am 1989; 12: 257–277.

55. Beutner K R, Conant M A, Friedman-Kien A E et al. Patient-applied podofilox for treatment of genital warts. Lancet 1989; 1: 831–834.

56. Friedman-Kien A E, Eron L J, Conant M et al. Natural interferon alfa for treatment of condylomata acuminata. JAMA 1988; 259: 533–538.

57. von Krogh G. HPV infection of the external genitals: Clinical aspects and therapy in dermatovenereology. In: Gross G, Jablonska S, Pfister H, Stegner H E, eds. Genital papillomavirus infections. Modern diagnosis and treatment. Berlin: Springer-Verlag, 1990: pp 157–179.

58. Beutner K R. Podophyllin in the treatment of genital human papillomavirus infection: A review. Sem Dermatol 1987; 6: 10–18.

59. Pamukcu A M, Yalciner S, Hatcher J F, Bryan G T. Quercetin, a rat intestinal and bladder carcinogen

present in bracken fern (*Pteridium aquilinum*). Cancer Res 1980; 40: 3468–3472.

60. Greenberg M, Rutledge L H, Reid R et al. A double-blind, randomized trial of 0.5% podofilox and placebo for the treatment of genital warts in women. Obstet Gynecol 1991; 77: 735–739.

61. von Krogh G, Hellberg D. Self-treatment using a 0.5% podophyllotoxin cream of external genital condylomata acuminata in women. Sex Trans Dis 1992; 19: 170–174.

62. Lassus A. Comparison of podophyllotoxin and podophyllin in treatment of genital warts. Lancet 1987; 2: 512–513.

63. Schwartz D B, Greenberg M D, Daoud Y, Reid R. Genital condylomas in pregnancy: Use of trichloroacetic acid and laser therapy. Am J Obstet Gynecol 1988; 158: 1407–1416.

64. von Krogh G. 5-Fluorouracil cream is the successful treatment of therapeutically refractory condylomata acuminata of the urinary meatus. Acta Derm Venereol (Stockholm) 1976; 56: 297–301.

65. Van Le L, Stern J L. Chemotherapeutic management of human papillomavirus infections. In: Winkler B, Richart R M, eds. Clinical practice of gynecology, vol 2. New York, NY: Elsevier Science Publishing, 1989: pp 245–255.

66. Scheuling M, Clemm C. Chromosomal aberrations in a newborn whose mother received cytotoxic treatment during pregnancy. New Engl J Med 1987; 317: 1666–1667.

67. Woodruff J F. Identifying and treating the acuminate wart. Contemp Obstet Gynecol 1976; 7: 125.

68. Krebs H B. Prophylactic topical 5-fuorouracil following treatment of human papillomavirus-associated lesions of the vulva and vagina. Obstet Gynecol 1986; 68: 837–841.

69. Sillman F H, Sedlis A. Anogenital papillomavirus infection and neoplasia in immunodeficient women. Obstet Gynecol Clinics North Am 1987; 14: 537–558.

70. Friedrich E G Jr. Vulvar disease. In: Major problems in obstetrics and gynecology, vol 9. Philadelphia: WB Saunders, 1983: p 194.

71. Stone K M, Becker T M, Hadgu A, Kraus S J. Treatment of external genital warts: a randomised clinical trial comparing podophyllin, cryotherapy and electrodesiccation. Genitourinary Med 1990; 66: 16–19.

72. Simmons P D, Langlet F, Thin R N T. Cryotherapy versus electrocautery in the treatment of genital warts. Br J Ven Dis 1981; 57: 273–274.

73. Jensen S L. Comparison of podophyllin application with simple surgical excision in clearance and recurrence of perianal condylomata acuminata. Lancet 1985; 2: 1146–1148.

74. Baggish M S. Laser therapy for genital warts. In: Winkler B, Richart R M, eds. Clinical practice of gynecology, vol 2. New York, NY: Elsevier Science Publishing, 1989: pp 187–213.

75. Duus B R, Philipsen T, Christensen J D, Lundvall F, Sondergaard J. Refractory condylomata acuminata: a controlled clinical trial of carbon dioxide laser versus conventional surgical treatment. Genitourinary Med 1985; 61: 59–61.

76. Peterson C S, Bjerring P, Larsen J et al. Systemic interferon alpha 2b increases the cure rate in laser treated patients with multiple persistent genital warts: a placebo-controlled study. Genitourinary Med 1991; 67: 99–102.

77. Sand P K, Shen W, Bowen L, Ostergard D R. Cryotherapy for the treatment of proximal urethral condyloma acuminatum. J Urol 1987; 137: 874–876.

78. Tyring S K. Interferon therapy of genital human papillomavirus infection. In: Winkler B, Richart R M, eds. Clinical practice of gynecology, vol 2. New York, NY: Elsevier Science Publishing, 1989: pp 233–244.

79. Condylomata International Collaborative Study Group. Recurrent condylomata acuminata treated with recombinant interferon alfa-2a: a multicenter double-blind placebo controlled clinical trial. JAMA 1991; 265: 2684–2687.

80. Schonfield A, Schattner A, Crespi M et al. Intramuscular human interferon-B injections in treatment of condylomata acuminata. Lancet 1984; 1: 1038–1042.

81. Vance J C, Bart B J, Hansen R C et al. Intralesional recombinant alpha-2 interferon for the treatment of patients with condyloma acuminatum or verruca plantaris. Arch Dermatol 1986; 122: 272–277.

82. Eron L J, Judson F, Tucker S et al. Interferon therapy for condylomata acuminata. New Engl J Med 1986; 315: 1059–1064.

83. Reichman R C, Oakes D, Bonnez W et al. Treatment of condyloma acuminatum with three different interferon-α preparations administered parenterally: a double-blind, placebo-controlled trial. J Infect Dis 1990; 162: 1270–1276.

84. Weiner S A, Meyskens F L, Surwit E A et al. Response of human papilloma-associated diseases to retinoids (vitamin A derivative). In: Howley P M, Broker T R, eds. Papillomaviruses. Molecular and clinical aspects. New York NY: Allan R Liss, 1985: pp 249–255.

85. Powell I C, Pollard M, Jinkins J L. Treatment of condyloma acuminata by autogenous vaccine. South Med J 1970; 63: 202.

12. Cytokine therapy of lower genital tract neoplasia

Richard Cirelli   Paul Rockley   Stephen K. Tyring

INTRODUCTION

The majority of lower genital tract tumors (benign and malignant) are related to infection by various human papillomaviruses (HPV). In fact, at least 20 of the more than 70 known types of HPV have been implicated in lower genital tract tumors. Traditional therapy of lower genital tract tumors has been surgical. If the tumor is malignant, treatment can also involve chemotherapy and/or radiation therapy. Alternatives to surgery for benign lesions include cryotherapy and topical chemotherapeutic agents. Such antitumor agents are used in an attempt to eliminate clinically apparent disease, but they do not eradicate the subclinical or latent reservoir of HPV remaining in adjacent, clinically normal-appearing skin and mucous membranes.[1] A multitude of cytokines have recently become available for clinical testing against various types of neoplasia. Thus far, however, the only cytokines even moderately well studied for treatment of lower genital tract neoplasia are the interferons (IFNs). The IFNs have been relatively well evaluated for therapy of benign and premalignant genital tract tumors.

Cytokines such as IFNs have the potential to eradicate, or at least reduce, this reservoir of HPV, but also act against malignant and premalignant cells via nonantiviral mechanisms. These activities of IFNs include immunomodulation and effects on proliferation, differentiation, oncogenes and antioncogenes. Although IFNα is approved for therapy of condyloma acuminatum, cytokine monotherapy of premalignant and malignant lesions has had limited activity. At this time the greatest potential for cytokine therapy of such tumors appears to be in combination with more tradi-tional therapies such as surgery, chemotherapy or radiation therapy.

CYTOKINE THERAPY OF CANCER

While many cytokines have been recognized and characterized, only four have been approved by the US Food and Drug Administration (FDA) for treatment of human disease. IFNα was the first cytokine approved, i.e., for hairy cell leukemia and is now also indicated for treatment of condyloma acuminatum, Kaposi's sarcoma in AIDS patients, hepatitis B and hepatitis C. IFNβ was approved for treatment of multiple sclerosis in 1993. IFNγ is approved for therapy of chronic granulomatous disease of children. Interleukin-2 (IL-2) was recently approved for the therapy of metastatic renal cell carcinoma.[2]

Other cytokines that have been tested in phase I/II trails include IL-4 (for renal cell carcinoma and melanoma), IL-6 (various malignancies) and tumor necrosis factor (various malignancies). The toxicities in these reports were dose limiting and monotherapy with any of these cytokines produced only rare therapeutic effects.

INTERFERON CHARACTERISTICS

A variety of stimuli including viruses, tumor cells and bacteria can elicit IFN production by several different cells.[3] IFNs comprise a multigene family of proteins first described by Isaacs and Lindenmann in 1957 who noted that supernatants from virus-infected cell cultures contained a protein that protected eukaryotic cells of the same species from viral infection.[4] This protein was called 'interferon' since it interfered with viral replication. Although IFNs are the body's first line of defense against viral diseases, these proteins also have antiproliferative and immunoregulatory properties. IFNs are classified into three major groups, IFNα, IFNβ and IFNγ, based on their biochemical, physiologic and genetic properties.[3]

Type 1 IFNs share a high degree of amino acid homology and include IFNα (leukocyte IFN) and IFNβ (fibroblast IFN). Type 1 IFNs are produced by virus-infected cells and are stable at pH 2 and at 56°C. Null lymphocytes and B-lymphocytes are capable of producing IFNα, while IFNβ is produced by fibroblasts and epithelial cells. Macrophages can produce both IFNα and IFNβ. IFNα is a multigene product containing at least 14 subtypes; IFNβ is a single gene product with at least two subtypes. IFNα and IFNβ share a 34% sequence homology and have similar biologic effects.

Type 2 IFN (immune IFN) is now termed IFNγ. It differs from IFNα and IFNβ both antigenically and functionally since its immunoregulatory activity is more prominent than its antiviral actions. It is a single gene product and is unstable at pH 2 or at 56°C. IFNγ is produced by T-lymphocytes and occasionally by natural killer cells as an anamnestic response to foreign antigens. Whereas IFNα and IFNβ share a cellular receptor, IFNγ has a unique receptor.

As cytokines, IFNs regulate cell proliferation, differentiation and immune function by binding to their specific cellular receptors which results in transmembrane signalling and synthesis of effector proteins. Inducible antiviral proteins include eIF-2a protein kinase, 2',5'-oligodenylate synthetase and Mx protein.[5,6] The eIF-2a protein kinase interferes with initiation of viral protein synthesis thus reducing translation of viral proteins. The 2',5'-oligodenylate synthetase pathway exerts its antiviral effects by enzymatically activating nucleases that degrade viral messenger RNA, which thus blocks viral replication. The Mx protein appears to interfere with viral replication by inhibiting transcription. IFNs can also affect glycosylation of viral proteins through an IFN-induced glycosyltransferase.[6]

In addition to their antiviral activities, IFN exerts direct antiproliferative effects on target tumor cells and makes the target cells more antigenically recognizable by the immune surveillance cells by enhancing expression of major histocompatibility antigens. Simultaneously, IFNs can activate host cytotoxic effector cells (e.g., macrophage, natural killer cells, cytotoxic T-cells) to more efficiently lyse tumor cells.[3] IFNs can modulate antibody production by plasma cells which may be important in enhancing antibody-dependent cellular cytotoxicity. IFNs can also regulate production of other cytokines and can affect cell membranes resulting in increased cell fluidity. Thus, IFNs have potential against tumors both of viral and of non-viral etiologies.[7]

IFN has been demonstrated to induce morphologic reversion with elimination of extrachromosomal HPV genomes in animal systems.[8] IFN inhibits the replication of HPV via antiviral proteins and interferes with the proliferation of virally infected wart cells. HPV-associated cell surface antigens are stimulated by IFN making the cells more antigenically recognizable by the immune system. Oncogenes and epidermal growth factor receptor genes are suppressed by IFN which inhibits differentiation of HPV-infected epithelial cells thus inhibiting epithelial cell proliferation. Furthermore, the recruitment, distribution and recirculation of lymphocytes in HPV infected skin can be regulated by IFNγ.[9]

INTERFERON FORMULATIONS

Virally infected cells produce picogram quantities of IFN. Therefore, early attempts to produce human IFN for therapeutic purposes from pooled human leukocytes were problematic and expensive.[10] Early clinical trials were conducted with partially purified IFN preparations, but genetic engineering now allows production of gram quantities of highly purified IFNs with comparable specific (biologic) activities. Peripheral blood mononuclear cells (PBMC) or 'immortalized' human lymphoblastoid cell lines[11] can be stimulated by viruses to produce multiple subtypes of IFNα in pharmacologic amounts. Recombinant IFNs are produced in large quantities using bacteria transfected with plasmids carrying genes for IFNα, IFNβ or IFNγ.[12,13] IFNαs produced via recombinant technology which are Food and

Drug Administration (FDA) approved in the US include IFNα2a (Roferon, Hoffmann-LaRoche) and IFNα2b (Intron, Schering), each representing a single subtype of IFNα. The only natural IFN available in the US is IFNαn3 (Alferon, Purdue Frederick), which is produced by virally stimulated PBMC. Both IFNαn3 and IFNα2b are FDA approved for treatment of benign anogenital HPV infections (i.e., condyloma acuminatum).

An international unit of IFN equals the reciprocal of the dilution of the preparation needed to decrease the viral yield in specified cell lines by 50%, The National Institutes of Health and the World Health Organization keep reference standards for each of the IFN types. Specific activities in the range of $1-2 \times 10^8$ IU/ml have been noted for purified preparations of IFN. Nanogram quantities of IFN produce measurable antiviral activities, while immunoregulatory and antiproliferative actions usually require higher concentrations.

INTERFERON PHARMACOKINETICS

The three major types of IFN differ in their pharmacokinetic properties.[14] IFNβ and IFNγ are rapidly inactivated in most body fluids while IFNα remains stable. The half-life of IFNα is prolonged in nephrectomized animals and in humans with renal insufficiency.[15,16] Parenteral administration of IFNα produces little or no detectable urinary IFNα concentration. These data support the renal metabolism and clearance of IFNα. Although no quantitative pharmacokinetic data are available for intralesional IFNα, detectable levels of IFNα appear in the plasma following this route of administration. In patients with normal renal function, plasma levels of IFNα peak within 4–8 h after subcutaneous or intramuscular administration and return to baseline within 24–48 h. When IFNα is given intravenously over a 30 min time period to persons with normal renal function, the IFNα levels peak by the end of the infusion and become undetectable within 4 h. Plasma levels of IFNα given subcutaneously or intramuscularly are dose related with a half-life of 10–14 h. Administration of IFNβ or IFNγ via either of these routes, however, does not produce detectable plasma levels

of IFN due to rapid inactivation and/or to increased tissue affinity. It is noteworthy, however, that the plasma concentrations of IFNs have not correlated well with their biological effects in clinical trials.

CLINICAL STUDIES WITH IFNs

While the majority of clinical trials using IFNs for the therapy of tumors of the lower genital tract have been for benign lesions, a variety of studies examined the efficacy or IFNα, IFNβ or IFNγ for the treatment of cervical intraepithelial neoplasia (CIN), vaginal intraepithelial neoplasia (VIN) or cervical cancer.

The first reported use of IFN in the treatment of lower genital tract tumors involved IFNα for topical therapy of condyloma acuminatum in 1975.[17,18] Despite early claims of high success rates, most subsequent studies demonstrated low efficacy rates.[19,20] When recurrence rates were provided, it was evident that wart clearance was often followed a few months later by a relapse.

Topical therapy (Table 12.1[21–29]) of CIN using natural IFNα was first reported in 1981.[21] In this study one million IU of IFNα ointment was applied daily for 2–3 weeks which resulted in a 54% (7/13 patients) complete response (CR) rate. A CR is defined as the disappearance of all clinically visible lesions as well as the prevention of new lesion formation during the follow-up period. No patient (0/18 patients) achieved a CR with the placebo ointment.

Similar efficacies were observed by Moller et al[23] in patients with CIN using natural IFNα at 0.06 million IU/0.5 cm^3 twice/week for 12 weeks. In this study 3 of 6 patients (50%) attained a CR, but no placebo treated patients were included.

Less impressive results were observed by Byrne et al[25] using natural IFNα at 0.4 million IU/2 cm^3 twice/week for 6–8 weeks. Only 3/13 CIN patients (23%) were observed with a CR following this IFNα treatment versus 2/13 (15%) patients treated with placebo. A similar CR rate, 22% (2/9 patients) was reported by Krause et al[26] in women with CIN who used natural IFNα (6.0 million IU) topically for 4 weeks continuously. No patients were treated with placebo in this report. Neither were recurrence rates (RR)

Table 12.1 Topical interferon monotherapy for condyloma acuminata, cervical intraepithelial neoplasia* and cervical cancer**

Reference	Preparation	Dose (MU)	Route/schedule	CR (%)		RR (%)	
				With interferon	With placebo	With interferon	With placebo
21*	IFNα (natural)	1.0	Top 1 ×/day for 2–3 weeks	7/13 patients (54%)	0/18 patients (%)	ND	ND
22**	IFNα (natural)	2.0	Top 1 ×/day for 3 weeks	2/6 patients (33%)	ND	0/2 patients (0%) at 11–34 months	ND
						0/1 patient (0%) at 11–34 months	ND
23*	IFNα (natural)	0.06 MU/0.5 ml	Top 1 ×/day and i.m. 1 MU/day for 3 weeks	1/9 patients (11%)	ND	ND	ND
			Top 2 ×/week for 12 weeks (intravaginal)	3/6 patients (50%)	ND	ND	ND
24*	IFNβ	ND	Top 1 ×/day for 4 weeks then IL for 4 weeks	18/18 patients (100%)	ND	ND	ND
			IL 1 ×/day for 4 weeks	7/7 patients (100%)			
19 (VIN) 1 or 2	IFNα (natural)	2.0 MU/g	Top four 2-week treatment courses 1 week apart (intravaginal)	3/8 patients (38%)	0/5 patients (0%)	3/3 patients (100%) at 1–2 months	ND
25*	IFNα (natural)	0.4 MU/2 ml	Top 2 ×/week for 6–8 weeks	3/13 patients (23%)	2/13 patients (15%)	ND	ND
26*	IFNα	6.0	Top continuously for 4 weeks	2/9 patients (22%)	ND	ND	ND
27*	rIFNα2c	10.0 MU/10 ml	Top 1 ×/day for 6–12 weeks women (intravaginal) Top 1 ×/day for 6–12 weeks men	5/8 patients (63%) 1/1 patient (100%)	ND	0/5 patients (0%) at 7.5 months (mean) 0/1 patient (0%) at 7.5 months	ND
28*	IFNα (natural)	9.0 MU/g	Top 1 ×/day 2-week courses 1 week apart	4/9 patients (44%)	7/10 patients (70%)	0/4 patients (0%) at 16 months	2/7 patients (29%) at 16 months
29 VIN 3	IFNα (natural)	1.0 ± 1% nonoxynol 9	Top 3 ×/day for 2–4 months	9/18 patients (50%)	ND	0/9 patients (0%) at 12 months	ND

with IFNα or with placebo reported in any of these four preceding studies.

Natural IFNα was used for the treatment of CIN by Yliskoski et al[28] who observed a 44% (4/9 patients) CR with topical IFNα at 9.0 million IU/gram when used daily in two 1-week courses separated by 1 week. Interestingly, the CR was 70% (7/10 patients) in the placebo treated women. None of four patients treated with IFNα available at 16 months follow-up were observed with a recurrence of CIN. In contrast the RR at 16 months in placebo treated women was 29% (2/7 patients).

Using IFNα2c at 10.0 million IU/10 cm³, Schneider et al[27] reported topical therapy once daily for 6–12 weeks resulted in a 63% (5/8 patients) CR of CIN. The RR at 7.5 months was 0% (0/5 patients). No patients were treated with placebo.

In another study[24] IFNβ was applied topically once daily to CIN for 4 weeks followed by intralesional IFNβ for another 4 weeks. The CR was 100% (18/18 patients) which was the same CR (7/7 patients) achieved with intralesional IFNβ (daily for 4 weeks) in another group of CIN patients without topical IFNβ. No patients were treated with placebo and no RR was given.

Natural IFNα[30] produced a 38% (3/8 patients) CR with VIN when applied topically (2 million IU/gram) for four 2-week treatment courses 1 week apart. No CR (0/5 patients) was observed with placebo. The RR following IFN, however, was 100% (3/3 patients) at 1–2 months.

Krusic et al[22] reported that natural IFNα, 2.0 million IU applied topically once daily for 3 weeks to cervical cancer resulted in a 33% (2/6 patients) CR. At 11–34 months follow-up the RR was 0%. No placebo treated patients were included.

Therefore the clinical efficacy of topical IFNs for CIN, VIN or cervical cancer appears to be modest and occasionally transient. In addition, few patients were included in any one study. One reason that topical IFN may have limited efficacy in these diseases is that insufficient IFN can reach the target calls via this route.

Although perhaps not as initially appealing to the patients, intralesional IFN therapy of condyloma acuminatum appeared more efficacious than the topical route.[31–39] When such data was re-ported, it appeared that recurrence rates following successful intralesional IFN therapy were relatively low.[31,33,34,37,38]

Somewhat greater efficacy also has been observed in the therapy of CIN and cervical cancer with the intralesional (i.l.) use of IFN (Table 12.2[40–51]) than via the topical route. Only 1 of 9 patients (11%) treated by Frost et al[47] with 2.0 million IU of IFNα2b three times per week for 5 weeks (i.l.) reached a CR. Dunham et al,[48] however, treated CIN with IFNα2b, 1.5 million IU twice weekly for 8 weeks (i.l.) achieving a 29% (2/7 patients) CR. No placebo treated patient (of 7 treated) reached a CR. Stellato et al[50] also using i.l. IFNα2b at 3.0 million IU three times per week for 3 weeks observed a very similar CR, 33% (8/24 patients with CIN). Hsu et al[43] noted that natural IFNα, 2.0 million IU twice weekly for 7–18 doses (i.l.) resulted in a 100% (3/3 patients) CR of CIN while IFNβ used in a similar manner did not result in a CR in the one treated patient. On the other hand, Choo et al[45] reported that natural IFNα 2.0 million IU given i.l. to CIN twice weekly for 4–6 weeks produced a 86% CR (6/7 patients) while IFNβ administered in an identical fashion resulted in a 40% CR (2/5 patients). The RR for IFNα treated patients was 50% (3/6 patients) at 12–24 months, but the RR for the IFNβ treated patients was not given. In other studies IFNβ was administered i.l. to CIN in doses ranging from 0.015 to 3.0 million IU in various combinations of daily and/or weekly schedules for 1–8 weeks. Relatively good CRs were reported: 100% (2/2 patients);[40] 60% (3/5 patients);[41] 54% (7/13 patients);[42] 80% (33/41 patients);[44] and 59% (19/32 patients).[51] No patients were treated with placebo in any of these studies.

IFNγ was administered i.l. to CIN[49] at 3.0 million IU twice weekly for 1–6 weeks which produced a 63% CR (5/8 patients) versus a 12% CR (1/8 patients) with placebo. None of 3 IFNγ treated patients (with a CR) available at 23–24 months follow-up nor the one placebo treated patient (at 3 months follow-up) was observed to have suffered a recurrence.

Using natural IFNα for the therapy of CIN and of cervical cancer, Vasilyev et al[46] gave i.l. injections (containing 0.02–3.0 million IU/treatment) 1–2 times daily for 10 days. This treatment re-

Table 12.2 Intralesional interferon monotherapy for cervical intraepithelial neoplasia* and cervical cancer**

Reference	Preparation	Dose (MU)	Route/schedule	CR (%)		RR (%)	
				With interferon	With placebo	With interferon	With placebo
40*	IFNβ	0.015–0.25	i.l. weekly for average of 8 weeks	2/2 patients 100%	ND	ND	ND
41*	IFNβ	2.0–3.0 ± 1.2	i.l. daily × 5 days/week for 1–3 weeks ± Top daily × 5 days	3/5 patients (60%)	ND	ND	ND
42*	IFNβ	2.0–3.0 ± 1.2	i.l. daily × 5 days/week for 2–3 weeks ± Top daily × 5 days	7/13 patients (54%)	ND	ND	ND
43*	IFNα (natural)	2.0	i.l. 2 ×/week (7–18 doses)	3/3 patients (100%)	ND	ND	ND
	IFNβ	1.0–2.0		0/1 patient (0%)	ND	ND	ND
44*	IFNβ	3.0	i.l. daily for 1 week then for 2 weeks	33/41 patients (80%)	ND	ND	ND
45*	IFNα (natural)	2.0	i.l. 2 ×/week for 4–6 weeks	6/7 patients (86%)	ND	3/6 patients (50%) at 12–24 months	ND
46*,**	IFNβ	2.0		2/5 patients (40%)	ND	ND	ND
	IFNα (natural)	0.02–3.0	i.l. 1–2 ×/day for 10 days	36/125 patients (29%)	ND	ND	ND
47*	rIFNα2b	2.0	i.l. 3 ×/week for 5 weeks	1/9 patients (11%)	ND	ND	ND
48*	rIFNα2b	1.5	i.l. 2 ×/week for 8 weeks	2/7 patients (29%)	0/7 patients (0%)	ND	ND
49*	IFNγ	3.0	i.l. 2 ×/week for 1–6 weeks	5/8 patients (63%)	1/8 patients (13%)	0/3 patients (0%) at 23–24 months	0/1 patient (0%) at 3 months
50*	rIFNα2b	3.0	i.l. 3 ×/week for 3 weeks	8/24 patients (33%)	ND	ND	ND
51*	IFNβ	1.0–3.0	i.l. daily × 5 days/week for 2 weeks	19/32 patients (59%)	ND	ND	ND

sulted in a 29% (36/125 patients) CR, but no RR was noted.

While the majority of these studies using intralesional IFNs for the treatment of CIN or cervical cancer suffer from small numbers of patients and/or from no reported recurrence rates, the CRs appear to be superior to those observed with topical IFNs. Unlike topical IFN, or even systemic IFN, self-therapy with i.l. IFN, however, would range from difficult to impossible.

In order to avoid the labor-intensive i.l. route of IFN administration and to enhance the patient acceptability of IFN therapy, numerous clinical trials have evaluated the systemic administration of IFN for condyloma acuminatum. These studies involved a variety of IFNα, β and γ preparations, dosages and schedules. In addition, few reports delineated the meaning of 'systemic,' i.e., whether the injection was given at a distant site such as the arm or locally such as the inguinal area. Due in part to these variables as well as to such patient characteristics as extent and location (i.e., genital versus perianal) of disease, complete clearance rates with systemic IFN therapy have ranged from 0 to 100%; most reports, however, have documented CRs of 20 to 70%.[52–69] The RR following a CR was provided for both IFN and placebo treatment groups in only four of these reports,[61–64] but the RR following successful IFN therapy was not superior to placebo.

The four reported studies with systemic IFN for therapy of CIN (Table 12.3[27,70–73]) differ from one another in the IFN preparation, in the dosage and in the treatment schedules. Schneider et al[27] treated CIN patients with 5.0 million IU of IFNα2c subcutaneously (s.q.) daily for an average of 6 weeks. Five of seven patients (71%) achieved a CR; none of these patients suffered a recurrence at an average 7.5 months follow-up. Five additional CIN patients were treated with 10.0 million IU of IFNα2c topically once daily for 6–12 weeks combined with s.q. injections of 5.0 million IU of IFNα2c given daily for a mean of 6 weeks. Only one patient cleared with this treatment (i.e., 20% CR), but this patient was still lesion free at her 7.5 months follow-up visit. Slotman et al[70] treated one CIN patient with 5.0 million IU of IFNα2b s.q. three times per week for 16 weeks. This person achieved a CR and had no recurrence

at her 18 months follow-up visit. Natural IFNα was used for s.q. treatment of CIN by Yliskoski et al[72] who reported a 49% CR (28/57 patients) following 1.5 million IU (later increased to 3.0 million IU) given three times per week for 7 weeks. Surprisingly the CR rate with placebo therapy was also 49% (25/51 patients). At 12 months follow-up the RR was 21% (6/28) and 16% (4/25) for the IFNα and the placebo treated patients, respectively. Costa et al[71] reported that 2.0 million IU of IFNβ given intramuscularly (i.m.) daily for 10 days for one or two treatment courses 1 month apart resulted in a 100% CR (6/6 patients) with CINII and a 25% CR (1/4 patients) with CINIII. The RR was 0% at 8–12 months follow-up for these seven patients.

Considering the low number of patients treated and that the only placebo-controlled study demonstrated no effect of IFN therapy, the efficacy of systemic IFN monotherapy for CIN appears questionable. The site of the IFN injection may have played a role in determining the efficacy since IFN given s.c. in the inguinal area may deliver higher concentrations of the drug to dysplastic cells than would an s.c. injection given into the arm. The site of the injection, however, was not provided for these published studies.

Many investigations combining IFN therapy with various nonantiviral treatments for the benign tumor, condyloma acuminatum, indicate that such combinations may have additive to synergistic therapeutic advantages over monotherapy.[27,57,67,74–82]

All of these studies used IFN following surgical (laser or electrocautery) removal of the warts. The only trial that combined surgical (laser) removal of warts followed by IFN that failed to produce a significant reduction in the RR was reported in 1993.[62] This group, however, gave s.q. rIFNα2a in the arm in contrast to the location of s.c. rIFNα2a injections given in trials which demonstrated successful combination therapy i.e. adjacent to the former site of the warts (e.g., Ref. 82). In contrast to the success of the majority of surgery plus IFN studies, however, neither combinations of IFN and cryotherapy[83,84] nor IFN and podophyllin[85] have been successful at reducing RR beyond that observed with monotherapy.

Table 12.3 Systemic interferon monotherapy for cervical intraepithelial neoplasia* and cervical cancer**

Reference	Preparation	Dose (MU)	Route/schedule	CR (%) W/IFN With interferon	With placebo or other TX	RR (%) W/IFN With interferon	With placebo or other TX
27*	rIFNα2c		10.0 MU/10 ml top 1 ×/day for 6–12 weeks and 5.0 MU s.c. daily × 6 weeks (mean)	1/5 patients (20%)	ND	0/1 patient (0%) at 7.5 months	ND
		5.0	s.c. daily × 6 weeks (mean)	5/7 patients (71%)	ND	0/5 patients (0%) at 7.5 months (avg)	ND
70*	rIFNα2b	5.0	s.c. 3 ×/week for 16 weeks	1/1 patients (100%)	ND	0/1 patient (0%) at 18 months	ND
71*	IFNβ	2.0 (CIN 2)	i.m. daily × 10 days for 1 or 2 treatment courses 1 month apart	6/6 patients (100%)	ND	0/6 patients (0%) at 8–12 months	ND
		2.0 (CIN 3)		1/4 patients (25%)		0/1 patient (0%)	
72*	IFNα (natural)	1.5 then 3.0	s.c. 3 ×/week × 1 week, then 3 ×/week × 6 weeks	28/57 patients (49%)	25/51 patients (49%)	6/28 patients (21%) at 12 months	4/25 patients (16%) at 12 months
73**	rIFNα2a	6.0 + oral 13-c retinoic acid (1 mg/kg)	s.c. daily × 2–3 months	1/26 patients (4%)	ND	ND	ND

Very little data, however, exists on combinations of IFNs (or other cytokines) plus traditional therapies for cervical cancer. Recently, Lippman et al[73] treated 26 patients with untreated, locally advanced squamous cell carcinoma of the cervix for at least 2 months with s.c. rIFNα2a (6 million IU/treatment) plus oral 13-*cis*-retinoic acid 13-cRA (1 mg/kg). While only one patient experienced a CR (4%), 12 (46%) other patients achieved major tumor regressions of ≥ 50% in association with resolution of symptoms. In the 13 nonresponders, the disease stabilized in nine and progressed in four patients. In addition to being active, this combination of IFNα2a and 13-cRA was well tolerated. These results are remarkable since 21 (81%) of the patients had stage II or higher cervical cancer. Therefore, this investigation provides one of the first clinical indications of the high therapeutic index that can be achieved in cervical cancer by combining cytokine therapy with another biological response modifier with a different mechanism of action.

ADVERSE EVENTS ASSOCIATED WITH IFNs

Side-effects of IFN therapy are dependent on the dosage of IFN as well as the route of administration and the schedule of treatment. Topical IFN is uncommonly associated with local side effects and very rarely produces systemic side effects. Administration of IFN at doses over one million IU/treatment, however, is commonly associated with a 'flu-like' syndrome regardless of whether the route is intralesional, s.c. or i.m. This flu-like syndrome may consist of any combination of symptoms such as fever, chills, headache, myalgias and malaise[13] and are much more frequent following the first treatment than after subsequent administrations of IFN. Typically this syndrome begins 4–6 h following therapy with IFN and will spontaneously resolve after 12–18 h. The incidence and severity of these symptoms, however, can be minimized by concomitant administration of acetaminophen (500–1000 mg). Acetaminophen can be repeated each 4–6 h as needed.[86] Even without acetaminophen, however, the side effects experienced following IFN at doses ≤ 5 million IU per treatment are usually mild to moderate and are well tolerated in most patients, especially following the second and subsequent doses. Late afternoon or evening administration of IFN is best tolerated.

Uncommon adverse reactions to IFN (at low to moderate doses) include dyspepsia, nausea, vomiting, somnolence and emotional lability. Laboratory abnormalities are occasionally observed and include mild cytopenias (anemia, leukopenia and thrombocytopenia) and liver enzyme elevations. These laboratory changes are usually mild and are rapidly reversible following discontinuation of IFN.

In certain patient populations, however, IFN should be used with caution or not at all. Although IFN is not a teratogen, it has antiproliferative properties which would preclude its use in pregnant patients. In addition, an increased incidence of menstrual irregularities and spontaneous abortions have been reported in primates receiving IFN.

Higher doses of IFN (i.e., >5 million IU/m^2 per day) have occasionally been associated with nausea, vomiting, diarrhea, hypotension, tachycardia, peripheral neuropathy, various rashes and moderate leukopenia and thrombocytopenia. Therefore, IFN therapy is relatively contraindicated in patients with significant preexisting cardiovascular diseases, renal dysfunction, neuropathy, psoriasis or in patients receiving myelosuppressive agents. Systemic IFN therapy has been associated with an increased rate of rejection in organ transplant patients and therefore may be contraindicated in such persons.[87] Since IFN has the capacity to upregulate various immune parameters, it can occasionally exacerbate certain autoimmune diseases.[88] Therefore, IFN should be used with caution in these patients, if at all.

IFN INDUCTION OF SERUM NEUTRALIZING FACTORS

Serum neutralizing factors have occasionally been detected in IFN treated patients, but their clinical significance remains unknown. Neutralizing antibodies appear to develop more frequently in response to recombinant IFNs than to natural IFNs.[89] In fact, Liao et al[90] determined that natural leukocyte-derived IFNα did not induce detectable neutralizing antibodies. Antonelli et al[91] reported a very low rate (i.e., 1.2%) of neutralizing antibody induction by another natural IFN (IFNαnl), but the induction rate by recombinant IFNs was much higher: rIFNα2a, 20.2% and rIFNα2b, 6.9%. This difference in induction rates by various recombinant IFNα preparations, however, had been proposed earlier by Spiegel et al,[92] but this group suggested that components other than IFNα in these preparations were actually responsible for these differences. Patients who fail to respond clinically to recombinant IFNs due to production of neutralizing antibodies can still be successfully treated with natural IFN since antibodies to one subtype of IFNα do not neutralize the activity of other subtypes of IFNα.

FACTORS AFFECTING THE EFFICACY OF IFN IN THERAPY OF LOWER GENITAL TRACT NEOPLASIA

Many variables have been determined to influence the efficacy of IFNs in treatment of condyloma acuminatum. These factors include anatomic location (genital versus perianal), site of injection, history of response to prior therapy, number and size of warts, etc. Which, if any, of these factors play a role in determining the response of lower genital tract neoplasia to IFN remains unknown. One reason for this lack of understanding is the low number of patients treated with IFN with the same dosage and via the same route and schedule. Whether the target lesion is benign or neoplastic, however, it appears that IFN injected into the tumor (or in close proximity) has greater efficacy that the same dose of IFN administered at a distant anatomical site.

Previous studies have demonstrated that IFN appears more effective in treatment of histologically benign warts than in dysplastic warts.[25] Closely associated with this observation is the report that lesions associated with HPV types 16 or 18 respond less well to IFN than do tumors associated with HPV types 6 or 11.[27] In addition, warts in patients infected with the human immunodeficiency virus (HIV) respond significantly less well to IFN than do warts in HIV negative

patients.[93] Since an intact immune system is needed for optimal response to IFN, dysplastic and neoplastic tumors in HIV positive persons would also be expected to respond poorly to IFN.

The role of the immune system in the response to IFN, however, remains incompletely understood. Cigarette smoking, for example, has been associated with an increased incidence of both genital warts and of anogenital neoplasia and may adversely affect patient response to IFN therapy. In otherwise healthy persons with condyloma acuminatum, cell-mediated immune defects have been documented both at the systemic level.[94,95] and at the local level.[96] Normalizations of at least some of these defects following clinically successful therapy of condyloma acuminatum with IFN have been observed both at the systemic[97] and at the local level.[98] Similar evaluations of immune function following IFN therapy of dysplastic or neoplastic tumors, however, have not been reported.

FUTURE ROLE OF CYTOKINE THERAPY IN LOWER GENITAL TRACT NEOPLASIA

Interferon monotherapy for lower genital tract dysplasia and neoplasia has thus far produced only modest results. Somewhat better rates of efficacy have been reported with IFN monotherapy of condyloma acuminatum, but these clearance rates were far from ideal. Several previously cited reports have documented that IFN in combination with traditional modes of therapy of genital warts produces additive to synergistic results in terms of reduced recurrence rates. By analogy, IFN and/or other cytokines in combination with surgery, radiation therapy and/or chemotherapy may produce enhanced cure rates in lower genital tract neoplasia. Other than the promising study of Lippman et al,[73] little clinical data exists to support this hypothesis. Data is rapidly accumulating on the superior therapeutic indices achieved in treatment of neoplasia of other organ systems using IFNs in combination with other cytokines and/or with more traditional therapeutic modalities.[2]

Clinical trials are presently being conducted which employ new classes of antiviral therapy such as antisense oligonucleotides for anogenital papillomavirus infections.[99] Gene therapy for neoplastic diseases is also being evaluated. Likewise, cytokine therapy is no longer restricted to administration of exogenous cytokines since inducers of endogenous cytokines are currently being studied in clinical trials. For example, imiquimod which induces a variety of cytokines such as IFNα, IL-1, IL-6, IL-8 and tumor necrosis factor is currently undergoing placebo-controlled clinical trials formulated as a topical cream in the therapy of external anogenital warts.[100]

Whereas little is known about the efficacy of cytokines other than IFNs in the therapy of lower genital tract neoplasia, it is unlikely that cytokine monotherapy will make a major clinical impact. The future of lower genital tract dysplasia/neoplasia therapy will likely involve cytokines (either exogenously administered or induced) in combination with other biological response modifiers such as retinoids and/or more traditional therapeutic modalities.

REFERENCES

1. Ferenczy A, Mitao M, Nagai N, Silverstein S J, Crum C P. Latent papillomavirus and recurring genital warts. New Engl J Med 1985; 313: 784–788.
2. Heaton K M, Grimm E A. Cytokine combinations in immunotherapy of solid tumors: a review. Cancer Immunol Immunother 1993; 37: 213–219.
3. Baron S, Tyring S D, Fleischmann R Jr et al. The interferons—mechanisms of action and clinical applications. JAMA 1991; 266: 1375–1383.
4. Isaacs A, Lindenmann J. Virus interference, I: the interferon. Proc Royal Soc Ser B 1957; 147: 258–267.
5. Pestka S, Langer J A, Zoon K C, Samuel C E. Interferons and their actions. Ann Rev Biochem 1987; 56: 727–777.
6. Samuel C E. Mechanisms of the antiviral action of interferons. Prog Nucleic Acid Res Molec Biol 1988; 35: 27–72.
7. Tyring S K. Antitumor actions of interferons: Direct, indirect, and synergy with other treatment modalities. Int J Dermatol 1987; 26: 549–566.
8. Turek L P, Byrne J C, Lowy D R, Dvoretzky I, Friedman R M, Howley P M. Interferon induces morphologic reversion with elimination of extrachromosomal viral genomes in bovine papillomavirus-transformed mouse cells. Proc Nat Acad Sci USA 1982; 79: 7914–7918.
9. Nickoloff B J. Role of interferon-γ in cutaneous trafficking of lymphocytes with emphasis on molecular and cellular adhesion events. Arch Dermatol 1988; 124: 1835–1843.
10. Cantell K, Strander H, Hadhazy G, Nevanlinna H R. How much interferon can be prepared in human leukocyte suspensions? In: Rita G, ed. The interferons. New York: Academic Press, pp 223–232.
11. Finter N B. An overview of wellferon (interferon alfa-N1): The product. Med Clinics North Am 1986; 70 (suppl): 13–18.
12. Pestka S. The human interferons — from protein purification and sequence to cloning and expression in bacteria: before, between and beyond. Arch Biochem Biophys 1983; 221: 1–37.
13. Trofatter K F Jr. Interferon treatment of anogenital human papillomavirus-related diseases. Dermatol Clinics 1991; 9: 342–352.
14. Cesario T C, Tilles J G. Inactivation of human interferon by body fluids. Tex Rep Biol Med 1977; 35: 443–448.
15. Bocci V, Pacini A, Muscettola M, Pessina G P, Paulesu L, Bandinelli L. The kidney is the main site of interferon catabolism. J Interferon Res 1982; 2: 309–314.
16. Tokazewski-Chen S A, Marafino B J, Stebbing S. Effects of nephrectomy on the pharmacokinetics of various cloned human interferons in the rat. J Pharmacol Exper Ther 1983; 227: 9–15.
17. Ikic D, Bosnic N, Smerdel S, Jusic D, Soos E, Delimar N. Double blind clinical study with human leukocyte interferon in the therapy of condylomata acuminata. In: Ikic D, ed. Proc Symposium Clin Use Interferon. Zagreb: Yugoslav Acad Sci Arts, 1975; pp 229–233.
18. Ikic D, Orescanin M, Krusic J, Cestar Z. Preliminary study of the effect of human leukocyte interferon on condyloma acuminata in women. In: Ikic D, ed. Proc Symposium Clin Use Interferon. Zagreb: Yugoslav Acad Sci Arts, 1975; pp 223–225.
19. Vesterinen E, Meyer B, Purola E, Cantell K. Treatment of vaginal flat condyloma with interferon cream. Lancet 1984; 1: 157.
20. Keay S, Teng N, Eisenberg M, Story B, Sellers P W, Merigan T C. Topical interferon for treating condyloma acuminata in women. J Infect Dis 1988; 158: 934–939.
21. Ikic D, Singer Z, Beck M, Soos E, Sips D J, Jusic D. Interferon treatment of uterine cervical precancerosis. J Cancer Res Clin Oncol 1981; 101: 303–308.
22. Krusic J, Kirhmajer V, Knezevic M et al. Influence of human leukocyte interferon on squamous cell carcinoma of uterine cervix: clinical, histological, and histochemical observations. J Cancer Res Clin Oncol 1981; 101: 309–315.
23. Moller B R, Johannesen P, Osther K, Ulmsteen U, Hastrup J, Berg K. Treatment of dysplasia of the cervical epithelium with an interferon gel. Obstet Gynecol 1983; 62: 625–629.
24. Marcovici R, Peretz B A, Paldi E. Human fibroblast interferon therapy in patients with condylomata acuminata. Israeli J Med Sci 1983; 19: 104.
25. Byrne M A, Moller B R, Taylor-Robinson J R W et al. The effect of interferon on human papillomaviruses associated with cervical intraepithelial neoplasia. Br J Obstet Gynaecol 1986; 93: 1136–1144.
26. Krause S, Philipsen T, Rank F, Stroyer I. Interferon and cervical dysplasia: CIN 3 treated with local

interferon application. Colposcopy Gynecol Laser Surg 1987; 3: 195–198.

27. Schneider A, Papendick U, Gissmann L, DeVilliers E M. Interferon treatment of human genital papillomavirus infection: Importance of viral type. Int J Cancer 1987; 40: 610–614.

28. Yliskoski M, Cantell K, Syrjanen K, Syrjanen S. Topical treatment with human leukocyte interferon of HPV 16 infections associated with cervical and vaginal intraepithelial neoplasias. Gynecol Oncol 1990; 36: 353–357.

29. Spirtos N M, Smith L H, Teng N N. Prospective randomized trial of topical alpha-interferon (alpha-interferon gels) for the treatment of vulvar intraepithelial neoplasia III. Gynecol Oncol 1990; 37: 34–38.

30. Vesterinen E, Meyer B, Cantell K, Purola E. Topical treatment of flat vaginal condyloma with human leukocyte infection. Obstet Gynecol 1984; 64: 535–538.

31. Geffen J R, Klein R J, Friedman-Kien A E. Intralesional administration of large doses of human leukocyte interferon for the treatment of condyloma acuminata. J Infect Dis 1984; 150: 612–615.

32. Hatch K D, Bart B J, Hansen R C, Millikan L E, Reichman R C, Berman B. Evaluation of interferon alpha₂ (SCH 30500) in the treatment of condyloma acuminatum. Colposcopy Gynecol Laser Surg 1988; 4: 187–196.

33. Friedman-Kien A E, Eron L J, Conant M et al. Natural interferon alfa for treatment of condylomata acuminata. JAMA 1988; 259: 533–538.

34. Eron L, Judson F, Tucker S et al. Interferon therapy for condylomata acuminata. New Engl J Med 1986; 315: 1059–1064.

35. Vance J C, Bart B J, Bart B, Welander C E, Smiles K A, Tanner D J. Effectiveness of intralesional human recombinant alfa-2b interferon (intron-A) for the treatment of patients with condyloma acuminatum. Clin Res 1986; 34: 993A.

36. Vance J C, Bart B J, Hansen R C et al. Intralesional recombinant alpha-2 interferon for the treatment of patient with condyloma acuminatum-verruca plantaris. Arch Dermatol 1986; 122: 272–277.

37. Boot J M, Blog B, Stolz E. Intralesional interferon alpha-2b treatment of condylomata acuminata previously resistant to podophyllum resin application. Genitourinary Med 1989; 65: 50–53.

38. Reichman R C, Oakes D, Bonnez W et al. Treatment of condyloma acuminatum with three different interferons administered intralesionally: A double-blind, placebo-controlled trial. Ann Int Med 1988; 108: 675–679.

39. Scott G M, Csonka G W. Effect of injections of small doses of human fibroblast interferon into genital warts. A pilot study. Br J Ven Dis 1979; 55: 442–445.

40. Uyeno K, Ohtsu A. Interferon treatment of viral warts and some skin diseases. In: Kono R, Vilcek J, eds. The clinical potential of interferons. Tokyo: University of Tokyo Press.

41. Stefanon D. Activity of interferon-beta in small condylomatous lesions of the uterine cervix. Cervix 1983; 1: 23–26.

42. De Palo G, Stefanon B, Rilke E, Pilotti S, Ghione M. Human fibroblast interferon in cervical and vulvar

intraepithelial neoplasia associated with papilloma virus infection. Int J Tissue React 1984; 6: 523–527.

43. Hsu C, Choo Y C, Seto W H et al. Exfoliative cytology in the evaluation of interferon treatment of cervical intraepithelial neoplasia. Acta Cytol 1984; 28: 111–117.

44. Penna C, Fallani M G, Gordigiani R, Sonni L, Taddei G L, Marchionni M. Intralesional beta-interferon treatment of cervical intraepithelial neoplasia associated with human papillomavirus infection. Tumori 1994; 80: 146–150.

45. Choo Y C, Seto W H, Hsu C et al. Cervical intraepithelial neoplasia treated by perilesional injection of interferon. Br J Obstet Gynaecol 1986; 93: 372–379.

46. Vasilyev R V, Bokhman J V, Smorodintsev A A et al. An experience with application of human leucocyte interferon for cervical cancer treatment. Eur J Gynecol Oncol 1990; 11: 313–317.

47. Frost L, Skajaa K, Hvidman L E, Fay S J, Larsen P M. No effect of intralesional injection of interferon on moderate cervical intraepithelial neoplasia. Br J Obstet Gynaecol 1990; 97: 626–630.

48. Dunham A M, McCartney J C, McCance D J, Taylor R W. Effect of perilesional injection of alpha-interferon on cervical intraepithelial neoplasia and associated human papillomavirus infection. J Royal Soc Med 1990; 83: 490–492.

49. Iwasaka T, Hayashi Y, Yokoyama M, Hachisuga T, Sugimori H. Interferon-γ treatment for cervical intraepithelial neoplasia. Gynecol Oncol 1990; 37: 96–102.

50. Stellato G. Intralesional recombinant alpha 2B interferon in the treatment of human papillomavirus-associated cervical intraepithelial neoplasia. Sex Trans Dis 1992; 19: 124–126.

51. Micheletti L, Barbero M, Preti M et al. I1 beta-interferone intralesionale nel trattamento delle CIN associate ad infezione da HPV. Minerva Ginecol 1992; 44: 329–334.

52. Einhorn N, Ling P, Strander H. Systemic interferon alpha treatment of human condylomata acuminata. Acta Obstet Gynec Scand 1983; 62: 285–287.

53. Trofatter K F, English P C, Hughes C E, Gall S A. Human lymphoblastoid interferon (Wellferon) in primary therapy of two children with condylomata acuminata. Obstet Gynecol 1986; 67: 137–140.

54. Gall S A, Hughes C E, Trofatter K. Interferon for the therapy of condyloma acuminata. Am J Obstet Gynecol 1985; 153: 157–163.

55. Olsen E A, Trofatter K F, Gall S A et al. Human lymphoblastoid alpha-interferon in the treatment of refractory condyloma acuminata. Clin Res 1985; 33: 673A.

56. Reichman R C, Micha J P, Weck P K et al. Interferon alpha-nl (Wellferon) for refractory genital warts: efficacy and tolerance of low dose systemic therapy. Antiviral Res 1988; 10: 41–57.

57. Weck P K, Buddin D A, Whisnant J K. Interferons in the treatment of genital human papillomavirus infections. Am J Med 1988; 85 (suppl 2A): 159–164.

58. Gross G, Ikenberg H, Roussaki A, Dress N, Schöpf E. Systemic treatment of condylomata acuminata with recombinant interferon-alpha-2a: low-dose superior to high-dose regimen. Chemotherapy 1986; 32: 537–541.

59. Gross G, Roussaki A, Schöpf E, DeVilliers E M, Papendick U. Successful treatment of condyloma acuminata and bowenoid papulosis with subcutaneous injections of low-dosage recombinant interferon-α. Arch Dermatol 1986; 122: 749–750.

60. Gall S A, Constantine L, Koukol D. Therapy of persistent human papillomavirus disease with two different interferon species. Am J Obstet Gynecol 1991; 164: 130–134.

61. Panici P B, Scambia G, Baiocchi G, Perrone L, Pintus C, Mancuso S. Randomized clinical trial comparing systemic IFN with diathermocoagulation in primary multiple and widespread anogenital condyloma. Obstet Gynecol 1989; 74: 393–397.

62. Condylomata International Collaborative Study Group. Randomized placebo-controlled double blind combined therapy with laser surgery and systemic IFN-α2a in the treatment of anogenital condylomata acuminatum. J Infect Dis 1993; 167: 824–829.

63. Reichman R C, Oakes D, Bonnez W et al. Treatment of condyloma acuminatum with three different interferon-α preparations administered parenterally: a double-blind, placebo-controlled trial. J Infect Dis 1990; 162: 1270–1276.

64. Schonfeld A, Nitke S, Schattner A et al. Intramuscular human interferon-beta injections in treatment of condylomata acuminata. Lancet 1984; 1: 1038–1042.

65. Kirby P, Wells D, Kiviat N, Corey L. A phase I trial of intramuscular recombinant human gamma interferon for refractory genital warts. J Infect Dis 1986; 86: 485.

66. Gross G, Roussaki A, Brzoska J. Low doses of systemically administered recombinant interferon-gamma effective in the treatment of genital warts. J Invest Dermatol 1988; 90: 242.

67. Fierlbeck G, Rassner G. Treatment of condylomata acuminata with systemically administered recombinant gamma interferon. Z Hautki 1987; 62: 1280–1287.

68. Kirby P K, Kiviat N, Beckman A, Wells D, Sherwin S, Corey L. Tolerance and efficacy of recombinant human interferon gamma in the treatment of refractory genital warts. Am J Med 1988; 85: 183–188.

69. Zouboulis C, Stadler R, Ikenberg H, Orfanos C E. Short-term systemic recombinant interferon-γ treatment is ineffective in recalcitrant condylomata acuminata. J Am Acad Dermatol 1991; 24: 302–303.

70. Slotman B J, Helmerhorst T J, Wijermans P W, Calame J J. Interferon alpha in treatment of intraepithelial neoplasia of the lower genital tract: a case report. Eur J Obstet Gynecol Reprod Biol 1988; 27: 327–333.

71. Costa S, Poggi M G, Palmisano L, Syrjanen S, Yliskoski M, Syrjanen K. Intramuscular β-interferon treatment of human papillomavirus lesions in the lower female genital tract. Cervix I.f.g.t. 1988; 6: 203–212.

72. Yliskoski M, Syrjanen K, Syrjanen S, Saarikoski S, Nethersell A. Systemic alpha-interferon (Wellferon) treatment of genital human papillomavirus (HPV) type 6, 11, 16 and 18 infections: double-blind, placebo-controlled trial. Gynecol Oncol 1991; 43: 55–60.

73. Lippman S M, Kavanagh J J, Paredes-Espinoza M et al. 13-cis-retinoic acid plus interferon α-2a: highly active systemic therapy for squamous cell carcinoma of the cervix. J Nat Cancer Inst 1992; 84: 241–245.

74. Gross G, Pfister H. Recurrent vulvar Buschke-Löewenstein tumor-like condylomata and Hodgkins disease effectively treated with recombinant interferon alpha 2c gel as an adjuvant to electrosurgery. J Cancer Res Clin Oncol 1988; 114s: 147.

75. Piccoli R, Santoro M G, Nappi C et al. Vulvo-vaginal condylomatosis and relapse: combined treatment with electrocauterization and beta-interferon. Clin Exper Obstet Gynecol 1989; 16: 30–35.

76. Tiedemann K H, Ernst T M. Combination therapy of recurrent condylomata acuminata with electrocautery and alpha-2-interferon. AKT Dermatol 1988; 14: 200–204.

77. Vance J C, Davis D. Interferon alpha-2b injections used as an adjuvant therapy to carbon dioxide laser vaporization of recalcitrant ano-genital condylomata acuminata. J Invest Dermatol 1990; 95: 146S–148S.

78. Hohenleutner U, Landthaler M, Braun-Falco O. Postoperative adjuvante therapie mit interferon-alfa-2b nach laserchirurgie von condylomata acuminata. Hautarzt 1990; 41: 545–548.

79. Erpenbach K, Derschum W, Vietsch H V. Adjuvant-systemische interferon-α2b-behandlung bei therapieresistenten anogenitalen condylomata acuminata. Urologe A 1990; 29: 43–45.

80. Petersen C S, Bjerring P, Larsen J et al. Systemic interferon alpha-2b increases the cure rate in laser treated patients with multiple persistent genital warts: a placebo-controlled study. Genitourinary Med 1991; 67: 99–102.

81. Davis B E, Noble M J. Initial experience with combined interferon alpha-2b and carbon dioxide laser for the treatment of condyloma acuminata. J Virol 1992; 147: 627–629.

82. Reid R, Greenberg M D, Pizzuti D J, Omoto K H, Rutledge L H, Soo W. Superficial laser vulvectomy V. surgical debulking is enhanced by adjuvant systemic interferon. Am J Obstet Gynecol 1992; 166: 815–820.

83. Handley J M, Horner T, Maw R D, Lawther H, Dinsmore W W. Subcutaneous interferon alpha 2a combined with cryotherapy vs cryotherapy alone in the treatment of primary anogenital warts: a randomized observer blind placebo controlled study. Genitourinary Med 1991; 67: 297–302.

84. Eron L J, Alder M B, O'Rourke J M, Rittweger K, DePamphilis J, Pizzuti D J. Recurrence of condylomata acuminata following cryotherapy is not prevented by systemically administered interferon. Genitourinary Med 1993; 69: 91–93.

85. Douglas J M Jr, Eron L J, Judson F M et al. A randomized trial of combination therapy with intralesional interferon alpha 2b and podophyllin versus podophyllin alone for the therapy of anogenital warts. J Infect Dis 1990; 162: 52–59.

86. Trofatter K F, Olsen E A, Kucera P R. Combination of NSAID and Wellferon: A controlled clinical trial of genital warts. In: Stewart W E II, Schellekens H, eds. The biology of the interferon system 1985. Amsterdam: Elsevier, 1986: pp 471–477.

87. Kovarik J, Mayer G, Pohanka E et al. Adverse effect of low-dose prophylactic human recombinant leukocyte interferon alpha treatment in renal transplant recipients. Transplantation 1988; 45: 402–405.

88. Ronnblom L E, Alm G V, Oberg K E. Autoimmunity after alpha-interferon therapy for malignant carcinoid tumors. Ann Int Med 1991; 115: 178–183.

89. Von Wussow P, Freund M, Block B, Diedrich H, Poliwoda H, Deicher H. Clinical significance of anti-IFN-α antibody titers during interferon therapy. Lancet 1987; 11: 635–636.

90. Liao M J, Axelrod H R, Kuchler M, Yip Y K, Kirkbright E, Testa D. Absence of neutralizing antibodies to interferon in condyloma acuminata and cancer patients treated with natural human leukocyte interferon. J Infect Dis 1992; 165: 757–760.

91. Antonelli G, Currenti M, Turriziani O, Dianzani F. Neutralizing antibodies to interferon-α: relative frequency in patients treated with different interferon preparations. J Infect Dis 1991; 163: 882–885.

92. Spiegel R J, Spicehandler J R, Jacobs S J, Oden E M. Low incidence of serum neutralizing factors in patients receiving recombinant alpha-2b interferon (Intron A). Am J Med 1986; 80: 223–228.

93. Douglas J M, Rogers M, Judson F N. The effect of asymptomatic infection with HTLV-III on the response of anogenital warts to intralesional treatment with recombinant α2 interferon. J Infect Dis 1986; 154: 331–334.

94. Carson L F, Twiggs L B, Fukushima M, Ostrow R S, Faras A J, Okagaki T. Human genital papilloma infections: An evaluation of immunologic competence in the genital neoplasia — papilloma syndrome. Am J Obstet Gynecol 1986; 155: 784–789.

95. Cauda R, Tyring S K, Grossi C E. Patients with condyloma acuminatum exhibit decreased interleukin-2 and interferon gamma production and depressed natural killer activity. J Clin Immunol 1987; 7: 304–311.

96. Arany I, Rady P, Tyring S K. Alteration in cytokine/antioncogene expression in skin lesions caused by "low-risk" types of human papillomaviruses. Viral Immunol 1993; 6: 255–265.

97. Tyring S K, Cauda R, Ghanta V, Hiramoto R. Activation of natural killer cell function during interferon-α treatment of patients with condyloma acuminatum is predictive of clinical response. J Biol Regulat Homeost Agents 1988; 2: 63–66.

98. Arany I, Rady P, Tyring S K. Interferon treatment enhances the expression of underphosphorylated (biologically active) retinoblastoma protein in human papillomavirus infected cells through the inhibitory TGFβ₁/IFNβ cytokine pathway. Antiviral Res 1994; 23: 131–141.

99. Cowsert L M, Fox M C, Zon G, Mirabelli C K. In vitro evaluation of phosphorothioate oligonucleotides targeted to the E2 mRNA of papillomavirus: Potential treatment for genital warts. Antimicrobial Agents Chemother 1993; 37: 171–177.

100. Spruance S, Douglas J, Hougham A, Fox T, Beutner K. Multicenter trial of 5% Imiquimod (IQ) Cream for the treatment of genital and perianal warts. 33rd Interscience Conference on Antimicrobial Agents and Chemotherapy. Washington: American Academy of Microbiology, 1993; p 381.

13. Vaginal intraepithelial neoplasia

Alberto Lopes   John M. Monaghan   Greg Robertson

INTRODUCTION

The first description of vaginal intraepthelial neoplasia (VAIN) appears to have been made at the Mayo Clinic in 1933 and reported by Hummer et al in 1970,[1] a century after vaginal carcinoma was first described by Cruveilhier in 1826.[2] Initially VAIN was thought to be a rare condition, Woodruff in 1981[3] reporting that less than 300 cases had been recorded in the literature. However, with the increasing use of routine cytological screening and colposcopy the frequency of its detection has increased. This combined with a probable increase in the condition itself means that in most colposcopy clinics today women with VAIN are being managed.

In general it is accepted that there is a need to treat these women because of a potential for progression to invasive carcinoma of the vagina. However controversy still exists over the rate of this progression and the efficacy of the numerous treatment options available both in eradicating the condition and in preventing subsequent malignant change.

EPIDEMIOLOGY

The true incidence of VAIN is difficult if not impossible to assess as it is an asymptomatic condition with the majority of patients being identified following an abnormal Papanicolaou (Pap) smear. As a result, the frequency of VAIN detection is in part related to the prevalence of cytology screening in a given population. In 1966 Timonen et al[4] identified 23 primary dysplasias of the vagina in 12 000 patients screened in 1 year giving an incidence of about 0.2% whilst Cramer and Cutler[5] in the 1970s reported an incidence of about 0.2 per 100 000 women. The true incidence probably lies somewhere within this thousand-fold variation in range.

Although the true incidence of VAIN is not known, it is far lower than that for cervical intraepithelial neoplasia (CIN). In a recent study of over 4000 women with CIN treated by laser vaporisation it was found that only 2.5% of the women had coexisting VAIN, i.e., extension of the intraepithelial lesion onto the upper vagina.[6]

The average age of patients with VAIN, quoted at 40–60 years, is greater than for those presenting with CIN. However ages have ranged anywhere between 19 and 86 years.[7-10] Patients with VAIN 1 and 2 tend to be younger than those with VAIN 3, Audet-Lapointe et al[10] reporting a 15 year age difference between the two groups. This may reflect differing etiological agents or indeed differing diseases.

ETIOLOGY/PREDISPOSING CAUSES

The etiology of VAIN has not been studied in great detail, but the major predisposing factor is likely to be the same as that of CIN, namely, exposure to sexually-transmitted carcinogenic agents. Currently the most likely agent is the human papilloma virus (HPV). The lower incidence of VAIN compared to CIN is explained by the fact that the vagina, unlike the cervix, lacks the metaplastic squamous epithelium of the transformation zone which is the putative target of the HPV.

The precise relationship between HPV and VAIN is unknown but as with other genital tract precancers, the development of VAIN, is probably a multistep process with various cofactors involved. These cofactors include sexual practices, other infectious agents, smoking, the patient's immune status and her fundamental genetic predisposition.

Schneider et al[11] in 1987 found the presence of HPV in the vagina of women posthysterectomy was associated with an increased incidence of VAIN. In their study 5% of HPV positive patients had VAIN, all associated with HPV 16. In the same year Bornstein et al[12] demonstrated HPV in five cases of VAIN in women exposed to diethylstilbestrol (DES) in utero. On this occasion HPV 16 was only detected in one case with HPV 6 being identified in the remaining four. This is unusual as HPV 6 is more often associated with condylomata acuminata than genital intraepithelial neoplasia.

Assuming a common etiology it is not surprising that VAIN is often found in conjunction with CIN. Between 36 and 48% of patients with VAIN have been found to have concomitant CIN[7,9] and as many as 51–62% have had previous treatment for cervical neoplasia, either intraepithelial or invasive.[8,9] Up to 25% of women with VAIN will have previously undergone hysterectomies for the treatment of CIN. Despite these figures the actual risk of developing VAIN following hysterectomy for CIN has been found to be less than 1% after 10 years follow-up.[13]

VAIN may also occur in women following hysterectomy for benign conditions and in some series approximately 40% of the preceding hysterectomies have been for benign reasons.[8] This apparently high incidence of previous hysterectomies has led some authors to the unlikely conclusion that hysterectomy on its own is a risk factor for the subsequent development of VAIN.[14,15]

Radiation treatment has also been cited as a cause of VAIN, with induced dysplasia occurring 10–15 years after radiotherapy for cervical cancer. It is thought that the intermediate or low-dose radiation may sensitize the epithelium for subsequent development of neoplasia.[16]

Immunosuppressed patients are at an increased risk of VAIN in keeping with their increased risk of developing all lower genital tract neoplasias.[17,18] In these patients VAIN is not only found more frequently but is also more often multifocal, persistent and aggressive. Again HPV probably plays a major role in this situation having been reported in many cases of genital intraepithelial neoplasia associated with immunosuppression.[17]

There have been reports that women exposed to DES in utero have an increased incidence of VAIN.[19,20] This may be due to the fact that up to 35% of these women have a transformation zone extending onto the vagina as a result of their in utero exposure. The age group at presentation of these women is younger than usual and as mentioned earlier HPV was identified in every case in Bornstein et al's series.[20] Interestingly recent data from Robboy (personal communication) no longer supports the increased risks of VAIN and CIN previously reported.

CLASSIFICATION

Numerous authors have classified VAIN based on its 'pathogenesis'.[10,20] These are essentially variations on that originally described by Woodruff.[21] The classification system used by Audet-Lapoint[10] is illustrated below.

1. de novo, or found alone without concomitant or previous CIN,
2. associated with CIN or invasive carcinoma, concomitantly or not,
3. postirradiation,
4. multicentric condition — associated with both CIN and VIN, and
5. incidental finding on a surgical specimen.

In a series of 76 patients with VAIN, Audet-Lapoint et al[10] found, as one would expect, the two main groups of VAIN were group 1, arising de novo (34%) and group 2, associated with CIN (33%). The remaining three groups had 13%, 5% and 15%, respectively.

These classification systems are far from ideal as they are an amalgamation of clinicopathological (groups 1, 2, and 4), etiological (group 3) and isolated (group 5) subdivisions. As the groups are not mutually exclusive, patients may fit into more than one group. For example, in the paper by Audet-Lapoint et al,[10] of the 10 patients placed in group 5 (incidental finding of VAIN on the surgical specimen), six were associated with CIN and three with invasive cervical tumors which could place them in group 2, but two had also had previous irradiation which could also place them in group 3.

If we consider that neither CIN, which is far more common, nor VIN are classified in this manner, it is probable that such a classification is unnecessary for VAIN. However, if one was to use a system it would appear more logical to create a clinicopathological classification with etiological subdivisions (see below). With the increasing incidence of immunosuppressed patients as a result of organ transplantation, HIV and other causes, a separate subdivision should probably be included for these patients.

Clinicopathological classification

1. De novo — found alone without concomitant or previous CIN or VIN.
2. Associated with CIN or invasive cervical carcinoma, concomitantly or not.
3. Associated with VIN or invasive vulval carcinoma, concomitantly or not.
4. Associated with both CIN, VIN, or their invasive counterparts, concomitantly or not. All four classifications have the following subdivisions:
   (a) postirradiation,
   (b) immunosuppressed, or
   (c) incidental finding on a surgical specimen.

PATHOLOGY

VAIN affects the upper third of the vagina in the majority of cases, the incidence being as high as 85–92.4% in some series.[8,10] Approximately half the cases are multifocal.[7–9] Rarely the whole vaginal epithelium may be involved particularly when associated with multifocal disease and immunosuppressed patients.

The microscopic features are similar to CIN with nuclear pleomorphism, loss of polarity, and the presence of abnormal mitoses. Traditionally as with CIN, VAIN has been divided into grades 1, 2 and 3. In VAIN 3, the neoplastic cells involve the full thickness of squamous epithelium whilst in VAIN 1 and 2 the cytoplasmic atypia is confined to the lower one-third or two-thirds. As with CIN it may be more useful to divide VAIN simply into low-grade (VAIN 1 and 2) and high-grade

(VAIN 3) lesions especially with regard to treatment and malignant potential.

CLINICAL FEATURES

VAIN is an asymptomatic condition and almost all patients are detected because of abnormal cytology. Colposcopic examination using acetic acid and Schiller's test (aqueous iodine) are essential in identifying the lesions. In post menopausal women and women previously irradiated, the application of local estrogen therapy daily for 2 weeks before colposcopy often clears any superimposed inflammatory changes and facilitates interpretation.

Colposcopy reveals areas of acetowhite epithelium with varying degrees of surface irregularity and accompanying punctation. These lesions are often more readily identified by their lack of iodine uptake. In women with a cervix present, the VAIN lesion is almost invariably an extension of a CIN lesion. In those women having undergone a hysterectomy, careful colposcopic examination of the 'dog ears' at the apex of the vault is essential as this may be the only site of VAIN. Colposcopic directed punch biopsies should be taken of any visible lesion to provide a histological diagnosis. Because of the multicentric nature of genital tract intraepithelial neoplasia it is important to colposcope the cervix and inspect the vulva in all cases of VAIN.

In patients presenting posthysterectomy, the epithelium sequestered above the suture line is not accessible to the colposcope. A careful bimanual examination is therefore essential following colposcopy as occasionally a tumour may be palpable above the suture line.

NATURAL HISTORY

The natural history of VAIN has not been clearly defined. The majority of low-grade lesions probably regress spontaneously without treatment and the risk of progression to an invasive lesion appears to be far less than for CIN. VAIN 3 lesions are thought to have a greater potential for malignant transformation than the low-grade lesions.

In a recent study of the natural history of VAIN, Aho et al[7] observed 23 women with VAIN for a mean period of 5.4 years (range 3–15 years). They performed colposcopy on a regular 6–12 monthly basis without treatment. They found that 78% of lesions regressed, 13% persisted, and 9% (two cases) went on to develop invasive cancer. Regression was more common in VAIN 1 lesions. Overall, lesions not associated with CIN or VIN showed a higher rate of regression (91%) than those associated with CIN or VIN (67%). Of the five VAIN 3 lesions in the study, four regressed and one progressed to cancer.

Even with treatment, VAIN may still recur irrespective of the treatment modality used (see below) and malignant change can develop in up to 5% of patients.[8]

TREATMENT

Numerous treatment modalities have been described for the treatment of VAIN ranging from observation to performing a total vaginectomy. Results are varied and conflicting. Irrespective of the mode of treatment it is essential to continue long-term review of these patients because of the risk of recurrence and the potential to undergo malignant change.

Observation

Currently it is our policy to observe patients with low grade lesions (VAIN 1 and 2) on a regular basis as a number of these will regress spontaneously. This has been shown recently by Aho[7] in a study of the natural history of VAIN (see above). When adopting this expectant policy it is important to repeat biopsies of the lesion to check there is no progression to VAIN 3.

Destructive methods

VAIN can be successfully treated by using various forms of local destructive techniques. Whichever method is used caution must be exercised because of the proximity of the bladder, urethra, rectum and in posthysterectomy cases, the ureters.

Cryocautery

Small VAIN lesions are suitable for cryocautery and a single freeze–thaw cycle is usually sufficient.

The surface area of the lesions treated should approximate that of the probe tip with larger lesions being subdivided to try and achieve this approximation. The ice ball should extend at least 3 mm onto colposcopically normal appearing epithelium. Scarring and contracture have not been found to be a problem with this technique.[22] An ileovaginal fistula has been reported following cryocautery for VAIN.[23]

Laser

In 1977 Stafl et al[24] reported the use of the CO_2 laser to treat 8 patients with VAIN, only one patient having residual disease after 1 years follow-up. Since then the CO_2 laser has been used extensively for the treatment of VAIN. The lesions are vaporised to a depth of 1–3 mm and with a lateral margin of at least 5–10 mm. Complications are uncommon with the procedure though the development of a vesicovaginal fistula has been reported.[25]

The cure rates quoted for treatment with the CO_2 laser have ranged from 42.9 to 100%. Disappointing results have been attributed to the lack of access to atypical epithelium in the 'dog ears' at the apex of the vaginal vault and to missing occult foci of VAIN.[26]

In one of the largest series of laser ablation for VAIN Sherman[25] reported only a 16% recurrence in 143 patients after one treatment and these were all successfully treated by repeat vaporization. He used a combination of wire sutures through the vaginal mucosa and infiltration of the submucosa with procaine HCl to provide retraction and ballooning of any recesses and scars in the vaginal vault. These maneuvers allow better exposure to the laser beam and probably account for the good results obtained. Unfortunately follow-up was short in this series.

Extensive multifocal disease may also result in a high failure rate for laser vaporisation but Jobson and Homesley[26] achieved satisfactory results in this situation by ablating the entire vaginal mucosa. The morbidity associated with this radical therapy makes it an unpopular option.

Latent HPV in seemingly normal mucosa has also been suggested as a cause for recurrence. Stuart et al[27] reported a recurrence rate of VAIN in 62.5% of patients who had evidence of HPV infection compared to 26.3% in patients without.

Invasive lesions occurring at the apex of the vaginal vault have been reported after laser ablation. These lesions probably arise from abnormal epithelium which has been sequestered above the suture line at the time of hysterectomy and would therefore be inaccessible to the laser.[28]

The consensus appears to be that laser ablative therapy does have a major role in the treatment of VAIN. However in posthysterectomy cases, VAIN involving the vaginal scar should be assessed carefully and surgical excision of these lesions may be more appropriate.[29]

Diathermy

Electrocautery has been used for the treatment of VAIN. In a small series Lenehan[8] reported a 25% failure rate after one treatment. With the introduction of loop electrosurgical excision procedure (LEEP) we can expect a possible resurgence in the use of electrocautery techniques in the treatment of VAIN.

Topical applications

Estrogen cream

In the postmenopausal woman cytological atypia on smears may arise as a result of atrophic changes in the vaginal mucosa without associated VAIN. With correction of the estrogen deficency using intravaginal estrogen therapy, the cytological atypia reverts to normal in a significant percentage of women.[30] For this reason it is important to exclude atrophic changes before investigating women in this age group for VAIN.

Estrogen cream has also been shown to be effective in eliminating histologically proven VAIN in postmenopausal women. Applying the cream twice a week for 3–6 months has been reported to result in normal colposcopy and cytology in up to half the women treated.[16] No lesions progressed to invasive cancer during this observation period.

5-Fluorouracil (5-FU)

The cytotoxic agent 5-FU is often used as a topical cream for the treatment of VAIN. In earlier studies it was used in a continuous regimen applied on a daily basis for anything from 5 to 14 days. This was repeated on a further two occasions at 1-weekly intervals. Unfortunately a major problem encountered with this regimen was that of chemical vulvovaginitis which cause severe irritation in many women.[31]

Stokes et al[32] were the first to suggest periodic vaginal applications of 5-FU. The cream, one-third of an applicator of 5% 5FU equivalent to 1.5 g, is inserted deeply into the vagina once weekly at bedtime for 10 consecutive weeks. To prevent vulval irritation the women are advised to apply a protective ointment such as petroleum jelly or zinc oxide to the introitus and vulva just before application of the 5-FU. Where the lesions only involve the upper half of the vagina, the insertion of a tampon into the vaginal introitus immediately after applying the cream further protects the vulval skin. Sexual intercourse must not take place on the night of treatment.

Using this regimen, cure rates of between 81 and 86% have been reported after a single 10-week course.[31,33] However, late treatment failures have been described and prophylactic maintenance therapy has been used to try and eliminate recurrences. Krebs[31] advised women to apply 1.5 g of 5-FU once every 2 weeks for 3 months after the initial treatment and found that 95% remained free of VAIN during a follow-up period of up to 7 years.

Side-effects during the treatment are usually minimal and consist of a sensation of vaginal burning and mild dyspareunia. Only rarely are these severe enough to cause delay in treatment. However in a study on the long-term sequelae of 5-FU therapy Krebs and Helmkamp[34] found that at colposcopic examination two to four weeks after treatment about 42% had signs of chemical mucositis of the vagina and/or cervix and 11.4% had an acute ulcer. In women treated with a single 10-week course, 5.7% developed chronic ulcers (lasting longer than 6 months) and this increased to 9.6% if they continued with prophylactic applications of 5-FU. The size of the ulcers varied from 0.5 to 7 cm with a mean of 2.5 cm. Almost 80% of the women were symptomatic as a result of the ulcers with a serosanguinous or watery discharge, postcoital or irregular bleeding or pain.

Only 50% of the ulcers healed spontaneously without treatment. The location of the ulcers was typically at the apex of the vagina and probably reflected pooling and retention of the cream within the fornices.

Because of the potential problems associated with 5-FU therapy, its use should probably be confined to treating extensive or multifocal high-grade VAIN.

2-4-Dinitrochlorobenzene (DNCB)

VAIN has been shown to regress after local exposure to DNCB treatment.[35] In this small study, six women were treated and all had normal cytology with 2–35 months follow-up.

Interferon

Recently there have been an increasing number of reports on the use of topically applied human leukocyte interferon cream or gel for the treatment of genital HPV infections and intraepithelial neoplasia.[36] Most of these reports have been small and without a control group. Clinical response rates have been poor at less than 50% in most series. This is probably due to the large molecular weight of interferon preventing adequate absorption through the dysplastic squamous epithelium.

Surgical excision

Surgery is probably still the most effective method of eradicating VAIN and has the advantage that the specimen is available for histological evaluation. Procedures include partial and total vaginectomy though wide local excision is often all that is necessary in patients with one or two discrete lesions.

VAIN occurring at the site of the hysterectomy vaginal scar should be treated by a partial vaginectomy due to the risk of an invasive lesion occurring in the vaginal epithelium sequestered above the scar.

A total vaginectomy, though rarely performed may be necessary when there is extensive multifocal disease involving the whole vagina. Both partial and total vaginectomies can be performed by either a vaginal or abdominal approach or a combination of the two.

The vaginal approach may be assisted by a Schuhardt incision to improve access though this is not essential. A 1 cm margin of normal-looking epithelium should be excised with the lesion. During the procedure care should be taken not to damage the ureters or bladder which lie in close proximity. Acute complications including bleeding, infection and accidental injury to the bladder are uncommon. In the long term, shortening and stenosis of the vagina may occur. Preventive measures include not closing the defect and using a dilator with or without estrogen cream in the early postoperative period. Using these measures the site of excision will have reepithelialized within 6 weeks. Covering the excised area with a skin graft is another alternative. A cure rate of 83% has been reported.[37,38]

An abdominal approach can also be used for performing a partial or total vaginectomy. The operation is complex and should only be undertaken by a surgeon experienced with the technique. The procedure involves reflecting the ureters, bladder and rectum off the vagina and occasionally may not be feasible because of extensive scarring. Those patients having a total vaginectomy should be offered a vaginal graft at the same procedure. In our own series of 32 patients,[28] morbidity was low and there were no cases of ureteric or vesicovaginal fistula. The main problem following the procedure has been bladder hypotonia and difficulty in initiating micturition.

Radiotherapy

Intracavity radiotherapy is a highly effective treatment for VAIN. No recurrences were reported in 48 patients treated in three different series despite the use of varying doses of absorbed radiation.[39-41] Short-term morbidity includes vaginal discharge, diarrhea and occasional cystitis. Despite the risk of vaginal stenosis, Woodman et al[41] reported the prevention of this problem by the use of vaginal dilators and early resumption of sexual activity. The median age of women in their series was 39 years and of the 10 women interviewed regarding sexual activity, nine continued to enjoy satisfactory sexual intercourse.

However six of the eight premenopausal women became estrogen deficient and required hormone replacement therapy.

In contrast Benedet and Sanders[42] reported significant complications in 63% of patients treated by irradiation. In our own small series, four women with VAIN were treated using selectron therapy to a surface dose of 60 Gy. The whole length of the vagina was treated. Two women developed vulval ulcerations and one of these has developed recurrent VAIN. One 39 year old developed vaginal stenosis which improved with the use of dilators.

Others

Interferon

There have been several studies investigating the use of human leukocyte interferon in the treatment of genital intraepithelial neoplasia and HPV infection.[36] The use of intralesionally- or perilesionally injected interferon has produced the best cure rates but these are still less than 50%.

Ultrasonic surgical aspiration

Recently ultrasonic surgical aspiration has been used to treat VAIN.[43] In this study, 26 patients with VAIN involving the upper vagina had the entire vaginal epithelium on the upper half of the vagina removed with the aspirator. The amplitude of the machine was set to give the tip an excursion of 175 µm in depth. The procedures were performed under general anesthesia and there were no complications reported. The pathology of the tissue obtained correlated well with cytology and punch biopsy. However 5 of the 26 (19%) recurred within a median follow-up of 45 weeks. Obviously the technique is new and further studies are required to assess its role in the treatment of VAIN.

SUMMARY

VAIN is an uncommon condition but appears to be increasing in incidence. Its etiology is closely linked to CIN with the human papilloma virus appearing the major predisposing factor. Overall the risk of malignant transformation appears small but real. The availability of numerous treatment modalities allows individualization of treatment. Whether treated or not these patients require long-term colposcopic assessment to exclude the development of cancer.

REFERENCES

1. Hummer W K, Mussey E, Decker D G, Docherty M B. Carcinoma in situ of the vagina. Am J Obstet Gynecol 1970; 108: 1109–1116.
2. Cruveilhier J. Varices des veines du ligament rond, simulant une hernie inguinale: Anomalie remarquable dans la disposition general du peritoine: Cancer ulcere de la paroi ante-rieure du vagin et du bas-sond de la vessie. Bull Soc Anat Paris 1826; 1: 199.
3. Woodruff J D. Carcinoma in situ of the vagina. Clin Obstet Gynecol 1981; 24: 485–499.
4. Timonen S, von Numers C, Meyer B. Dysplasia of the vaginal epithelium. Gynecologica 1966; 162: 125–138.
5. Cramer D W, Cutler S J. Incidence and histopathology of malignancies of the female genital organs in the United States. Am J Obstet Gynecol 1974; 118: 443–460.
6. Nwabineli N J, Monaghan J M. Vaginal epithelial abnormalities in patients with CIN: Clinical and pathological features and management. Br J Obstet Gynaecol 1991; 98: 25–29.
7. Aho M, Vesterinen E, Meyer B, Purola E, Paavonen J. Natural history of vaginal intraepithelial neoplasia. Cancer 1991; 68: 195–197.
8. Lenehan P M, Meffe F, Lickrish G M. Vaginal intraepithelial neoplasia: Biologic aspects and management. Obstet Gynecol 1986; 68: 333–337.
9. Mao C C, Chao K C, Lian Y C, Ng H T. Vaginal intraepithelial neoplasia: Diagnosis and management (English abstract). Chung Hua I Hsueh Tsa Chih 1990; 46: 35–42.
10. Audet-Lapointe P, Body G, Vauclair R, Drouin P, Ayoub J. Vaginal intraepithelial neoplasia. Gynecol Oncol 1990; 36: 232–239.
11. Schneider A, de Villiers E M, Schneider V. Multifocal squamous neoplasia of the female genital tract: Significance of human papillomavirus infection of the vagina after hysterectomy. Obstet Gynecol 1987; 70: 294–298.
12. Bornstein J, Kaufman R H, Adam E, Adler-Storthz K. Human papillomavirus associated with vaginal intraepithelial neoplasia in women exposed to diethylstilbestrol in utero. Obstet Gynecol 1987; 70: 75–80.
13. Gemmell J, Holmes D M, Duncan I D. How frequently need vaginal smears be taken after hysterectomy for cervical intraepithelial neoplasia? Br J Obstet Gynaecol 1990; 97: 58–61.
14. Brinton L A, Nasca P C, Mallin K, Schairer C, Rosenthal J , Rothenberg R, Yordan E Jr, Richart R M. Case-control study of in situ and invasive carcinoma of the vagina. Gynecol Oncol 1990; 38: 49–54.

15. Williams W C, Herman J M. Vaginal intraepithelial neoplasia: Methodological problems in a case controlled study. Family Pract Res J 1990; 10: 27–35.

16. Townsend D E. Intraepithelial neoplasia of vagina. In: Coppleson M, ed. Gynecologic oncology. Edinburgh: Churchill Livingstone, 1992: pp 493–499.

17. Sillman F, Stanek A, Sedlis A et al. The relationship between human papillomavirus and lower genital intraepithelial neoplasia in immunosuppressed women. Am J Obstet Gynecol 1984; 150: 300–308.

18. Halpert R, Butt K M H, Sedlis A et al. Human papillomavirus infection and lower genital neoplasia in female renal allograft recipients. Transplant Proc 1985; 17: 93–95.

19. Robboy S J, Noller K L, O'Brien P et al. Increased incidence of cervical and vaginal dysplasia in 3,980 diethylstilbestrol-exposed young women. JAMA 1984; 252: 2979–2983.

20. Bornstein J, Adam E, Adler-Storthz K, Kaufman R H. Development of cervical and vaginal intraepithelial neoplasia as a late consequence of in utero exposure to diethylstilbestrol. Obstet Gynecol Surv 1988; 43: 15–21.

21. Woodruff J D, Parmley T H, Julian C G. Topical 5-fluorouracil in the treatment of vaginal carcinoma in situ. Gynecol Oncol 1975; 3: 124–132.

22. Townsend D E. Cryosurgery. In: Coppleson M, ed. Gynecologic oncology. Edinburgh: Churchill Livingstone, 1992: pp 1139–1146.

23. Dini M M, Jafari K. Ileovaginal fistula following cryosurgery for vaginal dysplasia. Am J Obstet Gynecol 1980; 136: 692–693.

24. Stafl A, Wilkinson E J, Mattingly R F. Laser treatment of cervical and vaginal neoplasia. Am J Obstet Gynecol 1977; 128: 128–136.

25. Sherman A I. Laser therapy for vaginal intraepithelial neoplasia after hysterectomy. J Reprod Med 1990; 35: 941–944.

26. Jobson V W, Homesley H D. Treatment of vaginal intraepithelial neoplasia with the carbon dioxide laser. Obstet Gynecol 1983; 62: 90–93.

27. Stuart G C E, Flagler E A, Nation J G, Duggan M, Robertson D I. Laser vaporization of vaginal intraepithelial neoplasia. Am J Obstet Gynecol 1988; 158: 240–243.

28. Ireland D, Monaghan J M. The management of the patient with abnormal vaginal cytology following hysterectomy. Br J Obstet Gynaecol 1988; 95: 973–975.

29. Monaghan J M. Vaginal Cancer. In: Burghardt E, ed. Surgical gynecologic oncology. Stuttgart: Georg Thieme Verlag, 1993: pp 171–184.

30. Kaminski P F, Sorosky J I, Wheelock J B, Stevens C W Jr. The significance of atypical cervical cytology in an older population. Obstet Gynecol 1989; 73: 13–15.

31. Krebs H B. Treatment of vaginal intraepithelial neoplasia with laser and topical 5-fluorouracil. Obstet Gynecol 1989; 73: 657–660.

32. Stokes I M, Sworn M J, Hawthorne J H R. A new regimen for the treatment of vaginal carcinoma in situ using 5-fluorouracil. Case report. Br J Obstet Gynaecol 1980; 87: 920–921.

33. Kirwan P, Naftalin N J. Topical 5-fluorouracil in the treatment of vaginal intraepithelial neoplasia. Br J Obstet Gynaecol 1985; 92: 287–291.

34. Krebs H B, Helmkamp F. Chronic ulcerations following topical therapy with 5-fluorouracil for vaginal human papillomavirus-associated lesions. Obstet Gynecol 1991; 78: 205–208.

35. Guthrie D, Way S. Immunotherapy of non-clinical vaginal cancer. Lancet 1975; ii: 1242.

36. Yliskoski M, Cantell K, Syrjänen K, Syrjänen S. Topical treatment with human leukocyte interferon of HPV 16 infections associated with cervical and vaginal intraepithelial neoplasias. Gynecol Oncol 1990; 36: 353–357.

37. Hoffman M S, DeCesare S L, Roberts W S, Fiorica J V, Finan M A, Cavanagh D. Upper vaginectomy for in situ and occult, superficially invasive carcinoma of the vagina. Am J Obstet Gynecol 1992; 16: 30–33.

38. Curtis P, Shepherd J H, Lowe D G, Jobling T. The role of partial colpectomy in the management of persistent vaginal neoplasia after primary treatment. Br J Obstet Gynaecol 1992; 99: 587–589.

39. Hernandez-Linares W, Puthawala A, Nolan J F, Jernstrom P H, Morrow C P. Carcinoma in situ of the vagina: past and present management. Obstet Gynecol 1980; 56: 356–360.

40. Punnonen R, Gronroos M, Meurman L, Liukko P. Diagnosis and treatment of primary vaginal carcinoma in situ and dysplasia. Acta Obstet Gynecol Scand 1981; 60: 513–514.

41. Woodman C B, Mould J J, Jordan J A. Radiotherapy in the management of vaginal intraepithelial neoplasia after hysterectomy. Br J Obstet Gynaecol 1988; 95: 976–979.

42. Benedet J L, Sanders B H. Carcinoma in situ of the vagina. Am J Obstet Gynecol 1984; 148: 695–700.

43. Abbas F, Sert B, Fields A, Rosenshein N. The management of vaginal intraepithelial neoplasia by ultrasonic surgical apiration. Gynecol Oncol 1993; 49: 142 (abstract).

14. Minor cytological abnormalities

Mahmood I. Shafi

INTRODUCTION

The decision as to whether a woman should be referred for colposcopic assessment is based on several parameters, of which the cytological report is the most important. Consideration of a referral policy must take into account the scientific data available pertinent to the abnormality, the facilities that are available locally, and to the psychological impact of referral and possible treatment. These psychological sequelae of referral for colposcopy, with possible treatment, may be greater than the risk of serious disease developing from the abnormality that the smear identified. It must be remembered that as far as the screened population goes, the aim must be to do more good than harm to the population as a whole. Therefore, screening should not be used to turn people into patients and health into disease. The interests of the women must be served by a balanced approach that not only takes into account the most satisfactory clinical management, but also the most effective use of resources in terms of cost and manpower. Referral policies must allow some flexibility so that management may be tailored to an individual patient. Referral policies need to be continually reviewed in the light of new information with regards to the natural history of cervical intraepithelial neoplasia (CIN).

SIZE OF THE PROBLEM

A dramatic increase in the occurrence of abnormal cervical cytology and CIN has been noted in recent years, and has been referred to as an 'epidemic'.[1] In some areas up to 10–12% of all smears examined are abnormal to some degree.[2] Annually 4.3 million smears are performed in England, of which 2.4% are classified as borderline and 2.2% as mild dyskaryosis. Whilst these percentages relate to an average for all age groups, in younger women, minor cytological abnormalities account for up to 8% of smears performed. As the majority of smears are performed in the younger age groups, numerically this represents a considerable challenge. With an increasing trend towards a 'see and treat' management policy for abnormal cervical cytology, there is a growing desire to limit both physical and psychological trauma particularly in younger women. The Papanicolaou (Pap) smear remains a simple and relatively inexpensive test which is essentially free of risk and is easy to administer. This is important as asymptomatic women are approached for the screening program. Screening techniques require high sensitivity and specificity to be effective. Whilst this is satisfied at the more severe end of the cytological abnormality spectrum, this is not so at the minor cytological abnormality end. An important point about sensitivity and specificity is that there is a trade-off between them.[3] Some of the deficiencies of cervical cytology screening, particularly with regard to minor cytological abnormalities, may be attributable to collection errors and the rest to laboratory error. Quantitative disciplines have long recognized the need for quality control and accuracy is routinely assessed with standardized controls (e.g., biochemical investigations). The accuracy of Pap smears is more difficult to gauge because of its subjective nature and has only recently been addressed by quality assurance schemes run locally and nationally. Automation of the screening procedure may provide a more reliable and consistent diagnosis of smears than the personnel intensive procedures currently used.

CYTOLOGICAL CLASSIFICATION

Cytological abnormalities represent a continuum, which have arbitrarily been divided into the various diagnostic categories to make management simpler. The range of nuclear cytological abnormalities extends from 'borderline' changes to 'severe dyskaryosis, ? invasion.' The original description of the microscopic features of cervical cancer involved the aspiration of material from the vaginal fornix.[4] This was then fixed with equal parts of 95% of alcohol and ether, and stained with hematoxylin and cytoplasmic stains. The modern procedure of cervical cytology differs remarkably little from the original description and involves the examination of scrapings from the ectocervix and endocervical canal and/or aspirates which are collected and prepared in much the same manner.

In the UK, reporting of cervical cytology conforms to the guidelines of the British Society for Clinical Cytology; cytologists being encouraged to say precisely what abnormality is present in as many cases as possible.[5] Dyskaryosis is the cytological term used to denote abnormalities and literally means 'abnormal nucleus.' Irregularity of chromatin distribution is the most important change in nuclear morphology. This may be accompanied by irregularity of form and outline, multinucleation, further disproportionate nuclear enlargement, and hyperchromasia.

The minor cytological abnormalities include mild dyskaryosis and borderline changes. Mildly dyskaryotic cells usually have plentiful, thin, translucent cytoplasm with angular borders, resembling superficial or intermediate squamous cells. The nucleus occupies less than half the total area of the cytoplasm. Mild dyskaryosis correlates with cells from the surface of CIN 1. It is doubtful, however, if it can be reliably distinguished from the nuclear abnormalities associated with human papillomavirus (HPV) infection. Some cells will be on the borderline between the accepted definitions of normality and mild dyskaryosis, but the problem of classification can usually be resolved by the time the whole specimen has been examined. Despite this, an increasing number of smears are reported as 'borderline' necessitating further cytological or colposcopic intervention. In

women with minor cytological abnormalities, 95% will also have features of koilocytosis as HPV is preferentially seen in well-differentiated cells and is rarely reported with severe dyskaryosis.

HPV causes a variety of appearances in smears. Wart virus changes accompanied by dyskaryosis should be managed according to the degree of dyskaryosis and if no dyskaryosis is present, then the smear should be reported as being 'negative' and the patient screened as per agreed protocol for negative cervical cytology.

In the USA, cytological terminology has been revised and is now based on the 'Bethesda' system.[6–8] This incorporates categories for 'atypical squamous cells of undetermined significance (ASCUS);' 'squamous intraepithelial lesion (SIL)'; which encompasses the spectrum of squamous cell carcinoma precursors, divided into low-grade SIL (HPV-associated cellular changes, mild dysplasia, and CIN 1) and high-grade SIL (moderate dysplasia, severe dysplasia, and carcinoma-in-situ and CIN 2 and 3); and squamous cell carcinoma. The ASCUS category and low-grade SIL are comparable to the borderline and mild dyskaryosis categories as used in the UK.

Cytological screening can be beguiling and all screening programmes can potentially do more harm than good. It is often forgotten that the ratio of precancerous lesions of the uterine cervix to invasive cancer is at least 10 to 1, possibly even higher.[9] In other words, at the most, one in 10 precancerous lesions is likely to progress to invasive cancer if left untreated. This is because the cumulative incidence of preinvasive lesions far outweighs the expected incidence of invasive cancers of the cervix.[10] Our diagnostic impotence at predicting whether or not cases of CIN are potentially invasive, leads to unnecessary treatment of large numbers of patients for these abnormalities. In the UK, almost 300 000 smears are reported to be abnormal to some degree, whilst the incidence for invasive cervical cancer is approximately 4500 cases per annum.

RETROSPECTIVE STUDIES

Cross-sectional studies confirm that smears often underestimate the severity of the cervical lesions, as around 30% of women with mild cytological abnormalities have CIN 3.[11-13] In the study reported by Soutter et al,[11] the histological grade did not seem to be related to the number of times the abnormal smear had been repeated and was not confined to patients whose smears had been reported by only one laboratory. Age was not useful for predicting which women were at high risk of significant disease. Such studies have led to demands that any degree of dyskaryosis on a single smear justifies referral for colposcopy. Other studies show that careful repeat cervical cytology correlated closely with the histological grade of the lesion.[13,14] Repeat cytology was associated with an overall 24% false-negative rate, but most missed lesions were of low grade. Repeat cytology correctly identified 82% of all CIN lesions, and 93% of the most significant lesions (CIN 2 and 3).[13] In 46% of Robertson's large series the smear reverted to normal within 2 years, and none of these patients have developed invasive cancer; life table analysis showed that 75% of these women had not relapsed after a 14 year interval.[14] Relapse to abnormal cervical cytology was not related to age and relapses occurred throughout the whole follow-up period. This study concluded that cytological surveillance for minor cytological abnormalities was acceptably safe provided that biopsy is advised if cytological abnormalities persist. Thus although the first smear lacks diagnostic precision, this improved with subsequent smears. A further conclusion of the study confirmed that considerable experience is required for accurate colposcopy, and in Robertson's series more diagnostic errors resulted from colposcopy than from cytology. These diagnostic errors would be multiplied if colposcopy were adopted virtually as a screening procedure.

LESION SIZE

Many of the studies have neglected the effect of lesion size on the natural history of CIN and in the assessment of cytological screening. A positive association between lesion size and histological grade of CIN has been confirmed.[15] The size of the atypical transformation zone is also a major determinant of cervical cytology. Quantitative histological studies have confirmed a highly significant positive correlation between the grade

of a cervical smear and the size of the lesion for all grades of CIN.[16,17] Those patients that had CIN 3 and mild dyskaryosis or less had significantly smaller lesions than those with CIN 3 and moderate or severe dyskaryosis. Women with mild dyskaryosis may have small CIN 3 lesions but also have extensive areas of associated lower grade CIN, which is more likely to be sampled and yield mildly dyskaryotic cells. In this study, repeat cytology identified as severe dyskaryosis all those with large CIN 3 lesions. Lesion size therefore offers an explanation for the apparent discrepancies between cytological, colposcopic and histological assessment of progression of CIN. The smaller lesions may be at an earlier stage of progression or may be progressing more slowly, and so have a lower short-term risk of transformation to invasive cancer. Colposcopic assessment to identify those with CIN 3 associated with minor cytological abnormalities can only be justified if these lesions have truly comparable CIN 3 lesions to those with severe dyskaryosis and have the same high risk of developing invasive disease.

The size of CIN 3 measured histologically has been shown to be associated with invasive squamous cervical cancer.[18] The mean size for CIN 3 showing microinvasion was seven times greater than that for severe dyskaryosis without invasion and a 100-fold greater than with mild dyskaryosis. Invasive cervical cancer appears to arise in large CIN 3 lesions and these lesions are more often associated with severe dyskaryosis. The authors propose a model for the development of high-grade precancer as a small focus within low-grade precancer which then undergoes expansion in size, accompanied by apparent progression in cytological grade.

Much of the historical evidence of the risk of progression of CIN 3 to malignancy comes from studies of women who were initially detected cytologically as having severe dyskaryosis, and who presumably had larger CIN 3 lesions.[19] The small size of CIN 3 lesions associated with mild dyskaryosis may explain the discrepancy between the high rate of CIN 3 in a population presenting with mild dyskaryosis and the apparent low risk of progression to invasive disease, patients as often as not having had a colposcopic assessment.[14]

False-negative cytology also appears to be a determinant of lesion size and is increased in smaller lesions.[20,21] In a study by Giles et al,[21] none of the larger lesions of CIN (affecting more than two quadrants of the cervix) were associated with negative cytology. The false-negative rate for smaller lesions was 58%, and as these lesions were prevalent in 6% of the screened population (recruited from women attending their General Practitioners), studies of their clinical course are required. Local destructive or excisional therapy may well represent considerable overtreatment. Furthermore, in all cases of CIN 3, cytology was abnormal to some degree. If smaller lesions yielding negative results on cytology progress, then they too will be detected as the lesion increases in size or severity. Barton et al[20] looked at areas of acetowhite epithelium and area of atypical transformation zone, measuring them from cervicographs. Those women that had false negative cytology were found to have significantly smaller proportion of their atypical transformation zones affected by CIN. This factor can account for the sampling error which causes false-negative cervical cytology. These data suggest that the concentration of cells required to reach the threshold for detection may be directly related to the fraction of the atypical transformation zone affected by CIN.

The case for paying more attention to lesion size, and not just grade, appears to be very strong. Assessment of lesion size, whether clinically by colposcopy or cervicography, or histologically in excisional biopsies, is a requisite for advancing the understanding of both the natural history and the management of cervical precancer. The highest grade of CIN at a single point should be regarded as an inadequate endpoint in the study of CIN. Another question of major importance that has not been addressed is the likelihood of women with mild cytological abnormality proceeding to invasive cancer without progressing through the more severe degrees of cytological abnormality.[22] Repeat cervical cytology will detect women with larger and more severe CIN lesions. Minor lesions that progress should be detected when the lesions increase in size or severity.[21]

MANAGEMENT AND REFERRAL PATTERNS

The clinical management of mild cytological abnormalities is often narrowed down to either immediate colposcopic assessment and treatment or cytological surveillance. The answer to this can only be found through prospective longitudinal controlled trials, and these are currently under way. Punch biopsies may themselves influence the natural course of disease, and therefore observation studies without recourse to punch biopsy seem appropriate.[23] True progression and regression rates of mild cytological abnormalities can then be computed. Rather than using surrogate endpoints, appropriate outcome measures need to be defined to determine an optimal pathway through a combination of cytological surveillance, colposcopy and treatment within an economic framework. All studies should incorporate an assessment of lesion size in their study design, preferably using a technique that is quantifiable.

Until recently there were considerable variations in referral patterns in the UK.[24] Of those responsible for colposcopy services responding to a national postal questionnaire, 37% felt that the least cytological abnormality leading to referral for colposcopy was mild dyskaryosis on a single smear. Guidelines have recently been revised stating that smears showing borderline nuclear or mild dyskaryotic change in the presence of a macroscopically normal cervix should be repeated 6 months later and consideration given to colposcopic referral only if it is not then normal.[25,26] All protocols, including this one, require to be continually reviewed in the light of new scientific evidence.

Whilst immediate referral for colposcopic assessment would appear attractive at first, there is a hidden cost of immediate referral as interacting with colposcopy services is not a benign procedure. This is particularly true since the widespread introduction of large loop excision of the transformation zone (LLETZ) or loop electrosurgical excision procedure (LEEP) as a 'see and treat' strategy for the management of women with cytological abnormalities. In one large series of women with all grades of cytological abnormalities undergoing LLETZ, 27% had histological changes that were normal or showed koilocytic atypia.[27] Whilst immediate morbidity was acceptable and the cytological and histological success rates comparable with other local ablative and excisional techniques, it was associated with a cervical stenosis rate of 1.3% at the 6 month follow-up visit. The majority of patients destined to have cervical stenosis had LLETZ procedures exceeding 14 mm in depth. Whilst the cervical stenosis rate may be acceptable in those patients that have genuine cancer precursors, it would be deemed unacceptable in a group of patients with essentially normal cervices as assessed histologically. Therefore caution needs to be exercised in a 'see and treat' management strategy and more emphasis needs to be placed on patient demographic details and characterization of high-grade and low-grade lesions by thorough colposcopic assessment.

Many of the lesions in women with minor cytological abnormalities are associated with HPV infection. The much lower abnormality rate in older women suggests that many of these lesions will disappear with time.[28] The problem of managing these women is due to our limited knowledge of the natural history of mildly abnormal smears. Without prospective studies, evaluation of differing management protocols must be based on retrospective and epidemiological data. This makes validation of protocols more difficult and less decisive. Determinations of the accuracy of cytological testing are usually based on correlations with tissue punch biopsy diagnosis. This may be an inadequate surrogate endpoint, as there is considerable error when results of punch biopsy are compared with histology following diathermy loop excision of the transformation zone.[29] This may partly be explained by the considerable variation in the size of the lesions and often different grades of CIN are present together in the same biopsy.[17]

The economics of cervical cytology screening programs are in part determined by the referral threshold for colposcopy. Liberal criteria for referral to colposcopy clinics lead to an increased burden on these services and there is significant

psychological and psychosexual morbidity associated with this policy.[30] Advocates justify this approach, arguing that immediate colposcopy and biopsy lead to a prompt diagnosis, avoid possible default from cytological surveillance and may actually reduce psychological morbidity, by rapidly treating any underlying lesions and achieving a return to normal smears. Furthermore, should there be an underlying microinvasive or occult invasive lesion this will be diagnosed quickly.

Our inability to forecast whether or not cases of CIN are potentially invasive results in large numbers of patients being unnecessarily treated. From 1968 to 1978, it has been estimated that screening in Britain can be accredited with the prevention of approximately 500 deaths, at a cost of 100 000 cervices and about 20 million smears.[31] The question of whether to refer immediately for colposcopic assessment or cytological surveillance continues to generate debate from both protagonists. In a study to look at social criteria that may select patients for colposcopy, it was found that because of the high prevalence of CIN grades 2 and 3 in both the high-risk and low-risk groups, social factors were not useful for selecting women with minor cytological abnormalities that would benefit from early colposcopy.[32] In this study, smokers and those with more than one sexual partner were statistically more likely to have high-grade CIN but these could not be used to differentiate between high-risk and low-risk groups.

HISTOLOGICAL PROFILE AND RISK FACTORS

In our unit, patients referred with minor cytological abnormalities for colposcopic assessment have an entirely normal transformation zone in approximately 20%. In an ongoing study being conducted within our unit, 181 patients with minor cytological abnormalities have undergone treatment by LLETZ if they had an atypical transformation zone. Of these the histological profile was CIN 3 35 women (19.3%), CIN 2 8 women (4.4%), CIN 1 45 women (24.9%), koilocytic atypia 92 women (50.8%), no abnormality 1 woman (0.6%). This gives an overall rate of 23.7% high-grade lesions (CIN grades 2 and 3) in patients with minor cytological abnormalities. Univariate analysis of patient variables and histological grade identified increasing cigarette pack years (measure of smoking exposure), increasing number of livebirths, absence of cytological changes associated with HPV (koilocytosis), repeat cervical cytology result and the lesion size as statistically significant predictors of grade of abnormality in a univariate analysis. The lesion area may be measured either semiquantitatively or quantitatively.[33,34] When a multivariate analysis is performed (step-wise discriminant), this identifies three factors as important and independent variables associated with histological grade: lesion area (continuous variable), repeat cervical cytology result and number of livebirths. These variables can be used to develop models to predict the likelihood of high grade lesions in patients initially presenting with minor cytological abnormality.

FUTURE TASKS

Further basic scientific research may provide a means of determining those cases of CIN which have the potential to become invasive. This would allow considerable savings through the treatment of only potentially invasive lesions. If conservative approaches are utilised, computer-aided colposcopy can be useful, especially for image archiving and quantitative measurements of the various features of the images.[35]

With the lack of diagnostic capability of cervical cytology at the minor end of the cytological abnormality spectrum, there is an urgent need for a secondary screen with minimal intervention. Cervicography has been studied, but this has been hampered by the high sensitivity and low specificity inherent in this technique.[36,37] Detection of HPV, particularly the high-risk groups has been suggested as a secondary screen. The major problems lie in differing technologies and a lack of standardization between laboratories. Semiquantitation using the polymerase chain reaction (PCR) may offer some benefits. In a study by Cuzick, estimation of HPV 16 was performed in women referred for colposcopy because of abnormal cervical cytology.[38] An intermediate or high amount of HPV 16 DNA predicted the presence of high-grade CIN on colposcopic directed punch biopsy in almost 90% of patients. The use of HPV determinants to improve the specificity of cytology remains an important topic for future work. This technique needs further study to clarify whether it can identify those women with minor cytological abnormalities who harbor high-grade CIN. Other workers have failed to reproduce these results and have not found semiquantitation useful as a secondary screen.[39]

In conclusion, safety can only be achieved by full cooperation from the patients, a high standard of cytological assessment and colposcopy, and adequate follow-up administration.[40] There is a great need for controlled prospective studies to establish reliable baseline data before the introduction of management protocols of unproven effect.

REFERENCES

1. Wolfendale M R, King S, Usherwood M McD. Abnormal cervical smears: are we in for an epidemic? Br Med J 1983; 287: 526–528.
2. Jenkins D, Tay S K. Management of mildly abnormal cervical smears. Lancet 1987; i: 748–749.
3. Mant M, Fowler G. Mass screening: theory and ethics. Br Med J 1990; 300: 916–918.
4. Papanicolaou G N, Traut H F. The diagnostic value of vaginal smears in carcinoma of the uterus. Am J Obstet Gynecol 1941; 42: 193–206.
5. Evans D M D, Hudson E, Brown C L, Boddingtion M M, Hughes H E, Mackenzie E F D. Terminology in gynaecological cytopathology: report of the working party of the British Society for Clinical Cytology. J Clin Pathol 1986; 39: 933–944.
6. Anon. The 1988 Bethesda system for reporting cervical/vaginal cytologic diagnoses. JAMA 1989; 262: 931–934.
7. Kurman R J, Malkasian G D, Sedlis A, Solomon D. From Papanicolaou to Bethesda: The rationale for a new cervical cytologic classification. Obstet Gynecol 1991; 77: 779–782.
8. Broder S. The Bethesda system for reporting cervical/vaginal cytologic diagnosis — report of the 1991 Bethesda workshop. JAMA 1992; 267: 1892.
9. Koss L G. The Papanicolaou test for cervical cancer detection. A triumph and a tragedy. JAMA 1989; 261: 737–743.
10. Stern E, Neely P M. Carcinoma and dysplasia of the cervix. A comparison of rates for new and returning populations. Acta Cytol 1963; 7: 357–361.

11. Soutter W P, Wisdom S, Brough A K, Monaghan J M. Should patients with mild atypia in a cervical smear be referred for colposcopy? Br J Obstet Gynaecol 1986; 93: 70–74.

12. Bolger B S, Lewis B V. A prospective study of colposcopy in women with mild dyskaryosis or koilocytosis. Br J Obstet Gynaecol 1988; 95: 1117–1119.

13. Giles J A, Deery A, Crow J, Walker P. The accuracy of repeat cytology in women with mildly dyskaryotic smears. Br J Obstet Gynaecol 1989; 96: 1067–1070.

14. Robertson J H, Woodend B E, Crozier E H, Hutchinson J. Risk of cervical cancer associated with mild dyskaryosis. Br Med J 1988; 297: 18–21.

15. Shafi M I, Finn C B, Luesley D M, Jordan J A, Dunn J. Lesion size and histology of atypical cervical transformation zone. Br J Obstet Gynaecol 1991; 98: 490–492.

16. Jarmulowicz M R, Jenkins D, Barton S E, Goodall A L, Hollingworth A, Singer A. Cytological status and lesion size: a further dimension in cervical intraepithelial neoplasia. Br J Obstet Gynaecol 1989; 96: 1061–1066.

17. Jenkins D, Tay S K, McCanee D J, Campion M J, Clarkson P K, Singer A. Histological and immunocytochemical study of cervical intraepithelial neoplasia (CIN) with associated HPV 6 and HPV 16 infections. J Clin Pathol 1986; 39: 1177–1180.

18. Tidbury P, Singer A, Jenkins D. CIN 3: the role of lesion size in invasion. Br J Obstet Gynaecol 1992; 99: 583–586.

19. Mclndoe W A, McLean M R, Jones R W, Mullins P R. The invasive potential of carcinoma in situ of the cervix. Obstet Gynecol 1984; 64: 451–458.

20. Barton S E, Jenkins D, Hollingworth A, Cuzick J, Singer A. An explanation for the problem of false-negative cervical smears. Br J Obstet Gynaecol 1989; 96: 482–485.

21. Giles J A, Hudson E, Crow J, Williams D, Walker P. Colposcopic assessment of the accuracy of cervical cytology screening. BMJ 1988; 296: 1099–1102.

22. Woodman C B J, Jordan J A. Colposcopy services in the West Midlands region. Br Med J 1989; 299: 899–901.

23. Richart R M. Influence of diagnostic and therapeutic procedures on the distribution of cervical intraepithelial neoplasia. Cancer 1966; 19: 1635–1638.

24. Kitchener H C. United Kingdom colposcopy survey. British Society for Colposcopy and Cervical Pathology. Br J Obstet Gynaecol 1991; 98: 1112–1116.

25. Duncan I D. NHS Cervical screening programme: Guidelines for clinical practice and programme management. Oxford: National Co-ordinating Network, 1992.

26. Shafi M I, Luesley D M, Jordan J A. Mild cervical cytological abnormalities. Br Med J 1992; 305: 1040–1041.

27. Luesley D M, Cullimore J, Redman C W E et al. Loop diathermy excision of the cervical transformation zone in patients with abnormal cervical smears. Br Med J 1990; 300: 1690–1693.

28. Cuzick J. Cervical screening. Br J Hosp Med 1988; 39: 265.

29. Buxton E J, Luesley D M, Shafi M I, Rollason T P. Colposcopically directed punch biopsy: a potentially misleading investigation. Br J Obstet Gynaecol 1991; 98: 1273–1276.

30. Campion M J, Brown J R, McCance D J et al. Psychosexual trauma of an abnormal cervical smear. Br J Obstet Gynaecol 1988; 95: 175–181.

31. Knox E G. Cancer of the uterine cervix. In: Magnus K, ed. Trends in cancer incidence. Causes and practical implications. Washington: Hemisphere Pub Corp, 1982.

32. Anderson D J, Flannelly G M, Kitchener H C et al. Mild and moderate dyskaryosis: can women be selected for colposcopy on the basis of social criteria? Br Med J 1992; 305: 84–87.

33. Shafi M L, Finn C B, Luesley D M, Jordan J A, Dunn J. Lesion size and histology of atypical transformation zone. Br J Obstet Gynaecol 1991; 98: 490–492.

34. Shafi M I, Dunn J, Finn C B, Kehoe S, Buxton E J, Jordan E J, Luesley D M. Characterisation of high and low grade cervical intraepithelial neoplasia. Int J Gynecol Cancer 1993; 3: 203–207.

35. Crisp W E, Craine B L, Craine E A. The computerized digital imaging colposcope: Future directions. Am J Obstet Gynecol 1990; 162: 1491–1498.

36. Stafl A. Cervicography: A new method for cervical cancer detection. Am J Obstet Gynecol 1981; 139: 815–825.

37. Tawa K, Forsythe A, Cove J K, Saltz A, Peters H W, Warring W G. A comparison of the Papanicolaou smear and the cervigram: sensitivity, specificity, and cost analysis. Obstet Gynecol 1988; 71: 229–235.

38. Cuzick J, Terry G, Ho Linda, Holligworth T, Anderson M. Human papillomavirus type 16 DNA in cervical smears as predictro of high-grade cervical intraepithelial neoplasia. Lancet 1992; 339: 959–960.

39. Bavin P J, Giles J A, Deery A et al. Use of semi-quantitative PCR for human papillomavirus DNA type 16 to identify women with high grade cervical disease in a population presenting with a mild dyskaryotic report. Br J Cancer 1993; 67: 602–605.

40. Sprigg A I. Natural history of cervical dysplasia. Clin Obstet Gynecol 1981; 8: 65–79.

15. Management of cervical intraepithelial neoplasia

J. A. Jordan

CIN

Although the term cervical intraepithelial neoplasia (CIN) is relatively new the concept of premalignant disease of the cervix dates back to 1886 when Sir John Williams gave the Harveian Lectures in which he described how, on examining the cervix of a woman who had had a hysterectomy for menstrual problems, histological examination of the cervix showed a lesion which we would now refer to as a combination of microinvasive carcinoma and CIN.[1] He stressed that to naked eye examination the cervix had been completely normal and the woman was asymptomatic without any pain, bleeding or discharge. Following that report others also recognized the significance of the precancerous state[2] but there was no means of suspecting the existence of premalignant disease unless the cervix was removed: clearly there was no 'screening' which would allow the physician to suspect the presence of premalignancy. The turning point came in 1925 when Hinselmann[3] described the technique of colposcopy. As a young man Hinselmann had been appointed to the staff of the University Hospital in Hamburg and his task was to reduce the mortality from cervical cancer. He thought that if he could examine the cervix under magnification then he would see early, hopefully treatable, cancer as either a small ulcer or a small exophytic growth. He did in fact detect some preclinical cancers but the importance of his technique, which he named colposcopy, was to recognize premalignant disease.

Schiller[4] addressed the problem as a pathologist. He noted that mature normal squamous epithelium contained glycogen and would stain dark brown when iodine was applied to it: on the other hand, premalignant and malignant disease was relatively lacking in glycogen and, therefore, did not stain with iodine. As a result of this he suggested that all non-staining areas should be scraped carefully to permit the detection of abnormal epithelium. The solution used by Schiller contained iodine (2 g) potassium iodine (4 g) and distilled water to 300 ml. There is sometimes confusion in reporting of colposcopy findings in that the Schiller-positive test refers to an area which is nonstaining, whereas it is not uncommon to see inexperienced colposcopists (or clinicians who are not colposcopists) referring the Schiller-positive areas as those areas which stain with iodine. This of course should not be a source of confusion for the experienced colposcopist — a Schiller-positive test refers to an area which is nonstaining following the application of Schiller's iodine.

Although colposcopy and the Schiller test allowed some women with premalignant disease to be recognized the breakthrough in the detection of premalignant disease did not come until Papanicolaou and Traut[5] described their technique of exfoliative cytology.

COLPOSCOPY

Although there are many ways of treating CIN none should be used unless the patient has first been seen and assessed by a competent colposcopist. Because the distribution and type of disease varies from individual to individual, only colposcopy can show the clinician where the CIN is and, therefore, which tissue needs to be removed or destroyed. The most widely used form of colposcopy is the classical or extended technique of colposcopy as described and developed by Hinselmann but a technique referred to as the saline technique has also been described.

Classical colposcopy

With a few exceptions this is the method of colposcopy which is taught and practised. Colposcopy is an out-patient procedure. The patient is examined on a purpose-built colposcopy or urological couch and examined in a modified lithotomy position. The vagina should be assessed by a single finger examination to see what size and shape of speculum should be used and a warm speculum, covered with a small amount of lubricant, is then inserted to expose the cervix. The cervix is examined initially at low magnification ($\times$6 or $\times$10) and excess mucus or blood removed gently with a cotton wool swab moistened with normal saline. If it is felt necessary to take a cervical smear then it should be taken at this stage with great care being taken not to traumatize the cervix otherwise interpretation of the colposcopic image can be extremely difficult because of bleeding. Remember, however, that if the patient is presenting to the colposcopy clinic for the first time then it is usually because already she is known to have an abnormal cervical smear in which case the colposcopist should ask whether or not a repeat smear is really necessary, bearing in mind that the woman is there primarily for an accurate colposcopic assessment rather than for a repeat smear. Acetic acid (3% is the usual strength but many units use 5%) is then applied using a cotton wool swab. This will remove any residual mucus and CIN will appear as area or areas of whiteness. The whiteness of CIN is referred to as acetowhite (signifying that it is white only because acetic acid has been applied) and is to be distinguished from hyperkeratosis or leukoplakia, areas of epithelium which are white before the application of acetic acid. The reason why CIN appears white is not fully understood. Normal squamous epithelium remains pink following the application of acetic acid, the pinkness being due to a reflection from the underlying subepithelial capillaries. In other words it is pink because of the underlying vascularity which can be seen through the squamous epithelium. It is thought that the protein in the nucleus coagulates following the application of acetic acid so that in areas of high nuclear density such as CIN the resulting coagulation prevents the light from penetrating the epithelium and, therefore, the redness of the underlying capillaries is no longer visible, hence the overall appearance of 'acetowhiteness.' It should be stressed, however, that any area of high nuclear density such as immature metaplasia, congenital transformation zone, or regenerating epithelium will also appear acetowhite and sadly this is not often recognized by the inexperienced colposcopist with the result that many women with benign conditions are thought falsely to have an abnormality requiring treatment.

The Schiller iodine test can then be used following the acetic acid test. Most experienced colposcopists do not use the Schiller iodine test as a routine but sometimes it is useful, particularly when undertaking treatment in that it will outline very clearly the area of CIN. It is also useful for less experienced colposcopists in that sometimes they will be made aware of abnormality which otherwise may have been unrecognized. Care should be taken, however, when interpreting the results of the Schiller test because while false negatives are uncommon, false positives occur relatively frequently and can lead to overtreatment.

Saline colposcopy

This technique was first used in the Norwegian Radium Hospital in Oslo by Koller[6] (1963) and subsequently developed and popularized by Kolstad.[7] The technique is slightly different from the acetic acid technique in that it uses only saline. A saline-soaked cotton wool swab removes mucus from the cervix and moistens the epithelium to the extent that the subepithelial angioarchitecture can be seen in great detail. To do this the colposcopist needs to examine the cervix under high magnification (at least $\times$16 and $\times$25). The use of a green filter allows the redness of the subepithelial capillaries to stand out much more clearly and the colposcopist can then study the shape of the capillaries and the distance they are from each other. The saline technique is much more difficult to learn but on the other hand it teaches the would-be colposcopist the discipline of assessing with accuracy the underlying vascular pattern and will allow the experienced colposcopist to distinguish more readily between low- and high-grade lesions and metaplasia.

Digital imaging colposcopy

Like any technique which relies on the visual interpretation of different patterns, colposcopy is only as accurate as the experience of the person using the technique and even then interpretations will vary from day to day. The development of digital imaging technology has allowed the technique to be applied to colposcopy and Shafi[8] has described how digital imaging techniques can enhance, measure and assess the image as seen through the colposcope and by training the computer to recognize various patterns it is hoped that the interpretation of colposcopic images will become more standardized and, therefore, less open to interpreter error.

Diploma of colposcopy?

Although the introduction of colposcopy to all gynecological units is a source of pride to those who promoted colposcopy in the past, it has also resulted in concern that the overall standard of colposcopy will be lowered with obvious clinical repercussions. In the past colposcopists were 'enthusiasts' whereas now it has become part and parcel of what every young gynecologist should know and becomes no more than part of the general workload. Many believe that this is not good enough and to maintain confidence in the technique then some form of formalized program should be considered. The British Society for Colposcopy and Cervical Pathology (1994) has suggested that no one should call themselves an expert colposcopist unless they have had satisfactory training and as always the concern is that what may be deemed satisfactory training in one unit will be deemed inadequate training in another. The role of a Diploma would not be to banish colposcopy to the clinics of the enthusiast but rather that those who undergo proper formal training should be recognized. The BSCCP is

suggesting in simple terms that would-be colposcopists would see 50 first-time patients with abnormal cytology under the direct supervision of a tutor, following this by 100 or so cases alone but with the case notes and reports being seen and reviewed by the tutor. The program would also of course include teaching in cytology, histopathology and in all modern techniques for treatment of CIN and other premalignant disease of the lower genital tract.

Diagnostic criteria for colposcopy

Enough has been said to show that colposcopy is more than an ability to recognize acetowhite or Schiller positive epithelium because the colposcopist must be able to recognize those features which are suspicious of abnormality. These can be summarized as follows:

1. subepithelial vascular pattern
2. intercapillary distance
3. difference in color between normal and abnormal epithelium, and
4. surface pattern.

Of these criteria the most important are the vascular pattern and intercapillary distance. The vascular pattern which should be recognized can be summarized as follows:

1. *Punctation.* This is a pattern in which the tips of the capillaries approach the surface and the punctation or dot which is seen by the colposcopist is simply the tip of the afferent and efferent loops of the capillary as it lies immediately beneath the surface cells. With progressing degrees of CIN the average distance between the capillaries becomes greater and the capillaries themselves become more distinct.
2. *Mosaic.* In this pattern the capillaries are arranged parallel to the surface in a mosaic or 'crazy-paving' pattern. As in punctation the size of the vessels and distance between them increases as the lesion progresses from low-grade to high-grade CIN and subsequently to early invasive disease.
3. *Atypical vessels.* These are totally unlike either the punctation or mosaic vessel and

when present raise the suspicion of invasive disease. Typically they are irregular in size, shape and course and the greatest intercapillary distance is significantly higher than with the punctation or mosaic patterns.

For more information regarding the recognition of colposcopic images the reader is referred to one of the standard colposcopy atlases.[9–11]

MANAGEMENT OF CIN

Worldwide, cancer of the cervix is the second most common female cancer with approximately 460 000 occurring each year. Seventy-seven percent of these occur in the developing world and in these countries it is the most common female cancer with very high incidence rates being recorded in China, Latin America and the Caribbean. Sadly the majority of deaths from cervical cancer are avoidable if only it were possible to introduce planned cervical screening programs. The aim of any screening program is to detect the disease process either before it becomes malignant or at the stage of early invasion and in the cervix this means the detection of CIN which, for all practical purposes, carries a 100% cure-rate, and early invasive disease at a stage where a cure is likely. If one accepts that properly planned cervical cytology screening programs have resulted in a significant decrease in the incidence of cervical cancer and in the mortality and morbidity from the disease then the next question to be addressed is how women with premalignant disease should be managed, bearing in mind that with minor degrees of CIN to do nothing, i.e., no treatment, may be the preferred option. In 1982 the Royal College of Obstetricians and Gynaecologists stated "ideally, no patient with CIN should be treated unless there has been prior colposcopic assessment. If colposcopy is not available in a particular hospital then the patient should be referred to someone who can perform a colposcopic assessment following which proper treatment can be planned."[12] If this was being written today as compared with 1982 then the first word 'ideally' would be removed from the statement! Assessment by a skilled colposcopist is now accepted widely as a prerequisite to treatment, bearing in

mind that not all women with abnormal cytology require surgical intervention. Indeed a relatively high proportion of young women with abnormal cytology will be found to have no more than immature metaplasia, HPV changes or at most HPV with CIN I. The National Co-ordinating Network Guidelines[13] advise immediate treatment for high-grade lesions (CIN 2–3) whereas low-grade lesions (CIN 1) can safely be followed with cytology and colposcopy knowing that in many instances the epithelium responsible for the abnormal cells will revert to normal without treatment, particularly in the younger woman. While nontreatment is certainly an option in some women, it must be stressed, however, that if there is any minor abnormality of an ongoing nature then it should be removed.

Unfortunately there are still some areas in the world where no colposcopy service is available in which case the clinician has the problem of deciding whether or not the woman with abnormal cytology requires treatment and if so what sort of treatment is indicated and how much tissue should be removed. It is to be hoped, however, that where cytology is available then hand-in-hand with this service should be the development of colposcopy services and it cannot be emphasized enough that treating someone with abnormal cytology without prior colposcopic assessment is to be deprecated as being very much second class treatment. If, however, colposcopy is not available then a cone biopsy, aided by the use of the Schiller test, should be performed. It may be tempting to proceed immediately with hysterectomy but this would be a calculated risk for two reasons. First, in approximately 1–2% of cases the CIN will involve the upper vagina in which case a standard hysterectomy will not remove of all of the CIN. Second, occasionally the hysterectomy specimen will show occult invasive carcinoma in which case it can be argued that to have performed a simple hysterectomy, followed by radiotherapy, was not the ideal treatment for a woman with stage 1 cervical cancer. However, when colposcopy is practised then the clinician has available a variety of treatments all of which, in the right hands, can be equally efficacious. In simple terms management fall into two distinct groups, excision and destruction.

Surgical excision

Excision of CIN can either be local excision in which case the minimum amount of tissue is removed by conization or alternatively a more radical excision by hysterectomy. There are three ways in which cervical conisation can be performed, namely by knife, by laser excision and diathermy loop excision.

Cervical conization

When first introduced the aim of the cervical cone was to be diagnostic and to be followed by the appropriate hysterectomy depending on the histological findings. Although today cervical conization is well recognized as the standard treatment for CIN it was not really recognised as treatment until McLaren[14] reported that since 1952 he had been using 'a deep ring biopsy,' and later conisation to see if he could cure patients without resorting to hysterectomy. At the time of the 1960 report he said that only half of his

patients were cured and the other half required a hysterectomy. Following this report his standard treatment became a large cone biopsy, the intention of which was to remove most of the endocervical canal. His results were published in 1967 and he found that such a cone biopsy could be therapeutic in 93% of cases. In 1966 colposcopy was introduced into McLaren's department following which colposcopically directed cone biopsies tended on average to be much smaller, had fewer complications but were equally therapeutic[15,16] (Fig. 15.1).

When colposcopy is not available then the Schiller's iodine test should be used: this will give some help to the surgeon in deciding how much ectocervical tissue should be removed when excising the lesion but of course it does not tell the surgeon how far up the canal the lesion extends in which case he should remove most of the canal if he wishes the cone to be therapeutic as well as diagnostic. However, it is to be hoped that colposcopy is indeed available, certainly in major centers, in which case by determining the

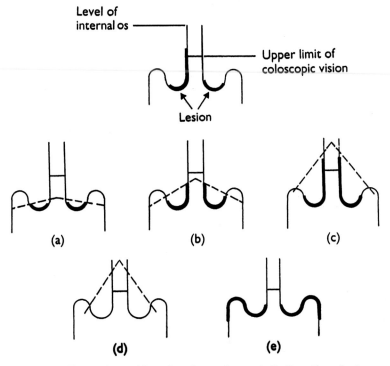

Fig. 15.1 Types of cone biopsy based on colposcopic findings (from Jordan 1976).

extent of disease on the ectocervix, and how far up the canal it reaches, the cone biopsy can be tailored to suit the needs of the individual woman (Fig. 15.1). If a colposcopically planned cone biopsy is performed, usually (particularly in younger women), most or at least a significant proportion of the endocervical canal can be left intact, and this is important for several reasons:

a. By minimizing the amount of tissue removed, primary and secondary hemorrhage is much less common.
b. Endocervical mucus is important for fertility so by leaving a reasonable amount of endocervical canal in place there should be no problem with the production of cervical mucus and thereby no problem with sperm transport from the vagina to the uterus.
c. An average sized cone biopsy will leave the internal os intact and so there will be no cervical incompetence in any subsequent pregnancy.

Figure 15.1 shows the various sizes and shapes of cone biopsy which can be performed depending on the extent of disease seen at colposcopy. In Fig. 15.1a a relatively small cone (often no more than a ring biopsy) is necessary whereas in 1c where the lesion extends beyond the upper limit of colposcopy it is necessary to remove the whole of the endocervical canal. When the lesion is not seen (Fig. 15.1d) then the surgeon should remove most of the endocervical canal knowing that if there is a lesion it will be high and close to the internal os. Finally, it is extremely important to recognise lesions which involve the vagina (Fig. 15.1e) because in such a case no type of cone biopsy will remove completely that part of the lesion which extends onto the vagina: in the event of the vagina being involved then it is perfectly acceptable to destroy the vaginal lesion (Co_2 laser vaporization is the best way to do this) or alternatively it may be felt appropriate to remove the uterus with a cuff of vagina either by vaginal or abdominal hysterectomy.

In an attempt to identify the extent of the lesion in the endocervical canal the microcolpohysteroscope can be used,[17] but most centers do not find this to be of any real practical value.

Knife conization. This is the traditional way of performing a cone biopsy and almost always requires a general anaesthetic. Some surgeons inject a vasoconstrictor (to reduce the incidence of secondary hemorrhage). Other surgeons simply insert two lateral sutures to maintain hemostasis while yet others cover the cone bed with Sturmdorf sutures: the use of sutures frequently results in partial stenosis of the cervix which can affect not only subsequent fertility but also the ability to perform satisfactory cytology and colposcopy follow-up afterwards. Probably the simplest way to perform a knife conization is to use a vasoconstrictor, employ diathermy to achieve hemostasis in the cone bed and to coat the cone bed with Monsel's solution (a hemostatic paste made up as described in Anderson et al[9]).

Laser excisional conization. Using the CO_2 laser under colposcopic direction it is possible to obtain a very satisfactory cone with minimal postoperative hemorrhage and virtually no postoperative stenosis. The technique is simply to outline the lesion and plan the size and shape of the cone using a colposcope. The cervix is then injected with a vasoconstrictor at four points (2, 5, 7 and 10 o'clock) to a depth of approximately 1 cm. An ordinary syringe and needle is not ideal and the operator will find the use of a dental syringe and needle will make the procedure much easier.

After allowing time for the vasoconstrictor to work (this usually takes about 3 min and corresponds to the cessation of bleeding from the injection sites) the CO_2 laser is used in the cutting mode. This entails turning the spot size to the minimum available (approximately 0.4 mm) and using the maximum wattage which the machine will allow. Using the laser in this mode the appropriate conization can be carried out under colposcopic direction, using a sharp pair of scissors or a knife to cut across the apex of the cone (this allows the pathologist to examine the apex of the cone for completeness of excision). The laser is then turned to coagulation mode by increasing the size of the spot to 1.7–2.00 mm still using the maximum wattage the machine will allow. The laser beam destroys the lower part of the remaining endocervical canal and then is used as a cautery to control bleeding on the cut surface of the cone bed. Once hemostasis has been achieved the cone bed is then coated with Monsel's solution. It is not necessary to pack the cone bed or the vagina, nor is it necessary to cover the procedure with an antibiotic (unless of course there is obvious cervicitis in which case it would be better, if possible, to clear this before performing a conization).

Large loop excision of the transformation zone. The technique of removing cervical tissue using a small diathermy loop was first described by Cartier.[10] Cartier's technique was modified by Prendiville[18] using a larger loop. In Europe the technique is known as LLETZ (large loop excision of the transformation zone) while in the US it is usually known as LEEP (loop electrosurgical excision procedure). Both techniques, however, rely on the same principle. The technique has rapidly become the treatment of choice for most patients with CIN, first because it is simple, cheap and easy to use and second because in most instances it can be performed under local anesthesia with a combination of local anesthetic agent and a vasoconstrictor being injected into the cervix. Although its use on an out patient basis is clearly important, its main advantage is that all of the tissue can be removed simply and easily for histological assessment (as compared with outpatient destructive methods which rely on one or more punch biopsies to assess the degree of CIN and to exclude invasion).

A management possibility which has been afforded by the introduction of LLETZ is that of 'see and treat' which means that at her first visit to the colposcopy clinic for assessment of abnormal cytology, treatment by LLETZ can if necessary be undertaken at the same time, thereby eliminating the need to bring the woman back on a subsequent occasion. However, Luesley et al[19] showed that although such management was simple and easy to introduce there was a major disadvantage. Of the women treated by them on a 'see and treat basis', 8% of specimens revealed no abnormality, 22% showed HPV only and 18% showed no more than CIN 1 with HPV, i.e., it could be argued that 48% of women treated in that series did not necessarily need to be treated at that time if at all (assuming that CIN 1 is of doubtful malignant potential). Luesley et al[19] also showed that the morbidity of LLETZ

was minimal and the complications tend to be related to the length of endocervical canal removed, i.e., the more of the canal removed the more likely there was to be a complication.

No matter what method of treating CIN is employed there is always concern about subsequent fertility. Bigrigg et al[20] found that there was no effect on subsequent fertility and pregnancy outcome but on the other hand Blomfield et al[21] found that when pregnancy occurred following LLETZ there was a higher incidence of babies with lower birth weights compared to controls even allowing for confounding variables.

Hysterectomy

Clearly, conization by one means or another is an excellent method of treating CIN and in general terms a properly planned cone will remove the lesion in its entirety in 94–96% of cases. If treatment by conization is so good, hysterectomy is clearly over-treatment for most women, but on the other hand can be regarded as the treatment of choice in certain circumstances:

a. Sometimes there is some other indication for hysterectomy such as menorrhagia, fibroids, or prolapse in which case the surgeon may feel that 'two birds can be killed with one stone' by performing a hysterectomy. While this may be so the surgeon should bear in mind that the woman may have occult invasive carcinoma which should be excluded histologically either by colposcopically directed biopsies or by a prior conisation.

b. In the postmenopausal woman with a narrow vagina and very short cervix then conization by knife, laser or LLETZ can be difficult, complicated by hemorrhage (because the cone extends into the lower part of the uterus) and finally postoperative stenosis. Under these circumstances it is perfectly reasonable to proceed directly to hysterectomy knowing that the morbidity of hysterectomy in such a woman is almost certainly lower than an excisional cone.

c. If the lesion involves the upper vagina then a hysterectomy (abdominal or vaginal) may be the treatment of choice bearing in mind of course that occult invasive disease should first be excluded. Under these circumstances an alternative to hysterectomy, for example in young women, would be to destroy the vaginal and intraepithelial neoplasia (VAIN) and treat the CIN by conization.

d. If following conization or destruction there is residual disease then hysterectomy may be the treatment of choice although the colposcopist always has the option of removing residual disease by conization. Local destruction of residual disease is also of course a possibility but since residual disease may in fact be due to occult invasive disease then destruction should only carried out by an experienced colposcopist after proper and careful assessment.

Local destruction of CIN

In its time local destruction of CIN was heralded, and indeed was, a major breakthrough in treatment. However, with the advent of simple and safe excisional methods, particularly LLETZ, the role of destruction has now to be questioned. Having said that it is still a method which, in good hands, can ensure good results. However, the margin of error is greater than with excision, but provided certain key criteria are strictly met the results are very acceptable:

a. The patient should be seen and assessed by a competent colposcopist.
b. The colposcopist should see the lesion in its entirety.
c. Colposcopically directed biopsy or biopsies should exclude invasive carcinoma.
d. There should be no suspicion either colposcopically or cytologically of abnormal columnar cells, because if there is then excision is obligatory.
e. The ablation should be carried out by the colposcopist.
f. There is adequate cytology and colposcopy follow-up.

The most commonly performed and successful methods of destruction are as follows:-

Radical electrocoagulation diathermy

This was developed in Australia.[22-23] For many years Chanen insisted that this should be performed under general anesthesia but more recently (personal communication) he feels that selected cases can be dealt with in the out patient clinic using local anesthesia. Chanen and Rome[23] claimed a 98.3% cure rate with a single treatment and concluded "a single application of electrocoagulation diathermy is a safe and effective means of treatment for most patients with premalignant disease of the cervix regardless of its extent or severity. The risk of subsequent invasive cancer in these patients has been virtually eliminated."

The technique is extremely simple and can be carried out with equipment available in any operating theatre throughout the world. The patient is first assessed as being suitable for destruction as outlined above. The cervix is first dilated, the lesion reviewed colposcopically, and if at this stage there is any doubt about the possibility of occult invasion then further biopsies should be taken. Using a needle electrode multiple insertions of the electrode to a depth of 1 cm are made into the whole of the transformation zone and into the columnar epithelium in the lower part of the endocervical canal. Next a ball electrode is used and by a process of fulguration and coagulation the whole surface area already subjected to the needle electrode is systematically diathermied.[24]

Cryocautery

Cryocautery of CIN was popularised in the USA and was the mainstay of outpatient treatment in the 1970s. It has the advantage that it can be carried out on an outpatient basis, under colposcopic direction, without anesthesia. The colposcopist assesses the size of the lesion and applies the appropriate cryocautery tip directly to the cervix. The freezing process usually takes 2–3 min and will destroy tissue to a depth of about 4 mm. The probe is defrosted and the cervix inspected colposcopically to ensure that the iceball has extended beyond the limits of the lesion. If the lesion is large then more than one application may be necessary. Most surgeons use a simple one-freeze technique but others advocate freeze–thaw–refreeze. Townsend[25] used a single freeze–thaw technique and concluded that elimination of CIN with a single treatment was successful in 88%. Of the 12% with residual disease a second cryosurgery was performed and this increased the cure rate to 95%. Townsend[25] concluded that the success rate depended not only on the skill of the colposcopist in excluding invasive disease but also on the size of the lesion. Small lesions were more likely to be cured with a single treatment but when the lesion covered most of the ectocervix (regardless of whether it was CIN 1, 2 or 3) there was a primary failure rate approaching 50%. Shafi et al[26] assessed the likelihood of success with a single LLETZ treatment and concluded, like Townsend, that the larger the lesion, regardless of the degree of CIN, the more likelihood there was of residual disease. This may be related to the observed fact that the larger the lesion the more likely there is to be high grade CIN.[26]

Sevin et al[27] described several cases of invasive carcinoma following cryotherapy but concluded that subsequent invasive disease was due largely to inadequate prior colposcopic assessment rather than the technique of cryocautery itself.

Cold coagulation

Duncan[28] and Gordon and Duncan[29] described how patients with CIN had been treated with the Semm 'cold' coagulator with an overall cure rate of 95%. Contrary to what its name implies the cold coagulator is not 'cold'. A applicator shaped like a cryocautery probe is applied to the cervical surface for 20 s and is heated rapidly to a temperature of 100°C. Using this technique it is possible to destroy the whole of the transformation zone, usually in five slightly overlapping areas, including the lower ectocervix, and Duncan finds that the usual treatment time is approximately 100 s. The technique is certainly simple and cheap and usually does not require local anesthesia.

Carbon dioxide laser

Laser is an acronym of light amplification by stimulated emission of radiation. The CO_2 produces energy at a wavelength of 10.6 μm. which is in the infrared portion of the spectrum where it is invisible to the naked eye. This compares with the Nd:YAG laser with a wavelength of 1.06 μm. and the Argon laser with a wavelength of 0.488–0.514 μm. The CO_2 energy by using a system of mirrors and lenses can be focused to a specific spot and at this focal point it releases its energy. Any tissue at the focal point is destroyed by vaporizing the water in the tissue at the speed of light. The spot size of the laser can be varied from 0.2 mm to 2.5 mm, i.e., the same laser can be used as a knife (with a small spot size) or in a vaporization mode (with a large spot size). When employing the technique of CO_2 laser vaporization the patient should be selected as mentioned above, i.e., a competent colposcopist should first exclude unsuspected invasive carcinoma and the treatment should also be carried out by a competent colposcopist. As with any destructive method the success of treatment depends not only on excluding occult invasive disease but on destroying tissue to a depth which will take into account that CIN frequently extends below the surface epithelium by growing into the subepithelial crypts or clefts, and failure to recognise this will result in inadequate treatment. With cryocautery the depth is easy to control (about 4 mm) and with radical diathermy the operator should be destroying to a depth of about 1 cm. With the laser it is very easy to fall into the trap of not destroying tissue deeply enough hence those using laser destruction for the first time will tend to have a relatively high failure rate. The histological study by Anderson and Hartely[30] showed that 99.7% of lesions extended less than 4 mm below the surface but since it is almost impossible to gage depth of destruction to exactly 4 mm a depth of 5–7 mm should be the aim of laser vaporization.[31] If laser vaporization is carried out correctly cure rates in excess of 95% can be expected.[31-33]

CONCLUSION

The diagnosis and treatment of CIN, will for all practical purposes, ensure that women will not die from squamous carcinoma of the cervix.

Various treatment modalities are available and the success of each method depends not so much on the skill of the surgeon but on the quality of the preoperative colposcopic assessment. It is fair to say that a competent colposcopist could employ any of the excision or destructive techniques and obtain excellent results. The key, therefore, is colposcopy.

It should be borne in mind, however, that not everyone with abnormal cervical cytology requires treatment. We recognize that there are low-grade and high-grade CIN lesions and that many so-called low-grade CIN lesions are nothing more than HPV infection which left to its own devices will resolve without any treatment whatsoever. It is important, therefore, that the colposcopist takes account of all factors otherwise a scenario will unfold in which many women, particularly young women, will be subjected to treatment which in retrospect is quite unnecessary.[34]

REFERENCES

1. Bigrigg M A, Haffernden D K, Shelhan A L, Codling B W, Read M D. Efficacy and safety of large loop excision of the transformation zone. Lancet 1984; 343: 32–34.
2. Rubin I C the pathological diagnosis of incipient carcinoma of the uterus. Am J Obstet Gynecol 1910; 62: 668–676.
3. Hinselmann H. Verbesserung der Inspektionsmoglichkeit von Vulva, Vagina and Portio. Munchener Medizinische Wochenschrift 1925; 77: 1733.
4. Schiller W. Jodpinselung und Abschabung des Portioepithels. Zentrablatt fur Gynakologic 1929; 53: 1056–1064.
5. Papanicolaou G, Traut H F. The Diagnosis of Uterine Cancer by the Vaginal Smear. New York: Commonwealth, 1943.
6. Koller O. The vascular patterns of the uterine cervix. London: Scandinavian University Books, 1963.
7. Kolstad P. Vascularisation. Oxygen tension and radiocurability in cancer of the cervix. London: Scandinavian University Books, 1964.
8. Shafi M I, Dunn J A, Chenoy R, Buxton E J, Williams C, Luesley D M. Digital imaging colposcopy, image analysis and quantification of the colposcopic image. Br J Obstet Gynaecol 1994; 101: 234–238.
9. Anderson M C, Jordan J A, Morse A, Sharp F. A text and atlas of integrated colposcopy. Chapman and Hall, 1992.
10. Cartier R. Practical colposcopy. Paris: Laboratoire Cartier, 1984.
11. Kolstad P, Stafl A. Atlas of colposcopy. Oslo: Universitetsforlaget, 1977.
12. Jordan J A, Sharp F, Singer A. Preclinical Neoplasia of the Cervix. Proceedings of the Ninth Study Group of the Royal College of Obstetricians and Gynaecologists, London. p 299.
13. Duncan I D. NHS cervical screening programme, guidelines for clinical practice and programme management. National Co-ordinating Network, Oxford: Oxford Regional Health Authority.
14. McLaren H C. Conservative management of cervical precancer. J Obstet Gynaecol Br Commonwealth 1967; 74: 487–492.
15. Jordan J A. Colposcopy in gynaecological practice. In: Jakob C A, Franco M A, eds. Proceedings of the First World Congress of Colposcopy and Cervical Pathology.

Argentina: Molachina Establecimiento, Grapio, Rosano, pp 131–113.
16. Jordan J A. The diagnosis and management of premalignant conditions of the cervix. Clin Obstet Gynecol 1976; 32: 295–315.
17. Soutter W P, Fenton D W, Gudgeon P, Sharp F. Quantitative microcolpohysteroscopic assessment of the extent of endocervical involvement by cervical intraepithelial neoplasia. Br J Obstet Gynaecol 1984; 91(7): 712–715.
18. Prendiville W, Cullimore J, Norman S. Large loop excision of transformation zone (LLETZ)): a new method of management for women with intraepithelial neoplasia. Br J Obstet Gynaecol 1989; 96: 1054–1060.
19. Luesley D M, Cullimore J, Redman C W E et al. Loop diathermy of the cervical transformation zone in patients with abnormal cervical smears. Br Med J 1990; 300: 1690–1693.
20. Bigrigg M A, Codling B W, Pearson P, Read M D, Swingler G R. Pregnancy after cervical loop diathermy. Lancet 1991; 337: 119.
21. Blomfield P I, Buxton J, Dunn J, Luesley D M. Pregnancy outcome after large loop excision of the cervical transformation zone. Am J Obstet Gynecol 1993; 169: 620–625.
22. Chanen W, Hollyock V E. Colposcopy and electrocoagulation diathermy for cervical dysplasia and carcinoma in situ. Obstet Gynecol 1971; 63: 623–628.
23. Chanen W, Rome R M. Electrocoagulation diathermy for cervical dysplasia and carcinoma in situ: a 15 year survey. Obstet Gynecol 1983; 61: 673–679.
24. Chanen W. Radical electrocoagulation. Diathermy. In: Coppleson M, ed. Gynecologic oncology. London, Churchill Livingstone, 1981; pp 821–825.
25. Townsend D E. Cryosurgery in gynecologic oncology. In: Coppleson M, ed. Gynecologic oncology. London, Churchill Livingstone, 1981: pp 809–815.
26. Shafi M I, Finn C B, Luesley D M, Jordan J A, Dunn J. Lesion size and histology of atypical transformation zone. Br J Obstet Gynaecol 1991; 98: 490–492.
27. Sevin B, Ford J H, Girtanner R D et al. Invasive cancer of the cervix after cryosurgery. Obstet Gynecol 1979; 45: 456.
28. Duncan I D. Treatment of CIN by destruction — "Cold coagulator". In: Jordan J A, Sharp F, Singer A, Preclinical carcinoma of the cervix. London: Royal College of Obstetricians and Gynaecologists, 1982; pp 197–202.

29. Gordon H, Duncan I D. Effective destruction of CIN 3 at at 100°C using the Semm cold coagulator: 14 years experience. Br J Obstet Gynaecol 1991; 98: 14–20.

30. Anderson M C, Hartley R B. Cervical crypt involvement by intrapeithelial neoplasia. Obstet Gynecol 1980; 55: 546–550.

31. Jordan J A, Woodman C B J, Mylotte M J et al. The treatment of cervical intraepithelial neoplasia by laser vaporization. Br J Obstet Gynaecol 1985; 92: 394–398.

32. Williams J. Cancer of the uterus. Harveian Lectures for 1886. London: H K Lewis, 1886.

33. Wright V C, Davies E, Riopelle M A. Laser surgery for cervical intraepithelial neoplasia: Principles and results. Am J Obstet Gynecol 1983; 145–181.

34. Jordan J A Minor degrees of cervical intraepithelial neoplasia. Br Med J 1988; 297: 6.

16. Human papillomavirus testing: major advance or scientific hoax?

Richard Reid   J. Thomas Cox

INTRODUCTION

Molecular probes for the detection of oncogenic human papillomavirus (HPVs) have been available since 1983.[1,2] From a research perspective, this molecular technology has yielded enormous benefits. More has been learned about the pathogenesis of cervical cancer within the last decade, than over all of preceding history. In this short time, the DNA sequences have been mapped, RNA transcription and protein translations have been partially elucidated, and rapid cost-effective viral tests have been developed. Paradoxically, interest in clinical application of these powerful and accurate tools remains stagnant. This chapter will begin by examining the misconceptions underlying this unusual turn of events. Current understanding of the relationship between HPV infection and cervical cancer will be reviewed, the rationale for HPV testing examined, and possible diagnostic and screening applications explored.

HISTORICAL INSIGHT: HOW THE MISCONCEPTIONS AROSE

Those who do not learn the lessons of history are destined to repeat past mistakes. This aphorism could not be more true than in the study of genital HPV infection. Initially, confusion about the relationship between HPV infection and cervical neoplasia was shared by scientists and physicians.[3] Why were these misconceptions so easily resolved by molecular geneticists but not by clinicians? The answer lies in dissecting the relevant medical literature into three discrete time periods.

Initial studies (1983–1986)

In 1983, Gissman et al[4] established that most benign condylomas contain HPV 6/11, and that this virus was distinct from the HPV types to be found in warts from nongenital skin. Soon afterward, HPV 16 and HPV 18 were cloned from stored cervical cancer biopsies.[1,2] The demonstration that 75% of this panel of 40 invasive cancers contained either HPV 16 or 18 introduced the concept of high-risk and low-risk types. Moreover, an association defined by histologic analysis of blinded hysterectomy specimens[5] was now equally discernible by molecular analysis. A period of overly optimistic expectations ensued, during which many presumed that viral testing of all women would replace cervical cytology. However, neither the plurality of HPV types nor the surprising prevalence of oncogenic HPV DNA amongst normal women had yet been appreciated. Even so, the suggestion that colonization by HPV 16 or 18 would inevitably lead to neoplastic sequelae was inherently simplistic. Other oncogenic DNA viruses (e.g., hepatitis B or Epstein–Barr) are characterized by large pools of latent infection, variable levels of clinical expression, and long lag times.[6,7] Why should it be different for HPV associated neoplasia?

The nihilistic period (1987–1990)

The concept that HPV 16 or 18 infection conferred a major risk of cervical carcinogenesis was quickly challenged. Low-risk HPV types were seemingly found in cervical cancers,[8,9] HPV 16 was soon suspected to be ubiquitous,[10,11] and clinicians became increasingly frustrated by endless reports of 'koilocytotic atypia' within minimally deranged biopsies.[12] Diagnostic and therapeutic excesses arose, creating an 'emotional blacklash' that further fueled growing scientific skepticism. However, much of the 'negative evidence' from the late 1980s is now known to represent laboratory error. A review of the testing modalities utilized in these studies clarifies how basic testing errors could occur on such a large scale.[13]

Limitations of filter in situ hybridization ('FISH')

Southern blot hybridization (SBH) was first described in 1975 and has been the 'gold standard' ever since.[14] This method has an analytic sensitivity of 95% and an analytic specificity of 98%.[15] Unfortunately, Southern blot is a process with about 30 steps, which takes about 3 weeks to complete. The test must be done by a scientist (rather than a technician), and is applicable only to individual specimens (rather than large batches). Hence, Southern blot is far too laborious and expensive for use in clinical situations.

Filter in situ hybridization (FISH) was developed in 1984 as a simple and rapid test for detecting HPV within cytologic specimens.[16] In essence, FISH bypasses the laborious early steps of SBH, by fixing an unprepared suspension of epithelial cells directly onto the nylon filter. A dot blot hybridization is then performed, to determine whether the test is 'positive' or 'negative.' FISH has only 10 steps, allows batched samples to be tested by a laboratory technician, and takes only 3 days to complete. When several large prospective studies were being planned in the mid-1980s, FISH was therefore the only economically acceptable choice. Unfortunately, FISH has several fundamental limitations, which were not appreciated until these studies were well underway or even completed. Accuracy of FISH depends upon two things. Any target DNA within the tested sample must bind sufficient ^{32}P molecules to produce an homogenous black spot on the underlying X-ray film (positive result). Conversely, for a clear-cut negative result, there must be no nonspecific binding of ^{32}P to impurities within the unprepared sample. In reality, neither of these stipulations is consistently met. First, the exfoliated cells may fail to lyse, or the lysed nucleic

acids may not bind to the filter; in either instance, any target HPV DNA within the sample is not available for detection. Hence, the sensitivity of FISH proved poor — generally of the order of 50%. Second, mucous and proteinaceous debris admixed with the exfoliated cervical cells can readily trap ^{32}P molecules, producing multiple false positives. Indeed, in many instances, even the testing endpoint was uninterpretable (Fig. 16.1).

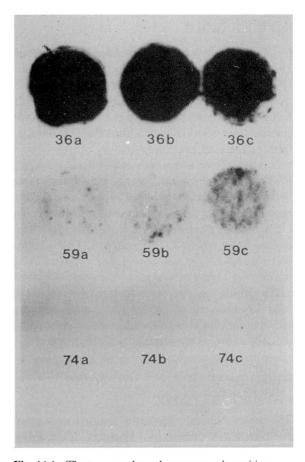

Fig. 16.1 The top row shows homogeneously positive blots, reflecting uniform release of any target HPV DNA by cell lysis, and successful binding of this target DNA to the underlying nylon filter. Conversely, the bottom row shows clearly negative blots, reflecting the fact that all of the unbound ^{32}P-labeled probe DNA was washed out of the sample. However, as shown in the middle rows, FISH blots are often completely uninterpretable. The stippled appearance of these middle blots could represent either virus positive samples showing patchy binding of the target HPV DNA or virus negative samples showing nonspecific trapping of the radiolabeled HPV DNA probe. Such ambiguity in test interpretation is the fundamental reason why studies based upon FISH gave invalid results.

Using FISH, Sutton et al[8] detected HPV 6/11 in 8 of 24 (33%) cervical cancers, and Reeves et al[9] reported HPV 6/11 in 129 of 756 (17%) such specimens. In hindsight, reports of HPV 6/11 in cancer are clearly attributable to testing artifact. Modern literature does not contain a single example of HPV 6/11 in invasive lesion, other than verrucous carcinomas of the vulva.[17,18] The frustration of having tested 20 161 samples from 11 667 women over 5 years is best expressed by Ethel de Villers,[19] who wrote "It became clear that this method [FISH] had several disadvantages. One disadvantage of this test was low sensitivity (a detection rate of at least 50 genome copies/cell) . . . a further limitation was that no true distinction could be made between 6/11 and 16/18."

Limitations of prototypic DNA–DNA in situ hybridization

DNA–DNA in situ hybridization (ISH) was first demonstrated in 1985. ISH differs from FISH in that the target is intranuclear HPV DNA within a histologic tissue section (rather than heterologously distributed granules within cellular material lyzed to a nylon filter) (Fig. 16.2). Because the end point is assessed microscopically, rather than macroscopically, DNA–DNA ISH is a moderately sensitive (90%) and highly specific (99%) method for detecting the presence of a replicating viral infection. Latently colonized cells contain few copies of the viral gene; hence radionucleotide binding often fails to reach a density sufficient for recognition through the light microscope. In many ways, this reduction in analytic sensitivity has been one of the strengths of ISH.

Intranuclear localization of HPV probe within the nuclei of koilocytotic or dysplastic cells is firm evidence that a given sample contains some form of HPV DNA. However, because of cross-reactivity between each of the HPV probes and background, typing data generated by this method are not reliable.[20] Syrjanen[21,22] used DNA–DNA ISH to study a group of 508 Finnish women with cervical HPV infection followed prospectively for a mean of 35 months. The reported progression to carcinoma in situ was 18% for HPV 6/11 versus 17% for HPV 16 and 18. However, these results are at variance with five recent cross-sectional[23–27]

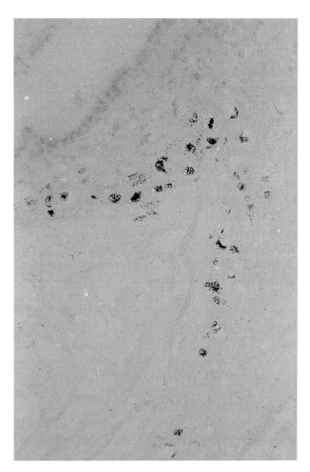

Fig. 16.2 A histologic section of a condyloma, which tested positive by DNA–DNA in situ hybridization. Localization of the ^{32}P grams to the nuclei of koilocytotic cells is clear evidence that this sample does contain some form of HPV DNA. However, attempts to type this sample by DNA–DNA–ISH are unreliable, because cross-reactivity between regions of partial nucleotide homology between HPV and any of the individual probes can produce erroneous results.

and three recent cohort studies,[28–30] all of which used more reliable analytical methods. Moreover, since it has been shown quite conclusively that HPV 6/11 lacks the ability to transform human keratinocytes in vitro, it is quite improbable that HPV 6/11 could exert an oncogenic effect in vivo.[31] Genuine but weak statistical associations do exist between herpes,[32] chlamydia,[33] gonorrhea,[34] and cervical cancer, reflecting sexual lifestyle similarities rather than a causal relationship. Any association between HPV 6/11 and cervical malignancy is likely to fit this model.

Amplification artifact in early polymerase chain reaction studies

Polymerase chain reaction (PCR) is a method for amplifying nucleic acid, such that trace amounts of HPV DNA can produce large quantities of target.[35] The clinical specimen is incubated with oligonucleotide primers for specific regions of the HPV genome. A polymerase is added, and the mixture is incubated through successive heating and cooling cycles. PCR can potentially detect as few as 10 copies of HPV DNA within 5×10^4 cells. However, signal amplification by 10 000 times or more is a two-edged sword. Just as happened with FISH, initial enthusiasm led to incorporation of this testing method in clinical studies before PCR had been adequately evaluated.

More than any other source of misinformation, naive results generated by improperly performed PCR have fueled the fallacy that HPV DNA is ubiquitous, and that HPV testing is therefore futile. This confusion can be traced to several mistakes which occurred during the 'learning curve'. The first source of error lay with unexpected contamination. Low levels of viral residues on clinic instruments or within laboratory dust presented a ready source of false-positive results. Some early PCR papers in which artifactual findings were clearly attributable to carry-over have already been retracted.[10,36] Other studies reporting upon the presence of HPV DNA in ovarian,[37] colon[38] or prostatic[39] cancers have been a subject of substantial scientific mirth (helped by amazing wisdom that hindsight can imbue). However, despite the jocularity with which molecular biologists view these early PCR excesses, most clinicians do not yet understand the joke!

Even the more recent PCR studies, which have employed better methodology, are not understood by gynecologists. PCR methods using extreme amplification will detect traces of HPV DNA in 30–50% of normal women.[40,41] However, the clinical relevance of such results requires qualification. First, most evaluations were done on college undergraduates. Such samples do not reflect the declining HPV DNA prevalence rates found in aging populations[42] and are therefore not representative. Second, several studies have docu-

mented that the risk of having cervical intraepithelial neoplasia is directly proportional to the viral load[24,43,44] rather than simple colonization. When amplification cycles are restricted, PCR detection rates in normal women fall to approximately 20%.[45] Third, of the 20% of women who test positive by restricted amplification, about half (10%) represent uncharacterized types.[41] Thus, even with skillfully performed PCR, only about 3–5% of normal women harbor oncogenic anogenital HPVs. Basically, it is only these results that are relevant to disease detection.

A second problem derives from ambiguities in the meaning attached to the words 'sensitivity' and 'specificity', depending upon whether these terms are being used by a molecular biologist or an epidemiologist. PCR has excellent molecular sensitivity (a positivity threshold as low as 10 target molecules per sample) and acceptable molecular specificity (probes directed against small and highly characteristic regions of the target nucleic acid).[46] However, these biochemical attributes threatened to destroy the clinical value of PCR testing for HPV, by making large numbers of virologically valid but clinically meaningless identifications of trace amounts of HPV DNA. Epidemiologic sensitivity and specificity are reciprocal ratios; hence an increase in epidemiologic sensitivity generally produces a compensatory reduction in the epidemiologic specificity.[47] For example, of 120 specimens tested by PCR and Southern blot, both methods detected HPV DNA in 85% of lavages from patients with cervical disease.[15] In contrast, PCR identified HPV in a much higher proportion of normal specimens (31 vs 11%), thereby eroding epidemiologic specificity (68 vs 89%). Recently, Goldsborough[48] demonstrated that PCR is most useful when molecular sensitivity approximates that of Southern blot hybridization (a positivity threshold of about 5×10^4 target molecules per specimen). At higher sensitivity levels, results were obscured by the fact that PCR detected HPV DNA (mainly uncharacterized types) in 60% of normal patients and in 35% of abdominal skin or air control swabs. Until reproducible methods have been demonstrated by formal validation trials, clinical studies tested by PCR must be interpreted with caution.[49]

The realistic period (1990–1994)

Now that molecular biologists have resolved the early sources of testing artifact, the presence of high levels of an oncogenic HPV DNA has proven to be highly predictive of cervical neoplasia. In contrast to the weaker, probably spurious associations between cervical cancer and other sexually-transmitted pathogens, the relationship of cervical cancer with HPV infection is strong, consistent, specific, and plausible. Given the volume of supporting experimental and epidemiologic evidence, such observations suggest a cause and effect relationship (Fig. 16.3).[50,51] It is now virtually certain that the basic cellular transformation that develops into cervical intraepithelial neoplasia is initiated by oncogenic HPV infection.[52,53] The early genomic region of the oncogenic HPVs (but not the nononcogenic HPVs), provides all the means for inducing cellular immortality and for evoking an aneuploid chromosome complement in tissue culture.[54,55] Transfection with oncogenic HPV DNAs can immortalize human keratinocytes in cell culture, and further growth of these immortalized cells on collagen rafts or in nude mice can produce histologic patterns essentially identical to CIN 3 (Table 16.1).[51–53,56] In clinical situations, the progressive potential of precursor lesions has been largely defined by HPV type.[28–30]

Whether these HPVs also play a role in promoting progression from the precursor state to invasive disease is less certain. There have been reports of HPV-immortalized cells acquiring invasive properties simply by continued growth in vitro for 2–4 years, without exposure to additional carcinogens.[56] Within naturally occurring cervical neoplasia and cancer-derived cell lines, the HPV genome is consistently transcribed,[57] albeit with striking differences at different points in the pathologic spectrum. Compared with the apparently 'balanced' transcription seen in low-grade lesions (where both early and late regions are represented), invasive cancer cells show increased expression of the two viral transforming genes (E6 and E7), but no detectable late gene expression. E6 and E7 proteins coded by the oncogenic HPV types antagonize the host tumor suppressor proteins, p53 and pRB, thereby deregulating cell growth.[57–59] Finally, the integration of HPV genetic sequences into the host genome usually occurs just as the cell develops invasive properties.[60] For integration to occur, the HPV episomes are linearized in a way that typically preserves E6/E7 expression but abolishes the negative regulatory effects of the E2 gene. The end result is a permanent mutation in the cellular genome, which is transmitted to all progeny cells during

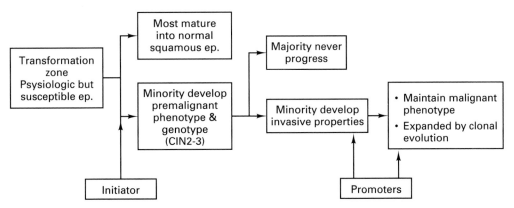

Fig. 16.3 A diagrammatic representation of the standard model for the pathogenesis of solid tumors. Initiators transform physiologic but susceptible squamous metaplasia into permanently altered precursor epithelium. In contrast, promoters act at various other points in this cascade, such as developing invasive properties, maintaining a malignant phenotype, or favoring clonal expansions. Reprinted with permission from: Reid R, Lorincz A. Should family physicians test for human papillomavirus infection? An affirmative view. J Family Prac 1991; 32: 183–192.[51]

Table 16.1 Evidence of HPV infection linked to pathogenesis of CIN 2–3*

1. Cancer-associated HPVs are found in 90% of CIN 2–3 vs 10% of normal women, yielding a relative risk estimate of 80:1.
2. CIN 1 is indistinguishable from condyloma, but viral cytopathic effect decreases with increasing levels of premalignant transformation.
3. Noninfected cervical epithelium becomes senescent after 10 passages in cell culture; however, cervical keratinocytes are immortalized by oncogenic HPV infection.
4. Histologic features of CIN 2–3 can be reproduced in vitro and in vivo by oncogenic HPV infection of previously normal human keratinocytes.
5. Progressive potential of minor cervical atypia is influenced by HPV type.

*Reprinted with permission from: Reid R, Lorincz A T. Should family physicians test for human papillomavirus infection? An affirmative view. Am J Family Pract 1991; 32: 183–192.[51]

subsequent mitotic divisions. Of course, malignant promotion from CIN 3 to invasive cancer probably involves multiple factors. Certainly the significant pool of chronic latent infection in otherwise healthy individuals and the low progression rate of untreated high-grade intraepithelial lesions indicate that this equation involves more than just the simple acquisition of an oncogenic HPV infection (Table 16.2).[50,61]

Table 16.2 HPV infection linked to progression from CIN 2–3 to invasive cancer*

1. Cross-sectional data show strong, consistent relationship between specific HPV types and both precursor and invasive disease.
2. HPV-immortalized human cells can eventually develop tumorigenic (invasive) properties with long-term culture.
3. Animal papillomaviruses of analogous genetic organization produce invasive cancers in several species.
4. Viral genome (especially E6 and E7) is continuously transcribed within cancer cells and cervix-cancer-derived cell lines.
5. E6 and E7 viral proteins bind two cellular 'antioncogenes' (p53 and pRB) that control cell growth rates.
6. HPV DNA is episomal in benign lesions, but integrated into the cellular genome of most cancer cells.
7. Integration destroys the viral negative control gene (E2) but preserves the transforming genes (E6 and E7).

*Reprinted with permission from: Reid R, Lorincz A T. Should family physicians test for human papillomavirus infection? An affirmative view. Am J Family Pract 1991; 32: 183–192.[51]

THE SCIENTIFIC BASIS FOR HPV TESTING

Testing for the presence of an etiologic factor is a long established principle in the management of infectious diseases. However, it could be argued that, if both condyloma and cancer contained the same HPV types, there would be no advantage to HPV testing. Fortunately, such is not the case. Given the strengths of the type specific relationships between HPV infection and varying grades of cervical disease, virus testing can provide substantial insight into the differing natural histories of morphologically similar lesions.[26,62]

Clinical groupings of mucosotropic HPVs

Anogenital HPVs can be subdivided into four main categories, based upon both nucleotide homology and type-specific disease associations (Fig. 16.4).[26]

HPVs 6/11, 42, 43 and 44

From the molecular perspective, HPV 6 and 11 are highly related, but were classified as separate viruses before their nucleotide similarities were truly known. Clinically, these subtypes are responsible for three main forms of disease. HPV 6/11 DNA is detectable in more than 90% of papillomas in the aerodigestive tract and upper airways, and in a similar proportion of benign exophytic condylomas in the anogenital tract. Thirdly, detection of HPV type 6/11 in minor lesions of the transformation zone fostered a mistaken belief that these types also accounted for the majority of minor cervical atypia. In reality, HPV type 6/11 probably causes only about 15% of flat condylomas or mild dysplasias.[63]

Included within this group are three recently cloned viruses, HPV types 42, 43 and 44, all of which are somewhat related to HPV 6/11 at the nucleotide level. HPV types 42, 43 and 44 are found in a small proportion of low-grade cervical, vulvar, and penile lesions, but have not been detected in an invasive cancer.

From the molecular perspective, HPV 6/11 does not appear to have an oncologic potential. Although the E6 and E7 proteins produced by

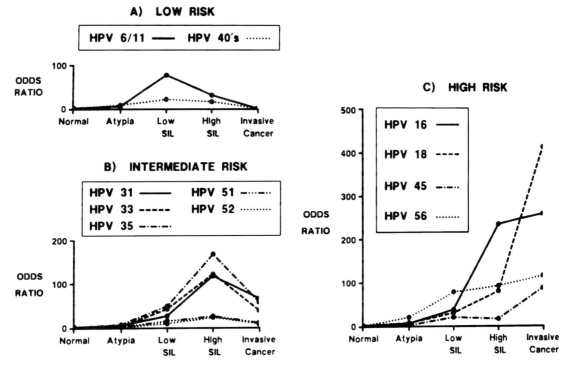

Fig. 16.4 Graphic profiles of the odds ratios for **A** low-risk, **B** intermediate-risk, and **C** high-risk human papillomavirus (HPV). Each graph is drawn to the same scale; hence, the pronounced variation in strengths of association is accentuated by the differences in the heights of the Y-axes. Reprinted with permission from Lorincz A T, Reid R, Jenson A B et al. Human papillomavirus infection of the cervix: Relative risk associations of 15 common anogenital types. Obstet Gynecol 1992; 79: 328–37.[26]

the HPV 6/11 group bind p53 and pRB, this binding is weak. Perhaps for this reason, this group of viruses cannot immortalize keratinocytes in vitro[31] or induce malignant transformation in vivo.[64] Moreover, HPV 6/11 appear unable to integrate their DNA into the human genome.[65] Epidemiologic studies demonstrating that HPV 6/11 are seldom (if ever) found in invasive cancer can therefore be accepted as firm evidence that this group can produce only benign mucosal lesions. Exceptions to this rule can arise through rare viral mutation,[66] or with concomitant exposure to radiation.[67]

HPV 16

Worldwide, HPV type 16 is the viral type detected in about 50% of high-grade intraepithelial neoplasia and invasive cancer. HPV 16 is predominantly associated with squamous cancer,

but is also present in about one third of adeno-carcinomas.[68] Elsewhere within the anogenital tract, HPV 16 is found in at least 85% of high-grade lesions (VIN, VAIN, PAIN, PIN).[69] Thus, from the clinical perspective, detection of HPV type 16 apparently identifies a patient at risk for the whole gamut of HPV-associated malignancies: namely squamous cancer of the cervical transformation zone, adenocarcinoma of the cervical canal, and squamous carcinomas of the vagina, vulva or anus and (for uncircumcised males) penis.

HPVs 18, 45 and 56

The distribution pattern for HPV 18 is different from HPV type 16. HPV 18 is the second most prevalent type (25%) in invasive cervical cancers but is relatively uncommon (5%) in minor-grade lesions. HPVs 45 and 56 are two rare types, which are closely related to HPV type 18 at the nucleotide level, and which share broadly similar clinical associations.[26]

The skewed distribution of HPVs 18, 45 and 56 within invasive rather than preinvasive lesions is difficult to explain, except by the suggestion that these particular viruses are associated with rapid-transit tumors. This tentative hypothesis is supported by several recent observations. First, HPV 18 was detected 2.6 times more frequently within invasive cancer occurring within 1 year of a negative smear (44 vs 17%); conversely, detection rates for HPV 16 were similar, regardless of whether the cancers arose in screened or unscreened women.[70,71] Second, Woodworth et al[53] showed that grafts of human keratinocytes transfected with either HPV 16 or 18 were equally effective in establishing tumors within nude mice, provided that these cultures were incubated in vitro for at least 40 cell generations. In contrast, if transplanted at an earlier stage, only HPV 18 transfected grafts formed tumors. Third, Cullen et al[60] found integrated viral sequences in 96% (25 of 26) of HPV 18/45/56-associated carcinomas compared with only 72% (31 of 43) in HPV 16, 31, 33 and 35-containing tumors. This disparity suggests that different groups of HPV infections may have different biologic mechanisms of cellular transformation. Finally, detection of HPV 18 within invasive cancer is an adverse prognostic factor. Compared with HPV 16-containing tumors, the average age of HPV 18 cancers is 8–12 years younger and recurrence rates are higher (45 vs 16%).[70]

HPVs 31, 33, 35, 39, 51, 52 and 58

These recently cloned types are often classified together as the intermediate-risk group. From the clinical perspective, this intermediate group presents certain similarities. This group of HPV types tend to be overrepresented (25%) in CIN 2–3 but underrepresented (10%) in invasive cancer.[26] Second, these more recently isolated viruses are usually found in squamous carcinomas of the cervix rather than in cervical adenocarcinomas or in other lower tract squamous cancers. From the molecular perspective, most of these intermediate-risk viruses resemble HPV type 16.[72]

PRIMARY SCREENING APPLICATIONS OF HPV TESTING

Virus testing of the general population

From the global perspective, cervical cancer is the second most common human malignancy, with an incidence approximating 450 000 cases per year.[73] In Asia, South America, and Eastern Europe, deaths from cervical cancer (mostly women under the age of 40 years) exceed the mortality rate for any cancer affecting both sexes. In the West, four decades of cytologic screening have reduced incidence rates to sixth among female malignancies.[74] Nonetheless, cervical cancer remains a disease of prime importance. Enormous sums are spent in running mass screening programs and in the diagnosis and treatment of patients with abnormal cells found on cytologic testing. Despite hefty public health expenditure, this entirely preventable cancer has not yet been eradicated in any community.

The overwhelming majority of cervical cancers begin as an HPV induced deviation of the otherwise physiologic process of squamous metaplasia; hence, some have suggested screening the general population for the presence of an oncogenic virus. However, this strategy contains a fatal flaw. About 3–5% of sexually active, but nondiseased, women harbor a latent infection by an oncogenic HPV type. Nonquantitative testing for the presence of HPV DNA cannot differentiate latent infection from active expression. That is, detection of HPV DNA in latent cervical infection is analytically correct but clinically misleading. In the future, this problem of latent infection may be solvable by testing for evidence of viral expression, rather than for simple DNA colonization. For example, exon-specific mRNA production by the E4 and L1 genes would indicate potential infectivity, while excessive E6 and E7 mRNA in basal cells might prove a reliable guide to the risk of neoplastic change. Likewise, assays for virus-specified protein production would establish that transcription and translation had occurred.

Despite the past achievements of Papanicolaou (Pap) smear screening, the ultimate goal of eradicating cervical cancer cannot be achieved by cytology alone. Moreover, 40 years of screening appear to have changed the natural history of cervical cancer. Slow-growing, less aggressive cases tend to be detected, while rapid transit, more aggressive cases are apt to fall through the screening net.[75,76] Epidemiologic evidence of this phenomenon is discernible in many countries. In the USA, for example, averaging the age-adjusted mortality for all age groups shows that cervical cancer mortality has fallen by about 18% over the last decade.[76] However, the mortality rate in women under 45 years has remained stable[77] or even increased slightly. Aside from the hope of improved screening performance, there is some evidence that future cytology-based programs may have difficulty in even maintaining the status quo.

Across the board, about 60% of cervical cancers arise in patients who have never had a Pap smear, or who have allowed their screening to lapse. Conversely, the other 40% represent *interval* cancers which occurred despite reasonable (if not optimal) Pap smear compliance. A recent population based survey by the Rhode Island Department of Public Health[79] pinpointed some interesting age differences. Among 81 cervical cancers occurring in that state over the preceding 5 years, two-thirds of cancers in women aged 40–69 were attributable to screening default. However, in women aged 20–39 years, this stereotype did not apply. Of these younger women, two thirds of the cases represented interval cancers which occurred despite adequate attendance (Table 16.3).[79] Whether such screening failures arose because of false negative interpretation of previous Pap smears or because of rapidly progressive disease remained an open question. In

Table 16.3 Circumstances associated with the occurrence of invasive cancer in a population-based survey of Rhode Island women*

Papanicolaou smear history	Percent aged 20–39 years (*n* = 33)	Percent aged 40–69 years (*n* = 48)
Never had smear, or interval between smears > 3 years	15	65
False-negative or rapid transit	67	35
Neglected positive smears	18	0
Total	100	100

*Data derived from Centers for Disease Control. Cervical cancer control — Rhode Island. MMWR 1989; 38: 659–662.[79]

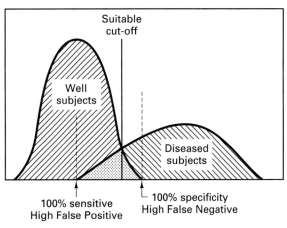

Fig. 16.5 Because the distribution of well and diseased individuals always overlaps, no single screening test can ever be perfect. Attempts to maximize sensitivity lead to loss of specificity and vice versa. Hence, actual cutoff points are a compromise. Reprinted with permission from: Reid R, Lorincz A. Should family physicians test for human papillomavirus infection? An affirmative view. J Family Prac 1991; 32: 183–192.[51]

a second study from the Victorian Cancer Registry in Australia,[80] which specifically looked at 138 cancers (out of 1044), arising in women who had one or more negative smears within the preceding 36 months, interval cancers were again common in younger women (21 vs 11%). Even more importantly, 38 of 223 (17%) with invasive adeno and adenosquamous cancers were diagnosed as interval cases, as compared to only 95 of 837 (11%) of squamous cancers.

In attempting to reappraise the Pap smear, it is essential to understand that screening tests can never be perfect — because the distributions of healthy and diseased individuals will always overlap (Fig. 16.5).[51] In practice, actual cut-off points are chosen to give the best compromise for the disease in question. Cut-off criteria for the Pap smear traditionally maximized specificity, for two principal reasons. First, in the days when diagnostic standards for the Pap smear were being framed, an abnormal report generally led to a somewhat injurious intervention (namely, cone biopsy). Second, since false positive results incur substantial fees, the cost–benefit ratio is tied to specificity not to sensitivity. Historically, imperfect sensitivity was compensated by the assumption that false negatives would be detected by repeat screening, before progression to invasive cancer could occur. In the 1990s, however, these assumptions are becoming increasingly hazardous, risking a calamitous illness for the patient and litigation for the physician.

After four decades of experience with exfoliative cytology, it seems doubtful that new advances can be secured by adaptations of the Pap smear alone. Rather, any further reduction of cervical cancer among screened women will probably depend on the incorporation of adjunctive measures. To test this hypothesis, we screened 1012 Michigan women from a sexually transmitted disease clinic using cytology, cervicography, and DNA hybridization.[81] Within this database, cytology alone detected only 12 (52%) of the 23 high-grade lesions, despite the expense of recalling 8.7% of the women. Any attempt to reduce triage expenses by recalling just patients with major cytologic lesions would have reduced sensitivity to just 35%. Similarly, attempting to bolster sensitivity by recalling all women with mildly dyskaryotic smears destroyed the specificity of the Pap smear. Recall rates would have risen to 16% of all women screened.

Cervicography and dot blot hybridization were also shown to be valid measures. Both were comparable to the Pap smear in overall accuracy; however, each test identified a different 60% of the high-grade disease present within these 1012 women (Fig. 16.6).[81] Thus, a simple combination of any two tests would have improved sensitivity. However, the flaw in this strategy is that any such simple combination provides two sets of false positive results, thereby eroding specificity. The key to incorporating multiple tests into a screening program is to differentiate between 'in parallel' and 'in series' strategies.

'In parallel' means applying all tests at the initial examination, and recalling any patient who had an abnormal result by an individual test (e.g., breast self-exam, physician breast exam and mammography for the detection of breast cancer). To safeguard against the economically disastrous effects of multiple false positives, the cut-point for each test within an 'in parallel' combination must be moved to the right (Fig. 16.5). Thus, in the example of the 1012 Michigan women, recalling only those with a high-grade positive from any of the three screening tests improved

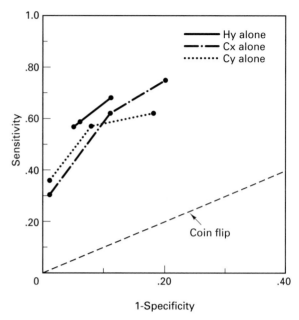

Fig. 16.6 Receiver operating characteristic curve comparing screening performance of cytologic testing, cervicography and hybridization, used alone. Reprinted with permission from Reid R, Greenberg M D, Lorincz A T et al. Should cervical cytologic testing be augmented by cervicography or human papillomavirus DNA detection? Am J Obstet Gynecol 1991; 164: 1461–1471.[81]

sensitivity (83 vs 52%) without increasing patient recall rates (7 vs 8.7%). However, a 1.7% reduction in patient recall would not be sufficient to pay for the extra costs of cervicography and virus testing.

'In series' means collecting a specimen at the initial visit, but only analyzing this sample if the primary screening result is not definitive. Hence, 'in series' tests do not contribute to sensitivity, but will protect specificity (e.g., FTA absorption antibody testing of a VDRL positive screen, before treating a patient for syphilis). Because so many low-grade histologic abnormalities reflect reparative/inflammatory atypia rather than oncogenic HPV infection, virus testing has great promise as an 'in series' test.

Primary screening of older women

Screening by cytology alone in peri- and postmenopausal woman is problematic for several reasons. First, the relative proportion of positive smears representing invasive cancer (rather than preinvasive disease) increases some 17 times in 40-year-old women, as compared to 20-year-old women.[82] Second, cytologic false-negative rates rise with age, due to the recession of the transformation zone into the cervical canal. Third, false-positives also rise with age, due to the confounding effects of estrogen deficiency.[83] Finally, decreasing need for contraception or obstetric care versus increasing need for general medical consultation tends to shift attendance patterns from obstetricians and gynecologists to internists, where less emphasis is placed on cervical screening. Hence, the availability of a valid and cost-effective adjunctive test would be of considerable value in this age group.

Genital HPV infections represent sexually-acquired colonizations, most commonly acquired during the late teens through early 30s. No more than 10% of such colonizations progress to clinically expressed cervical disease.[84] In the short term, most women manifest persistent latent infections. For example, in a population based study of Dutch women, Meijer et al[85] demonstrated that HPV colonization rates decline over time. As women reached menopause, prevalence halved in high-risk gynecology clinics (20% vs 10%) and fell by two-thirds in low-risk annual screening clinics (14 vs 5%). Moreover, preliminary findings from this Dutch study showed that none of the HPV negative patients developed dysplasia within a 2 year follow-up period. By comparison, persistence of HPV of any oncogenic type was highly associated with the presence of dysplasia. Thus, the predictive value of a positive HPV DNA test is so much higher in older women, that even primary population screening may prove cost-effective.

Expanded screening model

With modern emphasis on health care costs, even firmly established doctrines, like cervical cancer prevention are under scrutiny. The policy of offering Papanicolaou smears once a year was based upon traditional wisdom, rather than scientific data. There have been increasing demands to reduce screening frequency, by lengthening the interval to 2, 3 or even 5 years.[86] However, given the high false negative rate of Pap smears and the increasing importance of rapidly progressive disease in younger women,[87] the medico-legal risks of 3 or 5 year cytologic screening is unacceptable. An expanded screening model, providing both increased sensitivity (patient safety) and increased specificity (cost-savings), would provide a solution to this mounting dilemma.

Within our screening model of 1012 women,[81] optimal results were obtained by using cytology and cervicography 'in parallel' and virus testing 'in series.' Recall was therefore restricted to: (i) those women who had a high-grade morphologic abnormality on either cytology or cervicography, and (ii) patients with minor-grade aberrations in whom an oncogenic HPV type was detected. This strategy detected 96% of the high-grade lesions at the cost of recalling only 4% of the population (Fig. 16.7).[81] The reduction in recall for colposcopic triage and empiric therapy (88 vs 40 women) produced savings which more than offset the costs of the expanded screening profile.

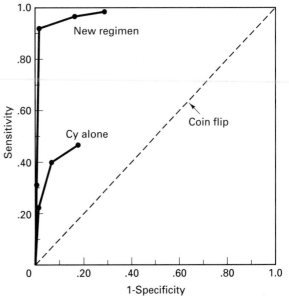

Fig. 16.7 Receiver operating characteristic curve showing the extreme sensitivity and specificity attainable with a three test regimen using one adjunctive test in parallel and the other in series. Reprinted with permission from Reid R, Greenberg M D, Lorincz A T et al. Should cervical cytologic testing be augmented by cervicography or human papillomavirus DNA detection? Am J Obstet Gynecol 1991; 164: 1461–1471.[81]

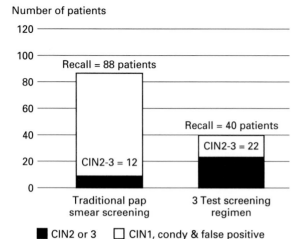

Number of patients

Fig. 16.8 Relative efficiencies of three-test regimen (40 recalls, detecting 22 cases of CIN 2–3) versus the traditional Papanicolaou smear regimen (88 recalls, detecting 12 cases of CIN 2–3). Reprinted with permission from Reid R, Greenberg M D, Lorincz A T et al. Should cervical cytologic testing be augmented by cervicography or human papillomavirus DNA detection? Am J Obstet Gynecol 1991; 164: 1461–1471.[81]

Moreover, since the three-test regimen detected 22 cases (vs 12 for cytology alone), the actual cost per case was 40% cheaper in the three-test model (Fig. 16.8).[81]

HPV TESTING AS A SECONDARY SCREEN

The Pap smear has been the greatest cancer screening device in the history of medicine. Nonetheless, cervical cytology is hampered by an inherent lack of sensitivity. Attempts to compensate by moving the cut-point to the left has increased sensitivity, but at the unacceptable cost of recalling too many women with equivocal changes. Likewise, although women with vulvar condylomas and women whose partners have penile condylomas manifest higher rates of cervical neoplasia, recalling patients solely on this basis produces more false positives than true positives. Hence, an effective 'in series' test could be used as a 'gatekeeper' to maximize the cost-effectiveness of colposcopic referral.

As explained above, primary screening for the presence of an oncogenic HPV DNA is counterproductive, principally because the prevalence of

Table 16.4 The predicted performance of a 90% sensitive, 95% specific viral test, used for primary screening of a general population with a 2% incidence of definite cervical disease and a 5% latency rate

| Virus testing | Cervical | Neoplasia | Total |
	Present	Absent	
Positive	18	96*	114
Negative	2	884	886
Total	20	980	1000

*95 = 49 latent infections (5% of 980) + 47 analytic false positives (5% of 931). Positive predictive value = 15.8%. Negative predictive value = 99.8%.

significant cervical disease within the general population is too low. However, in subsets of women known to be at higher risk, the same virus test can yield dramatic benefits. Consider a virus test with an analytic sensitivity of 90% and an analytic specificity of 95% (performance targets that are easily surpassed by modern techniques). Used as a primary screening tool in a general population containing 5% latent HPV infection and 2% occult cervical neoplasia, this test would have a positive predictive value of 14% (Table 16.4). That is, six out of every seven women with a positive virus test would represent false positives. However, using the same test as a secondary screening test in a subset with a 30% rate of occult cervical disease would raise the positive predictive value to 79% (Table 16.5). Even more important, the negative predictive value would exceed 98%, thereby providing an effective 'exit door' from what is otherwise a carousel of therapeutic excess. This concept is

Table 16.5 The predicted performance of a 90% sensitive, 95% specific viral test, used for secondary screening of patients with LGSIL/ASCUS Paps, of whom about 30% would be expected to have definite cervical disease: the latency rate would probably parallel the general population, at about 5%

| Virus testing | Cervical | Neoplasia | Total |
	Present	Absent	
Positive	270	68*	1338
Negative	30	632	662
Total	300	700	1000

*68 = 35 latent infections (5% of 700) + 33 analytic false positives (5% of 665). Positive predictive value = 79.9%. Negative predictive value = 95.5%.

supported by observed evidence, obtained under several different clinical circumstances.

Reducing recall rates of traditional colposcopic protocols

Colposcopic referral at the University of California, Santa Barbara Student Health Clinic included: (i) clinical evidence of HPV disease anywhere in the lower genital tract, (ii) a male partner with genital warts, (iii) patients previously treated for cervical dysplasia, and (iv) any suggestion of epithelial atypia on a current Pap smear. Each of these indications is a valid index of cervical disease; however, since each of the positive predictive values is < 50%, recalling women on these grounds is wasteful and intrusive. A group of 482 such referrals were therefore studied by repeat cytology, colposcopy, Virapap and (if indicated) cervical biopsy.[88] Not referring those with a negative repeat smear and a negative Virapap would have reduced colposcopic referrals by almost half (262 vs 482) at a cost of missing only 11 of 127 low-grade squamous intraepithelial

lesions (LGSILs) and 1 of 10 high-grade SILs (HGSILs) (Fig. 16.9). Even greater reductions would have occurred (178 vs 482), if repeat smears showing an ASCUS (atypical squamous cells of uncertain significance) pattern (in Virapap negative women) had also been followed by cytology alone. Major reductions in colposcopy costs would more than pay for the Virapap testing, yielding net savings of US$29 420 with 'Plan A' or US$57 820 with 'Plan B.'

Secondary screening of LGSIL cytology

Deciding to follow low-grade smears, based solely on cytologic assessment, is a hazardous practice. Cytology is fundamentally a screening test, designed to be reported as 'positive,' 'negative,' or (occasionally) as 'equivocal.' Attempts to subdivide positive smears into higher versus lower grades of abnormality are valid, but carry an inherent reduction in screening accuracy. In a series of 650 women seen with low grade cytologic abnormalities reported by Montz et al,[89] colposcopically directed biopsy detected a high

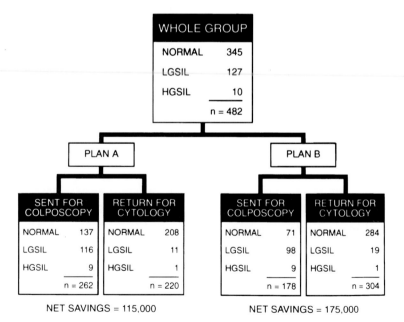

Fig. 16.9 Potential cost savings from using Virapap as a secondary screening test. 'Plan A' represents the most conservative approach, wherein patients were referred for colposcopy for (i) a positive Virapap, (ii) a repeat Pap smear showing SIL or (iii) a repeat Pap smear showing ASCUS changes. 'Plan B' is an even more cost-effective option, because repeat smears showing ASCUS changes were followed by cytology rather than going for colposcopic evaluation.

grade lesion in 18% of cases. Indeed, one patient in this group had an invasive cancer. Thus, under traditional triage rules, physicians who advocate follow-up of LGSIL are obliged to perform an initial colposcopy, in order to rule out the possibility of an occult high-grade lesion. In short, an LGSIL Pap must first be seen as a positive screening test, not a confirmed diagnosis.

A major problem associated with cervical cytologic screening has been the overzealous approach to women with minor grade lesions.[90] Each year approximately 2.3 million US women have a minor grade cervical lesion. It has been estimated that the cost of colposcopic evaluation and ablative therapy (currently considered the 'standard of care'), probably exceeds US$5 billion annually. Because more than 90% of high-grade lesions contain readily detectable levels of oncogenic HPV DNA (versus less than 5% in normal women), virus testing should prove to be a safe and reliable method for selecting which low-grade smears truly warrant colposcopic evaluation. Conversely, a negative HPV test in this population offers strong assurance as to the absence of an occult HGSIL. Hence, such women can be safely returned to cytological surveillance.

Measuring quantitative levels of any HPV DNA within patient samples may further increase predictive value of HPV testing as a detection tool for high-grade CIN.[78,88,89] For example, Cuzick et al[44] found that high levels of HPV 16 (measured by quantitative PCR) predicted the presence of CIN 2–3 with a 93% specificity. Conversely, low levels of HPV DNA were associated with high-grade dysplasias.

Secondary screening of ASCUS cytology

Hyperchromatism and nuclear enlargement produced by reparative or inflammatory changes are easily confused with the cytologic features of bona fide low-grade cervical intraepithelial neoplasia. This mimickery has been a thorny issue for cytologists. There is no clear-cut point between ASCUS and LGSIL. A group of 200 class II Pap smears, cytopathologists, produced from a community laboratory in Portland and then reread by three expert cytopathologists, generated 50 combinations of diagnoses.[91] All three experts

agreed in only 21 instances. For the purpose of data analysis, a consensus was generated by having the pathologists vote upon whether the smear was or was not likely to be SIL. A strong positive correlation was found between the consensus cytology opinion and the frequency with which oncogenic HPV DNA was found. Basically, these results were classical for the presence of an attenuated classification between the two variables. That is, there is both *diagnostic misclassification* (reflecting the fact that morphologic features span a continuum, without a clear cut-point), and *HPV testing misclassification* (reflecting incomplete probe panels, variable expression and sampling error). Significantly, virus testing was a more accurate predictor of occult disease than any of the expert cytopathologists.

Traditionally, only Pap smears showing unequivocal dysplasia were referred for colposcopic triage. Squamous atypia of uncertain significance were classified as a 'Class II Pap' and such patients were followed by repeat cytology. Since the introduction of the Bethesda system, the proportion of routine Papanicolaou smears flagged for colposcopy has essentially doubled, from 5% to about 10–12% now (Fig. 16.10). Of the 55 million smears done each year in the United States, at least 3 million are designated as ASCUS. In today's litigious society, these ambiguous reports often trigger colposcopic examination, perhaps followed by empiric destruction or loop electrosurgical excision procedure (LEEP) excision of

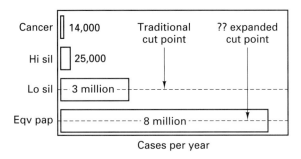

Fig. 16.10 Recent trends have lowered the 'cut-point', from 'definite CIN 1 versus condyloma,' down to 'ASCUS versus nonspecific reactive change.' Because prevalence rates have a pronounced pyramidal shape, the effect of this liberalization has been to overwhelm colposcopy clinics, for the sake of a small increase in detection rates for cancer or HGSIL.

the transformation zone. At an estimated minimum cost of US$1000–2000 per patient, these intrusive and unjustified interventions cost the national health care system another US$4 billion annually.[90]

Prior to the mid-1980s, no one was particularly alarmed by a 'Class II' report. However, about 5 years ago, public confidence was eroded by a series of articles in the lay press widely publicizing false-negative pap smears. Physician concern was further heightened by studies suggesting that colposcopic evaluation of even a single atypical Pap would detect a definite SIL in 15–25% of patients.[92–94] Mounting medicolegal pressure, the steadily rising incidence of genital HPV infection[84] and the effects of the newly introduced Bethesda system[95–97] have combined to create a health crisis. Because clinicians have become uneasy about managing squamous atypia by cytological triage, the nation's colposcopic services are overloaded to near breaking point.

From the theoretic perspective, the Bethesda system was correct in classifying ASCUS as a potential epithelial abnormality. However, from the practical perspective, the yield from colposcopic triage is too low to justify the physical, emotional and financial costs involved. Hence, the net effect of abolishing the old Pap Class 2 has been to remove a valuable buffer against overutilization of colposcopic triage and empiric transformation zone ablation.

ASCUS smears represent a heterogenous mixture of many entities, including non-specific reactive or inflammatory change, subtle cervical HPV infections and non-representative smears from a few well-developed precursor lesions. In a case control study of 2621 women subjected to viral testing, 270 ASCUS smears were associated with exfoliation of an oncogenic HPV type,[26] suggesting that virus testing could serve as a secondary screening test. The availability of a nonintrusive method for recognizing the small fraction of occult HGSILs and subtle oncogenic HPV infections would make the decision to follow the majority of ASCUS smears by repeat cytology a great deal safer. Although the original Virapap panel (HPVs 6, 11, 16, 18, 31, 33 and 35) was 78% effective, the availability of an expanded panel containing probes for seven additional genital HPVs (types 42, 43, 44, 45, 51, 52 and 56) increased the epidemiologic sensitivity to 91%.

In another study of 217 college students with minor screening abnormalities, referral of the entire group for colposcopy would have yielded a false positive rate of 76% (Fig. 16.11). Financially, this traditional protocol was also somewhat expensive, costing about US$1611.00 per SIL detected.[98] Conversely, using hybrid capture (a signal amplified, semiquantitative, liquid hybridization kit containing the 14 HPV probes) as a secondary screen would have reduced colposcopic referrals by 58% (91 vs 217). The sensitivity of this regimen was 87%, and cost per SIL detected fell to US$1051.00. Most importantly, 14 of 15

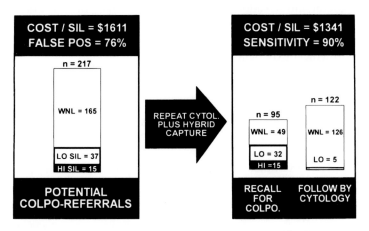

Fig. 16.11 Potential cost savings from using hybrid capture as a secondary screen.

high-grade lesions were detected by the hybrid capture kit; the single missed high grade lesion contained HPV 39 and 58, and would have been detected within further expansion of the above panel. Test specificity might be further improved by quantitation for example, restricting colposcopic referral to only those with hybrid capture levels above 5.0 would have decreased the number of colposcopic examinations by another 28%, without reducing detection rates for CIN 2–3. In contrast, repeating the cytology was of little benefit. Once licensed for general use, hybrid capture will provide a practical solution to the dilemma of either colposcoping large numbers of false positives (by recalling everyone) or eroding sensitivity by attempting triage with cytology alone.

POTENTIAL DIAGNOSTIC USES OF HPV TESTING

Once a health problem has been identified, the use of HPV testing is noncontentious, since it conforms to the basic philosophy of clarifying the nature and prognosis of any underlying disease.[99] Of course, many problems still remain. Optimal methods of cell sampling, intermittent patterns of exfoliation, and potential interaction with other clinical events still need clarification. Such difficulties, however, are simply obstacles to overcome, not reasons to abandon HPV testing. Of course, it would be desirable if any decision to apply routine testing was first evaluated in clinical trials rather than by sporadic introduction of the test. However, if such trials are not forthcoming, utilization patterns will have to be built up through judgement and accrued medical experience.

Management of equivocal histology

For the cytologist and the clinician, low grade SIL and ASCUS Paps fall at the bottom of the morphologic spectrum. Hence, there is often little to see by either method. For example, approximately 30% of patients who have colposcopic biopsy for a low grade smear will have negative or equivocal histology.[89] The question of whether to continue with triage and/or empiric treatment versus suspending the work-up and returning

the patient to cytologic follow-up is often a vexing one. In women who have been misdiagnosed as having 'HPV infection' on the grounds of low grade cytological atypia in a Pap smear, objective testing can save considerable psychological, physical and monetary costs. The combination of an essentially normal colposcopic examination and a negative virus test confers a negative predictive value greater than 98%. Virus testing obviates any clinical concern as to the presence of a significant cytocolphistologic discrepancy. Such women do not need to be considered for diagnostic conization. Rather, women with a negative HPV DNA test can be safely returned to cytologic follow-up.

Conversely, a positive HPV test will identify a subset of women in whom there is either an occult SIL missed at initial colposcopy, or an emerging lesion which will manifest within the succeeding year. In Nuovo's[100] series of 59 women with equivocal biopsies, a definite lesion elsewhere within the transformation zone was found in 71% of those with a positive HPV test versus only 20% of those with a negative HPV test. In a more recent study of women with unexplained abnormal cytology, Nuovo[101] reported that 55% of those with a positive Virapap developed definite SIL within 1 year, compared to only 11% of those with a negative Virapap.

Management of low-grade cervical disease

High-grade lesions represent an homogenous population of aneuploid lesions, most of which are induced by the same oncogenic HPVs as found in cancer (Fig. 16.12).[20] Since these lesions can

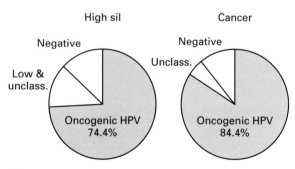

Fig. 16.12 Prevalence rates of oncogenic HPVs (solid) in high-grade SIL and cancer (data reflect results reported in Ref. 20).

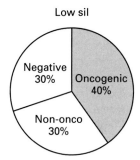

Low sil

Fig. 16.13 Prevalence rates for oncogenic HPVs (solid), nononcogenic HPVs (stippled) or HPV-negativity (according to diagnostic category) (data reflect results reported in Ref. 26).

be reliably recognized through the light microscope, virus testing has little to add. Conversely, LGSIL biopsies and ASCUS Pap smears comprise a hererogenous mixture of many different conditions, rather than a single pathologic entity (Fig. 16.13).[26] In essence, the histologic features represent a nonspecific tissue response to recent injury, be that infection by an oncogenic HPV virus or repair of a nonspecific injury. A multitude of natural history studies[102–116] have shown high rates of spontaneous regression — with a median of 48% if an initial biopsy is done and 33% if the low-grade lesion is simply diagnosed by cytology and colposcopy (Table 16.6).[28,102–116] Unfortunately, approximately 15% will progress to HGSIL, and at least 1% will eventually transform into cancer cells.[117,118] Indeed, several of these natural history studies[102,103,116,119] have been marred by progression to invasion (Table 16.7).[102,104,116,119] The policy of simply following LGSIL by repeat cytology carries a definite risk. Attempting to follow patients by cytology plus colposcopy is

safer, but impractical. The number of additional visits will overwhelm any large colposcopic service. Hence, traditional wisdom favored more pragmatic options. Namely, patients found to have definite minor grade lesions were managed by empiric destruction of the transformation zone, using relatively cost-effective office therapies. In reality, neither of these options is satisfactory. Long term cytologic follow-up of LGSIL represents systematic undertreatment and empiric destruction of all LGSIL's is systemic overtreatment.

The traditional policy of empiric transformation zone destruction has become particularly unrealistic

Table 16.6 Effect of biopsy upon natural history of CIN 1 lesions

Cytologic follow-up	Regression (%)	Progression (%)
Fox et al[102]	31	60
Hulka et al[103]	NS	36
Richart & Barron[104]	6	41
Svirannaboon et al[105]	33	30
Rummell et al[106]	40	17
McGregor & Lupen[107]	60	13
Campion et al[28]	11	26
Median	33	30

Biopsy confirmation	Regression (%)	Progression (%)
Peckham & Greene[108]	40	11
Rawson & Kroblich[109]	83	17
Figge et al[110]	26	9
Stern & Neely[111]	37	7
Hall & Walter[112]	45	17
Johnson et al[113]	50	6
Berget[114]	49	43
Nasiell et al[115]	60	11
Evans & Monaghan[116]	50	12
Reid (unpublished)	46	9
Median	48	12

Table 16.7 Natural history studies in which invasive cancer occurred during observation

Author(s)	Year(s)	Number of patients	Initial diagnosis	Regression rate (%)	Persistence rate (%)	Progression rate (%)	Invasive cancers
Richart & Barron[104]	1960–1966	557	Class III Pap smear*	6	53	20	3
Koss et al[117]	1963	93	CIN 3 (67) and CIN 1 (26)	29	60	11	10
Fox et al[102]	1967	278	Mild to moderate dysplasia	31	9	60	3**
Evans & Monaghan[116]	1981	50	Cervical warty atypia	50	38	12	1†

*Enrollees did not have initial histological studies (cytology only).
**Two microinvasive cancers and one invasive cancer.
†Microinvasive cancer.

since the introduction of the Bethesda system. Prior to the mid-1980s, LGSIL smears were subgrouped into 'flat condyloma' vs 'mild dysplasia.' Since 'flat condyloma' was often managed by repeat cytology, this artificial subdivision served to limit the number of colposcopic referrals. However, several studies have shown that attempts at cytologic[118] or histologic[120] distinctions between 'flat condyloma' and 'mild dysplasia' are not reproducible. Moreover, in applying Miesel's criteria[121,122] to a group of specimens of known HPV type, we found that many of the oncogenic HPV infections fell into the flat condyloma group.[123] Who would dispute that an HPV 18 containing flat condyloma represents a greater threat than an HPV 6/11 containing CIN 1 (Fig. 16.14)?[124]

Whereas pathologists cannot differentiate one cause of hyperchromatism from another, virus testing does not work under the same limitation.

Ample research has demonstrated that greater than 95% of HGSIL and cancers will contain an oncogenic HPV DNA, whereas very few non-specific inflammatory/reparative changes will be colonized by such viruses. On theoretic grounds, transformation zone destruction for LGSILs induced by an oncogenic HPV type would represent specifically indicated (rather than empiric) treatment.[28–30] This tenet certainly held true in a 4 year natural history study of 153 Michigan women, just completed by our group (Table 16.8) (Reid R, unpublished data).

QUALITY CONTROL

The clinician/pathology team can also look at their own correlations. The expected rate of an oncogenic HPV within each diagnostic compartment is now well defined. Second, because the ASCUS Pap smear category defines a transition

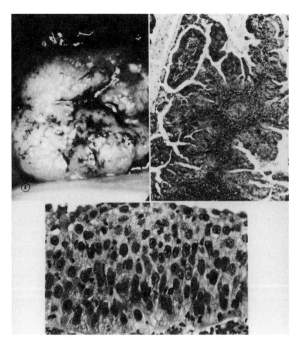

Fig. 16.14 An HPV 18 associated poorly differentiated adenosquamous carcinoma of the cervix diagnosed within 9 months of a negative smear. **A** Unmagnified photograph of cervix. **B** Photomicrograph showing adenocarcinomatous element. (H&E — Original magnification × 33). **C** Photomicrograph of squamous element. (H&E — Original magnification × 132). Despite having negative regional lymph nodes at subsequent hysterectomy, this 23-year-old nulliparous woman died of disseminated cancer within 16 months of diagnosis. Reprinted with permission from: Reid R, Greenberg M D, Jenson A B et al. Sexually transmitted papillomaviral infections I. The anatomic distribution and pathologic grade of neoplastic lesions associated with different viral types. Am J Obstet Gynecol 1987; 156: 212–222.[124]

Table 16.8   Association of HPV type with risk of progression or likelihood of regression in 153 women with LGSIL/ASCUS smears who were followed over 4 years

Virus testing	Disease outcome			
	Progressed to CIN 3	Persisted unchanged	Regressed spontaneously	Total
HPVs 16, 18 30s and 50s	11 (16.9%)	23 (35.4%)	31 (47.7%)	65
Unspecified HPV and virus negative	3 (4.1%)	40 (54.8%)	30 (41.1%)	73
HPV 6/11	0	6 (40%)	9 (60%)	15
Total	14	69	70	153

between very low levels of HPV DNA in normal women (e.g., less than 5%) and the very high level in the overtly diseased patients (e.g., 85%), one should expect some kind of intermediate level of positivity (e.g., 25%) in this group. Hence, if the HGSIL and LGSIL *diagnoses* by a particular pathologist show HPV DNA detection rates that are substantially below the accepted average, these categories must have been diluted by the upward migration of borderline or negative cases. Likewise, if the correlative study shows very low HPV positivity rates for the ASCUS category, it is clear that this buffer category is being diluted by the upward migration of too many reactive and inflammatory atypias.

In our ASCUS study, the chance occurrence of a change in the cytology laboratory exactly mid-way into the study confirmed this hypothesis. This change produced an approximate doubling in the rate of ASCUS (5.3% from Lab A vs 10% from Lab B). Consequently, the ASCUS category from Lab B showed a halving of the HPV DNA positivity rate (60–29.8%), a halving of the proportion found to have any grade of CIN (41–21.7%) and a greater than two-thirds reduction in the proportion of CIN 2–3 (12.5–3.7%).[98] When presented with these data Lab A identified some degree of cytologic undercall of HGSIL whereas Lab B clearly recognized substantial overcall of normal cytology.

The new generation of HPV tests

Recent studies have begun to delineate the proper role of HPV testing in the clinical management of patients. Obviously, indiscriminate use of HPV testing could further overwhelm both diagnostic and treatment services, thereby compounding ex-

isting problems with cervical screening. However, data from newer more accurate HPV tests within specific clinical settings have helped to reverse some of the misconceptions that arose through misleading, premature endorsement of prototypic HPV tests. The disciplined and systematic integration of this technology into clinical practice should deliver both improved screening efficiency and significant cost savings.

HPV testing will not become widespread until the available tests are able to detect a broad spectrum of HPV types quickly reliably and cheaply. Both consensus primer PCR (Roche Medical Systems, Branchberg, NJ) and Hybrid Capture (Digene Diagnostics, Silver Spring, MD) appear to fulfill these requirements and are likely to become available for general clinical use within the next 2–3 years.

Consensus primer PCR

PCR is a robust test, which can be used to analyze both fresh samples and formalin fixed tissues. Attempting to adapt the polymerase chain reaction for detection of HPV DNA within clinical samples has been impeded by two major drawbacks. First, the epidemiologic specificity of PCR is less than that of Southern blot hybridization, because of either (i) false-positive amplification of minuscule amounts of contaminating HPV DNA, or (ii) the over detection of very low viral copy number within latent or resolved HPV infections. Second, epidemiologic sensitivity can also be suboptimal, because of the presence of reaction inhibitors within certain clinical specimens.

There are several systems for detecting HPV DNA by polymerase chain reaction. Some systems use specific primers that detect a single HPV type. Hence, evaluation of a given clinical sample requires that this test be repeated with a panel of such probes. Alternatively, consensus primers can be used to detect many different HPV types within a single reaction. The most popular consensus primers are the MY09 MY11 primers and the GP primers, both amplifying a slightly different region of the L1 reading frame.[41] In contrast to type specific PCR, consensus primer PCR is unable to amplify all types equally. Consequently, certain HPV types (e.g., HPV 51) may not be detected in specimens infected by other HPVs. A second drawback of this variability in target amplification rate is that it is very difficult to quantify the amount of target HPV DNA originally present within the specimen.

Hybrid capture

Hybrid capture is a simple, nonradioactive solution hybridization test which is similar in principles to an immunoassay.[98] The target molecule is single stranded DNA which hybridize to RNA probes. These are dimers which are then captured on a plastic tube by immobilized antibodies specific for RNA–DNA hybrids. After washing the unreacted single stranded RNA and other nonspecifically bound material from the tubes, the remaining bound hybrids are reacted with an alkaline phosphatase RNA–DNA antibody. Chemoluminescent substrate is then cleaved by the alkaline phosphate to emit light that is directly proportional to the quantity of hybrid that is captured. Up to 16 different HPV types may be detected in a single reaction, with the same analytic sensitivity as for the detection of a single HPV type. Epidemiologic sensitivity and specificity are superior to Southern blot hybridization. In multicenter trials, reproducibility and precision of results was 95% or greater.[46] With adequate training of assay personnel the potential disadvantage of false-positive results can be eliminated.

REFERENCES

1. Durst M, Gissman L, Ikenburg H, zur Hausen H. A papillomavirus DNA from a cervical carcinoma and its prevalence in cancer biopsy samples from different geographic regions. Proc Nat Acad Sci USA 1983; 80: 3812–3815.
2. Boshart M, Gissman L, Ikenburg H et al. A new type of papillomavirus DNA, its presence in genital cancer biopsies and in cell lines derived from cervical cancer. EMBO J 1984; 3: 1151–1157.
3. Kitchener H. Commentary: Does HPV cause cervical cancer? Br J Obstet Gynaecol 1988; 95: 1089–1091.
4. Gissman L, Wolnik L, Ikenberg H et al. Human papillomavirus types 6 and 11 DNA sequences in genital and laryngeal papillomas and in some cervical cancers. Proc Nat Acad Sci USA 1983; 80: 560.
5. Reid R, Stanhope C R, Herschman B R et al. Genital warts and cervical cancer. I. Evidence of an association between subclinical papillomavirus infection and cervical malignancy. Cancer 1982; 50: 377–387.
6. Zur Hausen H. Viruses in human cancers. Science 1991; 254: 1167–1173.
7. Marx J L. How DNA viruses may cause cancer. Science 1989; 243: 1012–1013.
8. Sutton G P, Stehman F B, Ehrlich C E, Roman A. Human papillomavirus DNA in lesions of the female genital tract: Evidence for type 6/11 in squamous cell carcinoma of the vulva. Obstet Gynecol 1985; 70: 564–568.
9. Reeves W C, Brinton L A, Garcia M et al. Human papillomavirus infection and cervical cancer in Latin America. New Engl J Med 1989; 320: 1437–1441.
10. Tidy J A, Parry G C N, Ward P et al. High rate of human papillomavirus type 16 infection in cytologically normal cervices. Lancet 1989; 1: 434.
11. Young L S, Bevan I S, Johnson M A et al. Polymerase chain reaction: A new epidemiological tool investigating human papillomavirus infection. Br Med J 1989; 298: 14–18.
12. Reid R. Treatment of HPV-associated disease. Papillomavirus report. Leeds: Leeds University Press, 1991: 133–140.
13. Schiffman M H. Validation of HPV hybridization assays: Correlation of FISH, dot blot, and PCR with Southern blot. In: Munoz et al, eds. The epidemiology of human papillomavirus and human cancer. Lyon: IARC monograph, 1992: pp 169–179.
14. Southern E M. Detection of specific sequences among DNA fragments separated by gel electrophoresis. J Molec Biol 1975; 98: 503–517.
15. Schiffman M H, Bauer H M, Lorincz A T et al. Comparison of Southern blot hybridization and polymerase chain reaction methods for detection of human papillomavirus DNA. J Clin Microbiol 1988; 29: 573–577.
16. Wagner D, Ikenberg H, Boehm N. Identification of human papillomavirus in cervical smears by deoxyribonucleic acid in situ hybridization. Obstet Gynecol 1984; 64: 767.
17. Crowther M E, Shepherd J H, Fisher C. Verrucous carcinoma of the vulva containing human papillomavirus-11. Br J Obstet Gynaecol 1988; 95: 414–418.

18. Boshart M, zur Hausen H. Human papillomaviruses in Buschke–Lowenstein tumors: Physical state of the DNA and identification of a tandem duplication in the noncoding region of a human papillomavirus type 6 subtype. J Virol 1986; 58: 963–966.

19. de Villiers E M, Wagner D, Schneider A et al. Human papillomavirus DNA in women without and with cytological abnormalities. Results of a 5 year follow-up study. Gynecol Oncol 1992; 44: 33–39.

20. Chapman W B, Lorincz A, Willett G D, Wright V C, Kurman R J. Evaluation of two commercially available in situ hybridization kits for detection of human papillomavirus DNA in cervical biopsies: Comparison to Southern blot hybridization. Modern Pathol 1993; 6: 73–79.

21. Syrjanen K, Vayrynen M, Saarikoski S et al. Natural history of cervical human papillomavirus (HPV) infections based on prospective follow-up. Br J Obstet Gynaecol 1985; 92: 1086–1092.

22. Syrjanen K, Mantyjarvi R, Saarikoski S et al. Factors associated with progression of cervical human papillomavirus infections into carcinoma in situ during long term prospective follow-up. Br J Obstet Gynaecol 1988; 95: 1096–1102.

23. Becker T M, Wheeler C M, Gouch N M et al. Cervical papillomavirus infection and cervical dysplasia in Hispanic, Native American and Non-Hispanic white women in New Mexico. Am J Publ Health 1992; 81: 582–586.

24. Morrison E A, Ho G F, Vermund S H et al. Human papillomavirus infection and other risk factors for cervical neoplasia. A case control study. Int J Cancer 1991; 49: 6–13.

25. Munoz N, Bosch F X. International agency for research on cancer. The epidemiology of cervical cancer and HPV. Lyon: IARC, 1992: pp 271–281.

26. Lorincz A T, Reid R, Jenson A B et al. Human papillomavirus infection of the cervix: Relative risk associations of 15 common anogenital types. Obstet Gynecol 1992; 79: 328–337.

27. Cuzick J, Terry G, Ho L, Hollingworth T, Anderson M. Human papillomavirus type 16 DNA in cervical smears as predictor of high grade cervical intraepithelial neoplasia. Lancet 1992; 339: 959–960.

28. Campion M J, McCanee D J, Cuznik J, Singer A. Progressive potential of mild cervical atypia: Prospective cytologic and virologic study. Lancet 1986; 2: 237–240.

29. Koutsky L A, Holmes K K, Critchlow C W et al. A cohort study of the risk of cervical intraepithelial neoplasia grade 2 or 3 in relation to papillomavirus infection. New Engl J Med 1992; 327: 1272–1278.

30. Weaver M G, Abdul-Karim F W, Dale G, Sorensen K, Huang Y T. Outcome in mild and moderate cervical dysplasias related to the presence of specific human papillomavirus types. Modern Pathol 1993; 3: 679–683.

31. Woodworth C D, Waggoner S, Barnes W et al. Human cervical and foreskin epithelial cells immortalized by humanpapillomavirus DNAs exhibit dysplastic differentiation in vivo. Cancer Res 1990; 50: 3709–3715.

32. Nahmias A J, Sawanabori S. The genital herpes-cervical cancer hypothesis: 10 years late. Prog Exper Tumor Res 1978; 21: 117–139.

33. Schacter J, Hill E C, King E B et al. Chlamydia trachomatis and cervical neoplasia. JAMA 1982; 248: 2134–2138.

34. Furgyik S, Astedt B. Gonorrheal infection followed by an increased frequency of cervical carcinoma. Acta Obstet Gynecol Scand 1980; 59: 521–524.

35. Manos M, Wright D K, Lewis A J et al. The use of polymerase chain reaction amplification for the detection of genital human papillomavirus. Cancer Cells 1989; 7: 209–214.

36. Tidy J A, Farrell P F. Retraction: Human papillomavirus subtype 16b. Lancet 1989; II: 1535.

37. Kaufman R H, Bornstein J, Gordon A N et al. Detection of human papillomavirus DNA in advanced epithelial ovarian carcinoma. Gynecol Oncol 1987; 27: 340–349.

38. Kirgan D, Manalo P, Hall M et al. Association of human papillomavirus and colon neoplasms. Arch Surg 1990; 125: 862–865.

39. McNichol P J, Dodd J G. High prevalence of human papillomavirus in prostatic tissues. J Urol 1991; 145: 850–853.

40. Bauer H M, Ting Y, Greer C E et al. Genital human papillomavirus infection in female university students as determined by a PCR-based method. JAMA 1991; 255: 472–477.

41. Tham K M, Chow V T K, Singh P et al. Diagnostic sensitivity of polymerase chain reaction and Southern blot hybridization for the detection of human papillomavirus DNA in biopsy specimens from cervical lesions. Am J Clin Pathol 1991; 95: 638–646.

42. Schiffman M H. Recent progress in defining the epidemiology of human papillomavirus infection and cervical neoplasia. J Nat Cancer Inst 1992; 84: 394.

43. Terry G, Ho L, Jenkins D et al. Definition of human papillomavirus type 16 DNA levels in low and high grade cervical lesions by simple PCR technique. Arch Virol 1993; 128: 123–133.

44. Cuzick J, Terry G, Ho L et al. Type specific HPV DNA in smears as a predictor of high grade CIN. 1993 (manuscript submitted).

45. Evander M, Edlund K, Boden E et al. Comparison of one step and two step polymerase chain reaction with degenerate general primers in a population based study of human papillomavirus in young Swedish women. J Clin Microbiol 1992; 130: 987–992.

46. Lorincz A T. Diagnosis of human papillomavirus infection by the new generation of molecular DNA assays. Clin Immunol News 1992; 12: 123–128.

47. Campion M J, Reid R. Screening for gynecologic cancer. Obstet Gynecol Clinics North Am 1990; 17: 695–727.

48. Goldsborough M D, McAllister P, Reid R, Temple G, Lorincz A T. A comparison study of human papillomavirus prevalence by the polymerase chain reaction in low risk women and in a gynecology referral group at increased risk for cervical cancer. Molec Cell Probes 1992; 6: 451–457.

49. Lorincz A T. Diagnosis of human papillomavirus by the new generation of molecular DNA assays. Clin Immunol News 1992; 8: 123–128.

50. Schiffman M H, Bauer H M, Hoover R N et al. Epidemiologic evidence showing that human

papillomavirus infection causes most cervical intraepithelial neoplasia. J Nat Cancer Inst 1993; 85(12): 958–964.

51. Reid R, Lorincz A T. Should family physicians test for human papillomavirus infection? An affirmative view. Am J Family Pract 1991; 32: 183–192.

52. McCance D J, Kopan R I, Fuchs E, Laimans L A. Human papillomavirus type 16 alters human epithelial cell differentiation in vitro. Proc Nat Acad Aci USA 1988; 85: 7169–7173.

53. Woodworth C D, Doniger J, DiPaolo J A. Immortalization of human foreskin keratinocytes by various human papillomavirus DNAs corresponds to their association with cervical carcinoma. J Virol 1989; 63: 159–164.

54. Ray A F, Peabody D S, Cooper J L, Cram L S, Kraemer P M. SV40 T antigen alone drives karyotype instability that precedes neoplastic transformation of human diploid fibroblasts. J Cell Biochem 1990; 42: 13–31.

55. Schramayr S, Caporossi D, Mak I, Jelinek T, Bacchetti S. Chromosomal damage induced by human adenovirus type 12 requires expression of the E1B 55-kilodalton viral protein. J Virol 1990; 64: 2090–2095.

56. Hurlin P J, Kauer P, Snit P P et al. Progression of human papillomavirus type 18 immortalized human keratinocytes to malignant phenotype. J Proc Nat Acad Science USA 1991; 88: 570–574.

57. Stoler M H, Rhodes C R, Whitbeck A, Chow L T, Broker T R. Gene expression of HPV types 16 and 18 in cervical neoplasia. UCLA Symp Mol Cell Biol New Ser 1990; 124: 1–11.

58. Werness B A, Levine A J, Howley P M. Association of human papillomavirus types 16 and 18 E6 proteins with p53. Science 1990; 248: 76–79.

59. Barbosa M S, Shlegel R. The E6 and E7 genes of HPV 18 are sufficient for inducing two stage in vitro transformation of human keratinocytes. Oncogene 1990; 43: 1529–1532.

60. Cullen A P, Reid R, Campion M J, Lorincz A T. An analysis of the physical state of different human papillomavirus DNAs in preinvasive and invasive cervical neoplasia. J Virol 1991; 65: 606–612.

61. Koutsky L A, Galloway D A, Holmes K K. Epidemiology of genital human papillomavirus infection. Epidemiol Rev 1988; 10: 122–163.

62. Bergeron C. Human papillomaviruses associated with cervical intraepithelial neoplasia. Great diversity and distinct distribution in low- and high-grade lesions. Am J Surg Pathol 1992; 16: 641–649.

63. Reid R. Human papillomaviral infection, the key to rational triage of cervical neoplasia. Obstet Gynecol Clin North Am 1987; 14: 407–429.

64. Slagel et al. Papillomavirus in human cancer. Sem Virol 1990; 1: 297–306.

65. Story A, Pim D, Murray A, Osborn K, Banks L, Crawford L. Comparison of the in vitro transforming activities of human papillomavirus types. EMBO J 1988; 7: 1815–1820.

66. Di Lorenzo T P, Tamsen A, Abramson A L, Steinerg B M. Human papillomavirus type 6a DNA in the lung carcinoma of a patient with recurrent laryngeal papillomatosis is characterized by a partial duplication. J Gen Virol 1992; 73: 423–428.

67. Olofsson J, Bjelkenkrantz K, Grontoft O. Malignant degeneration of a juvenile laryngeal papilloma. A follow-up study. J Otolaryngol 1980; 9: 329–333.

68. Farnsworth A, Laverty C R, Stoler M H. Human papillomavirus messenger RNA expression in adenocarcinoma in situ of the uterine cervix. Int J Gynecol Pathol 1989; 8: 321–330.

69. McCanee D F, Clarkson P K, Dyson M et al. Human papillomavirus types 6 and 16 in multifocal intraepithelial neoplasia of the lower genital tract. Br J Obstet Gynaecol 1985; 92: 1101–1105.

70. Walker J, Bloss J D, Liao S Y, Berman M, Bergen S, Wilczynski S P. Human papillomavirus genotype as a prognostic indicator in carcinoma of the uterine cervix. Obstet Gynecol 1989; 74: 781–785.

71. Barnes W, Delgado G, Kurman R J et al. Possible prognostic significance of human papillomavirus type in cervical cancer. Gynecol Oncol 1988; 29: 267–273.

72. Van Ranst M, Kaplan J B, Burk R D. Phylogenetic classification of human papillomaviruses: correlation with clinical manifestations. J Clin Virol 1992; 73: 2653–2660.

73. Parklin D M, Stjernswang J, Muir C S. Estimates of the worldwide frequency of twelve major cancers. Bull WHO 1984; 62: 163.

74. American Cancer Society. Cancer facts and figures — 1994.

75. Kurman R J, Schiffman M H, Lancaster W D et al. Analysis of individual human papillomavirus types in cervical neoplasia: A possible role for type HPV 18 in rapid progression. Am J Obstet Gynecol 1988; 159: 293–296.

76. Centers for Disease Control. Chronic disease reports: Mortality trends — United States 1979–86. MMWR 1989; 38: 189–191.

77. Winkelstein W, Selvin S. Cervical cancer in young Americans [letter]. Lancet 1989; 1: 1385.

79. Centers for Disease Control. Cervical cancer control — Rhode Island. MMWR 1989; 38: 659–662.

80. Mitchell H, Medley G, Giles G. Cervical cancers diagnosed after negative results on cervical cytology: Perspective in the 1980s. Br Med J 1990; 300: 1622–1626.

81. Reid R, Greenberg M D, Lorincz A T et al. Should cervical cytologic testing be augmented by cervicography or human papillomavirus DNA detection? Am J Obstet Gynecol 1991; 164: 1461–1471.

82. Shingleton H. The significance of age in the colposcopic evaluation of women with atypical papanicolaou smears. Obstet Gynecol 1977; 49(1): 61–64.

83. Kaminski P F, Sorosky J I, Wheelock J B, Stevens C W. The significance of atypical cervical cytology in an older population. J Obstet Gynecol 1989; 73: 13–15.

84. Reid R. Human papillomavirus-associated diseases of the lower genital tract: implications for the laser surgeon. In: Keye W, ed. Laser surgery in gynecology and obstetrics, 2nd edn. Chicago, IL: Yearbook Medical Publishers, 1990.

85. Meijer C J L M, Van den Brule A J C, Snijders P J F et al. Detection of human papillomavirus in cervical

scrapes by PCR in relation to cytology: Possible implications for cervical cancer screening. In: Munoz N, Bosch F X, Shah K V, Meheus A, eds. The epidemiology of cervical cancer and HPV. Lyon, France IARC, 1992: pp 271–281.

86. Eddy D M. Screening for cervical cancer. Ann Int Med 1990; 113: 214–226.

87. Berkley A S, LiVolsi V A, Schwartz P E. Advanced squamous cell carcinoma of the cervix with recent normal Papanicolaou tests. Lancet 1980; 2: 375.

88. Cox J T, Schiffman M H, Winzelburg A J, Patterson J M. An evaluation of human papillomavirus testing as part of referral to colposcopy clinics. Obstet Gynecol 1992; 80: 389–395.

89. Montz F. Natural history of the minimally abnormal Pap smear. Obstet Gynecol 1992; 80: 385–388.

90. Herbst A L. The Bethesda system for cervical/vaginal cytologic diagnoses. Clin Obstet Gynecol 1992; 35: 22–27.

91. Sherman M E, Schiffman M H, Lorincz A T, Manos M et al. Towards objective quality assurance of cervical cytopathology: Correlation of cytopathologic diagnosis with detection of high risk human papillomavirus types. Am J Clin Pathol 1994; 102: 182–187.

92. Jones D E D, Creaseman W T, Dombroski R A, Lentz S S, Waeltz J L. Evaluation of the atypical Pap smear. Am J Obstet Gynecol 1987; 157: 544–549.

93. Lindheim S R, Smith-Nguyen G. Aggressive evaluation for atypical squamous cells in Papanicolaou smears. J Reprod Med 1990; 35: 971–973.

94. Himmelstein L R. Evaluation of inflammatory atypia. A literature review. J Reprod Med 1989; 34(4): 634–637.

95. The 1988 Bethesda System for Reporting Cervical/ vaginal cytologic diagnoses. JAMA 1989; 26: 931–934.

96. Rapid communication — The Bethesda system for reporting cervical/vaginal cytologic diagnoses — Report of the 1991 Bethesda Workshop. JAMA 1992; 267: 1992.

97. The Bethesda system for reporting cervical and vaginal cytologic diagnoses. ACTA Cytol 1993; 37: 115–124.

98. Cox J T, Schiffman M H, Winzelberg A J, Patterson J M. An evaluation of human papillomavirus testing as part of referral to colposcopy clinics. Obstet Gynecol 1992; 80: 389–395.

99. Feinstein A R. Clinical epidemiology — The Architecture of clinical research. In: Diagnostic and spectral markers. Philadelphia: WB Saunders, 1985: pp 597–631.

100. Nuovo G J, Blanco J J, Leipzig S et at. Human papillomavirus detection in cervical lesions nondiagnostic for CIN: Correlation with Pap smear, colposcopy, and occurrence of CIN. Obstet Gynecol 1990; 75: 1006.

101. Nuovo G J, Moritz J, Walsh L L et al. Predictive value of human papillomavirus DNA detection by filter hybridization and polymerase chain reaction in women with negative results of colposcopic examination. Am J Clin Pathol 1992; 98: 489.

102. Fox C H. Biological behavior of cervical dysplasia and carcinoma-in-situ. Am J Obstet Gynecol 1967; 99: 96–974.

103. Hulka B S. Cytologic and histologic outcome following an atypical cervical smear. Obstet Gynecol 1968; 101: 190–199.

104. Richart R M, Barron B A. A follow-up study of patients with cervical neoplasia. Obstet Gynecol 1969; 105: 386–393.

105. Svirannaboon S, Bhamanapravati N. Prevalence and outcome of dysplasia of the cervix in self-selected population of Thailand. J Med Assoc Thai 1974; 57: 35.

106. Rummel H H, Fick R, Heberling D et al. Cytologic follow-up of patients with suspicious Pap type 3D smear. Geburtahr Franenheilh 1977; 37: 521–526.

107. McGregor J E, Lupen S. Uterine cervical cytology and young women. Lancet 1978; i: 1029–1031.

108. Peckham B, Greene R. Follow-up of cervical abnormalities. Am J Obstet Gynecol. 1957; 74: 804–815.

109. Rawson A J, Knoblich R. A clinicopathologic study of 56 cases showing mild epithelial changes of the cervix uteri. Am J Obstet Gynecol 1957; 73: 120–125.

110. Figge D P, deAlvarez R R, Brown D V, Fullington W R. Long range studies of the biologic behavior of the human uterine cervix. Am J Obstet Gynecol 1962; 83: 643–647.

111. Stern E, Neely P M. Dysplasia of the uterine cervix. Incidence of regression, recurrence and cancer. Cancer 1964; 17: 508–512.

112. Hall J E, Walton L. Dysplasia of the cervix. Am J Obstet Gynecol 1968; 100: 662–665.

113. Johnson L D, Nickerson R, Easterday C L, Stuart R S, Hertig A T. Epidemiologic evidence for the spectrum of change from dysplasia through carcinoma in situ to invasive cancer. Cancer 1968; 22: 901–914.

114. Berget A. Epithelial dysplasia of the cervix uteri. Dem Med Bull 1974; 21: 169–171.

115. Nasiell K, Nasiell M, Vaclavinkova V et al. Follow up studies of cytologically determined pre-cancerous lesion (dysplasia) of the uterine cervix. In: Bostrom H et al, eds. Health control in detection of cancer. Stockholm: Almquist and Wiksell, 1976: pp 244–252.

116. Evans A S, Monaghan J M. Spontaneous resolution of cervical warty dysplasia. The relevance of clinical and nuclear DNA features: A prospective study. Br J Obstet Gynecol 1985; 92: 165–169.

117. Oster A G. Natural history of cervical intraepithelial neoplasia; a critical review. Int J Gynecol Pathol 1993; 12: 186–192.

118. Fletcher A, Metaxas N, Grubb C, Chamberlain J. Four and a half year follow up of women with diskaryotic cervical smears. Br Med J 1990; 301: 641–644.

119. Koss L G, Stewart F W, Foote F W, Jordan M, Bader M, Day E. Some histological aspects of behavior of epidermoid carcinoma in-situ and related lesions of the uterine cervix. Cancer 1963; 16: 1160–1211.

120. Robertson A J, Anderson J M, Beck J S et al. Observer variability in the histopathological reporting of cervical biopsy specimens. J Clin Pathol 1989; 42: 231–238.

121. Meisels A, Fortin R. Condylomatous lesions of the cervix and vagina. I. Cytologic patterns. Acta Cytol 1976; 20: 505–509.

122. Miesels A, Fortin R. Condylomatous lesions of the cervix and vagina. II. Cytologic, colposcopic and histopathologic study. Acta Cytol 1977; 21: 379–390.

123. Willett G D, Kurman R J, Reid R, Greenberg M D, Jenson A B, Lorincz A T. Correlation of the histologic appearances of intraepithelial neoplasia of the cervix with human papillomavirus types: Emphasis on low grade lesions including so-called flat condyloma. Int J Gynecol Pathol 1989; 8: 18–25.

124. Reid R, Greenberg M D, Jenson A B et al. Sexually transmitted papillomaviral infections I. The anatomic distribution and pathologic grade of neoplastic lesions associated with different viral types. Am J Obstet Gynecol 1987; 156: 212–222.

17. CIN in pregnancy

Patrick G. Walker

INTRODUCTION

Pregnancy is a common physiological condition and cervical intraepithelial neoplasia (CIN) a common pathological condition affecting women in the third and fourth decades of life. It is not surprising therefore, that the two conditions should from time to time, occur simultaneously, giving rise to the need for a management protocol for the supervising physician. In the UK, approximately 700 000 deliveries take place per annum, approximately 4 million women each year are screened for CIN, but no prevalence data exist for the coincidence of the two conditions. In the USA, Hacker et al[1] have estimated that CIN 3 occurs in 0.13% of pregnancies, i.e., there is one case of CIN 3 diagnosed in each 770 pregnancies. The subject of this chapter is CIN in pregnancy and not invasive cancer, but to keep the matter in perspective, Hacker et al again report the incidence of invasive carcinoma of the cervix in the USA to be 0.045% or approximately one case for each 2205 pregnancies, pregnancy coexisting with carcinoma of the cervix in approximately one in 34 cases of invasive carcinoma.

THE IDENTIFICATION OF WOMEN WITH CIN IN PREGNANCY

Should we take a smear in pregnancy?

In countries where a National Screening Program exists, such as the 3-yearly call and recall program in the UK, opportunistic smears should only be taken in the antenatal clinic when the woman has not availed herself of her screening smear at the appropriate screening interval, or if she has symptoms of contact bleeding or discharge that could be referable to an invasive cervical lesion, or a suspicious appearance to the cervix at speculum examination. In countries where the screening program is recommended to have an interval of only 12 months smears will be taken more frequently in the antenatal clinic. Physicians in the UK are increasingly being encouraged to desist from the practice of taking opportunistic smears in the antenatal clinic unless such smears are symptom directed or the patient requires one as part of the National Screening Program.

It has been argued that cervical smears performed in pregnancy are of limited value. There is an argument that the smear taker, being anxious to avoid bleeding from the more vascular pregnant cervix holds back in the performance of a thorough smear. The examiner may be reluctant to ensure that the Aylesbury spatula or endocervical brush garners a representative sample of the endocervix in the pregnant patient. Some others argue that the predominance of the intermediate cell pattern makes interpretation of the smear by the cytologist difficult. However, a properly obtained sample reviewed by an efficient Department of Pathology should allow that screening smears performed in pregnancy are representative of the true state of the cervix, be it with disease or without. It is important to remind patients that they may have a slight pink stain or spotting after the performance of a cervical smear in early pregnancy, that there will be the usual departmental reporting delay before they receive their results, that they should ensure that they confirm the results of the smear at a future clinic visit, but perhaps most importantly of all, they should be encouraged in the belief that should the smear be reported other than normal, this does not mean that they have cancer of the cervix or that their pregnancy is in any way threatened. Appropriate, gentle advice at the time of the performance of the smear will reduce the unprecedented level of anxiety that can be generated both in the pregnant and nonpregnant patient when the result of a smear is other than normal.

ACTION TO BE TAKEN ON RECEIVING AN ABNORMAL SMEAR REPORT IN PREGNANCY

Should we refer for colposcopy?

In the UK, the National Co-ordinating Network supervising the National Health Service Cervical Screening Programme[2] has recommended the following action to be taken on receipt of an abnormal smear report in the nonpregnant patient:

a. Borderline atypia or mild dyskaryosis, repeat in 6 months and consider referral for colposcopy if the smear is not at that time normal. If the repeat smear is normal, a further negative smear report should be obtained after 6 months before the patient rejoins the screening program.
b. All patients with smears suggesting moderate or severe dyskaryosis should be referred for colposcopy.

There is no biological evidence to support changing these recommendations for the pregnant patient. There is no evidence that CIN is accelerated by pregnancy and although reports have suggested that steroid hormones, notably, glucocorticoids might have a promoter effect in the etiology of cervical cancer,[3] no studies have demonstrated that the disease process itself is accelerated by pregnancy. Delay in investigating the abnormal smear in pregnancy and more importantly, delay in the treatment of a cervical intraepithelial abnormality because of pregnancy, will have implications for the natural history of CIN. However, it appears that the implication is only that the delay in treatment allows the condition to remain untreated for longer, not that progression is enhanced.

In receiving a smear report suggesting borderline atypia or mild dyskaryosis for the first time, the physician should arrange for the patient to be appropriately counseled and for a repeat smear to be performed postnatally. It is perhaps important to state at this point that the standard practice of performing a smear at the postnatal visit, i.e., 6 weeks postnatally is perhaps less than satisfactory. At this time, estrogen levels tend to be low because prolactin levels are high and the cytologist is faced with an atrophic smear to interpret. It is better, if there is no apparent disadvantage from a further slight delay, for the definitive postnatal smears, be they in patients with a previous abnormality, or those who have been treated, to be performed at between 8 and 12 weeks, possibly with an optimum of 10 weeks postnatally.

If a patient should receive a borderline or mildly abnormal smear report for the second time when the smear is performed in the early part of pregnancy then the patient should, like all those with moderate or severe dyskaryosis reported on their smears be referred for colposcopy.

COLPOSCOPY IN PREGNANCY — ADVANTAGES AND DISADVANTAGES

Should we take a biopsy?

The aim of colposcopy in pregnancy is to exclude invasive disease. There is no indication to treat cervical intraepithelial neoplasia in pregnancy. However, microinvasive disease and early invasive disease present the clinician and the patient with a range of difficult options to consider where intervention will be required. Colposcopy of the pregnant cervix is more complicated than colposcopy of the nonpregnant cervix. Changes in the consistency, shape and vascularity of the pregnant cervix together with an increased area and rate of squamous metaplasia of the exposed columnar epithelium can make interpretation of the changes within the transformation zone difficult, particularly for the inexperienced colposcopist. The primigravid pregnant cervix undergoes eversion due to changes in the collagenous tissue supports, under the influence of a rising estrogen; the multiparous cervix tends to gape during pregnancy. In both circumstances, the result is that a new area of columnar epithelium is exposed to the increasingly acid vaginal environment and it is thought that this gives rise to increased squamous metaplasia, both in area and rate.[4] For this reason it is essential that colposcopy of the pregnant patient is only performed by those who are expert in the art of colposcopy. This is not an examination that should be devolved to a junior member of the medical team.

When a patient has been referred for colposcopy because of a second borderline or mildly abnormal smear, the situation with regard to the pregnant patient will be similar to that in the nonpregnant patient. One-third of the patients will be found to have no colposcopic abnormality and will require simply a further cytology specimen; one-third will have changes consistent with minor grade disease and if they have been evaluated by an expert colposcopist and the examination is satisfactory in that the new squamocolumnar junction is visible to the colposcopist, then it is this author's view that a biopsy is unnecessary. The issue of biopsy involves more the one-third of women who will be found to have evidence of major grade disease at colposcopy[5] and of course, this situation will occur not only in one-third of those referred with borderline or mild abnormalities, but in a very large proportion of those referred because of moderate or severe dyskaryosis. In general terms, the more severe the cytology report, the more likely there is to be major grade disease present, such that if a smear report suggests severe dyskaryosis normal colposcopic findings are more likely to be explained by inexpertise or inaccessibility of the area to the colposcopist rather than any fault with the cytology laboratory. In the pregnant or the nonpregnant state it is a foolish clinician who ignores a severely dyskaryotic smear report.

In published accounts in the literature[1,6,7] there is almost universal overdiagnosis at colposcopy, usually by one grade in the pregnant patient. It is probable that the increased acetowhite appearance of the cervix and the vascular changes occurring in pregnancy convince the examining clinician that the changes are more severe than is the situation if a biopsy is taken. The question as to whether or not a biopsy should be performed will be governed by the experience of the colposcopist, the appearance of the cervix, the gestation of the pregnancy and the medicolegal framework within which the patient lives and the clinician practices.

COLPOSCOPIC BIOPSIES IN PREGNANCY

Should we or shouldn't we?

It is the view of this author, although it will be controversial, that if a patient has been assessed by an expert colposcopist, the entire transformation zone has been seen, the cytology and the colposcopic impression albeit either or both might suggest major grade disease but not evidence of microinvasion, that the logic of performing a colposcopically directed punch biopsy is flawed. The only aim of the biopsy is to exclude microinvasive or invasive carcinoma. The International Federation of Gynecology and Obstetricians (FIGO) definition of microinvasive carcinoma, states that this diagnosis should be based on a large biopsy, usually a wedge biopsy or a cone biopsy. It is exceedingly difficult to diagnose microinvasive carcinoma on a colposcopically directed punch biopsy and indeed, the changes of pregnancy itself may compound the diagnosis on a small colposcopically directed punch biopsy. In addition, the absence of evidence of microinvasion within a colposcopically directed punch biopsy comments only on the area that was biopsied itself and not on the rest of the transformation zone. If the clinician has a low threshold for proceeding either to a wedge biopsy or a conization to exclude microinvasive carcinoma, then colposcopically directed punch biopsies could be dispensed with when there is colposcopic evidence of minor grade or even major grade disease if there is no cytological or colposcopic evidence to suggest invasion.

Most publications[6,7] indicate that there is virtually no morbidity associated with a colposcopically directed biopsy despite the increased vascularity of the cervix. It has been suggested that colposcopically directed punch biopsies should be a routine in the evaluation of the pregnant patient.[4] In countries where it is necessary to do this in order to satisfy any potential medicolegal investigation the clinician may feel it is safer to perform one, but intellectual rigor suggests that for the formally evaluated patient, the logic of biopsy is flawed.

IS MICROINVASION OR INVASION PRESENT?

Wedge biopsy or cone biopsy?

For the small number of patients in whom either the cytology or the colposcopic impression suggests early invasive disease then the clinician has several options. One is to perform the standard wedge biopsy where the worst affected area of epithelium identified colposcopically is subject to a knife wedge biopsy. This will usually be performed under general anesthesia with the use of suture material for the wedge area and many colposcopists will like to use a solution of lidocaine and dilute epinephrine to aid hemostasis. Unfortunately, this technique again suffers from the fact that if microinvasion is ruled out on that particular wedge of tissue removed, there is no cast iron guarantee that it does not exist elsewhere on the badly affected cervix. For this reason, despite the potential for increased morbidity, some form of conization should be considered.

Many practitioners will prefer to continue using a standard cold knife cone biopsy technique with two laterally placed hemostatic sutures and intracervical lidocaine and epinephrine prior to knife cone, with diathermy to the base and vaginal pack with urinary catheter. This operation carries a morbidity and a mortality but will be effective for diagnosis and frequently for treatment. There may be, however, pregnancy-associated complications in the short term and the long term, such as miscarriage, premature labor or cervical stenosis in labor albeit that the majority of women undergoing the procedure will proceed to term and delivery without complication.

Laser cone biopsy allows a more precise excision of the transformation zone with less anatomical distortion to the cone base and the cervix itself and is therefore, less likely to be associated with medium and long-term complications after it has been performed.[8] In expert hands with a high power-density laser it should be as effective as cold knife cone biopsy for effecting simultaneous diagnosis and hopefully, treatment of the con-

dition. Unfortunately, laser cone biopsy appears to be associated with increased intraoperative blood loss, particularly with high grade early invasive lesions and this will be compounded by the increased vascularity of pregnancy. For this reason, some may prefer to use an electrical method of excision.

Diathermy loop excision can be an effective method of diagnosis for suspected early invasion in the pregnant cervix.

CASE HISTORY

Mrs RF was a 29-year-old prima gravid patient who booked at 14 weeks gestation. Her previous cervical smear had been three years prior to pregnancy and therefore, a booking smear was performed. This revealed severe dyskaryosis (Fig. 17.1) and the patient was referred for colposcopy.

Colposcoped at 23 weeks gestation, the colposcopic findings were suspicious for the possibility of a high-grade CIN 3 lesion or early microinvasion. The colposcopic examination was complete in that the new squamocolumnar junction could be visualized at colposcopy. The situation was discussed in detail with the patient and it was decided after careful consideration to repeat the colposcopy and smear at 28 weeks gestation at which point a definitive decision could be made with regard to further diagnosis and treatment at a time when the fetus might be viable should premature labor result.

Recolposcoped at 28 weeks, the findings were

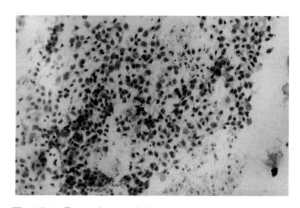

Fig. 17.1 Presenting cervical smear in pregnancy showing severe dyskaryosis.

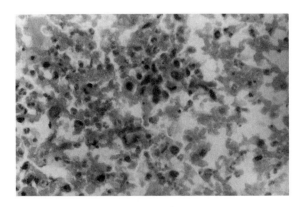

Fig. 17.2 Second cervical smear in pregnancy, suggests possibility of invasion.

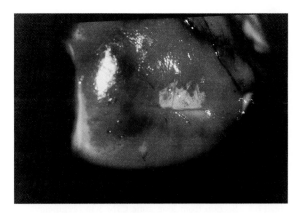

Fig. 17.4 Colophotograph CIN in pregnancy after iodine.

essentially unchanged, but a smear taken at this stage (Fig. 17.2) reported fiber cells suggesting either microinvasion or frank invasive carcinoma.

The patient was admitted for a loop cone excision of the transformation zone under general anesthesia. A solution of 2 ml of 1 in 80 000 epinephrine in 2% lidocaine administered via a dental syringe was used to aid hemostasis. The diathermy loop excision was performed without event (Figs 17.3–17.5) with roller ball coagulation to the cone base. A square of surgicel was placed within the cone bed (Fig. 17.6) and the patient observed over a 48 h period. No vaginal pack or catheter was used.

The histology reported CIN 3 (Fig. 17.7) with no evidence of invasion, but the lesion was incompletely excised. However, because the top of the transformation zone had been seen at colpos-

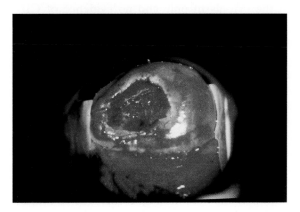

Fig. 17.5 Colophotograph CIN in pregnancy after loop excision.

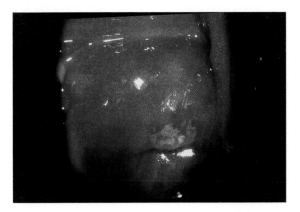

Fig. 17.3 Colophotograph CIN in pregnancy after acetic acid.

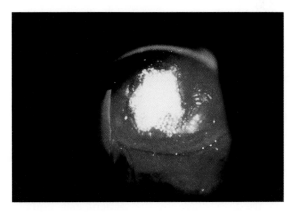

Fig. 17.6 Colophotograph CIN in pregnancy after surgicel.

copy, it was decided to continue a conservative expectant management.

At 34 weeks gestation the cervix had healed and the cervical smear showed keratinizing changes

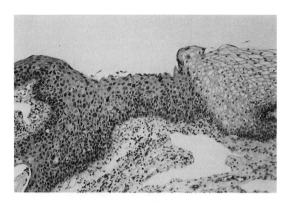

Fig. 17.7 Section from loop cone CIN 3 in pregnancy.

in the cytoplasm only and no evidence of CIN. The patient proceeded to an uncomplicated normal vaginal delivery.

Six weeks postnatally, the cervical smear suggested moderate dyskaryosis, the colposcopic appearances were of a small area of CIN 1–2 and a biopsy confirmed the latter diagnosis. Loop cone excision of the new central transformation was carried out under local anesthesia with no significant disease being discovered in the specimen.

The patient underwent colposcopy and smear 6 months following treatment both of which examinations were normal. A smear at 12 months postnatally was normal with endocervical cells present and the patient is now once again pregnant.

The blended cutting and coagulation current and the ability to adjust the levels of these modalities makes diathermy loop excision an attractive form of treatment for the patient in pregnancy with suspected CIN.

THE MANAGEMENT OF MICROINVASIVE CARCINOMA IN THE PREGNANT PATIENT

When microinvasion is present, the best outlook for the patient is if the conization procedure that was used to diagnose the patient has equally effected a cure. Under these circumstances, it would be necessary for the lesion to be budding rather than confluent, for there to be no endothelial space involvement and for the margins of the cone to be free of disease. Such patients will need to be kept under regular review for the rest of the pregnancy and be the subject of careful evaluation in the puerperium and thereafter, but there seems no logical clinical reason for not allowing such a pregnancy to continue. If there is endothelial space involvement or if the margins of the cone contain microinvasive disease or if the pattern of invasion is confluent rather than budding, then it must be assumed that the procedure has not been curative and the patient must be evaluated as a patient with early invasive carcinoma in pregnancy, a difficult clinical dilemma which we will return to later in this chapter.

TREATMENT OF CIN FOLLOWING PREGNANCY

The vast majority of patients who have an abnormal smear in pregnancy and are the subject of colposcopic evaluation with or without directed punch biopsy will be confirmed as having minor or major grade CIN and in the absence of any evidence of early invasive disease, may be managed conservatively in pregnancy. If a diagnosis of major grade disease is made early in pregnancy many practitioners will wish to repeat at least the cytological and possibly, also the colposcopic evaluation at 28 weeks of pregnancy indeed, some authors have suggested[6,7] that such evaluations should take place at 3, 5 or 6 weekly intervals throughout pregnancy although this seems to this author excessive. The key points at which to evaluate the patient would be at 28 weeks where clinical intervention, should it be necessary, may result in a viable pregnancy and equally, the choice of 34 weeks reflects the optimistic outcome for a fetus that has to be delivered, either as a result of a complication of investigation such as cone biopsy, or for the need to bring the pregnancy to an end in order to effect definitive treatment for an invasive lesion.

Following delivery, most clinicians will wish to treat major grade disease (CIN 2 or CIN 3) and many others would also encompass CIN 1 in their treatment program. It is probably preferable to repeat the colposcopic evaluation prior to definitive treatment, although those practising a 'see and treat' policy may feel that the puerperal arrangements for treatment can be effected at one visit. As with cervical cytology, colposcopic appearance of the recently delivered cervix is difficult to interpret. This is because of the recently distorted anatomy and the low estrogen level reflecting a high prolactin level in the breast feeding mother. For this reason, as with cytology, as mentioned earlier, colposcopic evaluation should, if a delay is not critical, be carried out at about 10 weeks postdelivery. If the patient is not breastfeeding and has returned to menstruation or the combined oral contraceptive pill whereby estrogen levels will be maintained and menstruation will occur, then treatment can be effected as soon as the final diagnosis is made. One group in whom caution should be displayed is in the breast feeding, high prolactin low estrogenized patient with major grade disease, requiring a fairly large area of either destruction or excision, It is in this group that even using loop diathermy excision or laser cone biopsy, stenosis may occur. It appears that the cervix requires preferably both high estrogens and menstruation to maintain the integrity of the functioning endocervical canal.

FOLLOW-UP OF PATIENTS TREATED FOR CIN IN SUBSEQUENT PREGNANCIES

If a woman has been treated for cervical intraepithelial neoplasia, pregnancy is not contraindicated in the follow up period, although common sense might dictate that it would be advisable for her to complete, if not the first year of follow-up, at least the first post-treatment follow up visit to be sure that there is not persistent disease present before embarking upon pregnancy. However, if pregnancy should supervene following treatment, but before the first follow up visit has been arranged no significant case can be made for altering the post-treatment management protocol or indeed, the conduct of the pregnancy.

The management protocol for women treated for CIN in the UK in the nonpregnant state is a cervical smear 6 months and 12 months following therapy, then annually for 4 years, at which point, if all smears have been normal, the patient may be returned to the cervical screening program.[2] Colposcopy may have an advantage in identifying persistent disease earlier if it is combined with the first post-treatment check up. There is no indication to alter the follow-up protocol because a patient finds herself pregnant following treatment, although many might feel that this is one of the circumstances where a colposcopy and cervical smear should be combined at the first post-treatment follow-up and a further, possibly additional cervical smear might be added 10 weeks postnatally if the first two follow-up visits have occurred during the course of pregnancy. Indeed, some may feel that if the first colposcopy and smear follow-up following treatment, carried out in early pregnancy is normal there may be some advantage in deferring the second follow-up visit until the postnatal period, rather than relying on a cervical smear performed in late pregnancy, which may be less reliable than one performed in the puerperium.

EARLY STROMAL INVASION AND INVASIVE CARCINOMA OF THE CERVIX

Whereas CIN and pregnancy frequently coexist, fortunately, invasive carcinoma and pregnancy is a rare combination. However, should early invasive malignant disease of the cervix be diagnosed in pregnancy, the clinician and the patient face difficult decisions about the appropriate management protocol. To a certain extent, the final decision will be based on the age and reproductive intentions of the mother, the stage of the carcinoma and the gestation of pregnancy. Other concerns that may need to be taken into account are any religious convictions the patient may have which would make it unacceptable for her to consider as one of the options for management, termination of pregnancy, either before or coincident with the treatment of the cancer.

If invasive cancer is diagnosed at the end of pregnancy, and this should only occur with a late booking patient or when the appropriate screening for and management of CIN in pregnancy has failed, many would opt for delivery by cesarean section, with or without coincident Wertheims hysterectomy, the timing of the procedure possibly being altered by up to 2 or 3 weeks in order to obtain maximum viability for the fetus. Others may prefer to perform a cesarean section and subsequently treat the patient with a combination of radiotherapy and surgery or surgery alone at an interval, but most would shy away from delivering the baby vaginally, because of fear of the theoretical risk of disseminating the carcinoma by vascular spread. It is fair to say, however, that the numbers in the literature are too small for there to be a comparative study of delivery by the vaginal versus the abdominal route and happily, the number of cases occurring are so small that a prospective randomised study would not be feasible.

In the first trimester, once the social and religious views of the patient and her family have been fully explored, many would suggest that termination of the pregnancy and definitive treatment of the carcinoma would offer the best outlook for the mother. Some might wish to effect a medical abortion, by external beam radiotherapy and then proceed to a Wertheims hysterectomy, others might wish to perform a Wertheims hysterectomy with the pregnancy intact in utero, a third option might be hysterotomy and subsequent definitive treatment. Again, as with management in late pregnancy many would avoid delivery of the products of conception per vaginam because of the theoretical risk of vascular dissemination.

Perhaps the most difficult time for definitive decisions to be made is in the mid-trimester. Clearly, the closer one approaches to the fetus being viable (this may now be as low as 24 weeks gestation), the greater will the temptation be to defer definitive treatment of the carcinoma to allow the fetus a significant chance of survival. The social, ethical and clinical decisions should be managed with a team approach, the ultimate decision being that of the patient after adequate information has been provided.

SUMMARY

The diagnosis and management of CIN diagnosed in pregnancy presents a challenge to the colposcoping obstetrician. At each point in the management pathway options exist but one successful protocol is summarized in the algorithm shown in Fig. 17.8.

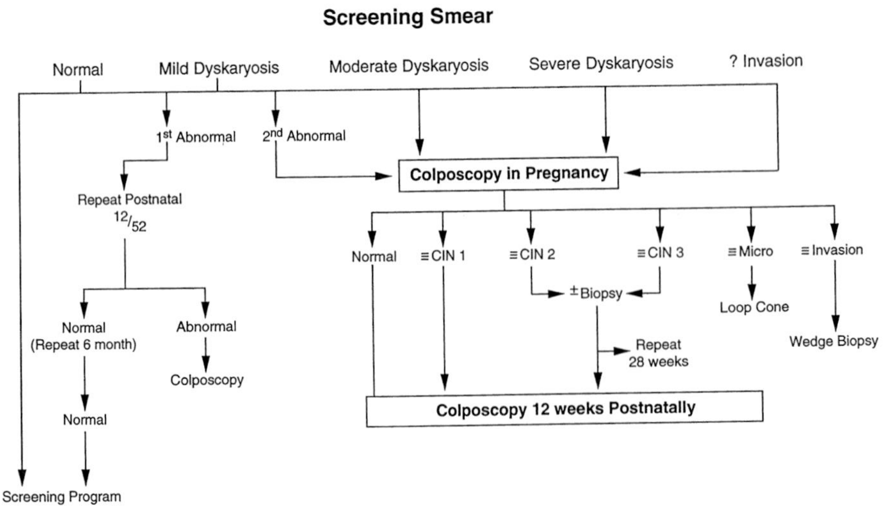

Fig. 17.8

REFERENCES

1. Hacker N F, Berek J S, Lagasse L D, Elsworth H C, Savage E W, Moore J G. Carcinoma of the cervix associated with pregnancy. Obstet Gynaecol 1982; 59: 735–746.
2. Duncan I D. Guidelines for Clinical Practice and Programme Management. National Health Service Cervical Screening Programme. Oxford: National Co-ordinating Network, 1992.
3. Pater M, Hughes G, Hyslop D, Nakshatri H and Pater A. Glucocortoid-dependent oncogenic transformation by type 16 but not type 11 human papilloma virus DNA. Nature 1988; 335: 832–835.
4. Singer A. Malignancy and premalignancy of the genital tract in pregnancy. In: Turnbull A, Chamberlain G, ed. Obstetrics. Edinburgh Churchill Livingstone, 1989: pp 657–672.
5. Giles T A, Deery A, Crow J, Walker P G. The accuracy of repeat cytology in women with mildly dyskaryotic smears. Br J Obstet Gynaecol 1989; 96: 1067–1070.
6. Benedict J L, Boyes D A, Nichols T M, Millner A, Colposcopic evaluation of pregnant patients with abnormal cervical smears. Br J Obstet Gynaecol 1977; 84: 517–521.
7. Lurain J R, Gallup D C. Management of abnormal Papanicolaou smears in pregnancy. Obstet Gynaecol 1978; 53: 484–488.
8. Hammond R, Edmonds D K. Does treatment for cervical intraepithelial neoplasia affect fertility and pregnancy. Br Med J 1990; 301: 1344.

18. The abnormal smear in postmenopausal women

M. E. L. Paterson   D. W. Sturdee

INTRODUCTION

The whole of the female genital tract is sensitive to estrogen and the cervix, in particular, undergoes various changes in response to different hormonal situations. At the menopause, there is a gradual reduction in circulating estrogen due to ovarian failure, and this also results in significant changes in the cervix and vagina. An appreciation of the embryology of this area is helpful in understanding these effects.

The urogenital sinus of fetal life develops into the vagina as well as the urethra and trigone of the bladder, but there is controversy about the development of the upper vagina. The cervix and upper four-fifths of the vagina may develop from the Müllerian duct,[1,2] but Bulmer[3] believes that the urogenital sinus forms all the vagina and the cervix. However, in late fetal life the columnar epithelium lining of the Müllerian duct covers the uterine cavity and extends downwards into the cervical canal where it comes into contact with the squamous epithelium of the urogenital sinus. The more caudal of the original columnar epithelium gradually becomes replaced by squamous epithelium due to the physiological process known as metaplasia. This process continues rapidly during late fetal life and on into adolesence as a result of the increasing estrogen levels. During pregnancy, this process is particularly prominent when estrogen levels are very high.[4] The process is maintained throughout adult life, but after the menopause with the decline in estrogen, the junction between the two epithelia — the squamocolumnar junction — tends to revert back into the endocervical canal.[5] Together with a general shrinking and atrophy of the cervix at this time, the squamocolumnar junction gradually becomes less easily visualized on colposcopy.[6,7]

In postmenopausal women the cervix is smaller (Fig. 18.1) and petechial hemorrhages may be a further feature of atrophic change. The vaginal epithelium also becomes thin and atrophic and there is reduced elasticity.

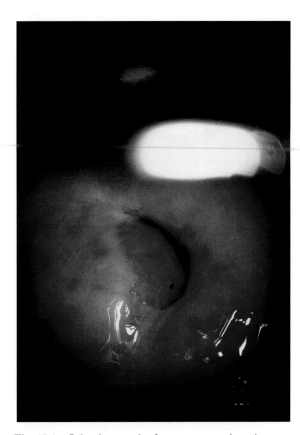

Fig. 18.1 Colp photograph of postmenopausal cervix showing atrophic changes and petechial hemorrhages.

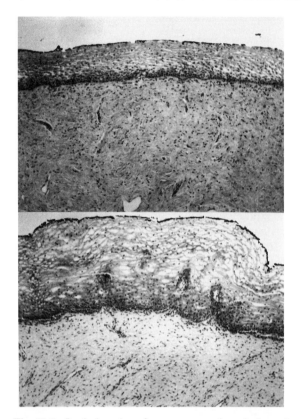

Fig. 18.2 Logical section of postmenopausal cervix (upper) and then after the same patient has been treated with estrogen therapy.

The effect of estrogen on the cervix can be clearly seen in histological sections before and after the menopause (Fig. 18.2). The epithelium becomes much thinner due mainly to the loss of cells in the superficial layers.

The squamous epithelium of the cervix is stratified and microscopically consists of five layers, originally described by Papanicolaou:[8]

Zone 1: The lower layer consists of a single layer of small cylindrical cells with relatively large nuclei referred to as a basal or stratum cylindricum.

Zone 2: This zone consists of several layers of polyhedral cells with fairly large nuclei and distinct intercellular bridges and is called the parabasal layer.

Zone 3: The cells in this layer begin to flatten and have glycogen-rich cytoplasm with frequent vacuolation. These are known as the intermediate cells.

Zone 4: This is a variable layer and often not recognised separately. It consists of a number of closely packed polyhedral cells and is called the intraepithelial zone.

Zone 5: This layer comprises the superficial layer of cells, which are elongated, flattened with small pyknotic nuclei containing a large amount of cytoplasm.

These groups of cells are recognized by the cytologist according to their characteristics and origin:[9]

a. Basal or parabasal cells which originate from the second zone.
b. Intermediate cells from the third zone.
c. Cornified or superficial cells from the fourth and fifth zones.

Smears from postmenopausal women have a high proportion of basal and parabasal cells (Fig. 18.3). A smear from the same woman after receiving estrogen reveals many more superficial cells (Fig. 18.4). The ratio of superficial to basal cells is described as the maturation index, and is a useful indicator of the hormonal status of the patient.

Not only do the basal and parabasal cells (Fig. 18.3) more closely resemble dyskaryotic cells (Fig. 18.5), but they do not exfoliate as readily as the superficial cells which makes the interpretation of such few cells much more difficult.

On scanning electron microscopy of a cervical

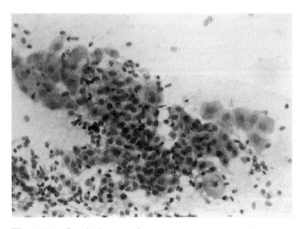

Fig. 18.3 Cervical smear from postmenopausal patient.

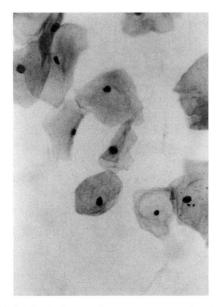

Fig. 18.4   Cervical smear from premenopausal patient.

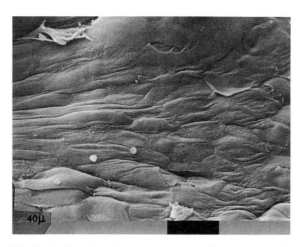

Fig. 18.6   Scanning electron microscopy of postmenopausal cervix.

biopsy from a postmenopausal woman (Fig. 18.6), the cells are closely adherent to each other, whereas examination of a biopsy from the same woman following estrogen therapy shows the cells are lifting away from each other (Fig. 18.7). Hence, it is easier to obtain more cells in a smear from a premenopausal woman, and in addition the vast majority are large superficial cells with plentiful cytoplasm and a relatively small nucleus.

THE INTERPRETATION OF SMEARS IN POSTMENOPAUSAL WOMEN

Cervical smears from postmenopausal women are much more difficult to interpret than from younger women, because the cells do not exfoliate so easily and are often from the basal and

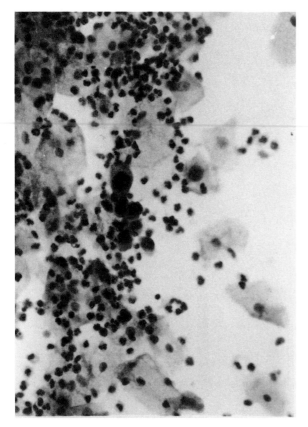

Fig. 18.5   Cervical smear from a patient with CIN 3 showing severely dyskaryotic cells.

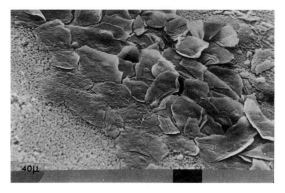

Fig. 18.7   Scanning electron microscopy on the same patient after receiving oestrogen treatment.

parabasal layers. The lack of satisfactory cellular material often means that the smears are unsatisfactory in interpretation. Three basic cytological patterns are found:

a. Early menopause
b. Crowded menopause
c. Atrophic or advanced menopause

Early menopause

There is a reduction in the number of superficial squamous cells. The squamous cells are smaller and it may appear to the casual observer that the nuclei are enlarged.

Crowded menopause

This type of smear from slightly older women is characterized by crowded clusters of intermediate and parabasal cells.

Atrophic or advanced menopause

The cells are of a size and degree of maturity corresponding to the parabasal cells. The nuclei are large and pale because of dryness. Endo-cervical cells are rare and when present are smaller than those found in smears from premenopausal women. Round or oval globules of inspissated blue-stained mucus, about the size of epithelial cells, may appear. It is generally agreed that these structures are of no significance except as a potential source of diagnostic error.

As a result of the features described above, smears from postmenopausal women can be much more difficult to interpret, and overreporting may result in high false positive rates. If there is insufficient cellular material, it may be impossible for the cytologist to be certain that there is no pathology in the cervix. Cytology is a cell-sampling technique, and the more epithelial cells that are in the smear, the greater the chance of assessing the state of the cervix correctly.

Among postmenopausal women with an abnormal smear the proportion that have significant pathology and especially invasive cancer is much greater than in smears from premenopausal women (Fig. 18.8).[10] It is also well recognized that invasive carcinoma of the cervix can be present despite a satisfactory but negative smear,

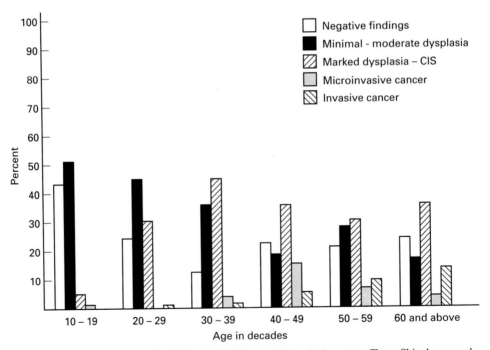

Fig. 18.8   Cervical pathology in 1197 women with atypical cervical smears. (From Shingleton et al (1977);[10] reprinted with permission.)

so if there is any clinical suspicion of malignancy further investigation, such as colposcopy, should be performed regardless of the cytology report. The mortality rate from cervical cancer in older women is not improving[11] and late diagnosis may be one of the reasons for this.

Tamoxifen

Breast cancer affects one in 12 women in the UK and increasing numbers of postmenopausal women are being prescribed tamoxifen either as prophylaxis or therapy following surgery. This drug has a variety of hormonal effects, and on the endometrium and cervix it seems to have an oestrogenic effect in postmenopausal women. Athanassiadou et al[12] reported a decrease in the karyopyknotic index in premenopausal women but a slight but significant increase in smears from postmenopausal women receiving tamoxifen. It is important, therefore, that the cytologist is informed about any hormone therapy that could affect the smear and its interpretation.

CYTOLOGY SCREENING IN POSTMENOPAUSAL WOMEN

Current cytology screening programs in the UK recommend 5-yearly smears on all women over the age of 35, but with no definite upper age limit at which screening may be discontinued. About half of all cases of invasive carcinoma of the cervix are registered in women after the menopause (Table 18.1), but the majority of these have never been screened. If a women has had regular screening, it seems reasonable to stop further smears after the age of 60 as the likelihood of developing cervical intraepithelial neoplasia (CIN) or carcinoma at this age is small. For this reason, Wijngaardn and Duncan[13] have questioned the value of cervical screening in women over 50 years. They found a low incidence of CIN in women over this age in Dundee and Angus (UK), and no cases occurring de novo in women over the age of 50 who had an adequate history of negative results on smear testing every 3 years. However, even in their region of Scotland, over half of the women above the age of 60 had never had a cervical smear. Hopefully with the wider uptake of

Table 18.1 Age–specific registrations and incidence of cervical cancer in the West Midlands 1985–1989 (Data kindly supplied by West Midlands Regional Cancer Registry)

	Registrations	Incidence per 100 000 population
0–4	0	0.0
5–9	0	0.0
10–14	1	0.1
15–19	0	0.0
20–24	34	3.2
25–29	140	14.4
30–34	271	32.0
35–39	276	30.7
40–44	229	25.8
45–49	204	28.0
50–54	179	25.8
55–59	163	23.1
60–64	245	34.7
65–69	196	29.3
70–74	140	24.6
75–79	103	21.6
80–84	65	20.5
85+	42	19.3
All ages	2288	17.4

cervical screening and improving efficiency of the call and recall systems, fewer women will be reaching the postmenopausal years who have not had regular smears, and in time the proposals of Wijngaardn and Duncan[13] may be appropriate. One of the benefits of cervical screening has been the reduction in the proportion of cases of advanced cervical carcinoma, and it will be interesting to see if this is maintained in postmenopausal women who have had regular cervical screening.

COLPOSCOPY IN POSTMENOPAUSAL WOMEN

The presentation of an abnormal cervical smear from a postmenopausal woman requires a different and considered response than for the younger woman. Not only is the likelihood of significant pathology much greater (see Fig. 18.8) but the clinician must also recognize that interpretation of the smear may be confounded by atrophic changes (see earlier) resulting in more false negative[14] and false positive reports so that the implications of a particular cytology report may be less certain. Colposcopy, however, is still the most appropriate method of assessment, though estrogen-deficiency changes resulting in shortening of the cervix, retraction of the squamocolumnar junction up the canal as well as uterovaginal prolapse can make this difficult. The technique of colposcopy is the same as for a premenopausal woman, and the use of acetic acid is helpful in differentiating abnormal areas, although the development of whiteness may take longer. In addition, the use of Lugol's iodine for a Schiller's test is also less satisfactory in postmenopausal women because of the lack of glycogen in the normal squamous cells of the vagina and cervix. A well estrogenized epithelium stains a dark-brown color, but with the lack of glycogen it may only stain a light-yellow color, and so the differentiation between CIN and normal squamous epithelium may be lost. Despite all these various problems, it may still be possible to assess the cervix adequately by colposcopy, that is to see clearly all the transformation zone, in a large proportion of patients.[15] Few studies, however, have documented this adequately, but from 120 postmenopausal women referred with abnormal cytology, Toplis et al[7] were able to assess the transformation zone completely in 47% and this was increased to 61% when some were given estrogen replacement therapy. Few colposcopists seem to consider using estrogen to help in the assessment of the postmenopausal woman. This may be because of the resulting delay in management and need for repeat colposcopy after an interval of treatment, but such measures may prevent unnecessary or more extensive surgical treatment.

THE VALUE OF ESTROGEN THERAPY

Only about 10% of postmenopausal women in the UK receive hormone replacement therapy, despite the overwhelming evidence of the benefits not only in relieving the acute climacteric symptoms, but especially the protective effect in the longer term on the cardiovascular system and skeleton. Every postmenopausal woman experiences atrophic changes in the genital tract, some of which have been described earlier, and estrogen will not only prevent the resulting symptoms but also make cytological and colposcopic assessment of the cervix easier and more accurate. The benefits of estrogen therapy in improving the interpretation of smears from an atrophic cervix

were initially reported by Keebler and Wied.[16] In their 'estrogen test' they gave about 5 days of high-dose oral or intramuscular injections of estrogen, and noted a dramatic improvement in the quality of the smear and the maturity of the desquamated cells 2–3 days later. The background became 'clean', free nuclei and degenerated cell changes were diminished, superficial and intermediate cells became the predominant cell types and previously present parabasal cells usually did not appear in the repeat smears. As a result, dyskaryotic and malignant cells became more clearly identified or excluded. Similar findings were reported by Paterson et al[6] in women examined before and after 3–12 months of oral sequential mestranol and norethisterone, but there were no further changes after the 3-month examination with continuation of therapy for up to 1 year. They also reported on the colposcopic and histologic changes of the atrophic cervix with hormone therapy, which is of particular importance to clinical practice. In their study of 12 women attending a colposcopy clinic who were at least 2 years postmenopause, initial colposcopy was unsatisfactory in six as the squamocolumnar junction was not visible. After 3 months hormone therapy, the junction was visible in each case, but it was not clear if this was due to a physical alteration of the site of the junction, or to increased elasticity of the vaginal epithelium and less patient discomfort, thus allowing the bivalve speculum to be opened further and the cervix to be everted. However, Coppleson et al[17] did not find evidence of eversion in 200 postmenopausal women given estrogen by suppository.

The vaginal epithelium seems to be more sensitive to estrogen than the cervix, and studies of vaginal blood flow have demonstrated a progressive improvement continuing throughout 24 months of estrogen replacement therapy.[18] This explains why dyspareunia may persist in the early months of estrogen therapy despite the return of hormonal and cytologic values to the premenopausal levels. The postmenopausal cervix, however, will never return morphologically to the premenopausal state with continuing estrogen therapy, though the cervical squamous epithelium will demonstrate a similar response to the vagina as shown by the cytology changes. (Figs 18.3

and 18.4). Histology of cervical biopsies before and during estrogen therapy show significant improvements in maturation, but assessment by scanning electron microscopy show the changes much more clearly (see Figs 18.6 and 18.7).[6]

Estrogen therapy clearly has a potential role in the assessment and management of the abnormal smear in postmenopausal women, though it may not be appropriate in every case. For some women, however, the estrogen deficiency changes can result in such vaginal dryness and discomfort that speculum examination and colposcopy are too uncomfortable. A delay for the symptomatic benefits of estrogen therapy would then be necessary in addition to achieving some of the other possible benefits already described.

ESTROGEN THERAPY

Various topical estrogen preparations are available for the relief of atrophic vaginitis, and for the benefits in colposcopic and cytologic assessment. Natural estrogens should be used rather than the older synthetic preparations, which can be associated with significant systemic absorption (Table 18.2).[19] The use of any of these preparations for 3–4 weeks will usually be sufficient, but longer therapy may be appropriate to maintain relief from the symptoms of estrogen vaginitis. Systemic estrogen therapy given by tablet, subcutaneous implant or transdermal patch or gel will also have the same effect on the vagina and cervix.

There is no evidence that estrogen therapy provokes or exacerbates cervical disease, and the incidence of cervical cancer is unchanged in women who have been taking long-term estrogen replacement therapy.[20]

MANAGEMENT

The majority of postmenopausal women presenting with an abnormal cervical smear will be within a few years of the menopause and some will be taking or have recently taken estrogen replacement therapy. The principles of management in such cases are the same as for younger women with colposcopic assessment being the optimum initial evaluation. For older women and those with marked atrophic changes such that the cervical os is stenosed and the squamocolumnar junction is not visible, estrogen therapy may give some benefit as previously described, and if subsequent cytology is normal, a repeat smear after an appropriate interval will be all that is required. For those with severe dyskaryosis on the initial smear or with persistent abnormality following estrogen, colposcopy may still be satisfactory and if the squamocolumnar junction is visible, management may be as already discussed for the premenopausal woman in Chapter 15. If no abnormality is seen or a lesion can be partly visualized in the cervical canal, further assessment by hysteroscopy, endocervical curettage or cone biopsy will be required (Fig. 18.9). Because of the much higher incidence of unsatisfactory colposcopy, a cone biopsy of the cervix will be necessary more often in older women to establish a diagnosis. Shingleton et al[10] found the need for conization increased with each decade of age, and was required in at least one-third of postmenopausal women following initial evaluation by colposcopy. Toplis et al[7] reported a cone biopsy rate of 71% in a group of 121 postmenopausal women.

Cone biopsy may be performed in the clinic using electrocautery or laser techniques with simple local anesthesia, and these techniques are

Table 18.2 Natural estrogen preparations for vaginal application

Product	Estrogen/strength	Recommended regimen
Ortho–Gynest	Estriol/0.1% cream or pessaries 0.5 mg	1 applicator daily 2–3 weeks then twice weekly
Ovestin	Estriol/0.1% cream	1 applicator daily 2–3 weeks then twice weekly
Premarin	Conjugated equine estrogens/0.625 mg per gram cream	1–2 g daily for 3 weeks then at 1 week intervals
Vagifem	Estradiol 25 µg	1 tablet daily for 2 weeks then 1 tablet twice weekly
Estring	Estradiol releasing 7.5 mg/24 h	Vaginal ring, change at 3 months

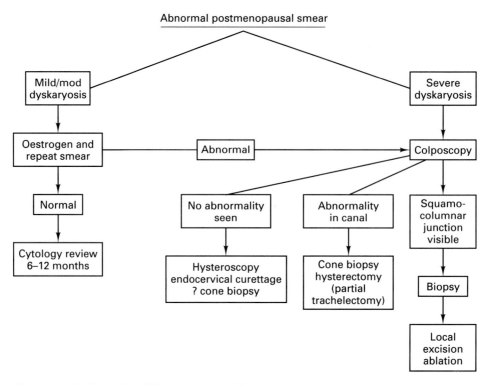

Fig. 18.9 Algorithm of possible management following abnormal smear in a postmenopausal woman.

described elsewhere, but for most cases it will be safer to perform such procedures in theatre with a general anesthetic. The main differences in the postmenopausal woman are that atrophy and reduced vascularity result in much less bleeding, but in addition the cervix may be too small or flush with the vaginal vault so that conization is not practical and there is a risk of damage to the bladder or uterine perforation. In such cases, hysterectomy may be the better option and if there are coincidental symptoms of prolapse or significant uterine descent, a vaginal hysterectomy may be appropriate.

Endocervical curettage is much more popular in North America than the UK as an additional evaluation prior to considering conization, but this is not always practical and can cause significant discomfort. Furthermore, in older women endocervical curettage often produces an inadequate tissue sample due to atrophy and stenosis of the canal.[7,10]

For the elderly woman with an atrophic and retracted cervix, an alternative management could be partial trachelectomy.[21] This procedure is performed under general anesthetic and briefly involves grasping the cervix with a tenaculum, making a circumferential incision through the vaginal skin which is dissected from the cervix with scissors. The cervix is pulled down as it is mobilized, and the descending cervical branch of the uterine artery on each side is ligated and divided. Mobilization is continued for 2–4 cm and the cervix is amputated. Sutures are inserted through the vaginal skin edge and cervical stump in order to cover the raw area in a similar manner to a Manchester repair.

Krebs and colleagues[21] reported on 26 elderly patients with a mean age of 69.6 years who were managed by this technique when cone biopsy was considered inappropriate and previous attempts at endocervical curettage and cervical biopsy had been unsatisfactory. Operative complications were few but included two uterine perforations. Twelve of the 26 patients, including four with severe dysplasia (CIN 3) and eight with invasive carcinoma received additional therapy, but 11 of

14 patients with CIN had clear surgical margins. They concluded that partial trachelectomy provides a specimen of sufficient length so that the incidence of positive surgical margin is low, and in the absence of carcinoma few will need further treatment. This technique has not been widely used in the UK, and neither author has any personal experience of it.

For those in whom colposcopy is considered satisfactory with full visualisation of the transformation zone, the management may be similar to that in the premenopausal woman. Cervical intraepithelial neoplasia can be removed by local excision or ablation techniques, but again care must be taken when the cervix is small that the treatment does not extend beyond the confines of the cervix.

ABNORMAL SMEAR FROM THE VAGINAL VAULT

Smears taken from the vaginal vault of women who have had a hysterectomy may also cause some difficulties in interpretation. Estrogen deficiency changes will be the same as previously described for the cervix. In addition, some women may have had radiotherapy and this can cause permanent changes in the epithelium resulting in cytological features which may be mistaken for dyskaryosis. Because vaginal vault cytology can be so misleading in such cases, we recommend that routine smears are not performed. Colposcopic examination can be helpful though it may not be possible to visualise all the vault satisfactorily, particularly when the vagina is short and narrow following a Wertheim hysterectomy, or if there are deep recesses in the vaginal angles. Selective punch biopsies will help to establish if there is abnormality present. Vaginal intraepithelial neoplasia (VAIN) at the vault can be difficult to erradicate. Laser vaporization, local excision, radiotherapy and application of 5-fluorouracil have been tried but none have been entirely satisfactory.

CONCLUSION

The significance of an abnormal smear in a postmenopausal woman is greater than for the younger woman, but it may be more difficult to evaluate and treat. The complicating effects of estrogen deficiency on smear interpretation and colposcopy assessment may be partly reversed by estrogen therapy, but there will still be many cases in which a diagnosis can not be established by colposcopy, and more invasive surgical procedures will be required. Nevertheless, the majority can still be managed in a colposcopy clinic.

REFERENCES

1. Koff A K. Development of the vagina in the human fetus. Contrib Embryol 1933; 24(1): 59–91.
2. Forsberg J G. In: Jordan J A, Singer A, eds Morphogenesis and differentiation of the cervicovaginal epithelium in the cervix. London: Saunders, 1976: pp 3–13.
3. Bulmer D. The development of the human vagina. J Anat 1957; 91: 165–168.
4. Singer A, Jordan J A. The anatomy of the cervix. In: Jordan J A, Singer A, eds. The cervix. London: Saunders, 1976: pp 13–36.
5. Singer A. The uterine cervix from adolescence to the menopause. Br J Obstet Gynaecol 1975; 82: 81–89.
6. Paterson M E L, Allen J, Jordan J A. Effects of the climacteric and sequential mestranol and norethisterone on the cervix and genital tract. Br J Obstet Gynaecol 1982; 89: 657–664.
7. Toplis P J, Casemore V, Hallam N, Charnock M. Evaluation of colposcopy in the postmenopausal woman. Br J Obstet Gynaecol 1986; 93: 843–851.
8. Papanicolaou G N. Atlas of exfoliate cytology. Cambridge, MA: Harvard University Press, 1954.
9. Papanicolaou G N, Traut H F, Marchetti A A. The epithelia of woman's reproductive organs. New York: Commonwealth Fund, 1948.
10. Shingleton H M, Partridge E E, Austin J M. The significance of age in the colposcopic evaluation of women with atypical Papanicolaou smears. Obstet Gynecol 1977; 49: 61–64.
11. Hussain O A N. Britain's failure to prevent deaths from cervical cancer. Br Med J 1984; 289: 50.
12. Athanassiadou P P, Kyrkou K A, Antoniades L G, Athanassiadou P H. Cytological Evaluation of the effect of tamoxifen in premenopausal and postmenopausal women with primary breast cancer by analysis of the karyopyknotic indices. Cytopathology 1992; 3: 203–208.
13. Wijngaardn W J, Duncan I D. Rationale for stopping cervical screening in women over 50. Br Med J 1993; 306: 967–971.
14. Roberts A D G, Denholm R B, Cordiner J W. Cervical intraepithelial neoplasia in postmenopausal women with negative cytology. Br Med J 1985; 290: 281.
15. Teaff N L, Malone J M, Ginsburg K A, Bartles L W, Haigler B B. Cervical dysplasia in the postmenopausal

female: Diagnosis and treatment. Int J Gynaecol Obstet 1990; 34: 145–149.

16. Keebler C M, Wied G L. The estrogen test: an aid in differential cytodiagnosis. Acta Cytologica 1974; 18: 482–493.

17. Coppleson M, Pixley E, Reid B. Colposcopy. Springfield, IL: Thomas, 1971. pp 93–99.

18. Semmens J P, Tsai C C, Semmens E C, Loadholt C B. Effects of estrogen therapy on vaginal physiology during menopause. Obstet Gynecol 1985; 66: 15–18.

19. Widholm O. The vaginal absorption of estriol and dienestriol in postmenopausal women. In: Abstracts XI World Congress of Gynaecology. Germany: Berlin, September, 1985.

20. Hunt K, Vessey M P, McPherson K. Mortality in a cohort of long–term users of hormone replacement therapy: an updated analysis. Br J Obstet Gynaecol 1990; 97: 1080–1086.

21. Krebs H–B, Wilstrup M A, Wheelock J B. Partial trachelectomy in the elderly patient with abnormal cytology. Obstet Gynecol 1985; 65: 579–584.

19. Psychological aspects of the investigation and treatment of abnormalities of the cervix

I. E. Doherty   P. H. Richardson

INTRODUCTION

The treatment of cervical intraepithelial neoplasia (CIN) has been regarded as a triumph of preventative medicine. The Papanicolaou (Pap) smear test together with colposcopy examinations have enabled the detection of early abnormal cell changes. Although not all abnormalities progress to invasive cancer and some in fact revert to normal,[1] the presence of CIN is regarded as a risk to the future health of the woman.[2] The degree of abnormality determines whether monitoring by further smear tests and/or colposcopy examinations or treatment is indicated. Local ablative techniques such as laser therapy, cold coagulation, and cryocautery are commonly used for the treatment of CIN together with, more recently, large loop excision of the transformation zone (LLETZ).[3] They have the advantage of minimal damage to the surrounding normal tissue and complications are relatively rare. The detection and treatment of CIN could therefore be viewed as a straightforward and minor procedure. From a medical perspective this perhaps is generally the case. However, it is only in recent years that the psychological impact on women of the process from cervical screening to further diagnostic procedures and treatment has been investigated and documented.[2,4]

This chapter examines research into the psychological effects of having a cervical smear test, receiving an abnormal smear result and undergoing the subsequent diagnostic and medical procedures. Strategies for reducing adverse psychological reactions are then examined.

PSYCHOLOGICAL ASPECTS OF CERVICAL SCREENING

It has been reported that the majority of women who present with invasive carcinoma of the cervix have not been previously screened.[5] Moreover, attendance for cervical screening programs varies from a 65% response rate[6] to as low as 33%.[7] Reasons given for nonattendance have included practical consideration such as poor organization of screening programs and inefficient recall systems[8] as well as a range of psychological factors which are discussed in greater detail below.

Although screening for a variety of conditions is now an integral aspect of many health care systems it cannot be assumed that it is free of psychological costs[9] not least because screening seeks signs of disease in the absence of overt clinical abnormality thereby making potential patients out of people who feel well. Despite several decades of cervical screening in many developed countries it has been suggested that women sometimes do not know what the test is for[5,10] or believe its purpose is to detect, rather than prevent cancer.[11-13] In a survey of 600 women in London 71% of respondents thought it was for detecting cancer with only 11% aware that the aim of cervical screening was to enables action to be taken to prevent cancer.[14] This confusion is understandable in view of the common use of the term 'cancer smear' in both medical and lay descriptions.[12] Many women do not ask for a smear test but are tested by their general practitioner as part of a more general examination[15] and are therefore more likely to think of the test as a diagnostic rather than preventative measure.[11] Words like 'cancer' or indeed 'cancer prevention' may provoke sufficient anxiety to discourage clinic attendance.[16] Moreover a diagnosis of cancer is thought to induce in many people a dread greater than that of other diseases carrying equally serious or worse prognoses.[11,17,18]

In addition to its association with the fear of discovering pathology, the pelvic examination itself is generally considered to be one of the most anxiety-producing of common medical procedures. Alexander & McCullough[19] describe the pelvic examination as requiring "the patient to undress and assume a supine position with legs elevated and spread as far apart as possible while an examiner inspects her genitalia. That this examination causes anxiety and embarrassment for some women needs little explanation as it necessitates behavior inconsistent with traditional values including modesty and respectability". It is therefore not surprising that research into women's attitudes to the pelvic examination has indicated a range of negative feelings including anxiety, vulnerability, humiliation, dehumanization[20] and feelings of degradation.[21] Gynecological visits are abhorred by many women,[22] dreaded, postponed and can be both physically and emotionally traumatizing.[23] One of the most frequent complaints of women is the overwhelming feeling of vulnerability and helplessness.[22] Physical discomfort and pain, particularly in connection with insertion of the speculum, are frequently cited accompaniments of pelvic examination.[24,25] Moreover, previous experience of the procedures does not necessarily reduce distress. It seems that women rarely overcome the feeling of personal intrusion, no matter how many prior examinations they have experienced.[26]

Various studies indicate that older women are less likely to attend for cervical screening than younger women.[7,27,28] A survey in Oxford found that menopausal and postmenopausal women felt they were no longer at risk of disease of the reproductive organs.[29] Older women in the same study were averse to the idea of an 'internal examination' despite having had children.[29] Other research however suggests that younger women are more likely than older women to state embarrassment as the reason for not having the test.[30]

Reasons given for nonparticipation in cervical screening by women of varying ages include embarrassment, unpleasantness or pain.[11,29–32] Social factors suggested are difficulties experienced by working women in finding time to attend,[33] heavy family commitments,[34,35] transport[34] and accessibility.[36] Eardley[5] suggests that any one of these factors taken individually may appear trivial but the cumulative impact of several of them may be considerable.

Research has tended to focus on the question as to why women fail to attend for cervical smear testing than on the reactions of those who do attend. In one of the few studies in this latter category 418 women were interviewed in the Netherlands after participating in a mass screening program but before they were informed of the results.[37] Negative experiences were reported by 30% of the women. These included 'bodily discomforts', 'objections against the screening room', 'too little privacy', 'too little personal attitude of screeners' and 'long waiting time'. Another study comparing participants and nonparticipants at a mass screening program indicated that nonparticipants considered gynecological examinations more unpleasant than did participants[32] implying that anticipation of the procedure is more aversive than the event itself. On the other hand it may be that nonparticipants had previously had more unpleasant experiences of cervical smears. In this respect a survey of women who had failed to respond to a computer-generated recall letter 3 years after a normal cervical smear reported that women who failed to respond were more likely to have 'disliked some aspect of the test and/or found it unpleasant and embarrassing'.[33]

REACTIONS TO AN ABNORMAL SMEAR TEST RESULT

For those women who do attend screening, an abnormal or positive smear result can have a very negative emotional impact. Initial feelings of shock and disbelief related to the prior expectation that there is nothing wrong have been reported together with anxiety associated with the belief that an abnormal smear indicates cancer with implications for future childbearing, the necessity of a hysterectomy and their own mortality.[2,38]

Adverse emotional effects were reported in the majority of women interviewed in one study[4] with 97% (n = 80) found to be at least 'a little' distressed; of these, 21% were 'moderately' distressed and 8% 'severely' distressed about their abnormal smear result. As part of a mass screening study in the Netherlands, Reelick et al[37] also noted that those women who had received a positive smear tended to feel more ill and became moodier than they were before the test when compared with a control group. However, these differences were no longer apparent at the follow-up which took place from 5 weeks to 6 months after treatment.

Although these findings indicated no long-term adverse effects, some worries may be tenacious and resistant to reassurance particularly during the diagnostic period between receipt of a smear result and medical interventions. In the Netherlands study 50% of women with a positive smear remained frightened or nervous after contacting their general practitioner for information prior to treatment.[37] Likewise Doherty[38] found that some women did not believe their general practitioner when told it was nothing to worry about. When informed it was 'just precancerous' they only heard the word 'cancer', the 'pre' did not register. In this respect, Palmer et al[39] suggested that 'once heard, the word cancer pervaded women's thinking'.

Doherty et al[4] were interested in examining the extent to which women were worried by various thoughts associated with an abnormal smear result. In Table 19.1 these worries are rank-ordered to show what it was that women were most concerned about.

Items concerning causality, outcome of treatment, perceived severity of the condition and perceived consequences of the condition were found to be the highest ranking worries.

Adverse psychosexual effects of an abnormal smear have been reported in several studies.[2,39,40] In a controlled investigation, Campion et al[40] found a significant increase in the frequency of negative feelings towards sexual intercourse and a reduction of spontaneous sexual interest subsequent to diagnosis and treatment of an abnormal smear result. Posner and Vessey[2] found that 'disturbed' sexual relationships were apparent in 43% of women interviewed (n = 150) during the diagnostic period and following treatment. 'Disturbances' included abstaining from, or not wanting to have sexual relations or painful intercourse resulting from tension. In addition to feelings of being 'dirty' and 'unclean', there were also fears that the condition (CIN) could be aggravated by sexual activity or that it could be transmitted to the sexual partner.[2] Similarly, Palmer et al[39] reported feelings of defilement together with detachment and loss of control of one's body.

These studies, together with several personal accounts recounting emotional trauma[41,42] suggest that for many women receipt of an abnormal smear result is not a minor medical event but one which threatens not only a woman's perceived

Table 19.1 Mean ($\bar{x}$) and standard deviation (SD) for distress scores of individual worries associated with an abnormal smear result ranked in order of magnitude

Rank	Worry	$\bar{x}$	SD	% of subjects moderately–very worried
1	What has caused the abnormal smear?	2.83	1.01	65
2	Will the treatment cure me?	2.79	1.09	63
3	Will the abnormal cells recur after treatment?	2.73	1.01	50
4	Have I got cancer?	2.68	1.09	53
5	Have I got something seriously wrong?	2.54	0.99	48
6	Will I need surgical treatment?	2.43	0.95	43
7	Will I get worse while waiting for appointments?	2.38	1.07	43
8	Will it affect having children?	2.15	1.16	33
9	Will I pass anything on to my partner?	1.80	1.07	26
10	Will it affect my sex life?	1.76	1.00	23
11	Have I caught something from my partner?	1.71	1.06	20
12	Will I need a hysterectomy?	1.56	0.91	16

health and life expectancy but her self concept, body image and sexuality. Moreover, partners may also be worried about an abnormal smear result, in some instances more so than the woman herself.[2]

PSYCHOLOGICAL EFFECTS OF A COLPOSCOPY EXAMINATION

To the clinician a colposcopy examination may appear to be a minor investigative procedure to detect abnormality which if found can be effectively treated. The prognosis is generally good. However, from the patient's perspective merely attending hospital can in itself be a stressful experience[38,43] — a consideration which may well be overlooked by health care professionals to whom hospitals are familiar places. Investigative and treatment procedures may well add to this distress.[4,43] In this respect, the findings presented in the previous section of this chapter imply that a pelvic examination may be considered as a stressful medical procedure for many women.

The term 'stressful medical procedure' encompasses different types of events and different levels of stress. Weinman and Johnston[43] have attempted to clarify what is meant by stressful medical procedures and have proposed two independent classifications. The first differentiates between procedures of an investigative or diagnostic nature (e.g., colposcopy) and those with a treatment function (e.g., radiotherapy). The second classification separates stress into procedural stress (associated with the immediate unpleasantness of the procedure) and outcome stress (associated with the long-term fears and concerns related to outcome of the investigative procedure or treatment). Women who have had an abnormal smear result (serving an investigative function) are then subjected to stressful medical procedures of both a diagnostic and treatment nature. Moreover, the colposcopy examination and subsequent treatment could, in principle, result in both procedural and outcome stress.

Investigations into the psychological effects of a colposcopy examination have reported high levels of anxiety prior to the procedure.[4,44–46] Lack of knowledge of both the purpose and procedural aspects of the colposcopy examination have also been found[2,4,44,45] in addition to concerns related to the outcome[2] which may well contribute to this anxiety. The fear that the procedure would be uncomfortable or painful[38,44] together with concern about the embarrassing and undignified nature of the examination[2] indicate a range of negative feelings associated with the colposcopy examination itself. Some research indicates that anticipation of the procedure can, however, be more stressful than the actual experience[38] as has been suggested with regard to the smear test examination.[32] In addition, anxiety prior to colposcopy has been found to be more related to fear about the procedure than to outcome, with no relationship between anxiety and the seriousness of the referred problem or perceived seriousness of problem.[4]

Although anxiety immediately prior to a colposcopy examination may be largely associated with procedural stress, the findings of a controlled study by Palmer et al[39] suggest that concerns relating to an abnormal smear result are very much in evidence even after a colposcopy examination. Palmer et al[39] interviewed women on the sixth or seventh days after receiving their diagnosis. Measures used included the Impact of Events Scale which looks at intrusive thoughts and avoidance[47] and the State Trait Anger Scale.[48] Women diagnosed as having CIN had significantly higher scores for intrusive thoughts, avoidance and state anger than women with a negative smear result supporting previous findings that a diagnosis of CIN is a traumatic experience.

PSYCHOLOGICAL EFFECTS OF OUTPATIENT TREATMENT OF CIN

Treatment is generally done on an outpatient basis with local ablative therapy including laser, cold coagulation and cryocautery or LLETZ. Documentation of the various methods from the patient's perspective is sparse. In terms of their physical effects, a study comparing laser and cold coagulation concluded that immediately after treatment (which included use of local anesthetic) women who had received laser ablation experienced significantly greater pain than patients receiving cold coagulation.[49] Posner & Vessey[2] reported that many women experienced pain both during and after treatment irrespective of whether cryocautery or laser techniques were used. In addition to the pain, 30% of women who had cryocautery complained of a watery discharge lasting up to 3–4 weeks after treatment. With regard to the relative psychological impact of various treatments, Posner & Vessey[2] comment that the word 'laser' had more frightening associations than cryocautery and was occasionally confused with radiotherapy.

Many of the psychological effects associated with the colposcopy examination apply equally to outpatient treatments. Negative feelings relating to the pelvic examination are evident[2] and high levels of anxiety similar to those before a colposcopy examination have been found prior to outpatient treatment with a subsequent post-treatment reduction[4,50] again suggesting procedural stress as a source of anxiety. With regard to worries associated with an abnormal smear result, Raju et al[50] found that although a significant pre- to post-treatment reduction emerged, women continued to report some worries at both post-treatment and at 6 month follow-up indicating that treatment did not provide complete reassurance. Similarly, Palmer et al[39] report high levels of intrusive thoughts, avoidance and state anger on the sixth to seventh day after treatment with scores comparable with those of people who have experienced a traumatic event. On the basis of interview data, they found that while many women mentioned 'being cured' as a benefit of treatment, further questions revealed doubt as fears of reoccurrence and progression of CIN to cancer were elicited. An additional finding by Palmer et al[39] was that treatment did not have a negative impact over and above that of diagnosis (postcolposcopy), i.e., both could be seen as traumatic events but treatment was no worse that diagnosis.

An advantage of LLETZ is that it is both a diagnostic and treatment technique and both functions can be performed at a patient's first visit to the colposcopy clinic[3] thereby reducing distress by eliminating a second stressful medical procedure. On the other hand, it has been argued that psychological adjustment may be greater if women are given the opportunity to consider their diagnosis and discuss treatment options.[51] It should be noted that some hospitals perform LLETZ treatment independently of the colposcopy examination and therefore this situation does not always arise and has not been the case in any of the studies discussed.

There appears to be a considerable body of evidence which demonstrates that the process from cervical screening to further diagnostic procedures and treatment frequently produces a range of adverse psychological reactions in many women. It is however worth keeping in mind that some women do not appear to be disturbed by either the diagnosis of abnormality or the subsequent medical procedures.[2]

METHODS FOR IMPROVING PSYCHOLOGICAL OUTCOMES

Information provision

Research on psychological preparation for surgery[52,53] and for a variety of other stressful medical procedures[54] has indicated that the provision of preparatory information can substantially reduce patient distress and improve various aspects of recovery. Information provision has been suggested as a way of reducing distress associated with cervical abnormalities and subsequent medical interventions.[5,44–46] Lower levels of anxiety were reported for women recalled for a repeat smear who had received an information leaflet advising them that most smears showing dyskaryosis do not indicate cervical cancer.[13]

Factors affecting the impact of information include the timing of information, modality (i.e., oral or written), communication skills of both clinicians and patients, readability of material and individual coping styles. With regard to when information should be given, Marteau[51] suggests that information should be provided at all stages of the screening process, i.e., prior to a smear test, when an abnormality is suspected and detected, and when referred for a colposcopy examination and treatment, with appropriate variations in the content. However, if information is given immediately before a medical procedure it may increase already high levels of anxiety.[55]

Both oral and written information are regarded as useful and complementary modalities. Ley[56] suggests that patients often feel they do not receive adequate information from health professionals and argues that this is because patients often do not understand or do not recall what they are told and are too diffident to ask for information when they do not receive it. Ley[57] further suggests that communication can be improved by supplementing oral communication with written information as well as altering the communicative behavior of the clinician and changing the behavior of the patient. It has been demonstrated in various health care settings that patients' understanding and memory for medical information, as well as their overall satisfaction with communications from clinicians may be predictive of the degree of anxiety experienced in relation to various aspects of diagnosis and treatment.[58] The provision of written information allows recipients to absorb it at their own pace; an important consideration for women with cervical abnormalities given that high levels of anxiety can interfere with the processing and recall of information.[51]

The communication skills of both clinicians and patients affects the quality and usefulness of information. Doctors often fail to elicit information from patients because of patients' diffidence, poor interviewing techniques on the part of the doctor and doctors' feelings of discomfort with the interview.[59] Interview training techniques used with doctors were shown to successfully increase the amount of useful information obtained by the interviewer.[60] Patient diffidence is frequently voiced as a reason for not obtaining information.[61,62] Roter[62] examined this problem by conducting an experimental investigation which included teaching patients how to word questions. Although the latter was found to be effective in reducing diffidence by increasing the number of questions asked it also led to an increase in anxiety and anger during the consultation, and high patient dissatisfaction.

Readability of written material has received considerable attention in both clinical and nonclinical contexts and there are numerous formulae intended to predict the ease with which a passage may be read and understood.[56] A widely used measure for health related material is the Flesch Index of Reading Ease[63] which uses the average number of syllables per word and the average sentence length per passage to assess the difficulty level of the text. Readability is expressed in terms of the level of education required to understand the material and the percentage of the adult population likely to understand it. Wolfe et al[46] used this formula to examine the readability of five information leaflets distributed by London teaching hospitals to patients who had an appointment for a colposcopy examination. All five were found to fall in the 'difficult' or 'fairly hard' category making them accessible to at most 52% of the patient population. The importance of information being understood is highlighted by Marteau[51] who reported less anxiety prior to a colposcopy examination in women who had received a booklet written in simple language than in those who were given a more complex one.

Although there appears to be a considerable body of evidence which suggests that patients want more information about their medical conditions, their treatment and the outcome[59] others would suggest that there are individual differences in preference for information which are associated with individual coping styles in response to stress.[64,65]

As a method of examining coping styles, Miller and Mangan[64] identified 'monitors' and 'blunters' on the basis of self-reported preference to seek or avoid information and involvement in stressful situations. Using the Miller Behavioral Styles Scale (MBSS) they interviewed a group of women attending hospital for a colposcopy examination and concluded that psychophysiological arousal was less when the amount of information given was consistent with the individual's coping style in that 'blunters were less aroused with low information and monitors were less aroused with high information'. They also found a significant interaction between coping style and psychological distress with 'blunters' in the low-information condition maintaining a lower level of tension/ anxiety throughout the procedure whereas 'blunters' in the high-information condition demonstrated a large increase in tension which decreased by the end of the procedure.

However, other research with women undergoing colposcopy found no relationship between the MBSS and information seeking and questions whether information-seeking behaviour is related to being designated a 'monitor' or 'blunter'.[65] Moreover, women in the Miller and Mangan[64] study were exposed to information immediately prior to the colposcopy examination which may have increased already high anxiety levels in 'blunters'. This point was discussed earlier with respect to timing of information provision which may be an important consideration rather than coping style per se.

Psychological interventions

In addition to the provision of information, a variety of psychological approaches have been used for patients undergoing invasive medical procedures based on the rationale that high levels of preprocedural fear are detrimental to patients' subsequent adaptation. These interventions include emotion-focused techniques, relaxation techniques, cognitive manipulations, behavioral instruction and counseling.[52] A criticism often leveled at studies which use a combinations of techniques is the inherent difficulty in separating out the effects of each technique. Moreover although research suggests that each of the various psychological interventions can be effective, methodological problems such as heterogeneity of sample characteristics and limited range of outcome measures prevent definitive conclusions.[66]

In this respect, using data from Mathews and Ridgway's[52] earlier review, Weinman and Johnston[43] reviewed the success of various interventions and concluded that whereas each of these approaches can be effective, interventions are not globally beneficial. Particular approaches were found to be more effective in relation to some responses than to others, e.g., relaxation was effective in dealing with physical discomfort and information provision reduced uncertainty. Behavioral instruction was found to be more helpful in coping with procedural distress.

Counseling is becoming an accepted intervention for psychological trauma such as the aftermath of large-scale catastrophes as well as for people afflicted by life-threatening diseases such as AIDS or cancer.[67] It may well be that if patients are given an opportunity to discuss their illness-related concerns with a health care professional then a variety of beneficial effects could accrue. As yet there has been little research on the potential benefits of counseling for women undergoing colposcopy and subsequent medical treatments.

Given the psychotherapeutic connotations sometimes associated with counseling and the possibility that these might be regarded as stigmatizing, a comparative study carried out by Wolfe et al[46] investigated the acceptability of the offer of counseling to women in the outpatient settings of a colposcopy clinic and a day surgery unit. The findings demonstrated that the use of the term 'counseling' did not lower the acceptability of the interview. Moreover, an overall uptake rate of 80% suggested that most of the women approached welcomed this service.

Only one study to date has examined the outcome of information provision alone with information provision in combination with counseling[50] In this study, the counseling interview which took place prior to colposcopy examination was based on cognitive-behavioral principles. This included clarification of information previously received, identification of additional information needs, identification of patients' expectations and concerns regarding diagnosis and treatment together with the use of cognitive coping strategies and brief relaxation training. Evaluation of the counseling suggested high levels of patient satisfaction with all aspects of the interview. However no statistically significant differences emerged between the counseling plus information group when compared with the information only group on any of the standard measures of psychological adjustment either immediately after colposcopy or at a 6 month follow-up interview. Various explanations were considered for these findings including the possibility that the consultation style of doctors in the subsequent colposcopy examination may have either enhanced or detracted from the effects of counseling. Unfortunately the design of the study did not allow for separation of 'counselor' and 'doctor' effects. It could well be that the application of sensitive interpersonal skills by doctors and other health care professionals (e.g., nurses) involved in the care of patients may reduce the necessity of employing dedicated counselors for stressful medical situations.

It has been established in other fields of health care research that perceived professional competence and personal qualities of the physician[68] together with physicians' emotional expressivity[69] are considered important attributes by patients whereas poor interviewing skills,[70] unresponsiveness to patients' concerns[71] and insensitivity to the psychological and social aspects of surgery[70] are viewed as detrimental to the patient's psychological well-being.

Finally, it may be that simple practical considerations relating to the way clinics and consultations are organized can also play a part in increasing or reducing anxiety associated with medical procedures. Having shorter waiting times between receipt of an abnormal smear result and attending for colposcopy and treatment can lead to improved outcomes by reducing unnecessary anxiety and uncertainty while greater privacy in the consultation room can facilitate communication between doctor and patient.[51] Reducing institutional practices in the waiting area and making it more consumer-friendly by, for example, arranging groups of chairs around coffee tables and having background music may also have a relaxing effect (personal communication from a former patient). However, as yet little research has been undertaken to examine which, if any, of the above considerations are useful in reducing trauma associated with attending hospital and undergoing medical procedures. There is, therefore, a need for systematic controlled research to answer these questions.

SUMMARY

The process from smear test and receipt of an abnormal smear result to further diagnostic and medical procedures has a considerable adverse psychological impact on many women. Much distress arises from lack of sufficient information about the nature of CIN which results in women assuming the worst. Further anxiety is associated with the diagnostic and treatment procedures which is not simply confined to physical pain but also concerned with feelings of vulnerability and personal intrusion. Fears and concerns about many aspects of these procedures can be reduced by the provision of adequate information both about the meaning of an abnormal smear result and what the subsequent medical procedures entail. Information given verbally is often more effective when accompanied by written information. However, written information is only likely to increase understanding and reduce anxiety if it is easy to read. A range of psychological interventions have been used to reduce stress associated with invasive medical procedures with some techniques more effective than others. Having an opportunity to speak to a health care professional such as a counselor, a doctor or a nurse may help to alleviate fears and concerns. However, if such an interaction is to be effective it is essential that the clinician has good communication and interpersonal skills. Last, but not least, attention to the organization and physical setting of the clinic may also be beneficial in reducing distress.

REFERENCES

1. Kinlen L J, Spriggs A I. Women with positive cervical smears but without surgical intervention. A follow-up study. Lancet 1978; 2: 463–465.
2. Posner T, Vessey M. Prevention of cervical cancer: the patients view. London: Kings Fund, 1988.
3. Prendiville W, Cullimore J, Norman S. Large loop excision of the transformation zone (LLETZ). A new method of management for women with cervical intraepithelial neoplasia. Br J Obstet Gynaecol 1989; 96: 1054–1060.
4. Doherty I E, Richardson P H, Wolfe C D, Raju K S. The assessment of the psychological effects of an abnormal cervical smear and subsequent medical procedures. J Psychosom Obstet Gynaecol 1991; 12: 319–324.
5. Eardley A, Knopf Elkind A, Spencer B, Hobbs P, Pendleton L, Haran D. Attendance for cervical screening — whose problem? Soc Sci Med 1985; 20 (9): 955–962.
6. Evans D, Hibbard B, Jones J et al. The Cardiff Cervical Cytology Study: enumeration and definition of population and initial acceptance rates. J Epidemiol Community Health 1980; 34: 9–13.
7. Doyle Y. A survey of the cervical screening service in a London district, including reasons for non-attendance, ethnic responses and views on the quality of the service. Soc Sci Med 1991; 32 (8): 953–957.
8. Cullum D E, Savory J N. Patient preferences for cervical cytology. Br Med J 1983; 287: 329–330.
9. Marteau T M. Psychological costs of screening. Br Med J 1989; 299: 527.
10. Gregory S, McKie L. Smear tactics. Nursing Times 1990; 86 (19): 38–40.
11. Knopf A. Changes in women's opinions about cancer. Soc Sci Med 1976; 10: 191–195.
12. King J. It's silly but I just don't want to know. Health Ser 1983 (March 11).
13. Wilkinson C, Jones J M, McBridge J. Anxiety caused by abnormal result of cervical smear test: a controlled trial. Br Med J 1990; 300: 440.

14. Schwartz M, Savage W, George J, Emohare L. Women's knowledge and experience of cervical screening: a failure of health education and medical organisation. Community Med 1989; 46: 499–507.

15. Sansom C D, Wakefield J, Yule R. Trends in cytological screening in the Manchester area 1965–1971. Community Med 1971; 126: 253–257.

16. Hulka B S. Motivation techniques in a cancer detection program. Public Health Rep 1966; 81: 1009–1015.

17. Senescu R A. The development of emotional complications in the patient with cancer. J Chronic Dis 1963; 16: 813–832.

18. McIntosh J. Process of communication, information seeking and control associated with cancer. Soc Sci Med 1974; 8: 167–187.

19. Alexander K, McCullough J. Women's preferences for gynecological examiners: sex versus role. Women Health 1982; 6(3/4): 123–134.

20. Weiss L, Meadows R. After office hours. Obstet Gynecol 1979; 54(1): 111–114.

21. Areskog-Wijma B. The gynaecological examination — women's experiences and preferences and the role of the gynaecologist. Psychosom Obstet Gynecol 1987; 6: 59–69.

22. Domar A D. Psychological aspects of the pelvic exam: Individual needs and physician involvement. Women Health 1985–6; 10(4): 75–90.

23. Olson B. Patient comfort during pelvic examination: New foot supports vs metal stirrups. JOGN-Nursing 1981; 10(2): 104–107.

24. Osofsky T. Women's reactions of pelvic examinations. Obstet Gynecol 1967; 301: 146–151.

25. Haar E, Halitsky V, Stricker G. Patients' attitudes toward gynaecology examination and to gynaecologists. Med Care 1977; 15: 787.

26. Debrovner C, Shubin-Stein R. Psychological aspects of vaginal examinations. Med Aspects Human Sexuality 1975; 9: 163–164.

27. Naguib S M, Geiser P B. Response to a program of screening in cervical cancer. Public Health Rep 1968; 83: 990–998.

28. Wookey B E P. Well-woman clinic in general practice. Br Med J 1971; 1: 296–398.

29. King J. Health beliefs, attributions and health behaviour. PhD thesis, University of Oxford, 1982.

30. Bailie R, Petrie K. Women's attitudes to cervical smear testing. NZ Med J 1990; 103: 293–295.

31. Davison R L, Clements J. Why don't they attend for a cytotest? Med Off 1971; 125: 329–331.

32. Hesselius I, Lisper H O, Nordstrom A, Anshelm-Olson B, Odlund B. Scand J Soc Med 1975; 3: 129–138.

33. Sansom C D, MacInerney J, Oliver V, Wakefield J. Differential response to recall in a cervical screening programme. Br J Prev Soc Med 1975; 29: 40–47.

34. Houghton J. Response to cervical screening. Med Off 1968; 122: 334–338.

35. Allman S T, Chamberlain J, Harman P. The National Cervical Cytology Recall System:report of a pilot study. Health Trends 1974; 6: 39–41.

36. Carruthers J, Wilson J M G, Chamberlain J et al. Acceptability of the cytopipette in screening for cervical cancer. Br J Prev Soc Med 1975; 29: 239–248.

37. Reelick N F, De Haes W F M, Schuurman J M. Psychological side-effects of the mass screening on cervical cancer. Soc Sci Med 1984; 18: 1089–1093.

38. Doherty I E. The psychological effects of an abnormal smear result and of the subsequent investigation and treatment. MSc thesis, University of East London, 1989.

39. Palmer A G, Tucker S, Warren R, Adams M. Understanding women's responses to treatment for cervical intra-epithelial neoplasia. Br J Clin Psychol 1993; 32: 101–112.

40. Campion M J, Brown J R, McCance D J, Atia W, Edwards R, Cuslick J, Singer A. Psychosexual trauma of an abnormal cervical smear. Br J Obstet 1988; 95: 175–181.

41. Britten N. A personal view. Br Med J 1988; 296: 1191.

42. Quilliam S. Positive smear. London: Letts, 1992.

43. Weinman J, Johnston, M. Stressful medical procedures: an analysis of the effects of psychological interventions and of the stressfulness of the procedures. In: Maes S, Defares P, Sarason I, Spielberger C, eds. Topics in first international expert conference on health psychology. Chichester: Wiley, 1988.

44. Marteau T M, Walker P, Giles J, Smail M. Anxieties in women undergoing colposcopy. Br J Obstet Gynaecol 1990; 97: 859–861.

45. Kincey J, Statham S, McFarlane T. Women undergoing colposcopy: their satisfaction with communication, health knowledge and level of anxiety. Health Educat J 1991; 50(2): 70–72.

46. Wolfe C, Doherty I, Raju K S, Holtom R, Richardson P. First steps in the development of an information and counselling service for women with an abnormal smear result. Eur J Obstet Gynecol Reprod Biol 1992; 45: 201–206.

47. Horowitz M, Wilner N. Alvarez W. Impact of Events Scale: A measure of subjective stress. Psychosom Med 1979; 41 (3): 209–218.

48. Spielberger C D, Johnson E H, Russel S F, Crane R J, jacobs G A, Worden T I. Assessment of anger: The State Trait Anger Scale. In: Spielberger C, Butcher J N eds. Advances in personality assessment NJ: Erlbaum, 1983.

49. Goodman J D S, Sumner D. Patient acceptability of laser and cold coagulation therapy for pre-malignant disease of the uterine cervix Br J Obstet Gynaecol 1991; 98: 1168–1171.

50. Raju K S, Wolfe C D, Richardson P H, Doherty I E. Controlled evaluation of the effects of information provision and counselling on the response of patients with abnormal smears. London: CRC, 1993.

51. Marteau T M. Psychological effects of an abnormal smear result. In: Prendiville W, ed. Large loop excision of the transformation zone: A practical guide to LLETZ. London: Chapman and Hall, 1993.

52. Mathews A, Ridgway V. Psychological preparation for surgery In: Steptoe A, Mathews A, eds. Health care and human behaviour. London: Academic Press, 1984.

53. Mumford E, Schlesingher H j, Glass G V. The effects of psychological intervention on recovery from surgery and heart attack: analysis of the literature. Am J Public Health 1982; 72: 141–151.

54. Ludwick-Rosenthal R, Neufeld R W J. Stress management during noxious medical procedures: an evaluative review of outcome studies. Psychol Bull 1988; 104(3): 326–342.

55. Shipley R H, Butt J H, Horowitz B, Farbry J E. Preparation for a stressful medical procedure: Effect of

amount of stimulus pre-exposure and coping style. J Consult Clin Psychol 1978; 46: 499–507.

56. Ley P. Psychological studies of doctor–patient communication. In: Rachman S, ed. Contributions to medical psychology, vol 1. Oxford: Pergamon Press, 1977.

57. Ley P. Memory for medical information Br J Soc Clin Psychol 1979; 18: 245–255.

58. Ley P. Communication with patients: Improving communication, satisfaction and compliance London: Croom Helm, 1988.

59. Ley P. Giving information to patients. In: Eiser J R, ed. Social psychology and behavioural medicine. New York: Joy, 1982.

60. Maguire P. Teaching essential interviewing skills to medical students. In: Osborne D, Gruneberg M M, Eiser J R, eds. Research in psychology and medicine. London: Academic Press, 1979.

61. Ley P. Complaints by hospital staff and patients: A review of the literature. Bull Br Psychol Soc 1972; 25: 115–120.

62. Roter D. Patient participation in patient–provider interaction. Health Educat Monogr 1977; 5: 281–315.

63. Flesch R. A new readability yardstick. J Appl Psychol 1948; 32: 221–235.

64. Miller S M, Mangan C E. Interacting effects of information and coping style in adapting to gynecologic stress: Should the doctor tell all? J Pers Soc Psychol 1983; 45: 223–226.

65. Barsevick A M, Johnson J E. Preference for information and involvement, information seeking and emotional responses of women undergoing colposcopy. Res Nursing Health 1990; 13: 1–7.

66. Anderson K O, Masur F T. Psychological preparation for invasive medical and dental procedures. J Behav Med 1983; 6: 1–40.

67. Fallowfield L J. Counselling for patients with cancer. Br Med J 1988; 297: 727–728.

68. Hulka B S. Patient–clinician interaction and compliance. In: Haynes R B, Taylor D W, Sacket D I, eds. Compliance in health care. Baltimore: Johns Hopkins University Press, 1979.

69. DiMatteo D R, Linn L S, Chang B L, Cope D W. Affect and neutrality in physician behavior. J Behav Med 1985; 8(4): 397–409.

70. Maguire P, Rutter D R. Training medical students to communicate. In: Bennett A E, ed. Communication between doctors and patients. London: Oxford University Press for the Nuffield Provincial Hospitals Trust, 1976.

71. Korsch B M, Gozzi E K, France V. Gaps in doctor–patient communication: Doctor–patient interaction and patient satisfaction. Pediatrics 1968; 42: 855–871.

20. Adenocarcinoma-in-situ and related lesions

John Cullimore

INTRODUCTION

The majority of cervical cancer is of the squamous variety. Cervical cancer has an easily detectable preinvasive phase, cervical intraepithelial neoplasia (CIN), and effective treatment of CIN will prevent progression to invasion. While squamous cancer accounts for the majority of cervical cancer, there is evidence that the absolute incidence of cervical adenocarcinoma is increasing[1,2] and the proportion of cervical malignancies which are glandular likewise shows an upward trend.[3,4] The more frequent application of mucin histochemistry to the histological assessment of cervical cancer indicates that malignant glandular elements may be present in approximately 40% of all cervical cancers.[5]

Cervical adenocarcinoma may be a preventable disease. It is recognized that there are histologically premalignant glandular lesions which are being diagnosed with increasing frequency in gynecological practice. However, while data are accumulating on the histopathological and cytological characteristics of these lesions, these are insufficient to provide an accurate model of the natural history of these lesions, and there is little follow-up data to assess the clinical usefulness of the various histological classifications.

HISTOLOGICAL CHARACTERISTICS

Adenocarcinoma-in-situ (AIS), also called high-grade cervical intraepithelial glandular neoplasia, was first described in 1953 by Friedell and McKay.[6] The histological characteristics of the lesion are listed below:

a. Cells show characteristic malignant features confined to the lining of the endocervical crypts, i.e., nuclear hyperchromasia, increase in nuclear to cytoplasmic ratio and mitotic activity. Cellular crowding gives rise to pseudostratification (Fig. 20.1).

b. There are characteristically abrupt transitions between abnormal and normal areas within the same crypt, and affected crypts can be found immediately adjacent to normal ones (Fig. 20.2).

c. Abnormal crypts do not usually extend below the deepest normal cervical crypt.

d. The lesion is described as being focal, or diffuse and continuous,[7] or less commonly multicentric within the endocervix.[8] There is a growing body of opinion which states that AIS is situated in close relation to the squamocolumnar junction extending in contiguity up the endocervical canal for a variable distance.[9,10]

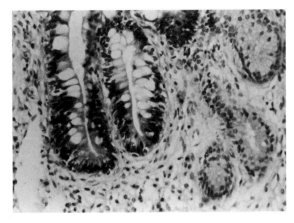

Fig. 20.1 A case of high-grade CIGN showing cellular pseudostratification and goblet cell (type 2) differentiation.

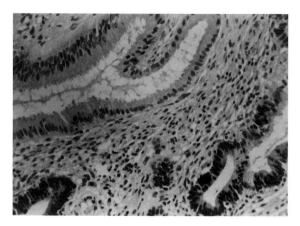

Fig. 20.2 Crypts showing high-grade CIGN are seen adjacent to a normal crypt (upper left of photomicrograph).

LESIONS OF LESSER HISTOLOGICAL GRADE THAN AIS

It has been postulated that there is a spectrum of preinvasive disease, with AIS representing the most cytologically and architecturally advanced form of premalignant glandular lesion.[8,11] Lesions of lesser histological grade than AIS were documented by Van Roon et al[12] who used the terms mild–moderate atypia, severe atypia and AIS. Similarly, Brown and Wells[8] called these lesions 'glandular atypia' (GA) and postulated low-grade (Fig. 20.3) and high-grade lesions based on morphological criteria. By reviewing 100 cases of CIN 3 diagnosed on conization specimens, they reported a 16% incidence of associated GA by critical review of glandular morphology. However, there have been no other reports of such a

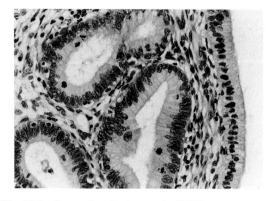

Fig. 20.3 Crypts showing low-grade CIGN are seen adjacent to a normal crypt (to right of photomicrograph).

high prevalence of GA. There would appear to be little difference between the definition of high-grade glandular atypia[3] and other definitions of AIS. Indeed it has been stated that the distinction may be artificial in terms of biological behavior.[8]

Gloor and Hurlimann[11] coined the term cervical intraepithelial glandular neoplasia, (CIGN). By direct analogy with Richart's classification of CIN,[13] they adopted a uniform terminology for glandular dysplasia and AIS. They applied mucin histochemistry and lectin binding procedures to 23 cases of CIGN and produced criteria similarly to those commonly applied to the evaluation of gastrointestinal dysplasias. The main histologic features of CIGN were observed to be nuclear abnormalities, mitoses, and reduction or complete absence of intracellular mucin. Grades of disease from 1 to 3 were described. Grade 3 represents the most atypical histological picture, and is believed to correspond to AIS.

CIGN was further subdivided into types A or B, on the basis of mucin histochemistry. Type A contained reduced quantities of mucin, the pattern of mucins being similar to normal endocervical tissue, with the presence of neutral mucins, and sulfomucins in excess of sialomucins. In CIGN type B, the columnar cells resembled intestinal goblet cells and there was virtual absence of sulfomucins. Absence of sulfomucins is believed by a variety of authors to indicate a functional disturbance of already preneoplastic cells prior to the appearance of morphological atypia.[14,15] Histological subtypes of AIS had been previously described,[16] types 1 and 2 corresponding to CIGN types A and B, respectively. Type 1 cases, which appear to be more common, showed mucin depletion. However, in type 2 cases, cells of goblet cell type were observed and these contained colonic type mucins (Fig. 20.1). It has been postulated that these different kinds of AIS could conceivably represent forerunners of differing histologic types of adenocarcinoma.

We have similarly observed a spectrum of intraepithelial disease (compare Fig. 20.1 with Fig. 20.3) and for the purposes of this discussion, premalignant glandular lesions will be classified as CIGN, without necessarily implying that there is any sort of progression through grades in any individual case.

ASSOCIATED PATHOLOGY

Squamous intraepithelial neoplasia

AIS coexists with CIN in approximately 70% of cases[7,17] (Fig. 20.4). It has been postulated that both these lesions have a common cell of origin, the subcolumnar reserve cell,[18] and this may be one factor which explains their association. However, why only a minority of intraepithelial neoplasias of the cervix are of glandular origin is unknown.

PREDISPOSING FACTORS

The etiology of CIGN is unknown. Its frequent occurrence with CIN (in approximately two-thirds of cases) suggests that there are shared etiological factors and a recent case control study conducted

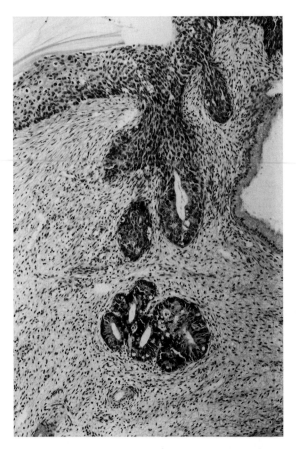

Fig. 20.4 There is CIN in combination with HPV effect in the surface epithelium and a crypt neck. High-grade CIGN is present in the underlying crypts.

by the author supports this hypothesis.[19] However CIGN also appears to have some unique risk factors; notably, low parity and a late age of onset of menarche, imply a possibly altered hormonal environment.[19] This is consistent with conclusions from other epidemiological studies of cervical adenocarcinoma.

There are few alternative data which explore this problem. The following areas have been researched.

The oral contraceptive pill (OCP)

CIGN and invasive adenocarcinoma have been noted to occur in patients taking the OCP.[20,21] However, the hypothesis that the OCP is causally related to the development of these lesions has not been formally tested. A small matched case control study has been carried out which compares women with both in situ and invasive adeno-carcinoma with CIN 3 and invasive squamous cancer controls. A history of OCP use was less frequently found in adenocarcinoma patients although the differences were not significant.[22]

Human papillomavirus

Recent research has indicated that this virus may have a role as a carcinogen or as a cocarcinogen in the female lower genital tract. Okagaki et al[23] have studied the presence of HPV subtypes in AIS, low-grade CIGN, early invasive adeno-carcinoma and microglandular hyperplasia (MGH) by in situ DNA hybridization techniques. Two-thirds of the AIS cases contained HPV DNA and a similar proportion of invasive adenocarcinomas stained positive for HPV. HPV was notably absent from MGH. Similar results were reported by other workers[24] using in situ hybridization. Using probes for HPV messenger RNA production, Farnsworth et al[25] demonstrated that 88.6% of their AIS lesions expressed HPV m-RNA. The majority of cases were positive for HPV 18. In this study, four cases of minor GA were negative for HPV expression. Similar findings were reported by Tase et al[26] implying that these lesions had less malignant potential. In a further comparison with squamous intraepithelial neoplasia, these workers found HPV DNA in 70% of AIS and 64%

of CIN 3 controls. HPV 18 was the preponderant type of DNA found in AIS and also in cases of microinvasive adenocarcinoma similarly studied. CIN which coexisted with AIS or early invasion contained the same type of HPV DNA as the associated glandular lesion, whereas CIN 3 controls all contained HPV 16 DNA. Stoler et al[27] analyzed 11 cases of AIS, some of which also had invasive adenocarcinoma, and 7/11 contained HPV 18, and 4 HPV 16, with all 11 demonstrating high levels of E6/E7 mRNA, the latter being implicated in the process of viral oncogenesis. Leary et al[28] found HPV DNA in 70% of their series of AIS, some of which had associated glandular or squamous invasive disease. HPV 18 was demonstrated in 37% and HPV 16 in 33%. Histologically normal glandular epithelium adjacent to these cases was always negative for HPV.

All the above data on the prevalence of putatively oncogenic HPV subtypes can be criticised on the grounds that normal controls have not been used in any of these studies, making the validity of the observed association between disease and HPV difficult to evaluate. Nevertheless, it is clear that HPV DNA is not universally found in AIS or lower grade glandular atypias. Hence, factors other than HPV must be involved in the genesis of the majority of these lesions.

The field change theory of carcinogenesis

Brown and Wells[8] postulated that there were transitional zones of epithelial atypia of lesser grade than AIS, intervening between areas of clear cut AIS and normal cervical crypts, implying that there may be a 'field change' of neoplastic potential. We have rarely observed such changes in cases of AIS but acknowledge this could merely reflect subjectivity in diagnosis. However, the assessment of AgNORs (markers of nuclear proliferation) in and adjacent to AIS, failed to support the presence of field changes.[29]

CERVICAL INTRAEPITHELIAL GLANDULAR NEOPLASIA: A PRECURSOR OF CERVICAL ADENOCARCINOMA?

There is strong presumptive evidence for the existence of a preinvasive phase of cervical adeno-

carcinoma although direct proof of the malignant potential of this lesion is lacking. This evidence rests largely on histopathological findings.

There is histological similarity between cells of invasive cancer and those of preinvasive lesions; the cells exfoliated by AIS lesions are indistinguishable from the cells of an invasive lesion. In situ lesions are often found adjacent to frankly invasive cancer.[30] In one series, this occurred in 43.9% of a series of adenocarcinomas.[31] There are difficulties in the differentiation of early invasive disease and AIS.

Direct progression from an in situ lesion to invasive cancer has been suggested. However, the evidence that this occurs is suspect, and much of this evidence is highly anecdotal.[32] A series of 18 patients with adenocarcinoma who had endocervical biopsies performed some time before the diagnosis of invasion was made is described.[18] In five of them, there was AIS which had been overlooked. Obata et al[33] reviewed cervical biopsies taken 1–3 years prior to the clinical presentation with adenocarcinoma, and found evidence of glandular dysplasias and/or AIS in a minority. However, biopsies such as those described give a very incomplete sample, assessment of stromal invasion is difficult[34] and a conization specimen is usually required to determine with confidence whether the disease is still in situ. Even then, this can be stated with conviction only if the disease appears fully excised.

The age specific prevalence of these apparently premalignant lesions supports the concept of progression towards malignancy. In the series of Qizilbash[35] the mean age of patients with AIS was 35.8 years, whereas those with early invasion had a mean age of 40.2 years suggesting that the in situ form precedes invasion by several years. Similar findings were reported by others[8] in relation to the gradient in age distribution of low-grade atypia, high-grade atypia and AIS, yet our data fail to confirm these findings.[36]

Further evidence of the invasive potential of lesions of lesser severity than AIS is extremely limited, being restricted to immunohistochemical studies linking GA to invasive adenocarcinoma.[37] A monoclonal antibody to HMFG1 (human milk fat globule antigen) was used to stain specimens of normal and abnormal cervices. The staining pattern found with cases of GA was similar to invasive adenocarcinoma, both of these staining patterns differing from normal cervical epithelium and microglandular hyperplasia of the cervix, a benign lesion which can be mistaken for CIGN by the inexperienced observer. There is no convincing evidence of progression of low degrees of endocervical atypia to higher grade lesions or to invasion.

'MICROINVASIVE'/EARLY INVASIVE ADENOCARCINOMA

While the existence of a microscopically invasive adenocarcinoma is not disputed, the concept and definition of a 'microinvasive' form of the disease has been much more difficult to substantiate than for squamous cancer. At this time, a universal definition of microinvasion does not exist, and current convention is not to use the term.[38]

In some cases where the term microinvasive adenocarcinoma has been used, the criteria used for arriving at this diagnosis have been unclear.[16] Qizilbash[35] regarded microinvasion to be present when there were foci in which there were back to back glands and gland extension below the normal depth of gland clefts, while others have stressed the importance of glandular budding with destruction of basement membrane and a stromal reaction.[32] None of these features are specific for invasive disease and even the presence of basement membrane can indicate malignancy. Teshima et al[10] defined 'early' adenocarcinoma as involving stromal invasion of 5 mm or less from the mucosal surface. However, radical hysterectomy was associated with recurrent disease in 1 of 30 patients where invasion was reported as 3 mm. Coppleson[39] has reported that 3 of 42 cases of 'early' invasive carcinoma (one with AIS and questionable superficial invasion, one with multifocal invasion <5 mm and the third with invasion to 1.8 mm) had either metastasized at diagnosis or experienced recurrent disease. The author has personally managed a case where the depth of penetration was reported as 2 mm, where lymph node metastasis had occured. Hence criteria for microinvasion based on depth of invasion appear to be inadequate either for diagnostic morphology or prognostication.

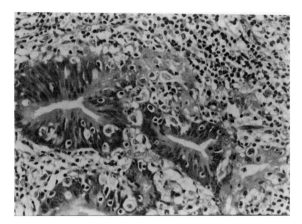

Fig. 20.5 A case of AIS/high-grade CIGN with foci of early stromal invasion.

It should be emphasized that difficulties often arise in the distinction between early invasive adenocarcinoma and AIS. This problem is usually encountered when AIS is florid, occupying most of the glandular field, and, in addition, when the specimen is difficult to orient or is insufficiently representative, e.g., punch biopsies.[40] We have observed features suggesting that there is an uncommon morphological equivalent of squamous early stromal invasion in glandular epithelium[41] (Fig. 20.5) though it seems unlikely that this morphological alteration precedes the development of most cases of invasive adenocarcinoma.

The clinician more than anyone else needs to understand that there may be subjectivity in the diagnosis of 'microinvasive' adenocarcinoma. In the absence of a uniform definition of early adenocarcinoma, clear guidelines on the management of these lesions are impossible to lay down at present. My personal practice is to manage these cases as if they were stage 1b carcinoma.

INCIDENCE

Unlike its squamous counterpart (CIN), comparitively little is known about the incidence of CIGN. However, it is an uncommon condition. Approximately 300 cases of AIS are described in the world literature. An incidence figure has not been calculated for this lesion; However, in an often quoted series,[16] the ratio of AIS to squamous carcinoma in situ was estimated as 1:239. Based on the experience of a single hospital laboratory with an interest in the condition, over the period 1983–1987 inclusive, the ratio of CIGN to CIN grades 2 and 3 was 1:88. (Buckley C H, personal communication) This somewhat lower ratio may be partly explained by the inclusion of lesser grades of atypia than AIS.

DETECTION OF CIGN

Cervical cytology

In the vast majority of cases described in the literature, the finding of AIS was an unexpected one following the treatment of women who had squamous dyskaryotic changes on cervical smears. Subsequent review of smears usually revealed some additional abnormalities thought to represent abnormal gland cells. The concept of cytologic screening for cervical adenocarcinoma was first proposed in 1976.[42] A retrospective examination was performed of the cervical smears of 13 women who had adenocarcinoma of the cervix. With the benefit of hindsight, it appeared that six of these women had abnormal smears at an interval of 2–8 years prior to diagnosis of invasion. This was assumed to provide evidence of a preinvasive lesion which is amenable to cytological detection.

Cytology appears to be the sole means of detecting this lesion, as it gives rise to no symptoms, and there are no accepted diagnostic colposcopic criteria.[17] Given the situation of CIGN within the endocervical canal (albeit close to the squamo-columnar junction) and the fact that many cervical smears fail to sample endocervical cells,[43] it appears that this lesion will be more difficult to detect than CIN using routine cervical cytology. Many will argue that if a cervical smear lacks the presence of endocervical or metaplastic cells, then the transformation zone has not been adequately sampled.[43] Accordingly, attention has been focused on endocervical columnar cells in cytologic smears. It is possible, though not proven, that a by-product of this awareness may be the detection of a higher rate of cytological abnormalities in glandular cells.[44] In Birmingham, between 1971 and 1978 there were 23 patients with a smear showing abnormal columnar cells of endo-cervical origin. Between 1980 and 1984, 119 such smears were encountered (unpublished data). The consensus view from the literature is that there is an undiagnosed reservoir of preinvasive disease.[8,17,45] which may be amenable to cytologic detection.

Krumins et al[46] described cytological criteria for the diagnosis of AIS in six cases. Later work[47] from the same center, described a larger series and modified the cytologic criteria for the diagnosis of AIS and 'early invasive' adenocarcinoma. These criteria were formulated on an experience of 19 cases of AIS, three cases of endocervical dysplasia, 19 cases of 'microadenocarcinoma' and 11 cases of overtly invasive adenocarcinoma.

To date, these diagnoses have been rarely made on cervical cytology in day to day practice, and although there are some data which support the existence of a clearly defined cytological diagnosis, the detection of such lesions by exfoliative cytology is not generally accepted. The exponents of cytodiagnosis[48] found one example of early endocervical adenocarcinoma or its precursors for every 12 000 smears examined. Just under half of these were from histologically confirmed AIS; i.e., approximately one case of AIS for every 25 000 smears examined. The rarity of this lesion explains why most of work supporting cytodiagnosis of glandular lesions is derived retrospectively, and there is a dearth of published work which apply cytologic criteria in prospective fashion.

The primary cytologic criteria for the diagnosis of AIS are:

a. the presence of short ribbons of tissue or clusters of cells, some showing glandular openings;
b. crowding of cells, with 'pseudostratification' of nuclei;
c. stripping of cytoplasm gives rise to an irregular edge to the sheets of cells — this is known as 'feathering.'

Using these criteria, 16/19 cases of AIS were correctly diagnosed. In a later publication from the same center,[49] it was stated that cytology made possible the distinction between well differentiated and poorly differentiated types of AIS on the basis of nuclear differences, and variant patterns of AIS were described. These were endocervical, endometrioid and intestinal. Cytology was said to correspond closely with histopathological findings. To date, no other group has reproduced these findings.

The Sydney group also believe that it is possible to distinguish cytologically between AIS and the conditions of endocervical dysplasia, early invasive and deeply invasive adenocarcinoma.[47,49] It must be recalled that the histological criteria of microinvasion are poorly defined, which makes for suspect cytological diagnosis. Even in expert hands, diagnostic accuracy appears to be less than 50%.[49] However, cytologic features associated with 'early invasion' appear to be abnormal chromatin clearing, nucleoli and occasionally a tumor diathesis. Obviously invasive tumors are characterized cytologically by: large cellular sheets, strips of tissue with marked crowding and loss of nuclear polarity. Large nuclei, oval or round with abnormal chromatin clearing and prominent nucleoli; tumor diathesis may be present.[48] In the series of Bousfield et al[12] by taking all 30 invasive lesions into consideration, only 43% were predicted correctly. An updated series[49] revealed an almost identical predictive value for diagnosis of a series of 'microinvasive' adenocarcinomas. These authors acknowledged that there was a tendency to overcall poorly differentiated AIS as invasive disease, and likewise in very inflammatory smears, difficulty in distinguishing neoplasia from reactive change was a problem. These findings tend to confirm the alternative opinion[32,50] that the exfoliative cytology of AIS and invasive glandular lesions does not differ in any major way.

Some smears demonstrate cytologic features intermediate between reactive changes and adenocarcinoma-in-situ. Goff et al[51] have defined these cases and investigated histopathological correlations. In the majority of cases, histological material was limited to colposcopically directed biopsies and endocervical curettage, which may significantly underestimate the prevalence of glandular lesions and no clinical follow up was presented. Clinically important cervical lesions were detected in 57%, ranging from mild dysplasia to microinvasive adenocarcinoma. Of the 51 women with cytological predictions of endocervical atypia, 26 had coexisting squamous abnormalities. In this subgroup, there was no cervical glandular pathology, but 70% had CIN. In the group with 'pure' endocervical atypia, 28% had glandular pathology, and 28% had CIN. There were no instances of glandular lesions of lesser grade than AIS. The overall incidence of glandular pathology in the study group was 11%, and 40% had CIN. Novotny et al[52] reported an increasing number of smears categorized as 'endocervical glandular dysplasia (EGD)', i.e., endocervical atypia less pronounced than AIS. These cases were temporally associated with the increased use of endocervical sampling devices. Fifty cases were reported, with histological follow-up which was comprehensive in 60% (i.e., cone biopsy or hysterectomy). In this subgroup, the most frequent histological finding was tubal metaplasia (66%). Glandular pathology was found in only 17% (invasion 7%, EGD/ AIS 10%) Based on this experience, these workers believed that reliable cytological criteria for AIS, invasion, and tubal metaplasia could be defined, which when applied to a blind reassessment of their material, led to a diagnostic accuracy of 93%. Specifically, tubal metaplasia was indicated by the presence of apical terminal bars with cilia. Cellular sheets appeared regular. Rosettes were rare, there was absence of feathering, and nuclei retained a basal location within cells. Mitoses were rarely observed and the smear background was typically clean. Other conditions which gave rise to an abnormal glandular smear included microglandular hyperplasia, CIN 3 with gland involvement, immature squamous metaplasia and reactive changes.

Further doubts concerning the specificity of diagnosis of glandular lesions have been expressed.[53] The Sydney group described their three false-positive diagnoses in a separate publication,[54] representing 2% of all their cytological diagnoses of CIGN or early invasive adenocarcinoma.

Some retrospective data are available from other centers. In the series of Nguyen et al,[32] 65% had a smear showing abnormal glandular cells. In a retrospective series from Birmingham,[17] the sensitivity of cytology was 71% for AIS and glandular atypia. The accuracy of a cytological prediction of AIS was assessed by Laverty et al.[55] Fifty-four predictions of AIS were made from 290 000 smears (1 case of AIS for every 5370 smears examined) and of these, 47 patients were fully investigated. Twenty cases of AIS were correctly predicted (positive predictive value 42.5%). However of the remaining 27 subjects, 14 had invasive adenocarcinoma, three adenosquamous carcinomas, one endometrial carcinoma and eight CIN 3 alone.

There is an obvious need for prospective studies of the cytological diagnosis of CIGN from more centers. Where attempts have been made at routine sampling of the endocervical canal with a brush smear in high risk patients, the effect has been to reduce the rate of inadequate and false negative smears.[56] In order to show an effect on the rate of diagnosis of CIGN much larger studies would be required.

Colposcopy

In a recent retrospective series[35] of CIGN, 27 patients were colposcoped. In 16 (59%) CIN only was suspected, in four colposcopy was thought to be normal; in five, invasion was suspected, and in two, the appearances were thought to be consistent with a glandular lesion, although diagnostic criteria were not specified. Colposcopic diagnosis in these two cases was likely to be biased by the cytologist's finding of glandular abnormality. On review of the literature, there are no established recognition criteria for these lesions[17,57] and it is likely that any associated colposcopic abnormalities are due to concomitant squamous CIN. Glandular epithelial dysplasias occur in an epithelium of single cell thickness. With this in mind, it seems unlikely that distinctive changes could be recognized with a low power microscope.

Some authors have employed endocervical curettage as a supplement to colposcopic examination. The diagnosis of AIS has rarely been made on endocervical curettage (ECC). Even a positive ECC result does not mean that all the affected tissue has been removed, and does not exclude the presence of an invasive lesion.

When a glandular lesion is suspected on cytology or limited cervical biopsy (punch biopsy) it is mandatory to proceed to a conization type biopsy of the cervix. It is often impossible to exclude the presence of invasion on the basis of lesser biopsies.[58]

MANAGEMENT

The majority of early studies advocate hysterectomy as definitive management of AIS. This recommendation is based on the belief that multifocal disease (i.e., skip lesions) can occur,[59] or that the proximal (uterine) portion of the endocervix can be a site for disease.[8] In addition, some concern has been voiced that lesions which were classified as in situ disease have in fact been invasive.[60] The clinician faced with a patient with cervical adenocarcinoma-in-situ has a considerable management dilemma, particularly if the patient is young and wishes to preserve her fertility.

Two groups of authors have argued that cervical AIS may be malignant despite its benign histological appearances.[60,61] Both recommend that pelvic lymph node sampling be carried out in the assessment of these lesions, quoting case histories of two patients who developed pelvic malignancy some years after hysterectomy which revealed only cervical AIS. It was hypothesized that occult lymphatic spread may have occurred despite apparently benign histology. The advocates of radical therapy are very much in a minority and their arguments are flawed when one considers that (i) there may have been an error in histological diagnosis: a recognized problem; and (ii) the patients in question may have had vaginal adenocarcinoma-in-situ in association with the cervical lesion.[62] Failure to recognize this lesion could in theory lead to pelvic 'recurrence' arising from failure to eradicate concomitant vaginal AIS, which progressed to invasion.

Qizilbash[35] reported that eight of his patients had disease-free margins at conization with no residual disease in hysterectomy specimens (one of these was a 'microinvasive' adenocarcinoma). Twelve patients in a later series[42] had conization prior to hysterectomy, and eight of these had residual disease in the hysterectomy specimen. However, these results failed to take account of cone biopsy dimensions or status of excision margins. Ostor et al[7] reported nine patients with AIS who had hysterectomy after conization. In six of these patients the margins of the cone were involved by disease, and four of these six had residual disease at hysterectomy. In three cases where conization demonstrated clear excision margins there was no residual disease at hysterectomy. On the basis of these data it was proposed that conization with disease-free margins may be adequate therapy for AIS. Luesley et al[17] reported 10 cases of hysterectomy following conization for AIS. In two cases with disease-free margins at conization, one specimen showed residual cervical disease. In eight patients with involved margins at conization, four instances of residual disease were found after hysterectomy. In this series, conization alone was successful management in 12 cases of AIS and GA after follow-up of 2–3 years. Hopkins et al[61] recognized that when cone biopsy margins were uninvolved, then residual disease was the exception. However, given that one of seven patients with disease-free margins on cone had residual disease in the subsequent hysterectomy specimen, they advocated hysterectomy. A meta-analysis of series reviewing the incidence of residual disease in hysterectomy specimens following conization is presented in Table 20.[7,9,17,35,36,44,57,58,61,63] Overall, there was a 15% incidence of residual disease at hysterectomy when cone margins were predicted as negative for AIS.

Recent evidence from histomorphometric studies indicates that cervical AIS is usually distributed in close relation to the cervical squamocolumnar junction[10,64–66] and 'skip' lesions are uncommon in the upper endocervical canal[51] and indeed multicentric disease is the exception[7,9] Nicklin et al[58] studied 34 cases of AIS and measured the proximal linear extent (PLE) of the lesion from the squamocolumnar junction. The mean PLE was 8.38 mm, range (1–25 cm) and the mean depth of involvement was 2.3 mm, range 0.5–6 mm. Interestingly the proximal extent of the lesion was positively correlated with age of the subject, with the majority of women under 36 years of age having < 10 mm PLE. This also implies that these neoplastic precursor lesions increase in volume prior to becoming invasive. These recent insights into the distribution of AIS lend support to the hypothesis that cone biopsy may be sufficient to eradicate the lesion in the majority of cases. Until recently, there have been no prospective data on the management of CIGN by conization, however we have recently reported the preliminary results of a prospective study of conization in the management of CIGN, which demonstrate that a cone biopsy with negative excision margins is associated with negative cytological follow-up in 83% of cases managed by conization alone after a median follow-up of 12 months.[36] Of those who developed abnormal

Table 20.1   Adenocarcinoma-in-situ: principle findings and recommendations for therapy

Reference	Number	Mean age	Margins (Cone biopsy)	Residual disease* (Hysterectomy)	Recommendation
63	5	46.7	5 free	1	Hysterectomy
35	7	35.8	0	0	Hysterectomy
45	16	42	Not reported	8/12	Hysterectomy
7	21	38	6/9 involved	4/6	Cone biopsy
			3/9 free	0/3	(Hysterectomy if cone margins involved)
17	31	36	8/10 involved	4/8	Cone ⩾ 25 mm
			2/10 free	1/2	length
9	5	—	1 involved	0/1	Cone biopsy
			4 uninvolved	0/4	⩾ 25 mm
61	18	37	5 involved	4/5	Hysterectomy,
			7 uninvolved	1/7	+lymph node sampling
57	36	36	4 involved	0/4	Cone biopsy
58	34	36.4	12 involved	5/11	Cone biopsy, 25 mm
			22 uninvolved	2/11	
36	51	35.7	8 involved	1/8	Cone biopsy, 25 mm
			42 uninvolved	0/2	
			1 indeterminate		

*Combined incidence of residual disease in hysterectomy specimens after cone with negative margins = 5/34 (15%).
Combined incidence of residual disease in hysterectomy specimens after cone with positive margins = 18/43 (42%).

cytology after apparent complete excision of CIGN, there has been one case of CIN 3, and one of CIN 1, but no glandular abnormalities. The findings clearly require confirmation by longer term follow-up.

CONCLUSIONS

Cervical adenocarcinoma may be assuming more importance because of postulated increases in incidence of this disease. The potential for diagnosis at the preinvasive stage exists. The natural history of the disease is by no means certain, yet there is considerable circumstantial evidence that high-grade intraepithelial lesions are premalignant. Cytological recognition is possible but more research is needed in order to validate and perhaps improve cytological recognition of this disorder, and it is clear that the outcome of this research will determine whether we can successfully screen for adenocarcinoma. Clinical management of in situ lesions is veering towards a more conservative approach, with conization being recommended increasingly frequently as primary therapy. This approach may be of most relevance to those wishing to preserve their fertility.

REFERENCES

1. Peters R K, Chao A, Mack T M, Thomas D, Bernstein L, Henderson B E. Increased frequency of adenocarcinoma of the uterine cervix in young women in Los Angeles county. J Nat Cancer Inst 1986; 76: 423–428.
2. Schwartz S M, Weiss N S. Increased incidence of adenocarcinoma of the cervix in young women in the United States. Am J Epidemiol 1986; 124 (6): 1045–1047.
3. Davis J R, Moon L B. Increased incidence of adenocarcinoma of the uterine cervix. Obstet Gynaecol 1975; 45 (1): 79–83.
4. Vesterinen E, Forss M, Nieminen U. Increase of cervical adenocarcinoma: a report of 520 cases of cervical carcinoma including 112 tumours with glandular elements. Gynaecol Oncol 1989; 33: 49–53.
5. Benda J A, Platz C E, Buchsbaum H, Lifshitz S. Mucin production in defining mixed carcinoma of the uterine cervix: A clinicopathologic study. Int J Gynaecol Pathol 1985; 4: 314–327.
6. Friedell G H, McKay D G. Adenocarcinoma in situ of the endocervix. Cancer 1953; 6: 887–897.
7. Ostor A G, Pagano R, Davoren R A M, Fortune D W, Chanen W, Rome R. Adenocarcinoma in situ of the cervix. Int J Gynecol Pathol 1984; 3: 179–190.
8. Brown L J R, Wells M. Cervical glandular atypia associated with squamous intraepithelial neoplasia; a premalignant lesion? J Clin Pathol 1986; 39: 22–28.
9. Bertrand M, Lickrish G M, Colgan T J. The anatomic distribution of cervical adenocarcinoma-in-situ: implications for treatment. Am J Obstet Gynecol 1987; 157: 21–25.
10. Teshima S, Shimosato Y, Kishi K, Kasamatsu T, Ohmi K, Uei Y. Early stage adenocarcinoma of the uterine cervix: histopathologic analysis with consideration of histogenesis. Cancer 1985; 56: 167–172.
11. Gloor E, Hurlimann J. Cervical intraepithelial glandular neoplasia (adenocarcinoma in situ and glandular dysplasia): A correlative study of 23 cases with histologic grading, histochemical analysis of mucins, and immunohistochemical determination of the affinity for four lectins. Cancer 1986; 58: 1272–1280.
12. Van Roon E, Boon M E, Kurver P J H, Baak J P A. The association between pre cancerous columnar and squamous lesions of the cervix; A morphometric study. Histopathology 1983; 7: 887–896.
13. Richart R. Natural history of cervical intraepithelial neoplasia. Clinical Obstet Gynecol 1967; 10: 748–784.
14. Ehsanullah M, Naunton-Morgan M, Filipe M I, Gazzard B. Sialomucins in the assessment of dysplasia and cancer risk patients with ulcerative colitis treated with colectomy and ileo-rectal anastomosis. Histopathology 1985; 9: 223–235.
15. Montero C, Segura D I. Retrospective histochemical study of mucosubstances in adenocarcinomas of the gastrointestinal tract. Histopathology, 1980; 4: 281–291.
16. Gloor E, Ruzicka J. Morphology of adenocarcinoma in situ of the uterine cervix; a study of 14 cases. Cancer 1982; 49: 294–302.
17. Luesley D M, Jordan J A, Woodman C B J, Watson N, Williams D R, Waddell C. A retrospective review of adenocarcinoma-in-situ and glandular atypia of the uterine cervix. British J Obstet Gynecol 1987; 94: 699–703.
18. Boon M E, Kirk R S, Rietveld — Scheffers P E M. The morphogenesis of adenocarcinoma of the cervix — a complex pathological entity. Histopathology 1981; 5: 565–577.
19. Cullimore J E. Prospects for primary and secondary prevention of cervical adenocarcinoma. M D thesis. University of London, 1991.
20. Dallenbach-Hellweg G. On the origin and histological structure of adenocarcinoma of the endocervix in women under 50 years of age. Pathol Res Practice 1984; 179: 38–50.
21. Valente P T, Hanjani P. Endocervical neoplasia in long term users of oral contraceptives: Clinical and pathologic observations. Obstet Gynecol 1986; 67: 695–704.
22. Jones M W, Silverberg S G. Cervical adenocarcinoma in young women: possible relationship to microglandular hyperplasia and use of oral contraceptives. Obstet Gynecol 1989; 73 (6): 984–989.
23. Okagaki T, Tase T, Twiggs L B L, Carson L F. Histogenesis of cervical adenocarcinoma with reference to humanpapillomavirus-18 as a co-carcinogen. J Reprod Med 1989; 34 (9): 639–644.

24. Tase T, Okagaki T, Clark B, Manias D A, Ostrow R S, Twiggs L B, Faras A J. Human papillomavirus types and localisation in adenocarcinoma and adenosquamous carcinoma of the uterine cervix: A study by in situ DNA hybridisation. Cancer Res 1988; 48: 993–998.

25. Farnsworth A, Laverty C, Stoler M H. Human papillomavirus messenger RNA expression in adenocarcinoma-in-situ of the uterine cervix. Int J Gynaecol Pathol 1989; 8 (4): 321–330.

26. Tase T, Okagaki T, Clark B, Twiggs L B, Ostrow R S, Faras A J. Human papillomavirus DNA in glandular dysplasia and microglandular hyperplasia: presumed precursors of adenocarcinoma of the uterine cervix. Obstet Gynecol 1989; 73 (6): 1005–1008.

27. Stoler M H, Rhodes C R, Whitbeck A, Wolinsky S M, Chow L T, Broker T R. Human papillomavirus type 16 and 18 gene expression in cervical neoplasias. Human Pathol 1992; 23 (2): 117–128.

28. Leary J, Jaworski R, Houghton R. In situ hybridisation using biotyylated DNA probes to Human Papillomavirus in adenocarcinoma in situ and endocervical glandular dysplasia of the uterine cervix. Pathology 1991; 23: 85–89.

29. Cullimore J E, Rollason T P R, Marshall T. Nucleolar organiser regions in adenocarcinoma in situ of the endocervix. J Clin Pathol 1989; 42 (12): 1276–1280.

30. Delgidisch I, Escay — Martinez E, Cohen C J. Endocervical adenocarcinoma: A study of 23 patients with clinical — pathological correlation. Gynecol Oncol 1984; 18: 326–333.

31. Abell M R A, Gosling J R G. Gland cell carcinoma (adenocarcinoma) of the uterine cervix. Am J Obstet Gynecol 1962; 83: 729–755.

32. Nguyen G K, Jeannot A B. Exfoliative cytology of in-situ and microinvasive adenocarcinoma of the uterine cervix. Acta Cytol 1983; 28 (4): 461–467.

33. Obata N, Sasaki A, Takeuchi S, Ishiguro Y. Clinico-pathologic study on the early diagnosis of cervical adenocarcinoma. Nippon Sanka Fujinka Gakkai Zasshi 1987; 39 (5): 771–776 (English abstract).

34. Fu Y S, Berek J S, Hilborne L H. Diagnostic problems of in situ and invasive carcinomas of the uterine cervix. Appl Pathol 1987; 5 (1): 47–56.

35. Qizilbash A H. In situ and microinvasive adenocarcinoma of the uterine cervix. A clinical, cytologic and histologic study of 14 cases. Am J Clin Pathol 1975; 64: 155–170.

36. Cullimore J E, Luesley D M, Rollason T P et al. A prospective study of conisation in the management of cervical intraepithelial glandular neoplasia (CIGN) — a preliminary report. Br J Obstet Gynaecol 1992; 99: 314–318.

37. Brown L J R, Griffin N R, Wells M. Cytoplasmic reactivity with monoclonal antibody HMFG1 as a marker of cervical glandular atypia. J Pathol 1987; 151: 203–208.

38. Yeh I, Tien Li, Volsi V A, Noumoff J S. Endocervical carcinoma. Pathol Res Practice 1991; 187: 129–144.

39. Coppleson M. Gynecologic oncology, vol 1. London: Churchill Livingstone, 1992; pp 643–644.

40. Pickel H, Natural history of adenocarcinoma of the cervix uteri. J Exper Clin Cancer Res 1990; 9 (1) (Supplement): L 172.

41. Rollason T R P, Cullimore J E, Bradgate M. A suggested columnar cell morphological equivalent of squamous carcinoma-in-situ with early stromal invasion. Int J Gynecol Pathol 1989; 8 (3): 230–236.

42. Boddington M M, Spriggs A I, Cowdell R H. Adenocarcinoma of the uterine cervix; Cytological evidence of a long pre-clinical evolution. Br J Obstet Gynaecol 1976; 83: 900–903.

43. Gondos B, Marshall D, Ostergard D R. Endocervical cells in cervical smears. American J Obstet Gynecol 1972; 110: 833–835.

44. Boon M E, Alons van Kordelaar J M, Rietveld — Scheffers P E M. Consequences of the introduction of the combined spatula and cytobrush sampling for cervical cytology. Acta Cytol 1986; 30 (3): 264–270.

45. Christopherson W M, Nealon N, Gray L A. Non-invasive precursor lesions of adenocarcinoma and mixed adenosquamous carcinoma of the cervix uteri. Cancer 1979; 44: 975–983.

46. Krumins I, Young Q, Pacey F, Bousfield L, Mulhearn L. The cytologic diagnosis of adenocarcinoma in situ of the cervix uteri. Acta Cytol 1977; 21 (2): 320–329.

47. Bousfield L, Pacey F, Young Q, Krumins I, Osborn R. Expanded cytologic criteria for the diagnosis of adenocarcinoma in situ of the uterine cervix and related lesions. Acta Cytol 1980; 24 (4): 283–296.

48. Ayer B, Pacey F, Greenberg M. The cytologic diagnosis of Adenocarcinoma in situ of the cervix uteri and related lesions. 1. Adenocarcinoma in situ. Acta Cytol 1987; 31 (4): 397–411.

49. Ayer B, Pacey F, Greenberg M. The cytologic diagnosis of Adenocarcinoma in situ of the cervix uteri and related lesions. 11. Microinvasive adenocarcinoma. Acta Cytol 1988; 32 (3): 318–324.

50. Betsill W L, Clark A H. Early endocervical glandular neoplasia; 1 Histomorphology and cytomorphology. Acta Cytol 1986; 30 (2): 115–126.

51. Goff B A, Atanasoff P, Brown E, Muntz H C, Bell D A, Rice L W. Endocervical glandular atypia in Papanicolau smears. Obstet Gynecol 1992; 79 (1): 101–104.

52. Novotny D B, Maygarden S J, Johnson D E, Frable W J. Tubal metaplasia. A frequent potential pitfall in the cytologic diagnosis of endocervical glandular dysplasia on cervical smears. Acta Cytol 1992; 1: 1–10.

53. Lee K R. False positive diagnosis of adenocarcinoma-in-situ of the cervix. Acta Cytol 1988; 32 (2): 276–277.

54. Pacey F, Ayer B, Greenberg M. The cytologic diagnosis of Adenocarcinoma in situ of the cervix uteri and related lesions. 111 Pitfalls in diagnosis. Acta Cytol 1988; 32 (3): 325–333.

55. Laverty C R, Farnsworth A, Thurloe J, Bowditch R. The reliability of a cytological prediction of cervical adenocarcinoma-in-situ. Aus NZ J Obstet Gynaecol 1988; 28 (4): 307–312.

56. Van Erp E J, Blaschek-Lut C H, Arentz N P, Trimbos J B. Performance of the cytobrush in patients at risk for cervical pathology: does it add anything to the wooden spatula. Eur J Gynecol Oncol 1988; 9 (6): 456–460.

57. Andersen E S, Arffmann E. Adenocarcinoma-in-situ of the uterine cervix; A clinico-pathologic study of 36 cases. Gynecol Oncol 1989; 35: 1–7.

58. Nicklin J L, Wright R G, Bell J R et al. A clinicopathological study of adenocarcinoma in situ of the cervix. The influence of cervical HPV infection and other factors, and the role of conservative surgery. Aus NZ J Obstet Gynaecol 1991; 31 (2): 179–183.

59. Wells M, Brown L J R. Glandular lesions of the uterine cervix: the present state of our knowledge. Histopathology 1986; 10: 777–792.

60. Buscema J, Woodruff J D. Significance of neoplastic abnormalities in endocervical epithelium. Gynecol Oncol 1984; 17: 356–362.

61. Hopkins M P, Roberts J A, Schmidt R W. Cervical adenocarcinoma in situ. Obstet Gynecol 1988; 71: 842–844.

62. Cullimore J E, Rollason T P R, Luesley D M, Waddell C, Williams D. A case of glandular intraepithelial neoplasia of the cervix and vagina. Gynecol Oncol 1989; 34 (2): 249–252.

63. Jaworski R C, Pacey N F, Greenberg M L, Osborn R A. The histologic diagnosis of Adenocarcinoma in situ and related lesions of the cervix uteri. Cancer 1988; 61: 1171–1181.

64. Matsukama K, Tsukamoto N, Tsunehisakaku N et al. Early adenocarcinoma of the uterine cervix. Its histologic and immunologic study. Gynecol Oncol 1989; 35: 38–43.

65. Tobon H, Dave H. Adenocarcinoma in situ of the cervix: Clinicopathologic observations of 11 cases. Int J Gynecol Pathol 1988; 7 (2): 139–151

66. Weisbrot I M, Stabinsky C, Davis A M. Adenocarcinoma in situ of the uterine cervix. Cancer 1972; 29 (5): 1179–1187.

21. Cervical disease in HIV-infected women: prevalence, pathogenesis, detection, and treatment

Thomas C. Wright

INTRODUCTION

Over the last decade, human immunodeficiency virus (HIV) infection has reached epidemic proportions in the USA and much of the world. Even though estimates of the prevalence of HIV infections are relatively inaccurate due to methodological problems relating to the acquisition and interpretation of the data, the magnitude of the problem is illustrated by recent World Health Organization (WHO) data estimating that 13 million men, women and children have been infected with the virus worldwide and that by the year 2000, this number will increase to almost 40 million.[1] WHO estimates that the number of infected individuals is increasing by 5000 per day. Currently, between 800 000 and 1 200 000 Americans are estimated to be infected with HIV, and women account for approximately 10% of those infected.[2,3] Women are the fastest growing segment of the HIV-infected population in both the USA and the world. In 1990, it was estimated that approximately 25% of those infected with HIV were women, whereby in 1992, it was thought to be at least 40%.[4] On a worldwide basis, it is expected that, in the near future, the number of women who are infected with HIV will surpass that of men.[5] The Center for Disease Control and Prevention, Atlanta, GA (CDC) has recently estimated that in the USA there will be 50 000–60 000 patients with acquired immunodeficiency syndrome (AIDS), as defined using the 1987 AIDS surveillance case definition in the USA in 1993, and an additional 120 000–190 000 people will have profound immunosuppression.[6,7] Using the new (1993) expanded case definition of AIDS, this latter group is also classified as having AIDS.[8] If 10% of these AIDS patients are female, there will be approximately 6000 cases of AIDS in women in 1993 as defined using the 1987 AIDS surveillance case definition. An additional 12 000–19 000 women will have profound immunosuppression.

The figures from New York City are even more alarming (Table 21.1). One percent of women enrolled in prenatal care in New York City in 1991 were estimated to be HIV infected. Other groups of women have an even higher rate of HIV infection. The prevalence of HIV infection has been estimated to be 3.3% in runaway teenage girls, 6.4% in women attending city-run STD clinics, 24% in women entering prison for the first time, and 53% in women enrolled in methadone maintenance programs in New York City (Table 21.1) (Chiasson M, personal communication).[9]

The prevalence of HIV seropositivity in the USA varies widely depending on geographic location. In the 1993 CDC AIDS Surveillance Report, the rates of AIDS per 100 000 women varied from 74.5 in the District of Columbia, 36 in Puerto Rico and 48.2 in New York state, to 0 per 100 000 women in North Dakota and 1.4 in Iowa and 1.5

Table 21.1 Prevalence of HIV-infection in selected groups of New York City women in 1991*

Population	Number tested	% HIV-infected
Prenatal care	32 896	1.1
Runaway youth	1928	3.3
STD patients	17 920	6.4
Entering prison	1065	24.1
Methadone maintenance	2223	53

*Table based on data obtained from Dr Mary Ann Chiasson, Bureau of Disease Intervention Research, New York City Department of Health.

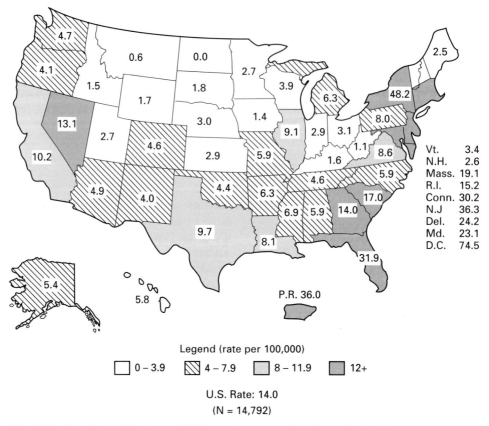

Fig. 21.1 Female adult/adolescent AIDS annual rates per 100 000 population, for cases reported October 1992 through September 1993, USA. Figure reproduced from the HIV/AIDS Surveillance Report, Issued October 1993, Vol. 5, No. 3.

in Idaho (Fig. 21.1). Moreover, within a given geographic location, the prevalence varies widely depending on race, ethnicity and the presence of other risk factors. The prevalence is greatest among minority women. Fifty-nine percent of the women diagnosed as AIDS in 1993 were black and 25% were Hispanic. AIDS continues to disproportionately affect inner-city minority and intravenous drug using women living in urban areas of the northeast. It is important to note, however, that in the USA, the current rate of increase in persons who become infected with HIV through heterosexual contact is greater than that of persons who become infected through either intravenous drug use or male homosexual or bisexual contact, and it is clear that HIV infection is no longer restricted to inner city, minority and i.v. drug-using women.[6]

IMMUNOSUPPRESSION AND CERVICAL CANCER

It is now well-established that women who are immunosuppressed for reasons other than for HIV infection are at increased risk for developing intraepithelial squamous neoplasia and invasive squamous cell carcinomas of the anogenital tract.[10] This has been best established for women taking immunosuppressive medications for organ transplantation, but has also been observed in women with lesser degrees of immunosuppression such as those with Hodgkin's disease. This has led to widespread concern that HIV-infected women will be at particularly high risk for developing anogenital neoplasia.[11–13] Moreover, many HIV-infected women would be expected to have other epidemiological risk factors for the development of invasive cervical cancer and human papillomavirus (HPV) infection, including multiple sexual partners, sex with high risk males, young age of first sex, smoking of cigarettes, low socioeconomic status, and poor compliance with recommended cytologic cervical cancer screening.[14] High rates of anogenital HPV infections and anal intraepithelial neoplasia (dysplasia) have also been reported in HIV-infected homosexual men and anal carcinomas may also be increased in this population.[15–18]

ASSOCIATIONS BETWEEN HIV-INFECTION AND CERVICAL DISEASE

The first report linking cervical intraepithelial neoplasia (CIN) to HIV infection to cervical disease in 11 women was published from a London HIV clinic in 1987.[19] In this study, cytologic screening was performed in 11 HIV-infected women and 8 (73%) had an abnormal smear. Colposcopy was performed on nine of the women and five had biopsy-proven CIN. Two of these cases were high grade. Subsequently, a number other studies were published reporting a high prevalence of CIN in HIV-infected women (Table 21.2). In these other studies, the prevalence of CIN ranged from 17% in women who had acquired HIV through either artificial insemination or blood transfusion to 27% in groups of i.v. drug users.[22] The significance of these early reports was unclear, however, since they were based on relatively small numbers of HIV-infected women, and these studies lacked appropriate control groups.[23]

Subsequently, an association between invasive cervical cancer and HIV infection was suggested

Table 21.2 Early studies assessing the prevalence of CIN in HIV-infected women*

Reference	Method	Number of HIV-infected women	Number (%) with CIN
Bradbeer et al.	Colposcopy	9	5 (56)
Byrne et al.	Cytology	15	4 (27)
Crocchiolo et al.	Colposcopy	24	6 (25)
Spurrett et al.	Colposcopy	6	1 (17)

* Table based on data from references (Bradbeer, 1987),[19] (Byrne et al, 1988),[20] (Crocchiolo et al, 1988),[21] (Spurrett et al, 1988)[22]

by two case reports of rapidly progressive invasive cervical cancers in young HIV-infected women. One of these reports described a 32-year-old woman who had a moderate to poorly differentiated, International Federation of Gynecologists and Obstetricians (FIGO) stage 2B, invasive squamous cell carcinoma. This 32-year-old developed a tumor relapse at a periclitoral site and disseminated carcinomatosis 2 months after radiation therapy.[24] Although she received chemotherapy with cisplatin, bleomycin, and mitomycin C, the patient died less than 5 months after beginning therapy. The other report described a 25-year-old woman with a FIGO stage 3B squamous cell carcinoma of the cervix, who, despite the fact she received neoadjuvant chemotherapy with vincristine, bleomycin, cis-platinum and an adequate course of external beam radiation therapy, died within 5 months of being diagnosed.[25] This patient also developed a metastasis to an unusual site, the iliopsoas muscle.

Soon after these two case reports appeared, Mitchell Maiman and coworkers at the State University of New York (SUNY) at Brooklyn published two separate papers on the prevalence of HIV infection among women under the age of 50 diagnosed with invasive cervical cancer at their institution. The prevalence of HIV infection was 19% in women under the age of 50 years who were diagnosed with invasive cervical cancer.[26] Although the HIV-seropositivity rate of women in their hospital's catchment area was not given, it would be expected to be considerably less than the 19% detected in the women with invasive cervical cancer. Another finding of concern was that many of the HIV-infected women were young and were asymptomatic with regards to their HIV infection. One of the patients was only 16 years old, but had a stage 2B squamous cell carcinoma. Many of the tumors in the HIV-seropositive group were high stage, bulky lesions and the patients had a poor outcome. Sixty-eight of the HIV-infected women died, and the mean interval until death was only 9.2 months. Taken together, the report from Brooklyn, as well as the individual case reports, confirm that invasive cervical cancer can develop in HIV-infected women. When these cancers develop, they tend to be high stage, aggressive lesions, and gynecological oncologists have observed that they respond poorly to therapy.

On the basis of these reports, the CDC recently included invasive cervical cancer as an AIDS case defining illness in the 1993 Expanded Surveillance Case Definition of AIDS. It should be noted, however, that those reports are from highly selected populations and may not be representative of the impact that cervical cancer is having on HIV-infected women as a whole. When considering the impact cervical cancer is having on HIV-infected populations, it should be noted that other studies, from both the USA and Africa, indicate that invasive cervical cancer is not a major cause of morbidity or mortality in HIV-infected women at the current time since the prevalence of cervical cancer appears to be quite low in various groups of HIV-infected women. Numerous studies (Table 12.3) have screened large groups of HIV-infected women for cervical cancer using either Papanicolaou (Pap) smears or colposcopy, and most have failed to detect invasive cervical cancer among the women who were screened. The studies from the USA have examined over 810 HIV-infected women, in aggregate, without detecting a single case of invasive cervical cancer. In our clinical experience with screening more than 500 HIV-infected women using colposcopy and Pap smears, we have not detected a single case of invasive cervical cancer although we have had a number of HIV-infected women with invasive cervical cancer referred to us for treatment. Similarly, the published studies from Africa involving over 288 HIV-infected women, as well as an Italian study that screened 161 HIV-infected women using colposcopy and Pap smears, found identical results.[32,35-37] The only study of this type that has detected invasive cervical cancers in the HIV-infected women who were screened was by Axel Schafer from Berlin.[33] This study found five cases of invasive cervical cancer among 111 women who were screened for cervical disease. It should be noted, however, that this study recruited women from among those hospitalized at a large Berlin teaching hospital for gynecological disease. This enrollment protocol may have produced a significant biasing of the sample towards women with cervical disease.

Other data also indicate that invasive cervical cancer is not currently affecting large numbers of HIV-infected women in Africa. In a study from Kenya, Rogo and Linge tested 200 consecutive women with invasive cervical cancer for HIV and found that only 1.5% were HIV-seropositive compared to 2% of other groups, such as Kenyan blood donors.[38] Similar findings have been reported from Tanzania where only 3% of women diagnosed with invasive cervical cancer were HIV-infected, compared to 13% of age-matched women attending the general gynecological clinics at the same hospital.[39] With respect to the USA, an analysis of death rates from invasive cervical cancer in northern New Jersey and New York state has failed to detect any increase in death rate from invasive cervical cancer through 1988. This represents a period of time during which the death

Table 21.3 Prevalence of cervical cancer in HIV-infected women*

Reference	Country	Population studied	Number of HIV-infected woman	Number of cancers
Carpenter et al.	USA	HIV clinic	100	0
Korn et al.	USA	HIV clinic	52	0
Provencher et al.	USA	Voluntary HIV testing	213	0
Vermund et al.	USA	Methadone maintenance	47	0
Wright et al.	USA	HIV and methadone clinics	398	0
Conti et al.	Italy	Former IVDU/s	161	0
Schafer et al.	Germany	Prostitutes	111	5
Smith et al.	UK	HIV and methadone clinics	43	0
Kreiss et al.	Kenya	Prostitutes	141	0
Laga et al.	Zaire	Prostitutes	41	0
Maggwa et al.	Kenya	Family planning	205	0

* Table based on data from references (Carpenter et al, 1991),[27] (Korn et al, 1994),[28] (Provencher et al, 1988),[29] (Vermund et al, 1991),[30] (Wright et al, 1994),[31] (Conti et al, 1993),[32] (Schafer et al, 1991),[33] (Smith et al, 1993),[34] (Kreiss et al, 1992),[35] (Laga et al, 1992),[36] (Maggwa et al, 1993)[37]

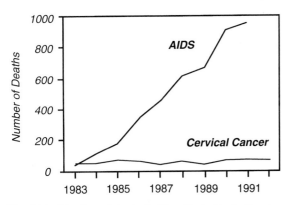

Fig. 21.2 Number of deaths in New York City in females 15 years or older attributed to AIDS or invasive cervical cancer. Data courtesy of Dr Mary Ann Chiasson, Bureau Disease Intervention, New York City Department of Health.

rate from other HIV-associated tumors such as non-Hodgkin's lymphoma and Kaposi's sarcoma was increasing in women.[40] Data from New York City have also failed to detect an increase in the number of deaths from invasive cervical cancer between 1980 and 1993, a time during which there was a dramatic increase in the number of female deaths attributed to AIDS (Fig. 21.2) (Chiasson M, personal communication).

There is considerably more data demonstrating an association between HIV infection and the development of CIN than there is for invasive cancer.[23] Despite the limitations of the early cytologic studies looking at associations between HIV infection and CIN, their conclusions were correct since they have now been confirmed by larger, controlled studies. One of the first of the large controlled studies on this subject compared the results of Pap smears in 201 HIV-seropositive women to those of 213 HIV-seronegative women

who had requested HIV serotesting (Table 21.4). This study which was published by Provencher et al[29] from Miami found that 63% of the HIV-infected group had an abnormal Pap smear whereas only 5% of the HIV-seronegative group had an abnormal Pap smear. In a review of cytologic findings in HIV-infected women, Marte et al[41] reported abnormal Pap smear rates that varied from 23 to 48% in HIV-infected women, with an overall abnormal Pap smear rate of 26% in the 135 women reviewed. Similarly, Vermund et al[30] studied HIV-infected and uninfected women enrolled from a methadone maintenance program in the South Bronx. They reported that 33% of the HIV-infected women had cytologic evidence of CIN, compared to 13% of the HIV-uninfected women. A high prevalence of cytologic abnormalities has also been reported in HIV-infected African women. Laga et al[36] found that 27% of HIV-infected prostitutes enrolled from Kinshasha, Zaire had an abnormal Pap smear, compared to 3% of a control group of HIV-uninfected prostitutes. A study from Nairobi, Kenya analyzed Pap smears from 4058 women enrolled in two family planning clinics, and found that 5% of the HIV-infected women had a cytological diagnosis of CIN, compared to 2% of HIV-uninfected women.[37]

Because the studies listed in Table 21.4 used cytology to determine whether or not cervical disease was present, they could have either underestimated the prevalence of cervical disease in the HIV-infected group, if the false-negative rate of cytology were unusually increased in the population, or alternatively, overestimated the prevalence of cervical disease in the presence of severe cervicovaginal infections in the HIV-infected

Table 21.4 Prevalence of cytologic abnormalities in HIV-infected women*

Reference	Country	Population studied	Number of seropositive women	% Abnormal smears	Number of seronegative women	% Abnormal smears
Marte et al.	USA	HIV clinics	135	26	Ambulatory clinics	6
Provencher et al.	USA	Requesting screening	201	63	213	5
Vermund et al.	USA	Methadone clinic	51	33	49	13
Smith et al.	UK	HIV and methadone	43	35	43	19
Laga et al.	Zaire	Prostitutes	41	27	41	3
Maggwa et al.	Kenya	Family planning	205	5	3853	2

* Table based on data from references (Marte et al, 1992),[41] (Provencher et al, 1988),[29] (Vermund, 1991),[30] (Smith et al, 1993),[34] (Laga et al, 1992),[36] (Maggwa et al, 1993)[37]

group, which could have resulted in the misinterpretation of reparative/inflammatory changes as CIN. To overcome these potential misclassification problems, two recent series have used colposcopy to determine the presence of cervical disease in HIV-infected women and compared the prevalence in the HIV-infected group to that of various control groups. Both of these studies have confirmed the results of the previous cytological studies in that a higher prevalence of CIN was detected in the HIV-infected women than in the control group. In the largest of these studies, which is a multicenter study based in the greater New York City area called the New York Cervical Disease Study, HIV-infected women were enrolled from a variety of clinical sites including HIV/AIDS clinics, STD clinics and methadone maintenance treatment programs. HIV-uninfected control women were enrolled from sexually transmitted disease (STD) clinics and methadone clinics. All women underwent colposcopy, a Pap smear and HPV DNA testing at their study visit. CIN was detected in 80 (20%) of 398 HIV-infected women enrolled in this study, compared to 15 (4%) of 357 HIV-uninfected women (odds ratio (OR), 5.7; $P < 0.001$) (Table 21.5).[31] Because colposcopy and cervical biopsy were used to determine whether CIN was present, the grade of CIN could be determined. Two-thirds of the HIV-infected women with CIN had low-grade CIN (CIN 1), and one-third had high-grade CIN (CIN 2–3). Another study from Italy that also used colposcopy in a cohort of 434 former i.v. drug users found an even higher percentage of biopsy-confirmed CIN than did the New York Cervical Disease Study. Thirteen (8%) of 161 HIV-uninfected women in

the Italian study had biopsy-confirmed CIN compared to 115 (42%) of the HIV-infected women.[32] Fifty-one percent of the CIN lesions were high-grade CIN (CIN 2–3) in the Italian study.

Taken together, the studies described above clearly indicate that an 'epidemic of invasive cervical cancer' has not yet developed among HIV-infected women and, that compared to opportunistic infections such as *Pneumocystic carinii*, invasive cervical cancer currently effects relatively small numbers of HIV-infected women. However, it is also clear that there is a very high prevalence of cervical cancer precursors (CIN) in this population and that many of these lesions are high grade. Therefore, the failure to detect invasive cervical cancers at the current time may be due to the fact that most HIV-infected women die of opportunistic infections before they can develop cervical cancer. This situation may change, however, as immunosuppressed HIV-infected women begin to live longer as a result of improved antiretroviral therapies and prophylaxis against opportunistic infections. As immunosuppressed HIV-infected women begin to live longer, cervical cancer may become more common.

PATHOGENESIS OF CERVICAL DISEASE IN HIV-INFECTED WOMEN

The pathogenesis of CIN in women in the general population is now established. Epidemiological studies have identified a number of possible risk factors for the development of CIN which include early age at first intercourse, early age of first pregnancy, large number of sexual partners, a history of cigarette smoking, prolonged interval

Table 21.5 Prevalence of biopsy-confirmed CIN in HIV-infected women enrolled in New York cervical disease study

Cervical disease status	Number (%) of HIV-seropositive women	Number (%) of HIV-seronegative women
No evidence of CIN	253 (64)	307 (86)
Indeterminate for CIN**	65 (16)	35 (10)
Low-grade CIN (CIN 1)	52 (13)	13 (4)
High-grade CIN (CIN 2–3)	28 (7)	2 (1)
Total number of women	398 (100)	357 (100)

* Table based on data from reference (Wright et al, 1994)[31]
** Indeterminate for cervical disease includes women with low-grade cytologic abnormalities who did not have any colposcopically observable lesions or who had a minor-grade cytologic abnormality and refused cervical biopsy.

since the last Pap smear and a history of abnormal Pap smears, as well as nutritional variables, immunosuppression and infection with specific types of human papillomavirus (i.e., types 16 and 18).[14,42,43] The two most important independent risk factors in recent case control studies of CIN have been history of cigarette smoking and lifetime number of sexual partners.[44,45]

To better define the pathogenesis of CIN in HIV-infected women, we have collected demographic information and information on the standard epidemiological risk factors for CIN and HPV DNA in 245 HIV-seropositive and 235 HIV-seronegative women enrolled in our ongoing New York City based study of cervical disease in HIV-seropositive women.[31,46] In this study, the overall prevalence of biopsy-confirmed CIN was approximately five times greater in the HIV-infected than in the HIV-uninfected women (Table 21.5). The HIV-seropositive and HIV-seronegative groups were similar with regards to age, race, income, education, gravidity, age at first intercourse, condom and oral contraceptive use, current smoking history and previous Pap smear screening history. There were, however, significant differences between the HIV-infected and HIV-uninfected groups with regards to number of lifetime sexual partners, history of i.v. drug use, prostitution and herpes simplex infections; all of which were increased in the HIV-infected women.[31,46]

The number of lifetime sexual partners, as well as other covariables that are a common feature of the population that has early, multiple sexual contacts, are now thought to act as surrogates for exposure to human papillomavirus, which is considered to be the primary etiologic agent in the multifactorial pathogenesis of both CIN and cervical cancer.[11,47] Therefore, we assayed cervicovaginal lavages from the women enrolled in our study for HPV DNA using polymerase chain reaction (PCR) and the L1 consensus sequence primers of Manos et al.[48] The presence of HPV DNA was found to be significantly associated with the presence of CIN in both the HIV-infected and HIV-uninfected groups. When a multiple logistic regression analysis was performed of all the standard epidemiological risk factors for CIN between the two groups of women, only four factors were found to be independently associated with CIN. These were HPV DNA positivity as detected using PCR (OR 9.83), HIV seropositivity (OR 3.45), CD4$^+$ T-cell count of < 200 cells/µl (OR 2.67) and age greater than 34 years (OR 2.01). Therefore, the variable most strongly associated with CIN was the detection of HPV DNA and the strength of the association between HPV and CIN in the HIV-seropositive group is similar to that reported by other recent studies of women in the general population.

A number of studies have analyzed HPV infections in HIV-infected women (Table 21.6). The first study to use molecular methods to analyze HPV infections in HIV-infected women was by Feingold et al from New York City.[49] Using Southern blot hybridization, HPV DNA was detected in 17 of 35 (40%) of the cervicovaginal lavages from HIV-infected women compared to 8 of 32 (25%) of the HIV-uninfected group. In HIV-infected women, HPV DNA positivity correlated with the degree of immunosuppression.

Table 21.6 Prevalence of HPV infections in HIV-infected and HIV-uninfected women*

Reference	Detection method	Total number of women	% HPV DNA positive	
			HIV-infected	HIV-uninfected
Laga et al.	ViraPap and Southern blot hybridization	95	38	8
Feingold et al.	Southern blot	67	40	25
Kreiss et al.	Dot blot and Southern blot hybridization	198	37	24
Vermund et al.	Southern blot	96	53	22
ter Meulen et al.	PCR	359	78	56
Wright et al.	PCR	669	60	36

* Table based on data from references (Laga et al, 1992),[36] (Feingold et al, 1990),[49] (Kreiss et al, 1992),[35] (Vermund, 1991),[30] (ter Meulen et al, 1992),[39] (Wright et al, 1993)[50]

HPV was detected in 1 of 13 (18%) of the cervicovaginal lavages from asymptomatic HIV-infected women but in 16 of 22 (73%) of those from symptomatic women. An unusually large number of the HIV-infected women in this study had HPV type 18 detected and infections with multiple types of HPV were quite common. Twenty-nine percent of the HIV-seropositive HPV DNA positive women had HPV type 18 and 35% were infected with more than one type of HPV. Another interesting finding of this study was that the HIV-seropositive women had a greater load of HPV genomes per unit amount of DNA isolated from the cervicovaginal lavages than did the HIV-seronegative women.

Other studies have now confirmed and extended these findings. Laga et al[36] used both the Viratype test and low-stringency Southern blots to detect HPV DNA and found that 38% of a group of HIV-seropositive prostitutes from Kinshasha, Zaire and 8% of a group of HIV-seronegative prostitutes were HPV DNA positive (Table 21.6). However, perhaps because of the small sample size, no statistically significant association between HIV infection, HPV infection, and demographic or behavioral features could be detected in these women. In a similar study, Kreiss et al[35] used dot blot filter hybridization and Southern blot hybridization to detect HPV DNA in cervical samples from HIV-seropositive and seronegative prostitutes from Nairobi, Kenya. HPV DNA was detected in 54 of 147 (37%) of the samples from HIV-seropositive prostitutes compared to 12 of 51 (24%) of those from HIV-seronegative prostitutes. However, this difference was not statistically significant. The failure to detect a significant difference in HPV DNA positivity between the HIV-seropositive and HIV-seronegative Nairobi prostitutes enrolled in this study may have been related to the fact that only one of the HIV-seropositive women had AIDS and that only nine had significant HIV-associated disease.

As part of our ongoing study of cervical disease in HIV-infected women we have assayed cervicovaginal lavages from 344 HIV-seropositive women and 325 demographically similar, HIV-seronegative women, for HPV DNA using the PCR and L1 consensus sequence primers that detect over 25 anogenital HPV types.[50] HPV of any type was detected in 60% of the cervicovaginal lavages from the HIV-seropositive group compared to 36% of the HIV-seronegative group (Table 21.6). Moreover, the prevalence of infection with multiple types of HPV or with high oncogenic risk HPVs such as 16 and 18 was greater in the seropositive group. Fifty-one percent of the HPV DNA positive samples from the HIV-infected women contained more than one HPV type compared to only 26% in the HIV-uninfected women. Similarly, 42% of HPV DNA positive samples from the HIV-seropositive groups contained high oncogenic risk HPV types 16 and 18, compared to only 22% of the HPV DNA positive samples from the uninfected group.

It is now well-established that specific types of HPV are associated with specific types of anogenital lesions in the general population.[12,51] The associations between specific types of HPV and CIN appear to be only minimally altered by HIV infection. 'Novel' HPV types were the most commonly detected types in women enrolled in the New York Cervical Disease Study who had no evidence of CIN, regardless of their HIV serostatus (Fig. 21.3).[50] Moreover, a similar percentage of HPV DNA positive samples in HIV-seropositive and HIV-seronegative women with no evidence of CIN contained the most commonly detected HPV types such as 6, 11, 16, 18 or the 30s (Fig. 21.3). Similarly there was no significant

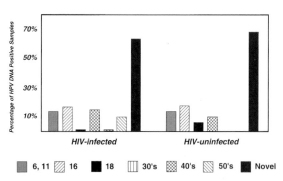

Fig. 21.3 Distribution of specific HPV types in HIV-infected and HIV-uninfected women who have no colposcopic or cytologic evidence of cervical disease. Percentages are expressed as the percentage of HPV DNA positive samples that contain a give HPV type. Since some samples contained more than one HPV type, the percentages do not equal 100. This figure is based on data from Sun et al (1995).[52]

difference between the HIV-infected and un-infected group with regards to the percentage of low-grade CIN (CIN 1) lesions that contained HPV 16 and the distribution of HPV types in HIV-seropositive women with high-grade CIN (CIN 2–3) was similar to that usually reported for the general population, since almost all cases were associated with HPV types 16, 18, 31, or 33. Low oncogenic risk HPV types such as 6, 11, 42 or the 'novel' HPVs of unknown oncogenic potential were rarely associated with high-grade CIN (CIN 2–3) in HIV-infected women. This finding may have important implications for both the detection and management of cervical disease in the HIV-infected patient, as well as for understanding the biology of HPV infections in general since it suggests that the relative restriction of these 'low oncogenic risk' viruses to women without cervical disease or to women with low-grade CIN (CIN 1) is due to an intrinsic lack of pathogenicity of these viruses which is independent of the host's immune response.

The one way in which associations between specific types of HPV and CIN appear to have been altered by HIV infection is in the percentage of low-grade cytologic abnormalities and CIN that are associated with HPV 18. HPV 18 is considered to be a particularly 'high oncogenic risk' virus since it is infrequently detected in women in the general population with low-grade CIN (CIN 1), but is frequently associated with high-grade CIN (CIN 2–3) and invasive cervical cancer. However, in the HIV-seropositive women in the New York City Cervical Disease Study, HPV 18 was detected in 47% of the 49 women with low-grade CIN (CIN 1).[50] This association is concerning since it suggests that these conditions which infrequently progress to high-grade CIN (CIN 2–3) or invasive cancer in women in the general population may have the potential for behaving more aggressively in HIV-infected patients.

The relative level of immunosuppression also appears to be a significant risk factor for both the development of CIN as well as for HPV DNA positivity. In a study of 111 HIV-infected prostitutes from Berlin, Schafer et al[33] found that 30% of the women with normal T-lymphocyte counts had CIN compared to 53% of those with CD4+ T-lymphocyte counts < 250 cells/μl. Although this difference was not statistically significant, highly significant differences were found when functional measures of immunosuppression were used. Functional immunosuppression in the HIV-infected women was assessed by assaying proliferation of lymphocytes isolated from peripheral blood when incubated with various mitogens including pokeweed mitogen, tetanus toxoid, and phytohemagglutinin. The prevalence of CIN was 12% in the 17 women who had normal lymphocyte blastogenic responses to these mitogens but was 63% in the 27 women who had reduced blastogenic responses to two of the mitogens and 80% in five women who had reduced blastogenic responses to all three mitogens. In aggregate cytologic data from three separate ambulatory sites, Marte et al[41] found a significant association between CD4+ cell count and the presence of a cytologic abnormality. Twenty-six percent of the HIV-infected women with CD4+ cell counts > 400 cells/μl had cytologic abnormalities compared to 45% of those with CD4+ T-lymphocyte counts < 400 cells/μl. Similarly, associations between cytologic abnormalities and HIV-associated symptomatic disease have been documented. Vermund et al[30] reported that 42% of symptomatic HIV-seropositive women had evidence of CIN on Pap smears compared to 17% of asymptomatic HIV-seropositive women. As part of the New York City Cervical Disease Study, we have analyzed associations between immunosuppression and the presence of both CIN and HPV infection in HIV-infected women. By multiple logistic regression analysis, immunosuppression as indicated by a CD4+ T-lymphocyte count was a significant, independent risk factor for both the presence of CIN as well as for HPV DNA positivity. Seventeen percent of the HIV-infected women with CD4+ T-lymphocyte counts of < 200 cells had biopsy-confirmed, low-grade CIN and 12% had biopsy-proven, high-grade CIN. In contrast, only 10% of the HIV-infected women with CD4+ T-lymphocyte counts of greater than 500 cells/μl had low-grade CIN and 6% had high-grade CIN.

DETECTION OF CERVICAL DISEASE IN HIV-INFECTED WOMEN

Pap smears are considered to be the standard

method for screening women for cervical disease throughout the world.[53-55] Mitchell Maiman and coworkers (from SUNY at Brooklyn, NY) recently suggested, however, that Pap smears are ineffective for detecting cervical disease in HIV-infected women and have recommended that all HIV-infected women undergo routine colposcopy.[56] This recommendation was based on a study in which 32 HIV-infected women underwent simultaneous colposcopy and Pap smear screening. Thirteen (41%) of the HIV-infected women had biopsy-confirmed CIN. However, only 1 (8%) of the 13 women had an abnormal Pap smear, giving a false-negative rate of 92%. The recommendation that all HIV-infected women undergo routine 'screening' colposcopy has caused considerable concern among both HIV-infected women, as well as those providing care to these women, since many HIV/AIDS clinics cannot provide this service due to either financial restraints or a lack of trained personnel. A critical review of the Downstate study, however, indicates that it had a number of limitations and potential problems. First, only 32 HIV-infected women were enrolled in the study. Second, the overall rate of abnormal Pap smears in the HIV-infected group was unusually low. Only 3% of the HIV-infected women had abnormal Pap smears, which is considerably lower than the 20–30% abnormal rate reported by almost all other studies of HIV-infected women in the USA. More recent studies have also analyzed the sensitivity of Pap smears in HIV-infected women, and all three have failed to confirm the exceptionally high false-negative rates reported by the Downstate group. Data from the New York City Cervical Disease Study indicates that the Pap smears in HIV-infected women is comparable to that previously reported for the general population.[31,50] In the New York Cervical Disease Study, study 398 HIV-infected women underwent colposcopy and had a Pap smear at the same visit. Only 13 of 68 HIV-infected women with CIN had Pap smears diagnosed as within normal limits. The false-negative rate of Pap smears was only 19%. Another study from Conti et al[32] found a cytologic false-negative rate of Pap smears of only 10% in 434 Italian former intravenous drug abusers (including 273 HIV-infected women) who underwent simultaneous colposcopic and cyto-

logic examinations. Taken together, these data indicate that Pap smears should be as effective in detecting cervical disease in HIV-infected women as in any other 'high-risk' population.[57]

It should also be noted that there are a number of other arguments against performing routine 'screening' colposcopy in HIV-infected women. One argument against, 'screening' colposcopy is the high cost of colposcopy which costs approximately US$300 to perform when the pathology charges are taken into account. This is considerably more expensive than the cost of obtaining a Pap smear at a routine office visit. In addition, on site colposcopic services are simply not available at many HIV/AIDS clinics and it is the experience of most clinicians working in these clinics that the attendence rate at off-site colposcopy clinics is quite poor. Another, more major problem with routine 'screening' colposcopy is that severe cervicitis is quite common in this population, and in our experience it can be difficult to distinguish between CIN and cervicitis (either colposcopically or histologically) in such patients. Therefore, 'screening' colposcopically may lead to the over diagnosis of CIN, and subsequently, to inappropriate treatment.

In light of the above arguments and data, the Centers for Disease Control and Prevention (CDC) has recommended in the 1993 STD Treatment Guidelines that all HIV-infected women be encouraged to have a Pap smear.[58] If the first smear is diagnosed as being within normal limits, at least one additional smear should be obtained within 6 months to insure that a CIN was not missed on the first smear. The STD Treatment Guidelines also recommends that if the first Pap smear has severe inflammation with reactive squamous cell changes, the smear should be repeated within 3 months. If the first Pap smear is diagnosed as having squamous atypical cells of undetermined significance (ACUS) or any degree of squamous intraepithelial lesion (SIL), the patient should be referred for further evaluation.

When considering these recommendations, it is important to keep in mind, however, that the prevalence of high-grade CIN is actually higher in the HIV-infected population than it is in many studies of women referred for colposcopy of low-grade abnormal Pap smears. Therefore, some clinicans continue to advocate routine colposcopy for HIV-infected women.

TREATMENT OF CIN IN HIV-INFECTED WOMEN

There is currently relatively little data on the safety and efficacy of standard therapies for treating CIN in HIV-infected women, such as cone biopsy, cryosurgery, laser ablation, or loop excision. The first study to compare outcomes after therapy for CIN in HIV-infected and uninfected women looked at outcomes after electrocautery and/or cone biopsy.[59] In this Italian study, no cases of recurrent/persistent disease were detected in 10 HIV-infected women with low-grade CIN who were treated with electrocautery, and, only one case of recurrent/persistent disease was detected in 8 HIV-infected women with high-grade CIN (CIN 2–3) treated using electrocautery or cold-knife cone biopsy (Table 21.7).[59]

The high success rate of electrocautery or cold-knife cone biopsy observed in this Italian study of HIV-infected women by Spinillo et al[59] was surprising, since previous studies of immunosuppressed transplant recipients had reported high rates of recurrent/persistent CIN after treatment with standard therapies.[60,61] More recent studies from the USA have all reported much higher rates of recurrent/persistent CIN after standard therapies in HIV-infected women. Adachi et al[62] treated 10 HIV-infected women with either cryosurgery or cold-knife cone biopsy and found a 50% failure rate in the HIV-infected women (Table 21.7). McGuiness and LaGuardia treated 18 HIV-infected women with cryosurgery and found a 78% failure rate.[63] Similarly, Maiman et al have found a 48% failure rate in HIV-seropositive women treated with cryosurgery, whereas the failure rate in seronegative women after cryosurgery was 1%.[64] The level and degree of immunosuppression as indicated by CD4[+] T-lymphocyte count was an important determinant of outcome in the HIV-infected women. Outcomes after either laser ablation or cold-knife cone biopsy in HIV-infected women have also been analyzed and somewhat better results than those obtained with cryosurgery have been reported.[64]

Recently, we have performed a retrospective chart review of HIV-infected women with CIN treated using loop electrosurgical excision.[65] We found a significantly higher rate of recurrent/persistent CIN after loop electrosurgical excision in women known to be HIV-infected compared to the other women who were of unknown HIV-serostatus but treated in the same clinic during the same time period. Recurrent/persistent CIN after loop electrosurgical excision was documented in 56% of the HIV-infected women compared to 13% of the women of unknown HIV serostatus. Outcome after loop excision was associated with level of immunosuppression as indicated by the absolute CD4[+] T-lymphocyte count, but not with grade of the lesion. The failure rate was 61% in HIV-infected women with CD4[+] T-lymphocyte counts of less than 500 cells/µl, but only 20% in the HIV-infected women with CD4[+] T-lymphocyte counts of 500 cells/µl or more.

The above reports of extremely poor outcomes after standard therapies for CIN in the immuno-

Table 21.7 Outcome after standard therapy for CIN in HIV-infected women*

Treatment method	Author	Number of patients	% Failure
Cryosurgery	McGuinness and La Guardia	18	78
	Maiman et al.	17	48
	Adachi et al.	5	50
Electrocautery	Spinillo et al.	10	—
	Agarossi et al.	32	69
Cold-knife cone	Spinillo et al.	8	15
	Adachi et al.	5	50
	Maiman et al.	8	13
Laser ablation	Maiman et al.	9	33
Loop excision	Wright et al.	34	56

* Table based on data from references (McGuinness et al, 1993),[63] (Maiman et al, 1993),[64] (Adachi et al, 1993),[62] (Spinillo et al, 1992),[59] (Wright et al, 1993)[65]

suppressed HIV-infected patient suggests that the currently available modalities for treating CIN in this population are relatively ineffective, and that alternative treatment approaches are probably called for. One example of an alternative treatment approach is the use of 5-fluorouracil (Effudex) as either a primary treatment modality for CIN in immunosuppressed patients or as an adjuvent therapy after standard therapy in these women to prevent recurrence of CIN.[60,61] It should noted, however, that 5-fluorouracil can cause nonhealing vaginal ulcers or superimposed infections.[66] Therefore, carefully controlled clinical trials will be required to determine whether such an approach is safe.

SUMMARY

This review indicates that there is a very high prevalence of CIN in HIV-infected women and that much of the CIN is high grade. However, it is also clear that to date an 'epidemic of invasive cervical cancer' in HIV-infected women has not yet developed and, that compared to opportunistic infections such as *Pneumocystis carinii*, invasive cervical cancer currently affects relatively small numbers of HIV-infected women. It is important to point out, however, that the failure to detect large numbers of invasive cervical cancers may simply reflect the fact that most HIV-infected women die of opportunistic infections before cervical cancer has a chance to develop. In transplant recipients, squamous cell neoplasia has a long latency period and develops, on average, 88 months after the onset of immunosuppression.[10] However, current data indicates that less than 20% of HIV-infected women survive 36 months after the diagnosis of AIDS.[67] Over the last several years improved prophylaxis against opportunistic infections and antiretroviral therapies has increased the survival of HIV-infected women. As immunosuppressed HIV-infected women begin to live longer, we may paradoxically observe an increase in the number of invasive cervical cancers developing in these women unless effective screening and treatment programs for CIN are established.

REFERENCES

1. CDC. World AIDS Day — December 1, 1993. Morbid Mortal Week Rep 1993; 42(45): 869.
2. Dondero T, StLouis M, Anderson J, Peterson J, Pappaioanou M. Evaluation of the estimated number of HIV-infected using a spreadsheet model and empirical data. Fifth International Conference on AIDS, San Francisco, CA, USA, 1989.
3. Vermund S. Changing estimates of HIV-seroprevalence in the United States. J NIH Res 1991; 3: 77–81.
4. AIDS in the world, 1992. JAMA 1992; 268: 445–446.
5. Specific HIV-related problems of women gain more attention at a price — affecting more women. JAMA 1992; 268: 1814–1815.
6. CDC. Projections of the number of persons diagnosed with AIDS and the number of immunosuppressed HIV-infected persons — United States, 1992–1993. MMWR 1992; 41: 18.
7. CDC. HIV/AIDS Surveillance Report. Atlanta: Centers for Disease Control.
8. CDC. 1993 Revised classification system for HIV infection and expanded surveillance case definition for AIDS among adolescents and adults. Morbid Mortal Week Rep 1993; 41: 1–20.
9. Des Jarlais D, Friedman S, Sotheran J et al. Continuity and change within an HIV epidemic. Injecting drug users in New York City, 1984 through 1992. JAMA 1994; 271: 121–127.
10. Penn I. Cancers of the anogenital region in renal transplant recipients. Cancer 1986; 58: 611–616.
11. Schiffman M H, Bauer H M, Hoover R N et al. Epidemiologic evidence that human papillomavirus infection causes most cervical intraepithelial neoplasia. J Nat Cancer Inst 1993; 85: 958–964.
12. Wright T C, Richart R M. Role of human papillomavirus in the pathogenesis of genital tract warts and cancer. Gynecol Oncol 1990; 37: 151–164.
13. zur Hausen H. Viruses in human cancers. Science 1991; 254: 1176–1173.
14. Brinton L A, Fraumeni J F. Epidemiology of uterine cervical cancer. J Chronic Dis 1986; 39: 1051–1065.
15. Bernard C, Mougin C, Madoz L et al. Viral co-infections in human papillomavirus-associated anogenital lesions according to the serostatus for the human immunodeficiency virus. Int J Cancer 1992; 52: 731–737.
16. Kiviat N, Critchlow C, Holmes K et al. Association of anal dysplasia and human papillomavirus with immunosuppression and HIV infection among homosexual men AIDS 1993; 7: 43–49.
17. Palefsky J, Gonzales J, Greenblatt R, Ahn D, Hollander H. Anal intraepithelial neoplasia and anal papillomavirus infection among homosexual males with group IV HIV disease. JAMA 1990; 263: 2911–2916.
18. Lorenz H, Wilson W, Leigh B, Crombleholme T, Schecter W. Squamous cell carcinoma of the anus and HIV infection. Dis Colon Rectum 1991; 34: 336–338.
19. Bradbeer C. Is infection with HIV a risk factor for cervical intraepithelial neoplasia? Lancet 1987; ii: 1277–1278.

20. Byrne M, Taylor-Robinson D, Harris J R W. Cervical dysplasia and HIV infection. Lancet 1988; i: 239.
21. Crocchiolo P, Lizioli A, Goisis F et al. Cervical dysplasia and HIV infection (letter). Lancet 1988; i: 238–239.
22. Spurrett B, Jones D S, Stewart G. Cervical dysplasia and HIV infection. Lancet 1988; i: 238–239.
23. CDC. Risk for cervical disease in HIV-infected women — New York City. Morbid Mortal Week Rep 1990; 39: 846–849.
24. Rellihan M A, Dooley D P, Burke T W, Berkland M E, Longfield R N. Rapidly progressing cervical cancer in a patient with human immunodeficiency virus infection. Gynecol Oncol 1990; 36: 435–438.
25. Schwartz L B, Carcangiu M L, Bradham L, Schwarz P E. Rapidly progressive squamous cell carcinoma of the cervix coexisting with human immunodeficiency virus infection: clinical opinion. Gynecol Oncol 1991; 41: 255–258.
26. Maiman M, Fruchter R G, Guy L, Cuthill S, Levine P, Serur E. Human immunodeficiency virus infection and invasive cervical carcinoma. Cancer 1993; 71: 402–406.
27. Carpenter C C J, Mayer K H, Stein M D, Leibman B D, Fisher A, Fopre T. Human immunodeficiency virus infection in North American women: experience with 200 cases and a review of the literature. Medicine 1991; 70: 307–325.
28. Korn A, Autry M, DeRemer P, Tan W. Sensitivity of the Papanicolaou smear in human immunodeficiency virus-infected women. Obstet Gynecol 1994; 83: 401–404.
29. Provencher D, Valme B, Averette H E et al. HIV status and positive Papanicolau screening: identification of a high-risk populations. Gynecol Oncol 1988; 31: 184–188.
30. Vermund S H, Kelley K F, Klein R S et al. High risk of human papillomavirus infection and cervical squamous intraepithelial lesions among women with symptomatic human immunodeficiency virus infection. Am J Obstet Gynecol 1991; 165: 392–400.
31. Wright T C, Ellerbrock T V, Chiasson M E, Sun X, Vandervanter N, New York Cervical Disease Study. Cervical intraepithelial neoplasia in women infected with human immunodeficiency virus: prevalence, risk factors, and validity of Papanicolaou smears. Obstet Gynecol 1994; 84: 591–597.
32. Conti M, Agarossi A, Parazzini F et al. HPV, HIV infection, and risk of cervical intraepithelial neoplasia in former intravenous drug abusers. Gynecol Oncol 1993; 49: 344–348.
33. Schafer A, Friedmann W, Mielke M, Schwartlander B, Koch M A. The increased frequency of cervical dysplasia–neoplasia in women infected with the human immunodeficiency virus is related to the degree of immunosuppression. Am J Obstet Gynecol 1991; 164: 593–599.
34. Smith J, Kitchen V, Botcherby M et al. Is HIV infection associated with an increase in the prevalence of cervical neoplasia? Br J Obstet Gynecol 1993; 100: 149.
35. Kreiss J K, Kiviat N B, Plummer F A et al. Human immunodeficiency virus, human papillomavirus, and cervical intraepithelial neoplasia in Nairobi prostitutes. Sex Trans Dis 1992; 19: 54–59.
36. Laga M, Icenogle J P, Marsella R et al. Genital papillomavirus infection and cervical dysplasia —

opportunistic complications of HIV infection. Int J Cancer 1992; 50: 45–48.
37. Maggwa B N, Hunter D J, Mbugua S, Tukei P, Mati J K. The relationship between HIV infection and cervical intraepithelial neoplasia among women attending 2 family planning clinics in Nairobi, Kenya. AIDS 1993; 7: 733–738.
38. Rogo K O, Linge K. Human immunodeficiency virus seroprevalence among cervical cancer patients. 1990; 37: 87–92.
39. ter Meulen J, Eberhardt H C, Luande J et al. Human papillomavirus (HPV) infection, HIV infection and cervical cancer in Tanzania, East Africa. Int J Cancer 1992; 51: 515–521.
40. Rabkin C, Biggar R, Baptiste M, Abe T, Kohler B, Nasca P. Cancer incidence trends in women at high risk of human immunodeficiency virus IHIV infection. Int J Cancer 1993; 55: 208–212.
41. Marte C, Kelly P, Cohen M et al. Papanicolaou smear abnormalities in ambulatory care sites for women infected with human immunodeficiency virus. Am J Obstet Gynecol 1992; 166: 1232–1237.
42. Brinton L A. Oral contraceptives and cervical neoplasia. Contraception 1991; 43: 581–595.
43. Parazzini F, LaVecchia C. Epidemiology of adenocarcinoma the cervix. Gynecol Oncol 1990; 39: 40–46.
44. Jones C J, Brinton L A, Hamman R F et al. Risk factors for in situ cervical cancer: results from a case-control study. Cancer Res 1990; 50: 3657–3662.
45. Parazzini F, LaVecchia C, Negri E, Fedele L, Franceshi S, Gallotta L. Risk factors for cervical intraepithelial neoplasia. Cancer 1992; 69: 2276–2282.
46. Ellerbrock T E, Wright T C, Chiasson M A, Bush T. Comparison of cervical intraepithelial neoplasia in human immunodeficiency virus-infected and uninfected women: prevalence, Pap smear validity and epidemiological risk factors. 9th International Conference on AIDS, Berlin, Germany, 1993.
47. Schiffman M H. Recent progress in defining the epidemiology of human papillomavirus infection and cervical neoplasia. J Nat Cancer Inst 1992; 84: 394–398.
48. Manos M M, Ting Y, Wright D K, Lewis A J, Broker T R, Wolinsky S M. Use of polymerase chain reaction amplification for the detection of genital human papillomaviruses. Cancer Cells 1989; 7: 209–214.
49. Feingold A R, Vermund S H, Burk R D et al. Cervical cytologic abnormalities and papillomavirus in women infected with human immunodeficiency virus. J AIDS 1990; 3: 896–903.
50. Wright T, Sun X, Ellerbrock T, Chiasson M. Human papillomavirus infections in HIV+ and HIV– women: prevalence, association with cervical intraepithelial neoplasia, and impact of CD4$^+$ count. 9th International Conference on AIDS, Berlin, Germany.
51. Lungu O, Sun X W, Felix J, Richart R M, Silverstein S, Wright T C. Relationship of human papillomavirus type to grade of cervical intraepithelial neoplasia. JAMA 1992; 267: 2493–2496.
52. Sun X, Ellerbrock T V, Lungu O, Chiasson M E, Bush T J, Wright T C. Human papillomavirus infections in women infected with human immunodeficiency virus. Obstet Gynecol 1995; (in press):
53. Koss L, Czerniak B, Herz F, Wersto R P. Flow cytometric measurements of DNA and other cell

components in human tumors; a critical appraisal. Human Pathol 1989; 20: 528–548.

54. Koss L G. Diagnostic cytology and its histopathologic basis. New York, 1992: J.B. Lippincott Company.

55. Sedlis A, Saigo P E. Cervicovaginal cytology: new terminology. Curr Prob Obstet Gynecol Fertil 1992; 15: 207–241.

56. Maiman M, Tarricone N, Vieira J, Suarez J, Serur E, Boyce J G. Colposcopic evaluation of human immunodeficiency virus-seropositive women. Obstet Gynecol 1991; 78: 84–88.

57. Shah P, Smith J, Kitchen V, Barton S. HIV Infection and the gynaecologist. Br J Obstet Gynecol 1994; 101: 187–189.

58. CDC. Sexually transmitted disease guidelines. Morbid Mortal Week Rep 1993; 42 (RR14): 90–91.

59. Spinillo A, Tenti P, Zappatore R et al. Prevalence, diagnosis and treatment of lower genital neoplasia in women with human immunodeficiency virus infection. Eur J Obstet Gynecol Reprod Biol 1992; 43: 235–241.

60. Sillman F H, Boyce J G, Macasaet M A, Nicastri A D. 5-Fluorouracil/chemosurgery for intraepithelial neoplasia of the lower genital tract. Obstet Gynecol 1981; 58: 356–360.

61. Sillman F H, Sedlis A. Anogenital papillomavirus infection and neoplasia in immunodeficient women. Obstet Gynecol Clinics North Am 1987; 14: 537–558.

62. Adachi A, Fleming I, Burk R D, Ho G Y, Klein R S. Women with immunodeficiency virus infection and abnormal papanicolaou smears: A prospective study of colposcopy and clinical outcome. Obstet Gynecol 1993; 81: 372–377.

63. McGuinness K, LaGuardia K. Cryotherapy in the management of cervical dysplasia (CIN) in HIV infected women. 9th International Conference on AIDS, Berlin, Germany.

64. Maiman M, Fruchter R G, Serur E, Levine P A, Arrastia C D, Sedlis A. Recurrent cervical intraepithelial neoplasia in human immunodeficiency virus-seropositive women. Obstet Gynecol 1993; 81: 170–174.

65. Wright T C, Koulos J, Schnoll F et al. Cervical intraepithelial neoplasia in women infected with the human immunodeficiency virus: outcome after loop electrosurgical excision. Gynecol Oncol 1994; 55: 253–258.

66. Krebs H B, Helmkamp B F. Chronic ulcerations following topical therapy with 5-fluorouracil for vaginal human papillomavirus-associated lesions. Obstet Gynecol 1991; 78(2): 205–208.

67. Ellerbrock T V, Bush T J, Chamberland M E, Oxtoby M J. Epidemiology of women with AIDS in the U.S., 1981–1990: a comparison with heterosexual men with AIDS. JAMA 1991; 265: 2971–2975.

22. Early invasive cervical carcinoma

Edgardo L. Yordan   George D. Wilbanks

INTRODUCTION

Implicit in the success of all screening, preventive, diagnostic, and therapeutic efforts aimed at the eradication of cervical intraepithelial neoplasia (CIN) is the avoidance of invasive carcinoma, more difficult to manage and more grave in prognosis. While the diagnosis of invasion carries with it the clinical frustration and chagrin of this implicit failure in preventive medicine, it also carries therapeutic opportunities in proportion to how early in the evolution of the disease the actual diagnosis can be established. This chapter is devoted to assisting the clinician in securing the basis for timely therapeutics of invasive carcinoma of the cervix through a better understanding of the pathogenesis, precise diagnostic definition, and clinical management of early invasive disease.

Over the past 50 years, continuing worldwide trends suggest diminishing incidence and mortality in cervical carcinoma (CA).[1,2] Mass population cytologic screening programs have undoubtedly played a contributory role in these decreasing trends, but since some of these statistics have preceded the institution of screening programs, the relative importance of their impact remains a matter of some controversy. Furthermore, in some countries the incidence has failed to decrease over time, and in some areas it is thought that changes in sexual behavior may in fact have brought about an increased incidence. Since CIN is not usually a reportable disease, the problem has been difficult to characterize.

Certainly, in the American, European, and Asian theaters the past 50 years have shown decreased mortality in cervical CA. Current 3-year and 5-year survival statistics in CA of the cervix are seen

Table 22.1 Carcinoma of the uterine cervix. Three and five-year survival rate by stage. Patients treated in 1982–1986*

Stage	Patients treated		Survival	
	N	%	3-Year (%)	5-Year (%)
I	12 143	37.9	86.9	81.6
II	10 285	32.1	69.5	61.3
III	8206	25.6	44.6	36.7
IV	1378	4.3	16.6	12.1
No stage	40	0.1	59.2	52.3
Total	32 052	100.0	68.4	59.8

*Reprinted with permission from Pettersson (1991).

in Table 22.1.[3] When analyzed stage by stage, however, salvage statistics in CA of the cervix show no dramatic trends (Fig. 22.1),[4] but overall survival has gradually improved as a relative distribution of cases by stage has progressively shifted in favor of early stage tumors (Fig. 22.2).[5] While relevant issues pertaining to the epidemiology, screening, immunology, and genetics of cervical CA are extensively discussed in other parts of the text, it is important to realize, in discussing early invasive CA, that concurrent with the dramatic reduction in the overall incidence and mortality rates for cervical CA are important increases in the relative incidence of premalignant and early invasive cancers.

PATHOPHYSIOLOGY

It is generally accepted that cervical dysplasia represents a continuum of gradually progressing grades of disease up to the most severe category, CIN grade 3, or carcinoma-in-situ. An intact basement membrane characterizes all grades of CIN, whereas penetration through the basement

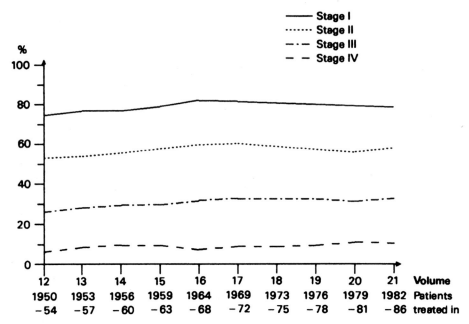

Fig. 22.1 Carcinoma of the uterine cervix. Five-year survival rates. Forty-four institutions collaborating in volumes 12 through 21 of the Annual Report. (Reprinted with permission from Pettersson, 1991.)

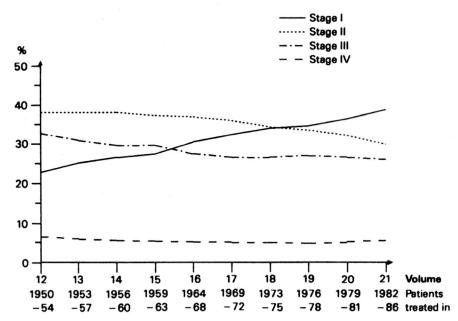

Fig. 22.2 Carcinoma of the uterine cervix. Distribution by stage percentages of total member treated. Forty-four institutions collaborating in volumes 12 through 21 of the Annual Report. (Reprinted with permission from Pettersson, 1991.)

membrane defines invasive CA. While spontaneous regression is commonly observed in the CIN process (including the increasingly higher grades, albeit less commonly), spontaneous regression is not observed after the process of invasion has been initiated, nor is an invasive lesion ever observed to revert into a CIN lesion. It is generally accepted that the conversion from CIN to invasive CA may take years.

Initiation of the process of early invasion requires acquisition by the cancer cell of the capacity to penetrate the basement membrane, a process which can be observed at the level of surface epithelial basement membrane or in the lymphovascular basement membrane, whether the cells are breaking through in the context of intravasation or extravasation. In crossing the basement membrane tumor cells are first observed to attach to the membrane matrix. The cells then acquire the capacity to degrade the membranous matrix by process of hydrolysis and proteolysis, creating a defect in the membrane. Finally, the cell is able to cross the membrane through the created defect. Following disruption of the integrity of the basement membrane, stromal invasion occurs at a variably progressive rate.

Stromal invasion seems to show a preference for the vicinity of the squamocolumnar junction. While the rate of progression is highly variable, early invasion is usually indolent and asymptomatic. Exophytic growth on the ectocervix may be sessile or polypoid, attracting little attention clinically unless contact bleeding occurs. As the malignant process penetrates the stroma, ulceration may occur by direct mucosal and stromal degradation or by infarction and sloughing as tumor necrosis develops secondary to overgrowth of the blood supply, infection, or both. The vaginal fornices may be obliterated by or incorporated into the infiltrative and ulcerative processes. The net symptomatic effect may be bleeding or seropurulent discharge. Depending on size and the anatomic direction of spread, the rate and pattern of growth can be highly variable and gross appearance can cover a broad spectrum, from the obviously malignant to the subtle and innocuous.

Alternately, disease can arise within the endocervical canal, sometimes high near the isthmus, in an endophytic process which may take some time to become clinically manifest. For cervical adenocarcinoma this is indeed the norm. An endocervical malignant polyp may distend the cervix or the tumor may actually infiltrate the endocervical stroma. Stromal infiltration, when nodular or asymmetrical, may distort the anatomy and clinically attract attention to the malignancy, but often diffuse symmetrical infiltration may progress insidiously and even reach the so-called 'barrel-shaped' configuration as it encroaches on the lower uterine segment and expands its diameter. This gradual and symmetrical growth may elude clinical detection until the size distortion is of such magnitude that the diagnosis becomes obvious. These endophytic lesions can likewise emerge and ulcerate on the forniceal surfaces, often with a necrotic appearance, but in the absence of ulceration and until such time as the sheer size of the cervix betrays the malignant process, the clinician may confuse it with insignificant forms of benign cervical hypertrophy.

Endophytic disease presumably has earlier access to stromal lymphatics than the purely exophytic form. With continued penetration of the stroma, and access thereby to the complex and extravagant cervical lymphatic network, tumor spread then begins to follow the lymphatic outflow pattern along the parametria, gradually infiltrating the cardinal and uterosacral ligaments. Because of the anatomic disposition of the lymphatic drainage along these ligaments and because of the relative impediment to direct anterior posterior tumor spread by the enveloping arrangement of the pubovesical fascia, there is a tendency for the early invasive growth to spare bladder and rectum from direct preferential penetration. But as tumor advances in volume, filling the pelvic basin and encroaching on the pelvic walls, bladder and/or rectal involvement may ensue and may even lead to vesicovaginal, ureterovaginal, or rectovaginal fistulation.

By a tumor embolic process, lymph nodes eventually become involved in metastatic spread, presumably in an orderly progression beginning with the parametrial lymph nodes and then progressing cephalad from the obturator to the external and internal iliac to the common iliac to the paraaortic and finally to the supraclavicular lymph nodes. In a collected series, Plentl[6] reported 17% internal iliac, 19% obturator, 23% external iliac, and 13% common iliac involvement. In his classic autopsy study, Henriksen[7] reported 27% obturator, 31% internal iliac, 27% external iliac, and 31% common iliac involvement among untreated cases.

With increasing stage of disease, the probability of lymphatic node metastasis increases and the survival decreases. The probability of lymphatic metastasis correlates well with tumor size and volume. In surgically treated patients direct correlation between lymph node status and survival can be demonstrated.[8] Tumor penetration to the vicinity of the ureters can result in obstructive nephropathy, and penetration to the serosal surfaces of uterus can result in intraperitoneal patterns of tumor spread. Although less frequent, hematogenous spread may be observed, resulting in metastatic patterns characteristically involving lungs, liver, and bone. In 10–30% of patients tumor extension into the lower uterine segment and the endometrial cavity can be observed, to the detriment of survival.[9]

PROGNOSIS

Many studies have sought to characterize cervical CA on the basis of different histopathologic features in attempts to define prognostic criteria. Grade of tumor differentiation, histopathologic type, depth of stromal invasion, lymph–vascular space involvement (LVSI), stromal reaction, and status of regional lymph nodes have been studied. In general, these morphologic criteria are problematic with respect to definition and reproducibility. The diagnostic challenge is further complicated by the frequent admixture of different variants, such that tumor sampling can become the critical factor.

Many histologic variants of cervical neoplasia have been described, the squamous variety comprising 85–90% of tumors. Several grading schemes have attempted a correlation between histologic morphology and the clinical behavior of these tumors.

Adenocarcinomas represent approximately 10–15% of the histologic variants reported. The endo-

cervical type is the most common and carries the best prognosis, while the endometrioid and adenosquamous types carry a worse prognosis. Other variants are considered rare and include clear cell adenocarcinomas, mucoid adenocarcinomas, neuroendocrine tumors such as oat cell carcinomas and carcinoid tumors, melanomas, sarcomas, lymphomas, and tumors metastatic to cervix.

Overall it would appear that squamous carcinoma carries a slight prognostic advantage over adenocarcinoma, but this relative advantage may disappear when other covariables are accounted for.[10] It has been argued that this advantage is more apparent than real because of delay in diagnosis caused by differences in tumor volume and anatomic distribution; the advantage may also relate to tumor grade considerations.

The Annual Report has shown over the years a consistent inverse relationship between increasing stage of tumors and decreasing survival.[3,4] The grading scheme initially proposed by Reagan et al,[11] based on cellular size and recognition of keratin in the tumor cells, has received the widest acceptance and, indeed, has been adopted by the World Health Organization (WHO). The large cell nonkeratinizing type is considered most well differentiated; the large cell keratinizing type is moderately differentiated; the small cell type is least differentiated. Prognosis has varied accordingly, and Wentz & Reagan[12] demonstrated significant survival differences with each category, the small cell type carrying the worst prognosis. Some have substantiated these observations, but generally speaking in studies where other covariables such as tumor volume were not critically controlled.[13] Others have demonstrated positive correlation between grade of differentiation and lymphatic involvement, but have not attached a survival advantage to grade.[14,15] Baltzer et al observed a relationship between survival and the grade of the tumor's invasive perimeter, as opposed to the grade of the tumor's central portion.[16] Observed tendency of cervical tumors toward wide variance and differentiation within the same tumor may well explain these inconsistencies. Reported data from the Gynecologic Oncology Group (GOG)[17] showed no correlation between histologic grade and the rate of nodal metastasis. Beecham et al[18] observed that histologic grade correlated neither with lymph node metastasis nor with survival in stage 1B cases.

Intravasation by tumor into the stromal lymphatic and vascular spaces may relate to lymph node metastasis and survival.[19,20] The GOG[21] demonstrated a positive correlation between LVSI and positive pelvic lymph nodes as well as survival; in fact, disease-free survival was related to LVSI even with negative pelvic lymph nodes. Stromal lymphocytic reaction may also correlate with better survival,[16,22,23] although this has not been consistently observed.[10] Boyce et al[24] demonstrated that depth of stromal invasion as well as LVSI correlated well with clinical outcome. As a descriptive criterion, depth of invasion alone may be deceptive, considering that a deep but focally invasive tumor may be of less adverse impact than a less invasive tumor over a broader front.

In a series of 150 cases Burghardt found increased pelvic lymph node metastases with increasing size of disease.[25] In a collaborative study totaling 718 surgical specimens, Baltzer found a similar relationship of lymphatic metastases and survival with tumor volume; he was also able to correlate survival with the volume of metastatic tumor in the lymph nodes.[16] In stage IB cervical carcinoma, several studies have demonstrated increased probability of lymphatic spread and decreased survival with increase in the size of the cervical lesion.[21,26-29]

In the final analysis, volume of tumor may be a better descriptive criterion, and therefore, a better prognosticator of clinical outcome, than depth of invasion. A series of studies correlating nodal involvement with painstaking calibration of cervical tumors have demonstrated a direct relationship between nodal involvement and tumor size, both as a function of surface area as well as of tumor volume.[16,25,30-32] Many other factors have been related to clinical outcome in both early invasive cervical CA as well as advanced tumors. Obviously, many of these factors are co-related with each other; therefore, multivariate analysis emerges as a useful tool in determining which of these many variables are indeed independently significant as prognostic factors.[21,33]

Cervical adenocarcinoma relates prognostically to grade, tumor volume, LVSI, lymph node status, and depth of stromal penetration.[34-36]

CLINICAL STAGING

Early attempts at clinical staging of cervical CA in the 1920s progressed to formal statements by the League of Nations and eventually to the first scheme by the International Federation of Gynecology and Obstetrics (FIGO) in 1950. With the first modification of staging criteria by FIGO in 1961, the concept of early stromal invasion was introduced. The staging criteria for cervical CA adopted by FIGO have become universally accepted as the basis for the standard classification system in current use among gynecologists. It was last revised in 1985.[37] Stage 0 is reserved for full thickness intraepithelial carcinoma without stromal invasion. In stage 1 tumors, carcinoma is confined to the cervix (regardless of extension to corpus). In stage 2, tumor extends beyond the cervix, but not to the pelvic wall, or tumor may involve the vagina, but not to the lower third. In stage 3, tumor extends to the pelvic wall or to the lower third of the vagina, or tumor is deemed to cause hydronephrosis or a nonfunctioning kidney. In stage 4, the tumor extends beyond the pelvis or involves bladder/rectal mucosa.

With specific reference to early invasive CA, clinical stage 1 tumors are subdivided into important and relevant subclassifications as follows:

Stage 1: Carcinoma strictly confined to the cervix.

Stage 1A: Microscopically diagnosed preclinical invasive carcinoma.

Stage 1A1: Minimal microscopically evident stromal invasion.

Stage 1A2: Lesions detected microscopically that can be measured. The measurement should not show depth of invasion of more than 5 mm taken from the base of the epithelium, either surface or glandular, from which it originates. A second dimension, the horizontal spread, must not exceed 7 mm. Larger lesions should be staged as 1B.

Stage 1B: Lesions of greater dimensions than stage 1A2 whether seen clinically or not.

Stage 2: Lesions extending beyond cervix but not to pelvic wall or lower third of vagina.

Stage 2A: Tumor with no obvious parametrial involvement.

Stage 2B: Tumor with obvious parametrial involvement.

The stage 2A subcategory accounts for surface spreading tumors invading the upper vagina. Under certain limitations of size and volume, some of the stage 2A tumors are suitably treated by methods similar to those for small size or low volume stage 1 tumors. In this sense, some stage 2 tumors can be considered early invasive and germane to the subject under consideration, although normally stage 2 lesions are not considered early invasive.

As part of FIGO's official promulgation of the current staging system, there are footnotes emphasizing important diagnostic definitional criteria. Particularly germane are those that relate to the diagnosis of microinvasive CA under the new scheme. Both stage 1A1 and 1A2 should be based on the microscopic examination of lesions removed in their entirety, preferably by conization. Stage 1A1 should be strictly limited to lesions with minute invasive loci that are only microscopically visible. Under stage 1A2, while the lesions should be *detected* microscopically, it should be measurable macroscopically. Upper dimensional limits are assigned: 5 mm in depth measured from the base of the epithelium, surface or glandular, and 7 mm of 'horizontal spread'. There are no lower limits set for horizontal spread. There are, in fact, no lower limits set for stage 1A2 in either of its dimensional criteria, surface extension or invasive depth, only that it should be macroscopically measurable, even if the pathologist has to rely on dots placed on the slide with microscopic assistance prior to macroscopic measurement. All other stage 1 cases should be relegated to stage 1B. Vascular space involvement, either intravenous or lymphatic is specifically interdicted as a staging parameter, although the specific recording of this feature is encouraged, acknowl-

edging that the information may prove useful in subsequent clinical management. Confluence of tumor projections is not addressed. The previously used '1B (occult)' category is specifically abandoned and superseded.

The staging process is based on careful clinical examination by an experienced observer, preferably under anesthesia. In case of ambiguity, the lower stage should be assigned; in case of disagreement the senior examiner should prevail. The cancer may be destined to cure or may subsequently progress or recur; but the assigned stage should never be 'restaged' or changed.

Since the purpose of staging is to facilitate comparison of results among different institutions or clinical settings, only diagnostic procedures generally available are permitted: palpation, inspection, colposcopy, endocervical curettage, hysteroscopy, cystoscopy, proctoscopy, intravenous urography (IVP), and X-ray examinations of the lungs and skeleton. Suspected bladder/rectal involvement should be histologically confirmed. In practice computerized tomography (CT) scans (either in lieu of intravenous urography or for evaluation of extrapelvic dissemination of tumor), magnetic resonance imaging (MRI), lymphangiography, arteriography, venography, laparoscopy, or 'staging' laparotomy are of frequent additional value in obtaining information useful in treatment planning; findings of such studies, however, should not serve as the basis for changing the clinical stage.

While staging of cervical CA is generally clinical, diagnosis and staging of the early invasive lesions relegated to stage 1 subcategories constitute a special situation in which staging is histologically based. The diagnosis must always derive from histologic evaluation of a cone biopsy, amputated cervix, or hysterectomy specimen. Implicit in the definitional criteria for stages 1A1 and 1A2, is that the histological specimen upon which the diagnosis is established should present surgical margins free of any tumor. Should 'microinvasion' be ambiguous, it should be relegated to stage 0 (CIN 3). Whenever hysterectomy or trachelectomy specimens are submitted as the expected basis for histologic staging, the clinician should request that pathology treat the specimen in a systematic, comprehensive process like that which conization specimens are subjected to. Unexpected cervical CA discovered in a simple hysterectomy specimen should be reported separately but never assigned a stage, even though the extent of disease can often be volumetrically defined in a properly evaluated specimen, as long as the margins of resection are clear of tumor.

The distinctions dictated by the 1985 FIGO classification require, at least ideally, that community pathology laboratories provide histological evaluation that in essence becomes a volumetric study of the early invasive tumor. This type of analysis is acknowledged to be tedious, painstaking, and difficult, even for select laboratories with an investigative interest in the matter. One of the criticisms of the current classification scheme is that perhaps it imposes unrealistic and therefore relatively irreproducible definitional criteria.

It should be understood that 'rules of staging' are intended to specify which subsets of data provide useful and permissible information for classification into stage categories, so that clinical results can be reasonably comparable. On the other hand, all available information about a tumor, from the standpoint of prognosis, extent of spread, and pathologic and biochemical behavior, is desirable for treatment planning and should not be ignored. Simply put, rules of staging define terms of classification but should not stifle meticulous, judicious, astute, and comprehensive thoroughness in clinical evaluation. Thus, the specialized or focused examinations previously mentioned, although invalid staging tools, often provide information about histology or relevant pathophysiology that is essential to treatment planning.

MICROINVASION

Originally introduced by Mestwerdt[38] in 1947, cervical microinvasion has been a subject of enduring clinical controversy until the present time. As the invasive process advances, tumor acquires increasingly greater access to the stromal lymphatic network; consequently, there is an increasing possibility of lymph node metastasis as an embolic phenomenon. The clinical significance of microinvasion, as a concept, is predicated on the desirability of defining a degree of invasiveness

such that the risk of lymph node or parametrial involvement is essentially nil. Thus, the prognostic implications for the patient should be no worse than CIN 3, despite the fact that the tumor is demonstrably invasive. The patient, then, can be theoretically treated in the same manner as CIN 3, without the need to undertake radical therapeutic modalities carrying inherently greater risks. Reaching consensus on a practical, reproducible, and consistent definition for microinvasion has proven elusive.

Measured depth of invasion seems to provide the most uncontested and reliable prognostic parameter. At 1 mm of invasion or less, the probability of lymphatic involvement is nil,[39,40] except for isolated case reports;[41] theoretically, therefore, treatment could be planned with disregard for the possibility of spread to lymph nodes and parametria. At 3–5 mm of invasion, the risk of lymphatic spread is small but clinically unacceptable in the range of 5–10%.[40,42–47] At 3 mm of invasion or less, lymph node involvement is less than 1%.[42,47]

In the past, some have relied on 5 mm as the working criterion for a definition of microinvasion. Because the degree of lymphatic metastasis at 5 mm has been unacceptable to many gynecologists, the Nomenclature Committee for the Society of Gynecologic Oncologists (SGO) undertook a definition of microinvasion, proposed in 1974 as an alternate to that of FIGO. The SGO set forth the following definitional criteria: invasion of the stroma in one or more places to a depth of 3 mm or less below the base of the epithelium; no demonstrable LVSI. The concept of confluent tongues of invasive neoplasia was not addressed by the SGO but was adopted in 1978 by the Japan Society of Obstetrics and Gynecology as an additional criterion in its respective definition of microinvasion.[48] The SGO definition has proved enduring, at least among American gynecologic oncologists.

Because the clinical outcome in the stage 1A subset of patients is so good, it would be exceedingly difficult to empirically obtain the clinical data on which to base irrefutable conclusions with regard to the optimal definitional criteria for microinvasion; with near-perfect clinical outcome, under any definition, the required caseload to demonstrate a statistically confident advantage for a particular definition of microinvasion would likely render any comparative study futile. At the very least, an attempted study of this magnitude would necessarily rely on the conjoint resources of a collaborative multi-institutional group and might therefore jeopardize the validity of its own conclusions, as the multiplicity of observers might result in loss of the exquisite discriminatory focus on which the distinction would hinge. Such difficulties were indeed apparent in an attempted collaborative study by the GOG.[42]

Perhaps, tumor volume would be a more reliable parameter to measure. Studies by Lohe et al[30] and by Baltzer et al[16] have shown a direct relationship between increasing tumor volume and probability of pelvic lymph node metastasis. Most importantly, they found no incidence of nodal involvement at tumor volumes of less than 500 mm³.

It should, of course, be emphasized that a diagnosis of microinvasion is never based on a punch biopsy of the lesion in question. Diagnosis should always be established on the basis of expert histopathologic evaluation of a cone, cervical stump, or hysterectomy specimen. Clear surgical margins are an absolute requirement, regardless of the specimen. Tissues should be subjected to serial segmental cuts at short intervals. One millimeter intervals would be ideal; this would imply that if tumor should happen to lie in-between cuts, a pathologist would, at worst, miss invasion of less than 1 mm size, well within clinically confident limits. Certainly, if one subscribes to 1 mm of invasion as the definition for microinvasion, 1 mm cuts are of the essence. At the very least, and consistent with definitional criteria used by most gynecologic oncologists, cuts should be obtained at 3 mm intervals, implying that, at worst, invasive tumor of only 3 mm could theoretically be overlooked. Deeper cuts are often necessary when morphologic criteria for invasion are ambiguous, and many pathologists recommend multiple histopathologic sections through each cut, as a routine. Volumetric histopathologic determinations are, of course, a suitable alternative, but would probably imply greater effort, commitment, and cost, and practically speaking would only be obtainable from a small number of laboratories throughout the world.

Pathologists have advanced morphologic criteria for proposed histologic definition of the notion of 'microinvasive' adenocarcinoma of the cervix. Use of a term so firmly vinculated to clinical considerations of conservative nonradical management in dealing with the squamous variety of tumor may have a misleading effect on clinicians if the implications of conization or simple hysterectomy as ample, sufficient, and reliable treatment are accepted uncritically. The fact is, however, that there is neither consensus nor consistency among pathologists as to the criteria for 'microinvasion' when it comes to adenocarcinoma. Furthermore, the ample clinical, empirical correlations on which are based the security of confident conservative management for squamous microinvasion are emphatically lacking as a basis for any reliable recommendation of conservative management in the case of 'microinvasive' adenocarcinoma. In the absence of any real consensus among gynecologic oncologists and gynecologic pathologists, and until such time as well-substantiated clinical correlations emerge to justify, in a practical sense, the notion of microinvasive adenocarcinoma, use of the term should simply be discouraged outside of an investigative setting. Although unspecified in FIGO rules of staging, it follows that perhaps cervical adenocarcinoma should not be assigned to stage 1A1, microinvasive disease being an undefined entity.

DIAGNOSIS

Overall, abnormal vaginal bleeding is the principal symptom leading to the diagnosis of cervical CA. It can present in the context of postmenopausal bleeding, polymenorrhea, hypermenorrhea, menometrorrhagia, or postcoital bleeding. Vaginal discharge is the second most common symptom and is often, but not necessarily, the herald of advanced disease. Asymptomatic presentation is seen approximately 10% of the time. Pelvic pain or pressure, with or without inguinal or sciatic radiation, usually suggests advanced disease. Less frequently, anuria, oliguria, dysuria, hematuria, or urinary frequency are the presenting symptom, again suggesting advanced stage disease. In rare instances, metastatic involvement of lung, bone, liver, or intestine, can lead indirectly to diagnosis of the cervical tumor.

The appearance on speculum or colposcopic examination of a lesion suspicious of invasive CA should prompt a directed punch biopsy or a small excisional biopsy ideally under colposcopic control. Avoidance of obviously necrotic areas should be emphasized. In the presence of grossly evident presumptive invasive lesions, a routine cervical cytology, for fear that a proper biopsy would cause active bleeding, should be discouraged because of an unacceptably high rate of false-negative readings, possibly resulting in diagnostic neglect or delay. Likewise, in the presence of a grossly obvious lesion, a cone biopsy should be frowned upon as an unnecessarily morbid and cumbersome means of histologic diagnosis. Occasional diagnostic problems, such as the question of fundal extension of tumor or the question of site of origin of an adenocarcinoma, endometrium versus endocervix, present the need for hysteroscopic evaluation, transvaginal ultrasonography, or fractional diagnostic dilatation and curettage (D and C). Fractional curettage of endocervix and endometrium may not be altogether helpful, since a curette, in the process of withdrawing endometrial tissue, can become 'contaminated' with passage through the endocervix, thereby procuring a false-positive report. With a grossly obvious lesion, colposcopy need not play the major role, although it may be of great value in defining the presence and extent of any significant dysplasia peripheral to the gross tumor; the information may play a role in treatment planning. With a diagnosis of primary early invasive cervical adenocarcinoma, concomitant squamous CIN is observed in a majority of cases. When adenocarcinoma or adenosquamous CA involves corpus as well as cervix it remains appropriate to consider the tumor endometrial in origin.

Colposcopy, of course, plays a far more important role in the symptomatic patient that presents without a grossly obvious lesion. Colposcopically directed biopsies may establish the diagnosis quite readily, although in the absence of a colposcopically visible lesion, endocervical curettage, endometrial biopsy, cervical conization, or D and C may prove expedient.

With respect to the early invasive lesions, whether squamous or glandular, the patient may well present with the usual symptoms of bleeding and discharge, but more often than not, diagnosis is established as a direct result of the clinical pursuit of abnormal cytology, as discussed elsewhere in this book. Conization is always indicated when colposcopically directed biopsies and endocervical curettage (ECC) fail to account for the cytologic suggestion of invasive CA.

Comprehensive and exhaustive sectioning of an expertly obtained conization specimen, of course, remains the diagnostic basis for the histologic characterization of early invasion. Once the histologic diagnosis is established, the patient can be evaluated, staged, and treated. A cone specimen positive for invasion may document parameters that clearly exceed the upper limits for stage 1A2; a stage IB is then assigned. Alternately, invasive tumor can be so overwhelmingly evident at the surgical margins of the cone that a stage 1B is assigned; characteristically, the margin may be heavily involved, or may be focally involved but in so many separate sections of the cone that the higher stage is prudently assigned. In a properly processed cone specimen with free margins, the distinction between stage 1A1 and stage 1A2 can usually be clearly established as the basis for treatment planning. Occasionally, a minimal focus of invasion is seen at or near a surgical margin in one of the sections of the cone, raising the question of excisional completeness as a prerequisite consideration for the appropriateness of conservative management; if the tumor would otherwise fit the criteria for a stage 1A1 or 1A2, endocervical curettage or a secondary conization may help resolve the issue of suitable treatment.

In those pathology laboratories where volumetric definition of a stage 1A2 is the norm, the clinician can be reasonably reliant on the absence of extracervical metastasis and select nonradical modalities of treatment. On the other hand, in those laboratories where bidimensional reports are the norm, it may be imprudent to proceed conservatively on the presumption of a stage 1A2, unless invasion is 3 mm or less, seen in one cut only, and without LVSI. If invasion is reported on two or more cuts at 3 mm intervals, one could entertain the theoretical possibility of exceeding the 7 mm of maximal surface extension and therefore exceeding the implied 250 mm^3 of tumor volume. Volumetric considerations aside, it must be emphasized that depth of stromal invasion is the principal consideration on which a diagnosis of microinvasion is established and, therefore, the most important element to be learned from histopathologic evaluation of the specimen.

In addition to morphometric considerations, it must be further emphasized that LVSI, confluence of multiple tongues of invasion, and multiple loci of minimal microinvasion remain adverse prognostic considerations in the minds of many, if not most, gynecologic oncologists and should receive due attention in treatment planning. This caveat is of particular gravity when we consider the absence of a true consensus among clinicians as to what defines microinvasion. The goal has been reliably and reproducibly to define that degree of early invasion below which we can remain confident that the invasive process carries no likelihood of extracervical extension; thus, treatment can be planned with the absolute certainty that conservative management will not carry the prognostic jeopardy of any added risk to the patient.

In the situation where the invasive lesion is quite incipient, perhaps early stromal invasion in a larger field of dysplasia, or perhaps a grossly invasive lesion with dysplastic areas along the tumoral perimeter, colposcopy may play an essential role in verifying that the biopsy site is indeed representative of the lesion at its worst. The importance of this cannot be overemphasized, since the most censurable error in colposcopic evaluation is the failure to detect invasive CA.

Occasionally, an obvious polypoid or papillary lesion within glandular portions of endocervix will yield an easy direct biopsy, establishing the diagnosis of cervical adenocarcinoma. Colposcopic visualization can occasionally facilitate early diagnosis of endocervical disease in the absence of grossly obvious features, but, unquestionably, endocervical colposcopy can be far more subtle and require far greater skill than ectocervical colposcopy. Practically speaking, endocervical adenocarcinomas may be colposcopically indistinguishable, at best, from their squamous ectocervical counterparts, but they are, at worst, subject to being overlooked because colposcopic visualization may seem normal in the presence of early invasive adenocarcinoma. Diagnosis of adenocarcinoma is an area of significant concern, not infrequently being a source of false negative

evaluations, both colposcopic as well as cytologic. Where adenocarcinoma is concerned, cautious mistrust of one's colposcopic prowess — even among experts, but certainly among the less experienced — is a suitably prudent clinical attitude. Liberal use of endocervical curettage and conization should be encouraged whenever endocervical abnormalities are visualized, whenever there are significant discrepancies between the histologic report and the degree of cytologic severity reported, whenever cytology reports glandular atypia or suggestion of adenocarcinoma, and especially when no ectocervical or vaginal lesions can be detected despite cytologic suggestion of invasive CA. Because of the difficulties of endocervical colposcopy in the stenotic postmenopausal cervix, and because of the propensity for disease to be found higher in the canal of postmenopausal women, due to physiologic retraction of the squamocolumnar junction, routine endocervical curettage should be attempted in this age group.

While routine endometrial curettage at the time of conization is usually nondiagnostic, most reported observations derive from treatment of younger women, or of women whose cone biopsies were indicated by the need to further evaluate cytologic dysplasia, most of which is, practically speaking, squamous. But when conization is indicated by failure to identify an overt lesion in the face of cytologic suggestion of invasive CA, particularly if the cytologic suggestion is adenocarcinoma or the patient is older, careful systematic endometrial curettage and careful adnexal palpation should be routinely undertaken at the time of conization. Furthermore, while the conization specimen may be narrow, it should generously sample the submucosal endocervical glands and should certainly be a reasonably deep specimen, striving for the upper reaches of the cervical canal, and hopefully precluding the unfortunate but occasional need for a second conization that can occur when the cone biopsy is nondiagnostic but the cytology remains positive.

TREATMENT

In general, advanced cervical CA is best treated by combined external radiation therapy and brachytherapy. Concomitant or sequential use of surgery, radiation therapy and chemotherapy in combinations considered theoretically complementary have gained increasing popularity in recent years, despite absence of conclusive evidence that survival is improved; however, any thorough discussion of the complexities and subtleties of combined modality treatment is beyond the scope of this chapter on early invasion.

For stage 1B and 2A squamous CA, radical surgery and radical radiation therapy have been considered equivalent alternatives. Comparable results can be expected, both in terms of survival as well as of complications, when either of these modalities is undertaken under circumstances of comparable clinical competence.[49]

Stage 1B

Although radiation and radical hysterectomy are considered equivalent therapeutic alternatives, many gynecologic oncologists have adopted a consensual bias restricting radical hysterectomy to the treatment of lesions 4 cm or less in diameter. The underlying assumption, a clinical view to which the majority subscribe, is that radiation therapy is best suited for lesions greater than 4 cm. While there is some clinical evidence that surgery, with or without postoperative tailored radiation therapy, provides results comparable to those obtained from radiation therapy alone,[50] most favor irradiation of the larger lesions.

With bulky stage 1B lesions penetrating into the lower uterine segment, the so-called 'barrel-shaped' lesions, the use of radiation therapy followed by an extrafascial adjuvant hysterectomy 4–6 weeks later has been demonstrated by some to improve survival.[51-53] In the absence of conclusive supportive data, the GOG has undertaken a randomized study (Protocol #71) to test this hypothesis; conclusions are pending.

It has become widespread clinical practice to offer adjuvant postoperative radiation therapy, with or without chemotherapy, following radical hysterectomy, when parametria or nodes have been clearly invaded or simply when the surgical margins are considered insecure, for reasons such as proximity of tumor to the margins, deep penetration into the cervical stroma, extensive LVSI, and high risk histological tumor types.

Current on-going GOG studies (Protocols #92 and #123) seek a better understanding of these issues through strictly controlled randomized trials.

Invasive cervical carcinomas are occasionally treated inadvertently by simple extrafascial hysterectomy because the clinician, for diverse reasons, failed to anticipate the possibility of invasive tumor. When this occurs, it may be prudent for the pathologist to treat the cervix with circumferential sequential sections in the manner of a cervical conization; thus, a proper tumor evaluation may be obtained, although technically, by convention, no stage will be assigned. Prognosis appears to vary with the extent of invasiveness, the worst prognosis being reserved for those true 'cut-through' situations where tumor is seen at the transected surgical margin, or perhaps even as gross residual tumor in the patient.[54-56] Postoperative radiation therapy of varying intensity is indicated in all of these cases, following suitable histologic evaluation, except for those cases where tumor conditions akin to stage 1A1 or stage 1A2 can be clearly reconstructed, and thus the clinical circumstances would make the patient otherwise eligible for conservative management.

Stage 1A

As previously discussed, the basis for assigning a stage 1A should always be a systematically analyzed conization specimen with clear margins, such that the critical elements of depth of invasion, growth pattern, and LVSI can be characterized with confidence.

Stage 1A1

With minimal focal invasion, and in the absence of LVSI, most gynecologic surgeons have felt confident that a simple extrafascial hysterectomy should provide suitable treatment. In recent decades, as the disease has come to affect younger and younger women who at the same time may voluntarily be delaying childbearing, the question has been increasingly raised as to the possible adequacy of conization alone as a therapeutic and not simply diagnostic measure. Multiple past conizations over the years have been considered successful therapeutically despite the plausible supposition that a small number of microinvasive carcinomas are likely to have simply escaped clinical detection and, therefore, gone unappreciated. With the increasing popularity of conization by loop electroexcisional procedure (LEEP) for diagnosis and management of cervical dysplasia, it has come to light that a small number of colposcopically undiagnosed microinvasive carcinomas are indeed detected only through histologic evaluation of the LEEP specimen;[57–59] these lesions, it seems, would simply have been treated conservatively in the past. Perhaps these past errors in detection are the underlying cause of the small, and possibly irreducible, but finite number of carcinomas seen following conservative treatment for apparent CIN that theoretically should have been successful. In 1981 Boyes and Worth[60] reported a 7% incidence of microscopic foci of invasive CA when simple routine additional cuts were obtained in the conization specimens.

To be sure, the clinical bias among most gynecologic oncologists, certainly in North America, has been that cervical conization is insufficient therapy for any form of invasive carcinoma, but it is also becoming clear that, as clinicians, we may have been treating inadvertently a small number of unappreciated microinvasive tumors by conservative conization without any apparent detriment to the clinical outcome. A number of studies from Europe, in fact, have demonstrated that conization can be advocated as a therapeutic option with relative safety, given meticulous and expert histopathological handling of the specimen.[30,61] While these data provide the basis for cautious and judicious acceptance of what has often been considered taboo, enough controversy surrounds the issue that it would seem imprudent and trivial for therapeutic conization, in this setting, to be promoted indiscriminately. It should rather be accepted as a suitable treatment alternative for those women who strongly wish to preserve their childbearing potential, as long as the proper caveats are well understood, particularly those referring to the possibility of cervical incompetence and, most importantly, to issues of careful .and meticulous follow-up with Pap smears and endocervical curettage, or at least careful cytology of the endocervical canal.

While recurrent cases of invasive CA are occasionally observed following conization with therapeutic intent, the relatively low incidence allows some leeway for clinical judgment, so that clinicians may balance the justification for conservative management and the demands of alert follow-up against the risks of recurrence and bad outcome, understanding that these risks are proportional to the observed incidence of LVSI and to the degree of microinvasiveness within that arbitrary spectrum ranging between 'early stromal invasion' and invasion to a depth of 5 min.[47]

Stage 1A2

The 1A2 FIGO classification is defined by morphometric parameters the clinical implications of which cover a broad spectrum. It has been mentioned that it is only at the level of 1 mm of invasion that the incidence of nodal or parametrial extension is, practically speaking, reduced to the level of absolute unlikelihood. At 3 mm of invasion this certainty is considered reasonable because of the extreme rarity of extrauterine disease, lymph nodes being positive in fewer than 1% of cases. At 5 mm of invasion, however, it is not altogether rare to find extrauterine spread, lymph nodes being involved in as many as 5–13% of cases. For this reason, the SGO in the USA proposed in 1974, and continues to advocate, a definition for microinvasion based on 3 mm of invasion and no LVSI, representing a level of invasion at which most gynecologic oncologists feel reasonably safe in applying conservative management criteria. It should, of course, be remembered that some gynecologic oncologists still advocate 1 mm of invasion as the definitional basis for microinvasion and are categorically unwilling to consider conservative treatment for anything beyond that depth of invasion. Recurrence of invasive CA would be unanticipated under either definition, but at a 3–5 mm degree of 'microinvasion' recurrence could be observed in as high as 11% of cases.[47]

Under the stage 1A2 category some very small microinvasive tumors are included, well under 3 mm of invasion, if only because they can be macroscopically measured. Extrafascial abdominal hysterectomy or vaginal hysterectomy should be considered appropriate treatment as long as no LVSI is detected. Clear conization margins are implicit in the assignment of stage 1A2; therefore, a cone biopsy should theoretically be therapeutic in this minimal disease category, but perhaps tumor-free margins are not as absolute a predictor of excisional sufficiency as we tend to assume. Studies[62,63] suggest a small but certainly not negligible likelihood of tumor persistence following conization in stage 1A2 cervical CA. Hence, therapeutic conization should remain an exceptional undertaking for this stage of disease, indicated only by strong desire for preservation of fertility and subject to stringent follow-up including frequent cytology and ECC. Under the category of 3–5 mm of invasion, however, radical hysterectomy or radical radiation therapy should be preferred. Likewise, when significant LVSI or cone margin involvement is detected, radical hysterectomy or radical radiation therapy should be advocated regardless of the measured level of invasion.

For medically inoperable cases of stage 1A squamous CA, intracavitary therapy with ^{137}Cs provides excellent results.[64] The external radiation therapy (ERT) complement need not be considered in those situations where conservative surgery would have sufficed but should be considered integral to the treatment plan in those situations (3–5 mm invasion, LVSI) where radical surgery would have been contemplated, unless outweighed by risk of morbidity.

Recommended treatment for cervical adenocarcinoma-in-situ includes hysterectomy and lymph node evaluation.[65] Adenocarcinoma-in-situ is likely an underdiagnosed entity.[66] Since adenocarcinoma-in-situ is so frequently found in contiguous association with frankly invasive adenocarcinoma, the diagnosis should be established by conization and never by office biopsy alone. Since adenocarcinoma-in-situ can precede invasive adenocarcinoma by approximately 10 years[66], it is frequently seen during the childbearing years. The question of clinically conservative management by conization and follow-up, therefore, occasionally arises. Conization margin status becomes a reasonably reliable predictor of residual disease. In a combined institutional and medical literature review, Hopkins reported residual disease in the hysterectomy specimen eight out of 12 times when the cone margin was involved but only two out of 32 times when the margin was uninvolved.[65]

While the therapeutic effectiveness of conization alone for adenocarcinoma-in-situ remains relatively undefined in view of limited numbers, preservation of fertility may serve as its justification in the young patient willing to subject herself to meticulous clinical follow-up observation. Outside of childbearing considerations, hysterectomy — whether abdominal or vaginal — is the preferred treatment. Considering that lymph node involvement carries such an adverse prognostic message in adenocarcinoma, that reported posthysterectomy recurrences have occurred at the pelvic wall, and that histologic diagnosis of adenocarcinoma can be relatively imprecise, lymph node sampling or imaging can be reasonably advocated.

Optimal treatment of cervical adenocarcinoma remains controversial. Best 5-year survival was reported by Hopkins in patients treated by radical hysterectomy.[34] A report of early invasive tumors by Eifel, on the other hand, failed to demonstrate a significant survival advantage when radical hysterectomy was compared to radiation or to combined surgery and radiation.[36] Furthermore, pelvic recurrence was reported as unacceptably high in tumors 3–4 cm in size when treated by radical hysterectomy alone. Whereas equivalent pelvic failure rates were observed in tumors less than 3 cm in size, Hopkins' study did not confirm significant adverse prognosis in tumor size greater than 3 cm.

For early invasive adenocarcinoma (tumor size < 3 cm), radical hysterectomy and radiation therapy probably offer equivalent efficacy in terms of survival and local control. Because of increased relative propensity for lymph node involvement by adenocarcinoma, brachytherapy without ERT for treatment of the seemingly very early invasive cases should only be weighed with extreme caution in those cases where external irradiation poses significant increase in the risk of complications. Hopkins' study would support ovarian conservation as a reasonable alternative for the young patient undergoing radical hysterectomy, but bilateral salpingo-oophorectomy should be considered preferable for the older patient.

For larger tumors (size 3 cm or greater), radical

hysterectomy and pelvic lymphadenectomy may provide the relative benefits of additional prognostic information, ovarian conservation when appropriate, and fewer delayed second primaries, but radiation therapy may secure improved local control; long-term survival is probably similar, perhaps because of similar rates of distant metastases. Adjunctive radiation therapy following radical surgery would be desirable for patients with tumor size greater than 3 cm, positive lymph nodes, LVSI, poorly differentiated lesions, or compromised surgical margins.

REFERENCES

1. De Vesa S S, Silverman D T, Young J L Jr et al. Cancer incidence and mortality trends among whites in the United States, 1947–84. J Nat Cancer Inst 1987; 79: 701.
2. De Vesa S S. Descriptive epidemiology of cancer of the uterine cervix. Obstet Gynecol 1984; 63: 605.
3. Pettersson F. Annual report on the results of treatment in gynecological cancer, vol. 21, FIGO. Int J Gynecol Obstet, 1991; 36 (supplement): 35.
4. Pettersson F. Annual report on the results of treatment in gynecological cancer, vol. 21, FIGO. Int J Gynecol Obstet, 1991; 36 (supplement): 33.
5. Pettersson F. Annual report on the results of treatment in gynecological cancer, vol. 21, FIGO. Int J Gynecol Obstet, 1991; 36 (supplement): 32.
6. Plentl A, Friedman E. Lymphatic system of the female genitalia. Philadelphia: W B Saunders, 1971: p 91.
7. Henriksen E. The lymphatic spread of carcinoma of the cervix and of the body of the uterus: a study of 420 necropsies. Am J Obstet Gynecol 1949; 58: 924.
8. Pettersson F. Annual report on the results of treatment in gynecologic cancer, vol. 21, FIGO. Int J Gynecol Obstet, 1991; 36 (supplement): 48.
9. Perez C A, Camel H M, Askin F, Breaux S. Endometrial extension of carcinoma of the uterine cervix: a prognostic factor that may modify staging. Cancer 1981; 48: 170.
10. Shingleton H M, Gore H, Bradley D H, Soong S-J. Adenocarcinoma of the cervix. I. Clinical evaluation and pathologic features. Am J Obstet Gynecol 1981; 139: 799.
11. Reagan J W, Harmonic M J, Wentz W B. Analytic study of cells in cervical squamous cell cancer. Lab Invest 1957; 6: 241.
12. Wentz W B, Reagan J W. Survival in cervical cancer with respect to cell type. Cancer 1959; 12: 384.
13. Underwood P B, Wilson W C, Kreutner A, Miller M C III, Murphy E. Radical hysterectomy: a critical review of twenty-two years' experience. Am J Obstet Gynecol 1979; 134: 889.
14. Sidhu G S, Koss L G, Barber H R K. Relation of histologic factors to the response of stage I epidermoid carcinoma of the cervix to surgical treatment: analysis of 115 cases. Obstet Gynecol 1970; 35: 329.
15. Chung C K, Nahhas W A, Stryker J A, Curry S L, Abt A B, Mortel R. Analysis of factors contributing to treatment failures in stages IB and IIA carcinoma of the cervix. Am J Obstet Gynecol 1980; 138: 550.
16. Baltzer J, Lohe K J, Köpcke W, Zander J. Histological criteria for the prognosis in patients with operated squamous cell carcinoma of the cervix. Gynecol Oncol 1982; 13: 184.
17. Lagasse L D, Creasman W T, Shingleton H M, Ford J H, Blessing J A. Results and complications of operative staging in cervical cancer: experience of the Gynecologic Oncology Group. Gynecol Oncol 1980; 9: 90.
18. Beecham J B, Halvorsen T, Kolbenstvedt M. Histologic classification, lymph node metastases, and patient survival in stage IB cervical carcinoma. Gynecol Oncol 1978; 6: 95.
19. Barber H R K, Sommers S C, Rotterdam H, Kwon T. Vascular invasion as a prognostic factor in stage IB cancer of the cervix. Obstet Gynecol 1978; 52: 343.
20. Van Nagell J R Jr, Donaldson E S, Wood E G, Parker J C Jr. The significance of vascular invasion and lymphocytic infiltration in invasive cervical cancer. Cancer 1978; 41: 228.
21. Delgado G, Bundy B, Zaino R, Sevin B-U, Creasman W T, Major F. Prospective surgical-pathological study of disease-free interval in patients with stage IB squamous cell carcinoma of the cervix: a Gynecologic Oncology Group study. Gynecol Oncol 1990; 38: 352.
22. Gusberg S, Yannopoulos K, Cohen C. Virulence indices and lymph nodes in cancer of the cervix. Am J Roentgenol 1971; 111: 273.
23. Boyce J. Fruchter R G, Nicastri A D, Ambiavagar P-C, Reinis M S, Nelson J H. Prognostic factors in stage I carcinoma of the cervix. Gynecol Oncol 1981; 12: 154.
24. Boyce J G, Fruchter R G, Nicastri A D et al. Vascular invasion in stage I carcinoma of the cervix. Cancer 1984; 53: 1175.
25. Burghardt E, Pickel H. Local spread and lymph node involvement in cervical cancer. Obstet Gynecol 1978; 52: 138.
26. Piver S, Chung W S. Prognostic significance of cervical lesion size and pelvic node metastases in cervical carcinoma. Obstet Gynecol 1975; 46: 507.
27. Van Nagell J R Jr, Donaldson E S, Wood E G, Parker J C Jr. The significance of vascular invasion and lymphocytic infiltration in invasive cervical cancer. Cancer 1978; 41: 228.
28. Alvarez R D, Soong S J, Kinney W K et al. Identification of prognostic factors and risk groups in patients found to have nodal metastasis at the time of radical hysterectomy for early stage squamous carcinoma of the cervix. Gynecol Oncol 1989; 35: 130.
29. Podczaski E S, Palumbo C, Manetta A et al. Assessment of pre-treatment laparotomy in patients with cervical carcinoma prior to radiotherapy. Gynecol Oncol 1989; 33: 71.
30. Lohe K J, Burghardt E, Hillemanns H G, Kaufmann C, Ober K G, Zander J. Early squamous cell carcinoma of the uterine cervix, II. Clinical results of a cooperative study in the management of 419 patients with early

stromal invasion and microcarcinoma. Gynecol Oncol
1978; 6: 31.

31. Zander J, Balzer J, Lobe K J et al. Carcinoma of the
cervix: an attempt to individualize treatment. Results of
a 20-year cooperative study. Am J Obstet Gynecol
1981; 13: 752.

32. Dargent D, Frobert J L, Beau G. V factor (tumor
volume) and T factor (FIGO classification) in the
assessment of cervix cancer prognosis: the risk of lymph
node spread. Gynecol Oncol 1985; 22: 15.

33. Stehman F B, Bundy B N, DiSaia P J, Keys H M,
Larson J E, Fowler W C. Carcinoma of the cervix
treated with radiation therapy: a multi-variate analysis of
prognostic variables in the Gynecologic Oncology
Group. Cancer 1991; 67: 2776.

34. Hopkins M P, Schmidt R W, Roberts J A, Morley G W.
The prognosis and treatment of stage 1 adenocarcinoma
of the cervix. Obstet Gynecol 1988; 72: 915.

35. Berek J S, Hacker N F, Fu Y-S, Sokale J R, Leuchter
R C. Lagasse L D. Adenocarcinoma of the uterine
cervix: histologic variables associated with lymph node
metastasis and survival. Obstet Gynecol, 1985; 65: 46.

36. Eifel P J, Burke T W, Delclos L, Wharton J T, Oswald
M J. Early stage I adenocarcinoma of the uterine cervix:
treatment results in patients with tumors ≤ 4 cm in
diameter. Gynecol Oncol 1991; 41: 199.

37. FIGO Committee on Gynecologic Oncology. Rules for
clinical staging and definitions of the clinical stages in
carcinoma of the cervix uteri. From Pettersson F.
Annual report on the results of treatment in
gynecological cancer, vol. 21, FIGO. Int J Gynecol
Obstet 1991; 36 (supplement): 27.

38. Mestwerdt G. Die frühdiagnose des collumkarzinoms.
Zentralbl Gynäkol 1947; 69: 198.

39. Averette H E, Nelson J H, Ng ABP, Hoskins W J,
Boyce J G, Ford J H. Diagnosis and management of
microinvasive (stage 1A) carcinoma of the uterine
cervix. Cancer 1976; 38: 414.

40. Maiman M A, Fruchter R G, DiMaio T M, Boyce J G.
Superficially invasive squamous cell carcinoma of the
cervix. Obstet Gynecol 1988; 72: 399.

41. Collins H S, Burke T W, Woodward J E, Spurlock J W,
Heller P B. Widespread lymph node metastases in a
patient with microinvasive cervical carcinoma. Gynecol
Oncol 1989; 34: 219.

42. Sedlis A S, Sall Y, Tsukada Y et al. Microinvasive
carcinoma of the uterine cervix: a clinical–pathologic
study. Am J Obstet Gynecol 1979; 133: 64.

43. Van Nagell J R Jr, Greenwell N, Powell D F,
Donaldson E S, Hanson M B, Gay E C. Microinvasive
carcinoma of the cervix. Am J Obstet Gynecol 1983;
145: 981.

44. Creasman W T, Fetter B F, Clarke-Pearson D L,
Kaufmann L, Parker R T. Management of stage 1A
carcinoma of the cervix. Am J Obstet Gynecol 1985;
153: 164.

45. Simon N L, Gore H, Shingleton H M, Soong S-J, Orr
J W, Hatch K D. Study of superficially invasive
carcinoma of the cervix. Obstet Gynecol 1986; 68: 19.

46. Tsukamoto N, Kaku T, Matsukuma K et al. The
problem of stage Ia (FIGO, 1985) carcinoma of the
uterine cervix. Gynecol Oncol 1989; 34: 1.

47. Sevin B-U, Nadji M, Averette H E, Hilsenbeck S,
Smith D, Lampe B. Microinvasive carcinoma of the
cervix. Cancer 1992; 70: 2121.

48. Noda K, Taki I, Takeuchi S et al. A new proposal
regarding criteria for stage Ia cancer of the uterine
cervix. Gynecol Oncol 1979; 8: 353.

49. Morley G W, Seski J C. Radical pelvic surgery versus
radiation therapy for stage I carcinoma of the cervix
(exclusive of microinvasion). Am J Obstet Gynecol
1976; 126: 785.

50. Alvarez R D, Gelder M S, Gore H, Soong S-J,
Partridge E. Radical hysterectomy in the treatment of
patients with bulky early stage carcinoma of the cervix
uteri. Gynecol Obstet 1993; 176: 539.

51. Durrance F Y, Fletcher G H, Rutledge F N. Analysis of
central recurrent disease in stages 1 and 2 squamous
cell carcinomas of the cervix on intact uterus. Am J
Roentgenol 1969; 106: 831.

52. Rutledge F N, Wharton J T, Fletcher G H. Clinical
studies with adjunctive surgery and irradiation therapy
in the treatment of carcinoma of the cervix. Cancer
1976; 38: 596.

53. Gallion H H, Van Nagell J R Jr, Donaldson E S et al.
Combined radiation therapy and extrafascial
hysterectomy in the treatment of stage IB barrel-shaped
cervical cancer. Cancer 1985; 56: 262.

54. Durrance F Y. Radiotherapy following simple
hysterectomy in patients with stage I and II carcinoma
of the cervix. Am J Roentgenol Radium Ther Nucl Med
1968; 102: 165.

55. Hopkins M P, Peters W A, Andersen W, Morley G W.
Invasive cervical cancer treated initially by standard
hysterectomy. Gynecol Oncol 1990; 36: 7.

56. Roman L D, Morris M, Eifel P J, Burke T W,
Gershenson D M, Wharton J T. Reasons for
inappropriate simple hysterectomy in the presence of
invasive cancer of the cervix. Obstet Gynecol 1992;
79: 485.

57. Bigrigg M A, Codling B W, Pearson P, Read M D,
Swingler G R. Colposcopic diagnosis and treatment of
cervical dysplasia at a single clinic visit. Experience of
low-voltage diathermy loop in 1000 patients. Lancet
1990; 336: 698.

58. Chappatte O A, Byrne D L, Raju K S, Nayagam M,
Kenney A, Histological differences between colposcopic-
directed biopsy and loop excision of the transformation
zone (LETZ): a cause for concern. Gynecol Oncol
1991; 43: 46.

59. Howe D T, Vincenti A C. Is large loop excision of the
transformation zone (LLETZ) more accurate than
colposcopically directed punch biopsy in the diagnosis
of cervical intraepithelial neoplasia? Br J Obstet
Gynaecol 1991; 98: 588.

60. Boyes D A, Worth A J. Treatment of early cervical
neoplasia: Definition and management of preclinical
invasive carcinoma. Gynecol Oncol 1981; 12: S317.

61. Kolstad P. Follow-up study of 232 patients with stage
1A1 and 411 patients with stage 1A2 squamous cell
carcinoma of the cervix (microinvasive carcinoma).
Gynecol Oncol 1989; 33: 265.

62. Burghardt E, Girardi F, Lahousen M, Pickel H,
Tamussino K. Microinvasive carcinoma of the uterine
cervix (International Federation of Gynecology and
Obstetrics stage 1A). Cancer 1991; 67: 1037.

63. Greer B E, Figge D C, Tamimi H K, Cain J M, Lee
R B. Stage 1A2 squamous carcinoma of the cervix:
difficult diagnosis and therapeutic dilemma. Am J
Obstet Gynecol 1990; 162: 1406.

64. Grigsby P W, Perez C A. Radiotherapy alone for medically inoperable carcinoma of the cervix: stage 1A and carcinoma in situ. Int J Radiat Oncol Biol Phys 1991; 21: 375.

65. Hopkins M P, Roberts J A, Schmidt R W. Cervical adenocarcinoma in situ. Obstet Gynecol 1988; 71: 842.

66. Boon M E, Baak J P A, Kurver P J H, Overdiep S H, Verdonk G W. Adenocarcinoma in situ of the cervix: an underdiagnosed lesion. Cancer 1981; 48: 768.

23. A critical appraisal of screening and diagnostic techniques

W. P. Soutter

SCREENING TECHNIQUES

INTRODUCTION

The objective of a screening program is the reduction of morbidity and mortality from a disease. This requires both efficient detection and successful management of the condition in question. The first section of this chapter looks at the basis of the established cytological technique for cervical screening and upon ways in which it might be improved. Alternative screening techniques are then examined. Important factors such as the design, implementation, cost and benefits of a screening program are discussed elsewhere in this book (Chapter 5).

REQUIREMENTS FOR A SUCCESSFUL CANCER SCREENING PROGRAM

Long premalignant phase

If cancer screening is to be effective, the disease itself must have a long premalignant or readily curable invasive phase. This will allow a large window of opportunity in which the condition may be detected before it has become incurable. The larger this window, the less frequently must the screening test be repeated.

In practice, tests that must be repeated more frequently than every year are likely to be prohibitively expensive and excessively demanding on the screened population, leading to reduced compliance. Ideally, tests would be required only once every few years over a relatively narrow age range.

Reliable and acceptable test

The screening test must reliably detect the disease at these early stages and must be both inexpensive and acceptable to the population who will be screened. The accuracy of a test is measured by its sensitivity — the proportion of cases correctly identified, and by its specificity — the proportion of normals correctly identified. The false negative rate is the inverse of the sensitivity and the false positive rate the inverse of specificity.

No test is completely accurate and so a cut-off value has to be chosen that will detect the maximum number of cases of the disease (a high sensitivity) with the smallest possible number of false positive results (a high specificity). The cut-off value chosen must also take into account the prevalence of the condition in the population being screened. If the condition is very uncommon, high specificity is required to avoid undue anxiety for large numbers of healthy people even if this means accepting a slightly lower sensitivity and more false negative results (Fig. 23.1). This is even more true if the condition progresses slowly because there will be an opportunity to detect the abnormality at a subsequent screen.

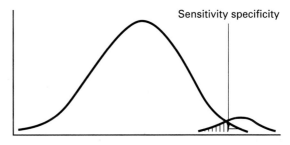

Fig. 23.1 Because CIN are relatively uncommon, any screening test must have high specificity to avoid undue anxiety for large numbers of healthy people. This means accepting a slightly lower sensitivity and more false negative results which will be detected at a subsequent screen.

Simple and effective investigation and treatment of abnormalities

All of the abnormalities found must be investigated promptly and effectively. The investigations must be as noninvasive and nontraumatic as possible because some of these people will have no lesion. There will always be uncertainty about the degree of risk of invasion developing in individual cases and so treatment of premalignant disease must carry a low morbidity. If treatment is to be applied widely it must be cheap. In particular, it must be substantially cheaper than the treatment of established invasive disease. The treatment must be shown to be highly effective, not just in eliminating the premalignant lesion, but also in reducing the incidence of invasive disease in these subjects.

DOES SCREENING FOR CERVICAL DISEASE MEET THESE CRITERIA?

Length of premalignant phase

For ethical reasons, there are few studies of untreated women with unequivocal cervical intraepithelial neoplasia (CIN) but those which have been described all suggest that at least 30% of women with CIN 3 will develop invasive disease over a period of 20 years.[1,2] Thus it would seem that cervical cancer does have a prolonged preinvasive phase in most cases making detection possible with 3–5-yearly testing. The same conclusion was drawn from a study which looked at the incidence of invasive cervical cancer in relation to the screening interval.[3]

Cost and acceptability of cervical cytology

Cervical cytology is a relatively cheap test and requires little in the way of special equipment in the clinics where the samples are collected. Staff taking smears need training not only in the mechanics of taking the smear and preparing the slides but also in the counseling of the women having the smears done. The counseling is important to avoid undue anxiety if the test should prove to be abnormal; the woman should not think that this means that she has cancer. It is also important that the woman should not have un-

realistic expectations of the test. Many still believe that it will detect ovarian and endometrial cancer. In particular, it is important to say that, while the test is very effective in reducing the risk of squamous cancer, it is much less useful in preventing the uncommon adenocarcinoma of the cervix (see below).

The acceptance of cervical cytology is good on the whole but certain sections of the population are slow to take up screening. This tends to be the older women and racial and cultural minorities.[4-6]

Inaccuracies of cervical cytology

A subjective technique like cytology cannot be completely accurate. There are bound to be differences in the interpretation of smears between observers and between the same observer at different times.[7,8] The same is true of histopathology.[9] With so much observer variation, it is most unlikely that the severity of the smear result will correspond exactly with the histological grade of the lesion and substantial overlap is inevitable. For these reasons, it is unwise to predict from the smear result the severity of the lesion on the cervix.

From studies using a variety of methods, estimates of the false positive rate range from 7.4 to 27% and the false negative rate from 1.5 to 30%.[10-14] The low estimates in these figures were derived from studies using cytology data only and are likely to underestimate substantially the real error rate. The error rates are higher in all studies where follow-up histology has been obtained, or the regional cancer registry searched for subsequent records of cancer in the study population.

A more reliable way of determining the accuracy of cervical cytology is to examine an apparently healthy population of women with cervical smears and colposcopy with biopsies taken from any suspicious areas. This allows independent confirmation of the presence or absence of disease. One such study reported a false negative rate for cytology of 48% and a false positive rate of 6%.[15] Two other similar studies have been reported in abstract form only and broadly confirm these results.[16,17]

Although these are high false negative rates, they must be seen in the context of the relatively long premalignant phase of cervical neoplasia and the policy of taking smears at three to five year intervals. In UK, the majority of women who develop cervical cancer have either never had a smear or have not had one for many years.[18]

Screening does reduce incidence and mortality from cervical carcinoma

Population-based studies

Several population-based studies have demonstrated a reduction in the incidence and mortality following the introduction of cervical screening. A cancer register study in Finland, which has a screening program, and Estonia, which does not, showed that the age-standardized incidence and mortality rates of cervical cancer had fallen very much faster in Finland. By 1987 the incidence rates in Finland and Estonia were 3.8 and 14 per 100 000 and the mortality rates were 1.6 and 6.0 per 100 000 respectively.[19] A study of the trends in mortality from cervical cancer in the Nordic countries showed that the rate of fall in mortality was proportional to the intensity of the screening program.[20] A Danish cancer register study indicated that the 5-year risk of developing cervical cancer was 48% lower in women with one previous negative smear than in an unselected population of unscreened women.[21] The 5-year risk for women with two to four previous negative smears was 69% lower than that for unscreened women.

Case-control studies

Although there are potential problems with case control studies of screening[22] much interesting and valuable information has been obtained from this type of study. A study of screening in rural China found a relative risk* of cervical cancer of 0.33 in women with three or more smears compared with women with one or less smears.[23] In the same study, the risk of cervical cancer was 11.4 times greater 8 or more years after the last

smear than in the first 2 years after a smear. A Dutch study found that their screening program resulted in an odds ratio of 0.22 (95% CI = 0.07–0.69) for invasive cancer 5 years after the last smear.[13]

A case-control study was conducted in Miyagi Prefecture, Japan, to evaluate the effectiveness of mass screening for invasive cervical cancer.[24] The smear histories of 109 cases with invasive cervical cancer diagnosed in the years 1984–1989 were compared with those of 218 age and area-matched controls. The odds ratio for 98 cases with squamous cell carcinoma for screened versus never screened women was 0.14 (95% CI = 0.080–0.253).

A case control study in Milan that used hospital controls showed that compared with no smear, three or more cervical smears decreased the risk of invasive cervical cancer by about 90%. The relative risk was about 60% lower in women reporting their smear within 2 years compared with women screened 6 or more years ago.[25] A study in Florence using carefully chosen controls from the community showed that even one smear reduced the risk by about 70% (odds ratio 0.29, 95% CI = 0.15–0.55).[26] The reduction was even greater for those screened twice or more. However, they were not able to show an increasing risk with increasing interval since last test.

A case control study in Maryland used both neighborhood controls and random controls and found similar relative risk rates of 0.23 and 0.30.[27] A Danish case control study, which separated women who had their smears taken because of symptoms from those who were asymptomatic, found that regular screening reduced the relative risk of cancer to 0.25.[28] When only asymptomatic women were considered, the relative risk was 0.15 in those screened every 3 years. Even those screened more than 5 years previously had a relative risk of 0.67 compared with those who had never had a smear.

A large case control study using data from 10 centers in eight countries estimated a 91% reduction in the risk of developing invasive cervical cancer with a programme of 3-yearly smears from 20 to 64 years of age.[3] Oortmarssen and his colleagues calculated that screening gave even more protection against of dying of cervical cancer.[29] In

---

*In the context of cervical screening, the relative risk and the odds ratio for invasive disease may be regarded as virtually identical. A relative risk for invasive disease of 0.20 in screened women means that they have a five times lower risk of developing invasive cancer than the control, unscreened population.

women with two negative smear results estimates of protection against cervical cancer were about 50% higher when death from invasive cancer was used as the criterion rather than incidence.

Conclusion

This wealth of information testifies to the value of cervical cytology in preventing both the morbidity and the mortality of invasive squamous cervical carcinoma. No randomized, controlled trial has ever been undertaken and none is likely ever to be performed. No controlled trial was needed to demonstrate the value of penicillin and the huge weight of evidence derived from so many different sorts of investigation attests to the value of conventional cervical cytology.

Screening has little effect on adenocarcinoma of the cervix

While there is good evidence of the protective value of cervical cytology screening in squamous carcinoma of the cervix, most of the data available suggest that it is relatively ineffective in adenocarcinoma.

A report of abnormal glandular cells is quite uncommon but upto 36% of such smears may be associated with invasive disease.[30] This is usually located on the cervix but may be endometrial or, rarely, ovarian.

False positive rate

There are few data on the false positive rate. One group found that it was only 2%[30] but everyday clinical experience and other investigators suggest that the rate is usually much higher.[31,32] The Hammersmith (London, UK) colposcopy clinic experience has been that 57% had no apparent lesion. However, most of the remainder had CIN 3, adenocarcinoma-in-situ (AIS) or invasive squamous cancer.

False negative rate

The false negative rate is hard to establish with certainty but a study of the cytological histories of 375 women with cervical carcinoma within 3 years of the diagnosis showed that, even after reviewing the smears, 30% of the 40 adenocarcinomas had negative smears compared with 13% of the squamous cancers.[34] A study of the cytology results of both endometrial and cervical adenocarcinomas and adenosquamous carcinomas reported that 20% of the initial cytological diagnoses were negative and failed to indicate the need for further investigation.[35]

A comparison of the rates of adenocarcinoma in two successive rounds of screening the same population of Dutch women showed a clear reduction in squamous cell carcinoma but no effect on adenocarcinoma.[36] The Japanese case control study which demonstrated a protective effect against squamous cancer showed that the Papanicolaou (Pap) smear was less effective as a screening procedure for adenocarcinoma of the cervix than for squamous cell carcinoma.[24] Of 11 cases with adenocarcinoma, 81.8% were screened, compared with 90.9% of controls. The odds ratio was 0.45 — not significantly different from 1.0 (95% CI = 0.054–3.719).

WAYS OF IMPROVING CYTOLOGY SCREENING

It is clear from the discussion above that there is room for improvement in cytology screening.

Alternative sampling devices

For the past 20 years many people have devoted enormous energy and considerable resources to designing and testing different devices for obtaining samples of cervical squames for cytology. The objective of all the different devices has been to improve the pick up rate (specificity) of abnormalities. Sadly, the net benefit of all this effort has been small.

Published studies show little or no advantage

Many studies do show that some devices more frequently obtain endocervical or metaplastic cells,[37] but the objective is to detect dyskaryosis more often. In young women, different samplers do not seem to make much difference.[38,39] Nor do combinations of a spatula and a brush improve detection rates over a brush alone.[39] One study of a new sampler that appeared to offer better results, and which also suggested benefits from combining an Ayre spatula and a cytobrush[40] used an inappropriate method of statistical analysis.[41] When the data were reanalyzed properly, there was no hint of a difference.

A study based in a colposcopy clinic which allowed the cytology detection rate to be compared to the histology, showed no advantage from combined cytobrush/spatula smears and only a slight advantage for the Aylesbury sampler over the Ayre's spatula in the detection of moderate dyskaryosis or worse and CIN 2 or worse.[42] However, the detection rates (sensitivity) for both devices were not high (Ayres 42%, Aylesbury 58%).

In the largest controlled comparison of the Aylesbury with the Ayre spatula, including 17 781 women from the general population, the Aylesbury spatula detected 21% more smears with dyskaryotic cells (age adjusted rates: 3.5 vs 2.9%), a difference which was not statistically significant.[43]

Possible advantage in older women

Many of these studies have contained a preponderance of young women in whom the theoretical advantages of the cytobrush and other devices designed to obtain cells from a squamocolumnar junction in the endocervical canal would not apply. Any advantage in the older women would be masked by the lack of benefit in the much larger numbers of younger subjects. Reexamining the crude data shown in the paper by Wolfendale et al,[43] there does seem to be a larger difference in the women 40 years and older in whom the rate of abnormality was 42% greater with the Aylesbury spatula (1.6 vs 1.1%) by comparison with a 25% difference in the younger women (4.0 vs 3.2%).

Conclusion

The Aylesbury spatula is widely used in the UK because of its marginal advantages. There is no place in routine screening for the cytobrush alone or in combination with a spatula. However, it may have advantages in women in whom the squamocolumnar junction is known to be in the

canal. At the end of the day, the relatively small differences between different sampling methods are probably much less important than the skill and experience of the operator.[44]

Management of mild cytological disorders

Mild dyskaryosis is common and often associated with high-grade CIN

Another way of improving the results of cytology screening would be to make the management of mild cytological disorders more effective. About 2% of smears in England and Wales are reported as mild dyskaryosis[45] and 50% of these may be expected to have CIN 2–3.[46,47] In 1990, 25% of women in Tayside Region found to have CIN 3 were diagnosed because of a mildly dyskaryotic smear (Duncan I, personal communication). It has been said that many of these lesions are small and less likely to progress to invasion.[48] Certainly, there is a trend for larger lesions to be associated with early invasive disease but small lesions do get bigger and there are no data to show that small CIN 3 lesions are innocuous.

Mild lesions become a larger problem as coverage improves

As a the coverage of a screening program improves, so the proportion of women who develop invasive disease in spite of having had a smear will increase. Two centers with high population coverage have recently reported that their incidence of cervical cancer has stopped falling and remains at a disappointingly high rate.[49,50] Both reports identify their policy of cytological follow up of women with mild abnormalities as contributing to the problem.

Referral to colposcopy is frequently required

Referral of these women to colposcopy is still a controversial subject largely because of the financial implications. It is often said that cytological surveillance allows most women with mild abnormalities to avoid colposcopy. An analysis of all the recent studies of cytological surveillance undertaken in the UK has shown that the cumulative referral rate to colposcopy after 4–4½ years ranged from 14 to 64%.[51] The two studies with the lowest referral rates had the highest rates of invasion.

Incidence of invasion is high with cytological follow-up

One of the main measures of the success of cervical screening is the incidence of invasive cancer. In one retrospective study of cytological surveillance of women with mild dyskaryosis which has been widely quoted as reassurance of the safety of this approach, 10 of the 1781 patients developed invasive cancer.[52] Excluding the three carcinomas which occurred in the 434 women who were lost to follow-up, this represents an annual incidence of invasive cancer of 143 per 100 000 women — hardly a reassuring statistic![51] Subsequently, a similar study in North London found an annual incidence of invasive disease of 420 per 100 000, a rate 60 times greater than the age-adjusted background rate.[53] An analysis of all the recent, large studies of cytological surveillance of women with mild cytological abnormalities undertaken in the UK showed that the annual incidence of invasive cancer in these women ranged from 143 to 420 per 100 000.[31] The average rate of all six studies was 208 per 100 000.

The women in these studies were mainly in the age group 15–34 years. They had a 16–47-fold greater incidence of invasive disease than women of the same age group in the general population in whom the incidence of invasive cancer was 9 per 100 000 in England and Wales in 1985 (Fig. 23.2). These data do not include cancers that may have occurred in women lost to follow-up. Given that all of these women had been screened, and that 80% of invasive cancers at that time occurred in women who had never had a smear, the real increased risk is likely to be even greater.

Decision analysis suggests a reduced risk of invasion

A recent decision analysis of this problem, concluded that repeating the smear would be almost as effective as referral to colposcopy in reducing the rate of invasive cancer.[54] However, they calculated the cancer risks in a very indirect way which

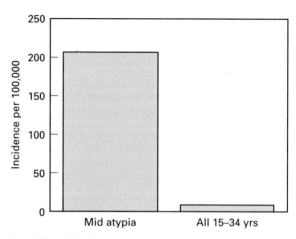

Fig. 23.2 This figure compares the incidence of invasive cancer in women with mild dyskaryosis followed cytologically with that of women aged 15–34 years in England and Wales. (Soutter 1994[53a]).

underestimates the rate in women followed cytologically. Furthermore, prevalence data rather than incidence rates were used in the calculations. Substituting 5-year cumulative incidence rates in their calculations, suggests that immediate referral to colposcopy would result in a 54–84% reduction in the risk of invasion.[51]

Immediate colposcopy is less expensive than deferred colposcopy

Because well over 50% of these women will eventually need colposcopy, the choice for most is immediate colposcopy versus deferred colposcopy. The objections made to immediate referral for colposcopy are the cost, lack of resources and the psychological impact on women. One comparison of the cost of colposcopy with that of multiple repeated smears has suggested that immediate colposcopy would be cheaper.[54] In my experience, many women with mildly abnormal smears ask for colposcopy even when cytological surveillance has been recommended to them. There is no doubt that colposcopy does induce a great deal of anxiety but that can be reduced substantially by explanatory leaflets sent out with the appointment.[55] I do not know of any published study comparing the levels of anxiety in women being followed cytologically with those attending for immediate colposcopy. This is obviously an important area that requires investigation.

Conclusion

These data provide compelling evidence that women with mild dyskaryosis often have CIN 2–3. If followed cytologically, they are at high risk of developing invasive cancer. While there has been no prospective, randomized comparison of cytological follow-up with immediate colposcopy in the management of these women, it would seem prudent to refer this high-risk group of women for colposcopy after the first abnormal smear. Many will have no abnormality, will not require biopsy and may be reassured quickly and returned to the screening program. Those who do have abnormalities can be treated effectively in the outpatient clinic with only mild discomfort and little or no risk to their fertility or fecundity.

NEW SCREENING METHODS

Methods based on Feulgen hydrolysis

It is well known that nuclear changes are a feature of many malignant cells. This is the basis of cytology. It would seem reasonable to use methods which measure the amount of DNA to identify abnormal cells objectively.[56] Feulgen hydrolysis has been used in this way by several workers.[57] Indeed, a modified Feulgen hydrolysis which measures only the rapidly hydrolyzable fraction of acid-labile DNA appears to reveal alterations in morphologically normal cells in smears from women with CIN.[57,58]

This suggests that it might well be suitable for cervical screening. A study of 237 normal controls from a family planning clinic and 419 women with CIN or invasive cancer from a colposcopy clinic suggested that a sensitivity of 87.1% and a specificity of 99.2% might be achieved.[59] Unfortunately, attempts in my own unit to reproduce these results using both microdensitometry and image analysis were unsuccessful.

Image analysis

The idea of computerized image analysis of cytological preparations is attractive but there are considerable technical difficulties to be overcome. One of the most vexed is the development of suitable cell preparations which minimize or abolish clumping of overlapping of cells as this can cause problems for the computer.[60,61] Some have attempted to develop new methods of cell preparation such as laying separated cells onto glass slides coated with the cationic polyelectrolyte poly-L-lysine,[62] while others have sought to develop computer algorithms to segment the image and reject artifacts.[61]

There are two broad approaches to automation.[63] In the first, the samples are prepared by an instrument which aims to provide a dispersed sample. Such systems may use either a conventional Pap stain[64] or one of the alternative staining methods. A recently evaluated system, using a gallocyanin DNA-stochiometric dye, appeared to have a similar false negative rate to routine screening as judged by rescreening of the same slides by three other observers.[65]

The false negative error rate was 5% for high-grade cases, 17% for mild dyskaryosis and 29% for borderline smears. The 'false positive rate' was 34%. In spite of this high proportion of slides which would have required further evaluation, the authors felt that the system was potentially cost-effective. However, the error rates do seem rather high.

The second approach is to use conventional cervical cytology smears and Pap stains. These identify slides that require further examination by a technician and require varying degrees of interaction. One system uses a neural network as well as conventional image analysis algorithms. There are no results of large-scale testing for any of these systems.

It must be recognized that machines cannot achieve morphological distinctions which human experts cannot define. Nor can they remove an intrinsic overlap in features between the normal and abnormal populations. The way ahead may lie in the use of different markers combined with morphology, exploiting the ability of the computer to combine information from different signal systems to provide better discrimination. One such system might use infrared spectroscopy.[66]

Cervicography

The method is similar to colposcopy

The combination of cytology and colposcopy increases the accuracy of detection of CIN and cervical cancer[67] but colposcopy is too costly to use as a screening tool in most circumstances. Cervicography is a technique which attempts to reproduce colposcopy photographically.[68] A photograph of the cervix is taken with a specially designed camera after the application of acetic acid. The camera incorporates a light source and is designed to minimize problems of focus or movement artifact. Since neither an expensive colposcope nor a highly trained colposcopist are required, cervicography can be performed by any doctor or nurse who is able to insert a speculum and visualise the cervix. The photographs obtained are sent to an expert for interpretation. By projecting the images onto a screen, a magnification and resolution similar to colposcopy are obtained and interpretation can be performed far more quickly than in a colposcopic examination.

Studies in selected populations are encouraging

Several studies have compared cervicography with cytology in selected populations. Tawa and associates,[69] in a study of 3271 routine gynaecological patients, showed the cervigram to be significantly more sensitive than the Pap smear — over five times as many cases of CIN were diagnosed by cervicography. The sensitivity and specificity of cervicography were 0.89 and 0.91, respectively, with 11.2% technically defective cervigrams. Gundersen et al[70] studied 274 gynecological patients and found a sensitivity of 0.90 and specificity of 0.83 with 8.8% technically defective. In two studies of women with 'atypical' smears the estimates of sensitivity were 0.78 and 0.87 and of specificity were 0.50 and 0.65.[71,72]

Lack of independent confirmation of disease status

However, another paper comparing the use of cervical cytology, cervicography and HPV DNA detection illustrates clearly the difficulties faced by most studies which attempt to determine the specificity and sensitivity of tests for cervical premalignancy.[73] Almost one-third of the women studied had an equivocal result in one of the three tests and nearly a quarter of these were not reevaluated with colposcopy. No further tests were performed on the women with negative results, raising the possibility that further pathology may exist in the apparently negative population. The true prevalence of CIN in that study population remains unknown.

Studies which determine the disease status with colposcopic biopsy

This important limitation was avoided in a recent study of an asymptomatic screening population by performing colposcopy on all of the study population.[15] To limit the impact of errors in colposcopic interpretation, biopsies were taken liberally from any atypical areas. Thus the true prevalence of CIN and invasive cancer was established histologically with the help of a technique which is independent of the screening tests being evaluated. This study confirmed the previously suspected low sensitivity of cervical cytology (0.52) and the significantly better sensitivity of cervicography (0.89). Both tests had a similar specificity (0.94, 0.92). Technically defective cervigrams were reported in 5.5% of cases. Two other studies of cervicography evaluated in a screening population who also underwent colposcopy have been reported in abstract form only.[16,17] They confirm the results reported by Kesic et al.[15]

Conclusion

The excellent results of cervicography in these studies may be due in part to the cervigrams being taken by gynecologists. It remains to be shown that nursing staff or nongynecological medical staff can maintain this low rate of defective photographs. Stafl's report[68] is reassuring with only 3.8% technically defective cervigrams in a study in which the great majority of photographs were taken by nurse practitioners or resident physicians. Experience with the technique has shown that the lithotomy position is essential because of the pistol grip on the camera.[74] This and the expense of the instrument required are disadvantages of cervicography which may make it more difficult to provide in a family doctor's surgery. Although cervicography is more sensitive than cytology and only slightly less specific, its true role has still to be determined. In a cost-conscious health service, it may find a place as a secondary screening test of women with minor cytological abnormalities.

Testing for human papilloma virus (HPV)

Testing for the presence of HPV types known to be associated with CIN and invasive cancer is an attractive idea. The modern tests are highly specific and very sensitive (see Chapter 16 for a discussion of the older test methods). The high sensitivity is a problem in itself because it makes false positive results from contamination more likely unless elaborate precautions are taken. In addition, with PCR techniques that can detect as little as one copy of the genome, it is more likely that unaffected women will test positive because they were exposed to the virus some time in the past but did not develop CIN. False negative results will inevitably occur with those lesions which are not associated with the HPV types detected by the test. This can be reduced but not eliminated by increasing the number of probes in the test.

Nonquantitative HPV testing in combination with cytology and cervicography

A study of 1021 women aged 18–35 years underwent a smear test and cervicography, and a sample was taken for HPV testing by Southern blot using probes for 14 different HPV types.[73] Of 298 patients recalled for colposcopy because one of the three tests was abnormal, 68 could not be traced or would not come leaving the final diagnosis in doubt in these women. On the evidence available, three were classified as having high-grade lesions and 14 as low grade but their real disease status remains unknown. The sensitivity of cytology for high-grade lesions was only 0.52 with a specificity of 0.92 and both cervicography and HPV testing had a sensitivity of 0.61 with specificity values similar to cytology. By trying different, post hoc combinations of the data, it appeared that the best results might have been achieved by referring for colposcopy: women with high-grade cytology results; or positive cervicography results; plus any woman with an atypical smear and a positive HPV test for an 'oncogenic' virus probe (sensitivity 0.96, specificity 0.96). The

authors concluded that the increased screening costs would be offset by the reduced need for referrals.

The results of cervicography in this study are disappointing by comparison with the studies quoted above and illustrate the potential difficulties with this technique. The major problem with the authors' suggestions is that the recommended combination of tests was derived by a retrospective examination of the dataset. The validity of these conclusions would need to be determined by applying these criteria to another population.

Quantitative PCR

In order to overcome the problem of false positive results due to the high sensitivity of PCR tests for HPV, a semiquantitative PCR test has been advocated.[75,76] Indeed, two relatively small studies of women referred for colposcopy have given encouraging results. In the first study of 200 women referred with mild dyskaryosis, 56% of the women with CIN 1 or less had some detectable HPV compared with 70% of those with CIN 2–3.[77] However, when low HPV results were regarded as negative, 25% of the normal or low-grade group tested positive compared with 56% of the high grade. In the second study of 133 women referred with a range of cytological abnormalities, the quantitative HPV test for HPV 16 only had a 93% positive predictive value and a 53% sensitivity for high-grade disease.[78] By including HPV 18, 31, 33 and 35 the positive predictive value was reduced to 79% but the sensitivity rose to 84%. Combining the cytology and the HPV results appeared to give still better sensitivity but the authors cautioned against overinterpretation of post hoc analysis of these data.

Conclusions

These studies all provide interesting information which should stimulate further research. Much larger studies of the general screening population, including older women, are required for the next phase. Colposcopic examination of all subjects with any degree of abnormality in any of the tests and biopsy of any abnormalities will be essential.

DIAGNOSTIC TECHNIQUES

Cervical cytology is not a diagnostic tool. When a smear is abnormal, when the cervix looks suspicious or when a woman complains of worrying symptoms such as postcoital bleeding or intermenstrual bleeding, she should be referred for an appropriate diagnostic test to rule out cervical pathology.

DIAGNOSTIC COLPOSCOPY

Prior to the introduction of colposcopy, the only way of excluding a diagnosis of CIN or preclinical carcinoma was to perform a biopsy. This was often a cone biopsy but multiple, blind punch biopsies and ring biopsies were used in an attempt to reduce the trauma to the cervix of what were usually young women.

Colposcopic technique

A detailed description of colposcopic technique is beyond the scope of this chapter and the reader is referred to other textbooks for further information.[79] There are two slightly different methods in widespread use. In one, sometimes referred to as the 'Saline Technique,' the blood vessel pattern of the cervix is examined through a green filter after the application of normal saline. The vascular architecture and the intercapillary distance are examined carefully. Abnormal punctation, mosaic and atypical vessels are sought. The second technique relies more on the results of applying acetic acid and, sometimes, iodine (Table 23.1). It is

often said that the vascular markings are obscured by acetic acid but I seldom find that to be the case. In reality, most experienced colposcopists use a combination of the two 'techniques,' looking closely at the vascular markings and the surface contours before applying acetic acid. Sometimes an application of saline or use of the green filter will help this part of the examination.

Colposcopy is subjective

No matter what method is used, it is clear that colposcopic inspection is a every bit as subjective as cytology and most colposcopists emphasize the importance of directed biopsies in confirming the colposcopic diagnosis. There have been few studies which have examined directly the accuracy of colposcopy but these confirm the difficulties of this subjective technique. A study of 161 women referred because of a smear showing mild dyskaryosis compared the repeat smear, colposcopy and colposcopically directed biopsy.[80] The sensitivity and specificity in detecting CIN of any grade with cytology were 0.77 and 0.53. The results for colposcopy were little different at 0.71 and 0.61. In the study of cervicography mentioned above, the unpublished results for sensitivity and specificity of the colposcopic diagnosis of CIN were 0.77 and 0.94.[15] Differences in these results may be due to different prevalences of high-grade disease which is easier to identify.

The difficulties of colposcopy are greatest at the two extremes: differentiating between CIN 1 and metaplasia or HPV changes; and identifying cases of early invasion in women who appear to

Table 23.1 The modified Reid colposcopic score (modified from Reid 1987[79a] and reprinted from Soutter 1993[79] with permission)*

Feature	Zero points	1 point	2 points
Margin	Condylomatous or micropapillary contour. Indistinct acetowhite edge. Flocculated or feathered edge. Angular or jagged edges. Satellite lesions.	Regular Smooth Straight	Rolled, peeling edges. Internal demarcations between areas of different appearance. (lesion within a lesion.)
Colour	Shiny, snow-white colour. Indistinct acetowhite.	Shiny grey.	Dull, oyster white.
Vessels	Fine-caliber vessels, poorly formed patterns. Capillary loops in micropapilli.	No vessels.	Definite punctation or mosaic.
Iodine	Minor iodine negativity.	Partial stain.	Negative uptake.

*A score of 0–2 = subclinical wart virus infection or CIN 1; 3–5 = CIN 1–2; 6–8 = CIN 2–3.

have CIN 3. The difficulty at the mild end of the spectrum is hardly surprising given the problems that even histopathologists have in this area.[9] This causes a therapeutic dilemma made more acute by the relative unreliability of punch biopsy (see below). Some solve this predicament by leaving 'mild lesions' untreated but this imposes a considerable burden of review cases. Others prefer to treat these uncertain cases as the quickest way of returning the smear to normal and the woman to routine screening. Given the low morbidity of most outpatient treatments, the latter would seem to be a reasonable approach provided the woman is aware that she may be being treated 'unnecessarily.' Much of the problem at the severe end of the spectrum has been solved by the wide availability of outpatient excisional treatments which should certainly be used for all severe lesions and probably be adopted as the treatment of choice for any degree of CIN.[81–83]

Pitfalls of colposcopy

The squamocolumnar junction in the canal

However, difficulties in diagnosis of high-grade or invasive disease remain. The colposcopist must recognize the limitations of the technique and the pitfalls that await the unwary.[79] It is fundamental to colposcopy that the squamocolumnar junction is visualized clearly and that any visible lesion be seen in its entirety. A lesion which extends up the endocervical canal can be very difficult to evaluate because it cannot be viewed at right angles. This makes the colposcopic diagnosis suspect. It also means that it is difficult to assess the length of the endocervical canal involved because of the foreshortening of the image that occurs when an object is viewed obliquely.

The false squamocolumnar junction caused by an abrasion

The squamocolumnar junction (SCJ) must be identified by observing *the lower limit of normal columnar epithelium* not the upper limit of squamous epithelium.[79] This is because CIN and metaplastic epithelium can be detached very easily from the underlying stroma by an examining finger, by the insertion of a speculum or by the taking of a smear. An abrasion may persist for several months so it is impossible to say when the epithelium was removed or by what. When an abrasion occurs at the SCJ, the unwary may mistake the upper limit of acetowhite change for the true SCJ.

The previously treated cervix

Because colposcopy depends upon an intact, unadulterated transformation zone to give reliable results, the interpretation of colposcopy findings in women who have been treated previously must be made with great care.[79] Areas of metaplasia, CIN or invasive disease in the canal or in cervical glands may have escaped destruction and may persist as isolated 'iatrogenic skip lesions.' These may lie on the surface of the endocervical canal surrounded by the columnar epithelium which grew over the area destroyed, or may be buried in the stroma.

Glandular lesions

Finally, the rules of colposcopy do not apply to women with adenocarcinoma or AIS because it is not possible to identify these lesions reliably with the colposcope.[84] Consequently, women who have abnormal glandular cells in their smear require a cone biopsy to determine the diagnosis. The saving grace of this situation is that about 65% of women with AIS also have CIN and it is this which is detected both cytologically and colposcopically.[84,85] The glandular lesion is often discovered incidentally in the histological samples. Indeed the common coexistence of CIN and AIS and the difficulties which pathologists often have in distinguishing adenocarcinoma of the cervix from squamous cancer raise the possibility that both may be different morphological versions of the same disease.

PUNCH BIOPSY

Missing invasive disease

The difficulties of colposcopic diagnosis are not entirely resolved by punch biopsy. There is considerable concern that early invasive lesions may be missed by colposcopically directed punch biopsy and then treated inappropriately by ablation.[86–88] A review of 1609 women with carcinoma-in-situ reported higher rates of recurrence and of death among women in whom the diagnosis was based only upon a small biopsy.[89] The authors concluded that this was due to inadequate diagnosis and a failure to detect invasive disease with punch biopsy.

False negative punch biopsy

The punch biopsy will often underestimate the severity of the lesion. False negative rates of 41–54% have been reported.[90–92] These results were not as good as those described by Kirkup et al.[93] However 92% of their material was CIN 2 or worse, the area where observer variation is least. In addition, punch biopsies may well not detect glandular abnormalities. An awareness of these problems led to the development of outpatient excisional methods of treatment. However, even cone biopsy may give a false negative result because of handling artifacts caused by clinician or pathologist, or sampling error when the pathologist cuts the blocks.

Working diagnosis

It is necessary to come to a working diagnosis in order to decide what should be done next. A histological diagnosis based upon an adequate biopsy is the 'gold standard' in spite of the problems of observer error. However, in view of the relative unreliability of punch biopsies, a working diagnosis cannot always be based solely on the result of this investigation.[79]

CONE BIOPSY

Diagnostic cone biopsy

Cone biopsy with a knife, laser or loop diathermy is probably the most reliable diagnostic method available. Because these are used so often for treating lesions identified with colposcopy, their diagnostic role is sometimes forgotten. This is particularly true in the management of women with an abnormal smear and unsatisfactory colposcopy.[79] If CIN is visible lying partly on the ectocervix but disappearing into the canal, a cone biopsy is required to determine the diagnosis and to excise the lesion. In this situation the operator knows that the woman has CIN at least and there is no question of an 'unnecessary' cone biopsy.

Unsatisfactory colposcopy and cone biopsy

Even when the ectocervix is normal, if the squamocolumnar junction is out of sight, CIN or invasive disease may lurk up the canal. If the smear shows moderate or severe dyskaryosis, the risk of a significant lesion in the canal is substantial (Fig. 23.3) and cone biopsy is required to determine the diagnosis.[79,94]

When the cytological abnormality is mild, the likelihood of finding no pathology in the cone biopsy increases (Fig. 23.3) and some alternative management is needed. All of the diagnostic problems encountered in postmenopausal women may be alleviated by giving estrogen therapy, either topically or orally, and repeating the colposcopy in 6 weeks. This may resolve the problem by bringing the squamocolumnar junction into view and by improving the quality of the smear. If doubt persists at a repeat examination

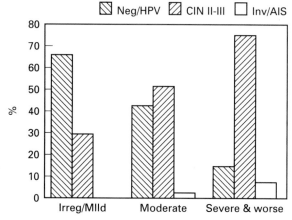

Fig. 23.3 This chart shows the histological findings in cone biopsies performed because of abnormal cervical cytology and unsatisfactory colposcopy. The likelihood of significant CIN (CIN 2–3) or of invasive disease or adenocarcinoma-in-situ (Inv/AIS) increased with increasing severity of the smear. (After Ref. 94). However, even with mild cytologic abnormalities, a substantial proportion of the cone biopsies in this study contained significant pathology and, in my own experience, can even contain unsuspected invasive disease. (Reproduced with permission from Ref. 79.)

after oestrogen replacement, a further review in 6 months may be justifiable but cone biopsy is often necessary in the end.

False negative and false positive results in cone biopsy

However, cone biopsy is not without its own problems. Missing epithelium as a result of surgical trauma or handling in the laboratory may make it impossible to determine the diagnosis or the completeness of excision. It is often worth taking deeper sections in a block in case the problem is confined to the edges of the block. The thermal artifact from laser or diathermy may make it difficult to determine the completeness of excision but the main diagnosis is impaired only in exceptional circumstances.

If the cone biopsy is large, many blocks may need to be cut and examined to avoid sampling error. While some laboratories cut 50 to 60 blocks, this is unnecessary in most cases and blocks cut 3 mm thick are more than adequate for the largest cone biopsies. The pathologist must be alert to the problem of carry over, in which a piece of abnormal epithelium is displaced from one part of the specimen (or from another specimen altogether) and appears as a focus of apparent invasive disease. Orientation of the biopsy is important, especially when considering whether transversely cut glands with CIN are loci of early invasion or lymph-vascular space involvement. Finally, lymph-vascular space involvement is always a difficult diagnosis to make with certainty. The more assiduously it is sought, the more often it is found and the less important it becomes in the prognosis.

CONCLUSIONS

The optimum screening program involves the close collaboration of public health physician, cytologist, histopathologist and colposcopist. The limitations of all the techniques being used must be recognized and steps taken to minimize their impact.

REFERENCES

1. Petersen O. Spontaneous course of cervical precancerous conditions. Am J Obstet Gynecol 1956; 72: 1063–1071.
2. McIndoe W A, McLean M R, Jones R W, Mullins P R. The invasive potential of carcinoma in situ of the cervix. Obstet Gynecol 1984; 64: 451–458.
3. IARC Working Group on Evaluation of Cervical Cancer Screening Programmes. Screening for squamous cervical cancer: duration of low risk after negative results of cervical cytology and its implication for screening policies. Br Med J 1986; 293: 659–664.
4. Schwartz M, Savage W, George J, Emohare L. Women's knowledge and experience of cervical screening: a failure of health education and medical organization. Community Med 1989; 11: 279–289.
5. Nicoll P M, Narayan K V, Paterson J G. Cervical cancer screening: women's knowledge, attitudes and preferences. Health Bull Edin 1991; 49: 184–190.
6. Ciatto S, Cecchini S, Bonardi R, Venturini A, Ciacci R. Attendance to a screening program for cervical cancer in the city of Florence. Tumori 1991; 77: 252–256.
7. Husain O A N, Butler B B, Evans D M D, Macgregor J E. Quality control in cervical cytology. J Clin Pathol 1974; 27: 935–944.
8. Kern W H, Zivolich M R. The accuracy and consistency of the cytologic classification of squamous lesions of the uterine cervix. Acta Cytol 1977; 21: 519–523.
9. Robertson A J, Anderson J M, Swanson Beck J et al. Observer variability in histopathological reporting of cervical biopsy specimens. J Clin Pathol 1989; 42: 231–238.
10. Beilby J O, Bourne R, Guillebaud J, Steele S T. Paired cervical smears: a method of reducing the false-negative rate in population screening. Obstet Gynecol 1982; 60: 46–48.
11. Yobs A R, Swanson R A, Lamotte L C Jr. Laboratory reliability of the Papanicolaou smear. Obstet Gynecol 1985; 65: 235–244.
12. Goes-Junior J S, Goes J C, Lemos L B et al. Practical approaches to screening for cervical cancer. Cancer Detect Prevent 1987; 10: 265–277.
13. The Evaluation Committee. Population screening for cervical cancer in The Netherlands. A report by the Evaluation Committee. Int J Epidemiol 1989; 18: 775–781.
14. Pairwuti S. False-negative Papanicolaou smears from women with cancerous and precancerous lesions of the uterine cervix. Acta Cytol 1991; 35: 40–46.
15. Kesic V I, Soutter W P, Sulovic V, Juznic N, Aleksic M, Ljubic A. A comparison of cytology and cervicography in cervical screening. Int J Gynaecol Oncol 1993; 3: 395–398.
16. Campion M J, diPaola F M, Vellios F. The value of cervicography in population screening. J Exper Clinic Cancer Res 1990; Supplement 9: FC 107.
17. Miloiu A, Guernier C, Andry M et al. Correlation between the Pap smear and a new screening approach. The cervicograph — the Belgian experience. J Exper Clin Cancer Res 1990; Supplement 9: FC 108.
18. Chamberlain J. Failures of the cervical cytology screening programme. Br Med J 1984; 289: 853–854.

19. Aareleid T, Pukkala E, Thomson H, Hakama M. Cervical cancer incidence and mortality trends in Finland and Estonia: a screened vs. an unscreened population. Eur J Cancer 1993, 29A: 745–749.

20. Läärä E, Day N E, Hakama M. Trends in mortality from cervical cancer in the Nordiccountries: association with organised screening programmes. Lancet 1987; 1: 1247–1249.

21. Lynge E, Poll P. Incidence of cervical cancer following negative smear. A cohort study from Maribo County, Denmark. Am J Epidemiol 1986; 124: 345–52.

22. Moss S M. Case-control studies of screening. Int J Epidemiol 1991; 20: 1–6.

23. Zhang Z F, Parkin D M, Yu S Z, Esteve J, Yang X Z, Day N E. Cervical screening attendance and its effectiveness in a rural population in China. Cancer Detect Prevent 1989; 13: 337–342.

24. Makino H, Sato S, Yajima A, Fukao A. Case control study of the effectiveness of mass screening in reducing invasive cervical cancer. Nippon Sanka Fujinka Gakkai Zasshi 1991; 43: 1226–1232.

25. Parazzini F, Negri E, La-Vecchia C, Bocciolone L. Screening practices and invasive cervical cancer risk in different age strata. Gynecol Oncol 1990; 38: 76–80.

26. Palli D, Carli S, Cecchini S, Venturini A, Piazzesi G, Buiatti E. A centralised cytology screening programme for cervical cancer in Florence. J Epidemiol Community Health 1990; 44: 47–51.

27. Celentano D D, Klassen A C, Weisman C S, Rosenshein N B. Duration of relative protection of screening for cervical cancer. Prev Med 1989; 18: 411–422.

28. Olesen F. A case-control study of cervical cytology before diagnosis of cervical cancer in Denmark. Int J Epidemiol 1988; 17: 501–508.

29. Oortmarssen G J van, Habbema J D, Ballegooijen M van. Predicting mortality from cervical cancer after negative smear test results. Br Med J 1992; 305: 449–451.

30. Laverty C R, Farnsworth A, Thurloe J, Bowditch R. The reliability of a cytological prediction of cervical adenocarcinoma in situ. Aus NZJ Obstet Gynaecol 1988; 28: 307–312.

31. Lee K R. False positive diagnosis of adenocarcinoma in situ of the cervix. Acta Cytol 1988; 32: 276–267.

32. Lee K R, Manna E A, Jones M A. Comparative cytologic features of adenocarcinoma in situ of the uterine cervix. Acta Cytol 1991; 35: 117–126.

33. Feldman M J, Seeve C C, Srebnik E. False positive cervical cytology: an important reason for colposcopy. Am J Obstet Gynecol 1977; 129: 141–144.

34. Kristensen G B, Skyggebjerg K D, Holund B, Holm K, Hansen M K. Analysis of cervical smears obtained within three years of the diagnosis of invasive cervical cancer. Acta Cytol 1991; 35: 47–50.

35. Costa M J, Kenny M B, Naib Z M. Cervicovaginal cytology in uterine adenocarcinoma and adenosquamous carcinoma. Comparison of cytologic and histologic findings. Acta Cytol 1991; 35: 127–134.

36. Boon M E, de Graaff Guilloud J C, Kok L P, Olthof P M, van Erp E J M. Efficacy of screening for cervical squamous and adenocarcinoma — the Dutch experience. Cancer 1987; 59: 862–866.

37. Woodman C J B, Yates M, Williams D R, Ward K, Jordan J, Luesley D. A randomised controlled trial of two cervical spatulas. Br J Obstet Gynaecol 1991; 98: 21–24.

38. Goorney B P, Lacey C J N, Sutton J. Ayre v Aylesbury cervical spatula. Genitourinary Med 1989; 65: 161–162.

39. Szarewski A, Cuzick J, Nayagan M, Thin R N. A comparison of four cytological sampling techniques in a genito-urinary medicine clinic. Genitourinary Med 1990; 66: 439–443.

40. Boon M E, de Graaf Guilloud J C, Reitveld W J. Analysis of five sampling methods for the preparation of cervical smears. Acta Cytol 1989; 33: 843–848.

41. Sasieni P D. Cervical samplers. Br Med J 1991; 303: 313.

42. Beeby A R, Keating P J, Wagstaff T I et al. The quality and accuracy of cervical cytology: a study of five sampling devices in a colposcopy clinic. J Obstet Gynaecol 1993; 13: 276–281.

43. Wolfendale M R, Howe-Guest R, Usherwood M M, Draper G J. Controlled trial of a new cervical spatula. Br Med J 1987; 293: 33–35.

44. Wolfendale M R. Cervical samplers. Br Med J 1991; 302: 1554–1555.

45. Soutter W P. Report on Workshop on Mild Dyskaryosis — National Coordinating Network and United Kingdom Coordinating Committee for Cancer Research. Oxford: National Coordinating Network, 1992.

46. Soutter W P, Wisdom S, Brough A K, Monaghan J M. Should patients with mild atypia in a cervical smear be referred for colposcopy? Br J Obstet Gynaecol 1986; 93: 70–74.

47. Bolger B S, Lewis B V. A prospective study of colposcopy in women with mild dyskaryosis or koilocytosis. Br J Obstet Gynaecol 1988; 95: 1117–1119.

48. Jarmulowicz M R, Jenkins D, Barton S E, Goodall A L, Hollingworth A, Singer A. Cytological status and lesion size: a further dimension in cervical intraepithelial neoplasia. Br J Obstet Gynaecol 1989; 96: 1061–1066.

49. Sigurosson K, Aoalsteinsson S, Tulinius H, Ragnarsson J, Snorradottir M. The value of screening as an approach to cervical cancer control in Iceland 1964–88. J Exp Clin Res 1990; 9: Supplement FC/276.

50. Bjerre B. Invasive cervical cancer in a thoroughly screened population. J Exp Clin Res 1990; 9: Supplement FC/276.

51. Soutter W P, Fletcher A. Invasive cancer in women with mild dyskaryosis followed cytologically. Br Med J 1994; 308: 1421–1423.

52. Robertson J H, Woodend B E, Crozier E H, Hutchinson J. Risk of cervical cancer associated with mild dyskaryosis. Br Med J 1988; 297: 18–21.

53. Fletcher A, Metaxas N, Grubb C, Chamberlain J. Four and a half year follow up of women with dyskaryotic cervical smears. Br Med J 1990; 301: 641–644.

53a. Soutter W P. The management of a mildly dyskaryotic smear: immediate referral to colposcopy is safer. Br Med J 1994; 309: 591–592.

54. Johnson N, Sutton J, Thornton J G, Lilford R J, Johnson V A, Peel K R. Decision analysis for best management of mildly dyskaryotic smear. Lancet 1993; 342: 91–96.

55. Wilkinson C, Jones J M, McBride J. Anxiety caused by

abnormal result of cervical smear test: a controlled trial. Br Med J 1990; 300: 440.

56. Strang P, Stendahl U, Frankendal B, Lindgren A. Flow cytometric DNA patterns in cervical carcinoma. Acta Quant Cytol Histol 1986; 25: 249–254.

57. Millett J A, Husain O A N, Bitensky L, Chayen J. Feulgen hydrolysis hydrolysis profiles in cells exfoliated from the cervix uteri: a potential aid in the diagnosis of malignancy. J Clin Pathol 1982; 35: 345–349.

58. Sincock A M. Semi-automated diagnosis of cervical intraepithelial neoplasia grade 2 by the measurement of acid labile DNA in cytologically normal nuclei. Cancer 1986; 58: 83–86.

59. Partington C K, Sincock A M, Steele S J. Quantitative determination of acid-labile DNA in cervical intraepithelial neoplasia. Cancer 1991; 67: 3104–3109.

60. Rosenthal D L, Manjikian V. Techniques in the preparation of a monolayer of gynecologic cells for automated cytology. An overview. Anal Quantit Cytol Histol 1987; 9: 55–59.

61. Bengtsson E. The measuring of cell features. Anal Quantit Cytol Histol 1987; 9: 212–217.

62. Watts K C, Husain O A, Tucker J H et al. The use of cationic polyelectrolytes in the preparation of cell monolayers for automated cell scanning and diagnostic cytopathology. Anal Quant Cytol 1984; 6: 272–278.

63. Industrial Developments in Automated Cytology as submitted by their Developers. Anal Quantit Cytol Histol 1993; 15: 358–370.

64. Geyer J W, Hancock F, Carrico C, Kirkpatrick M. Preliminary evaluation of Cyto-Rich: an improved automated cytology preparation. Diagnost Cytopathol 1993; 9: 417–421.

65. Husain O A, Watts K C, Lorriman F et al. Semi-automated cervical smear pre-screening systems: an evaluation of the Cytoscan-110. Anal Cell Pathol 1993; 5: 49–68.

66. Wong P T T, Wong R K, Caputo T A, Godwin T A, Rigas B. Infrared spectroscopy of exfoliated human cervical cells: evidence of extensive structural changes during carcinogenesis. Proc Nat Acad Sci USA 1991; 88: 10988–10992.

67. Navratil E, Burhardt E, Bajardi F et al. Simultaneous colposcopy and cytology of the cervix. Am J Obstet Gynecol 1958; 75: 1292–1296.

68. Stafl A. Cervicography: a new method for cervical cancer detection. Am J Obstet Gynecology 1981; 139: 815–821.

69. Tawa K, Forsythe A, Cove K J, Saltz A, Peters H, Watring W G. A comparison of the Papanicolaou smear and the cervigram: sensitivity, specificity and cost analysis. Obstet Gynecol 1988; 71: 229–235.

70. Gunderson J H, Schauberger C W, Rowe N R. The Papanicolaou smear and the cervigram: a preliminary report. J Reprod Med 1988; 33: 46–47.

71. Spitzer M, Krumholz B A, Chernys A E, Seltzer V, Lightman A R. Comparative utility of repeat Papanicolaou smears, cervicography and colposcopy in the evaluation of atypical Papanicolaou smears. Obstet Gynecol 1987; 69: 731–735.

72. Darnell-Jones D E, Creasman W T, Dombroski R A, Lentz S S, Waeltz J L. Evaluation of the atypical Pap smear. Am J Obstet Gynecol 1987; 157: 544–549.

73. Reid R, Greenberg M D, Lorincz A et al. Should cervical cytologix testing be augmented by cervicography or human papillomavirus deoxyribonucleic acid detection? Am J Obstet Gynecol 1991; 164: 1461–1471.

74. Soutter W P, Chaves J, Gleeson R, Lim K, Segall S, Skehan M. Cervicography in a colposcopy clinic. J Obstet Gynaecol 1991; 11: 218–220.

75. Cuzick J, Terry G, Ho L, Hollingworth T, Anderson M. Human papillomavirus type 16 DNA in cervical smears as predictor of high-grade cervical cancer. Lancet 1992; 339: 959–960.

76. Morrison E A, Goldberg G L, Kadish A S, Burk R D. Polymerase chain reaction detection of human papillomavirus: quantitation may improve clinical utility. J Clin Microbiol 1992; 30: 2539–2543.

77. Bavin P J, Giles J A, Deery A et al. Use of semi-quantitative PCR for human papillomavirus DNA type 16 to identify women with high grade cervical disease in a population presenting with a mildly dyskaryotic smear report. Br J Cancer 1993; 67: 602–605.

78. Cuzick J, Terry G, Ho L, Hollingworth T, Anderson M. Type-specific human papillomavirus DNA in abnormal smears as predictor of high-grade cervical intraepithelial neoplasia. Br J Cancer 1994; 69: 167–171.

79. Soutter P. A practical guide to colposcopy. Oxford: Oxford University Press, 1993.

79a. Reid R. A rapid method for improving colposcopic accuracy. Colposcopy Gynaecol Laser Surg 1987; 3: 139–146.

80. Maggi R, Zannoni E, Giorda G, Biraghi P, Sideri M. Comparison of repeat smear, colposcopy and colposcopically directed biopsy in the evaluation of a mildly abnormal smear. Gynecol Oncol 1987; 35: 294–296.

81. Partington C K, Turner M J, Soutter W P, Griffiths M, Krausz T. Laser vaporisation versus laser excision conisation in the treatment of cervical intraepithelial neoplasia. Obstet Gynaecol 1989; 73: 775–779.

82. Prendiville W, Cullimore J, Norman S. Large loop excision of the transformation zone (LLETZ). A new method of management for women with cervical intraepithelial neoplasia. Br J Obstet Gynaecol 1989; 96: 1054–1060.

83. Murdoch J B, Grimshaw R N, Morgan P R, Monaghan J M. The impact of loop diathermy on management of early invasive cervical cancer. Int J Gynecol Cancer 1992; 2: 129–133.

84. Andersen E S, Arffmann E. Adenocarcinoma-in-situ of the uterine cervix: a clinico-pathologic study of 36 cases. Gynecol Oncol 1989; 35: 1–7.

85. Nicklin J L, Wright R G, Bell J R, Samaratunga H, Cox N C, Ward B G. A clinicopathological study of adenocarcinoma in situ of the cervix. The influence of cervical HPV infection and other factors and the role of conservative surgery. Aus NZ J Obstet Gynaecol 1991; 31: 179–183.

86. Grundsell H, Alm P, Larsson G. Cure rates after laser conisation for early cervical neoplasia. Annales Chirugiae Gynaecologica 1983; 72: 218–222.

87. Anderson M C. Are we vaporising microinvasive lesions? In: Sharp F, Jordan J A, eds. Gynaecological laser surgery. New York: Perinatology Press, 1986: pp 127–132.

88. Pearson S E, Whittaker J, Ireland D, Monaghan J M. Invasive cancer of the cervix after laser treatment. Br J Obstet Gynaecol 1989; 96: 486–488.

89. Burghardt E, Holzer E. Treatment of carcinoma in situ: evaluation of 1609 case. Obstet Gynecol 1980; 55: 539–545.

90. Byrne P, Jordan J, Williams D, Woodman C. Importance of negative result of cervical biopsy directed by colposcopy. Br Med J 1988; 296: 172.

91. Skehan M, Soutter W P, Lim K, Krause T, Pryse-Davies J. Reliability of colposcopy and directed punch biopsy. Br J Obstet Gynaecol 1990; 97: 811–816.

92. Howe D T, Vincenti A C. Is large loop excision of the transformation zone (LLETZ) more accurate than colposcopically directed punch biopsy in the diagnosis of cervical intraepithelial neoplasia? Br J Obstet Gynaecol 1991; 98: 588–591.

93. Kirkup W, Singer A, Hill A S. The accuracy of colposcopically directed biopsy in patients with suspected intraepithelial neoplasia of the cervix. Br J Obstet Gynaecol 1980; 87: 1–4.

94. Lopes A, Pearson S E, Mor-Yosef S, Ireland D, Monaghan J M. Is it time for a reconsideration of the criteria for cone biopsy? Br J Obstet Gynaecol 1989; 96: 1345–1347.

24. Retinoids in differentiation and prevention of malignant transformation

Nadine Darwiche   Luigi M. De Luca

INTRODUCTION

Retinoids are essential for maintenance of normal epithelial morphology and function[1] in the adult and for the control of morphogenesis in the embryo.[2,3] Nearly 70 years ago Wolbach and collaborators[4] established that deficiency of vitamin A causes squamous metaplasia and keratinization of most columnar epithelia of the body. Common targets of squamous metaplasia are the sites of neoplastic disease, including the bronchus,[5,6] trachea,[7] stomach,[8,9] prostate, urinary bladder[10] and the cervical columnar epithelium.[11,12] Squamous metaplasia is considered, in some tissues, to be a preneoplastic lesion in the development of squamous cell carcinoma and retinoids became of interest to cancer researchers because they offered a way to control epithelial differentiation and to prevent tumorigenesis by inhibiting squamous metaplasia and inducing cells to differentiate normally. Early studies have shown that retinoids could in fact inhibit tumorigenesis in the skin and in the respiratory, buccal, stomach, mammary and cervical epithelia.[13,14] As an introduction to the role of retinoids in differentiation and prevention of malignant transformation, it is crucial to understand how retinoids modulate the expression of epithelial phenotypes.

Retinoids and modulation of epithelial differentiation

Figure 24.1 suggests that a simple columnar epithelium can become pseudostratified, squamous metaplastic and stratified keratinizing due to vitamin A depletion. The endocervical epithelium, a typical simple columnar epithelium, becomes pseudostratified and eventually stratified squamous metaplastic and stratified epidermoid keratinizing as vitamin A deficiency progresses. The concentration of retinoids in different epithelia, therefore, appears to be an important determinant of phenotypic expression.

In addition, steroid hormones are known to be involved in the maintenance of normal morphology and function of the cervical and vaginal epithelia and an antagonistic action between estrogen/androgen and all-*trans* retinoic acid (RA) has also been characterized in these epithelia.[15,16] Estrogen induces the keratinizing phenotype during the estrus phase of the menstrual cycle in squamous stratified nonkeratinizing epithelia and progesterone and RA antagonize this effect.[17,18] Kahn investigated the interaction of vitamin A and estrogen on the vaginal epithelium.[17] He found that topical application of vitamin A inhibited the induced keratinization of the vaginal epithelium as shown by the vaginal smear assay.[19] The vaginal epithelium acquired the epidermoid keratinizing phenotype 72 h after exposure to estrogen and the same keratin genes were expressed in the vagina and epidermis.[20] Vitamin A deficiency and estrogen induced the same epidermoid differentiation in the vaginal and ectocervical epithelia as judged by histological and keratin profile. Because of these findings we are presently investigating the effect of vitamin A status on estrogen receptor expression in the vaginal and cervical epithelia.

Due to their powerful effect on cervical epithelial differentiation, retinoids have been used as chemopreventive agents of cervical dysplasia and neoplasia.

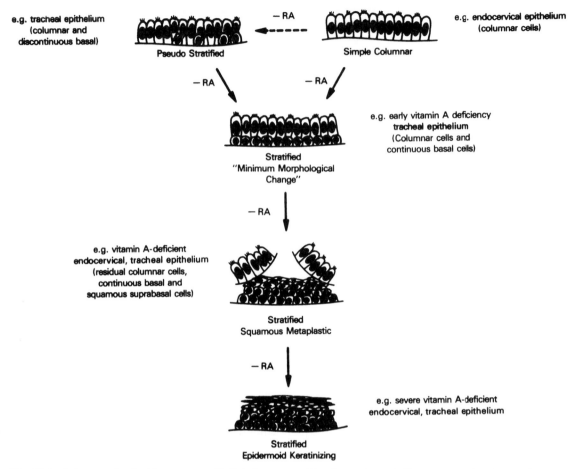

Fig. 24.1 Influence of retinoid status on epithelial phenotypes. The chart schematically represents the phenotypic conversion caused by vitamin A deficiency in the endocervical and tracheal epithelia. A simple columnar epithelium, e.g., the endocervical epithelium, is gradually converted to a stratified keratinizing phenotype resembling the epidermis under severe vitamin A deficient conditions. Similarly, a pseudostratified epithelium, e.g., the tracheal epithelium, is gradually transformed into a stratified epidermoid keratinizing epithelium. These changes are fully reversible in the presence of retinoic acid (RA). (Reproduced from Ref. 1 with permission.)

Chemoprevention of cervical dysplasia and neoplasia by retinoids

As discussed previously, deficiency of vitamin A has long been known to induce squamous metaplasia of the cervical epithelium. Romney and associates[21] and others[22,23] demonstrated a possible correlation between low dietary levels of vitamin A and the development of cervical intraepithelial neoplasia (CIN). Furthermore, it was suggested that dietary β-carotene, or a vegetable-rich diet, is protective against invasive cervical cancer.[23] A decreased intake of β-carotene by women having cervical dysplasia was reported in a nutritional survey.[23] In addition, plasma β-carotene levels were significantly lower in women with cervical dysplasia or cancer compared to the control.[24] These observations have suggested that retinoids might prevent cervical squamous metaplasia and reverse dysplasia and CIN. In fact, phase 1 and phase 2 clinical trials of RA for CIN have shown that RA can reverse cervical dysplasia in some patients.[25–29] Topical application of RA via a collagen sponge/diaphragm insert in grades 2 and 3 CIN resulted in reduced intraepithelial lesion in six of 18 patients and complete resolution of disease in two patients.[30] This was followed by a phase 1 trial of RA for mild or moderate CIN in 35 patients, resulting in cervical alterations in 50% of patients, however without complete resolution of preneoplastic conditions.[27] In addition, topical application of retinyl acetate has also been suggested as a treatment for cervical dysplasias.[31] Recently, there has been renewed interest in the antioxidant properties of vitamins, when in a cross-sectional study, it was reported that significantly reduced plasma levels of β-carotene and α-tocopherol were observed in 116 women with histopathologic lesions of cervical dysplasias or cancer.[24] Also there was a strong association between smoking status and plasma β-carotene levels, independent of any cervical pathology.[24] Further studies have shown significantly decreased β-carotene levels in plasma and in exfoliating epithelial cervicovaginal cells in 105 women with CIN and cervical cancer as compared with the controls.[32] Oral supplementation with β-carotene resulted in increased β-carotene levels in cervicovaginal cells in 79% of the patients.[32]

Deficiency of other nutrients like ascorbic acid and α-tocopherol has been suggested to play a role in the histogenesis of CIN or cervical cancer. Furthermore, possible synergistic interactions of β-carotene, vitamins A, C, and α-tocopherol have been suggested in reducing the risks of human cancers. We will focus on retinoids in this review.

STRUCTURE OF NATURAL RETINOIDS AND THEIR BIOLOGICAL ACTIVITIES

Vitamin A (retinol) is introduced in the diet either as retinyl esters from animal tissues (e.g., liver) and animal products (e.g., milk and eggs) or as its precursor β-carotene (Fig. 24.2) from green and yellow leafy vegetables.[33] This carotenoid and other similar structures are converted to retinal by the enzyme 15,15′-dioxygenase which generates two molecules of retinal from one molecule of β-carotene. Other carotenoids usually yield one molecule of retinal and one molecule of a derivative of retinal without known biological function in mammalian tissues. Although β-carotene is the most effective precursor of retinal and of the retinoids, other carotenoids may be equally important to epithelial tissues because they may function as antioxidants, and as such may perform vital protective functions. Retinal is either oxidized to RA or reduced to retinol (vitamin A). Retinol is stored in the liver as retinyl esters and it reaches concentrations from 2×10^{-6} M to as high as 1×10^{-4} M. The delivery of retinol to the circulation

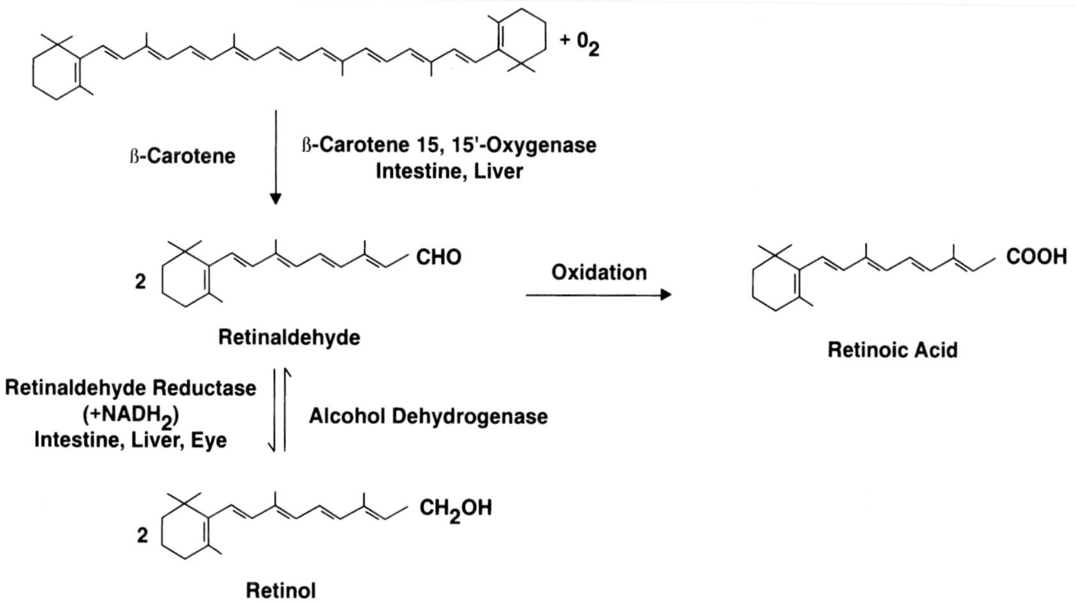

Fig. 24.2   Conversion of β-carotene to retinal and formation of retinol and retinoic acid.

is regulated strictly by homeostatic mechanisms which are by and large unknown.[34] The result is that a constant blood concentration of approximately 10^{-6} M is maintained, even when liver retinyl esters reach very high or fairly low concentrations. However, if dietary high retinol intake is continued for long periods of time, blood concentration also increases and retinyl esters are found in blood.

Under normal conditions blood retinol is found in complex with the retinol binding protein (RBP) which, in turn, forms a 1:1 complex with trans-thyretin (TTR), a protein that binds thyroxine.[35,36]

The implications, if any, of the existence of such a complex, although not understood, may not be trivial for the functioning of the cell, particularly if one considers the heterodimeric interaction between the thyroid hormone receptor (TR) and the RXR receptor for 9-cis-retinoic acid (C-RA). These interactions and their importance in regulating gene expression will be discussed later.

The structure and function of naturally occurring retinoids is presented in Fig. 24.3. All retinoids are derived from the parent compound retinol (vitamin A) of which RA is the major derivative.[37] At variance with retinol, RA is not stored by tissues in any appreciable amounts and it is present in concentrations usually two orders of magnitude smaller than retinol. Its synthesis and metabolism is the subject of intense investigation because RA is the active metabolite of retinol. It is in fact capable of inducing growth in vitamin A-deficient animals, which otherwise would loose weight and eventually succumb to the deficiency due to a variety of reasons including increased risk of infection. RA is also active as a protective agent of epithelial tissues, because it maintains normal epithelial phenotypic expression. This is one of the reasons why this compound has been considered a potentially useful chemopreventive agent against epithelial cancer.

Vitamin A metabolites, such as RA and 3,4-didehydroretinoic acid (dd-RA) may function in morphogenesis.[38,39] The wing bud of the chick embryo responds to the application of low concentrations of RA by forming a set of supranumerary digits in the mirror image of the original set.[40] RA exerts this activity by inducing the formation of cells similar to the inductive cells of the zone of polarizing activity (ZPA).[41,42] In this system RA has been shown to be metabolized to the dd-RA.[43] This retinoid is listed in Fig. 24.3 as one of the four naturally occurring retinoic acids. It is derived from 3,4-di-dehydroretinol or vitamin A_2 that is also found in the epidermis.[44]

Of the other retinoids listed in Fig. 24.3 we need to mention the interesting properties of the derivative of retinol 4,14-dihydroxyretroretinol (4,14-HRR). The sole precursor for this compound is retinol and the compound cannot be converted to RA. Nevertheless, it is able to stimulate the division of T-lymphocytes which are refractory to RA. Retinol also stimulates T-lymphocytes to divide, probably through the action of the 4-HRR metabolite.[45] Therefore pathways of gene activation other than RA-dependent ones probably exist.

This brief introduction to the retinoids should also emphasize that these substances are usually found in complex with proteins, which may have protective as well as functional roles. A detailed discussion of these retinoid binding proteins is not within the scope of this chapter, but Table 24.1 gives a summary of them and their presumed or established function.[46] The latest to join this list are the nuclear receptors for RA and C-RA respectively termed RARs and RXRs.[2,47,48] In the following section we will give a brief summary of the different types of retinoid receptors and of their target genes.

RETINOID RECEPTORS

A few years ago orphan receptors of the steroid-thyroid hormone receptor superfamily were found to bind RA in a specific manner.[49,50] At that time since target genes had not yet been identified, chimeric molecules were constructed containing the DNA-binding domain of the estrogen receptor for known target genes and the ligand-binding domain of the RAR in order to demonstrate cis activation. In this manner RA activity could be demonstrated with constructs containing reporter genes fused with promoter sequences of estrogen target genes. Using this ingenious assay, RA was demonstrated to be the ligand of RARs and this development opened up the way for further

STRUCTURE

FUNCTION

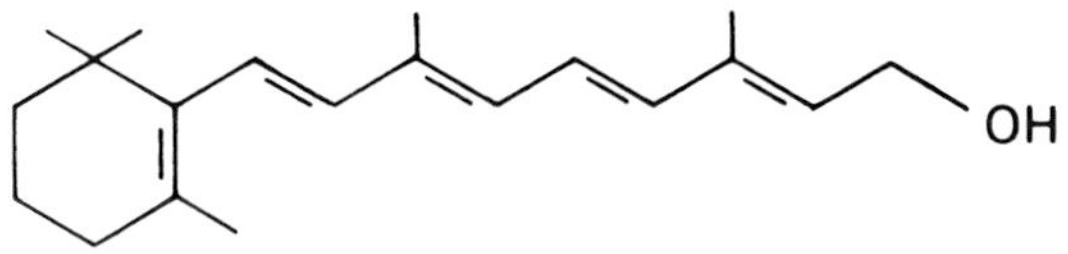

all-trans Retinol (Vitamin A)

Growth, differentiation, vision, reproduction.

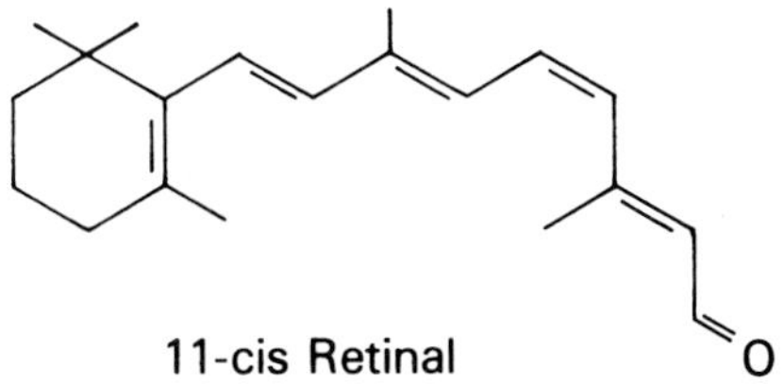

11-cis Retinal

All-trans and 11-cis retinal are chormophores of rhodopsin. Fulfills all vitamin A functions because it converts to retinol. 13-cis Isomer is chromophore of bacteriorhodopsin.

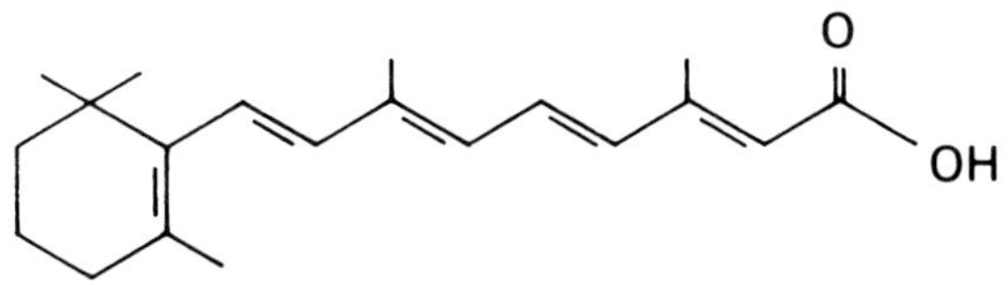

all-trans Retinoic Acid

Not reduced to retinol. Has all functions of vitamin A except vision and reproduction. Ligand of RARα,β,γ.

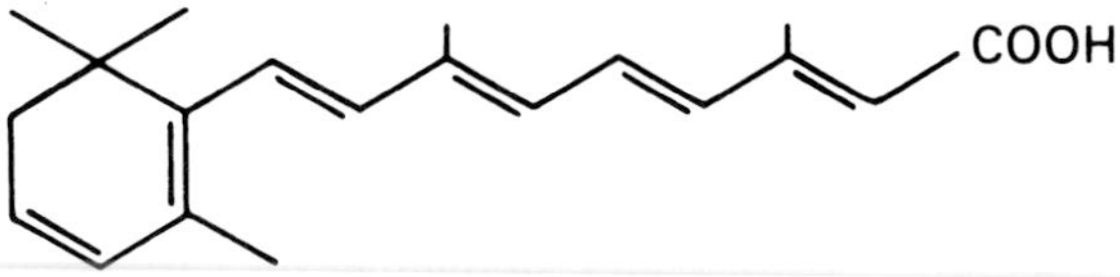

3,4-Didehydroretinoic Acid

Metabolite active in embryonic development. Ligand for RAR.

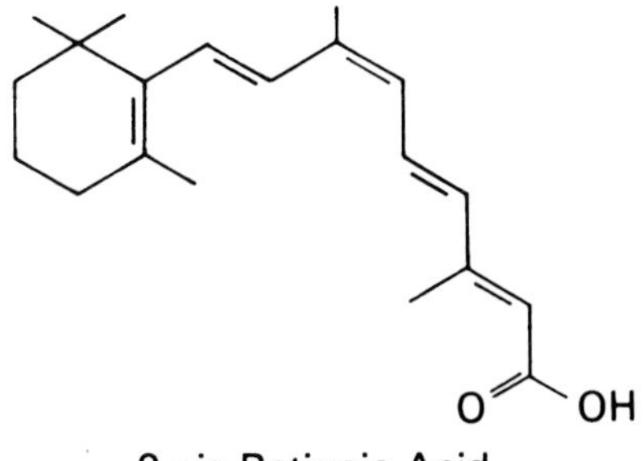

9-cis Retinoic Acid

Specific ligand for RXR.

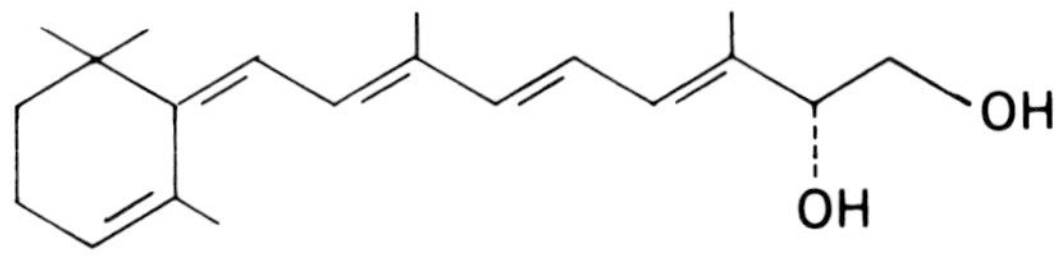

14-Hydroxy-4,14-retroretinol

Functions as mitogen in lymphocytes.

Fig. 24.3   Structure and function of natural retinoids.

Table 24.1 Retinoid-binding proteins and nuclear receptors*

Protein	Approximate mass (kDa)	Main ligand	Suggested function
RBP	21	Retinol	Blood plasma transport
IRBP	140	Retinol, retinal	Intercellular transport in visual cycle
Four proteins secreted from pig uterus	22	Retinol	Transport to the fetus
Two luminal proteins in rat epididymis	20	RA	Intercellular transport
CRBP 1	16	Retinol	Donor for esterification, intracellular transport
CRBP 2	16	Retinol	Donor for esterification
CRBP 3 from fish eye	15	Retinol	
CRABP 1	16	RA	Intracellular transport, regulates free RA
CRABP 2 from neonatal rat	15	RA	Intracellular transport, regulates free RA
CRABP 2 from embryonal chick	16	RA	Intracellular transport, regulates free RA
CRALBP	36	Retinal	Enzymatic reactions in the visual cycle
RARα (7 isoforms)	48	RA	Ligand-dependent transcription factors
RARβ (4 isoforms)	48	RA	Ligand-dependent transcription factors
RARγ (7 isoforms)	48	RA	Ligand-dependent transcription factors
RXRα, β, γ	48	9-cis-RA	Ligand-dependent transcription factors

* Adapted from Ref. 34, with permission.

understanding of the mode of action of RA in transcriptional regulation. The field of retinoid receptors has been reviewed recently.[48,51,52] These receptors have a multidomain structure (domains A to F) based on amino acid sequence homology between the RARs and other members of the nuclear receptor superfamily and each domain possesses a different function.[53] Of these domains, the DNA-binding domain, or C region, is the most conserved (93–95% identity among RARs) and it is 66 amino acids long.[53,54] The ligand-binding domain, or E region, is the second most conserved (85–90% identity among RARs). This region has a role in receptor dimerization and a RA-dependent transcription activation function.[55] The most amino and carboxy terminal ends, A and F regions, respectively, are highly variable among the RARs. Though no function has yet been determined for the D and F regions, the A and B domains were shown to contain a promoter specific transactivation function that is ligand independent.

Retinoic acid and retinoid X receptors

Two families of nuclear retinoic acid receptors, each consisting of three receptor types (α, β, and γ) have been cloned. The retinoic acid receptors (RARs)[56] bind both RA and C-RA with high affinity and the retinoid X receptors (RXRs)[57,58] specifically interact with C-RA under physiological conditions. Six different genes that are located on different chromosomes code for RARs (α, β, γ)[59] and RXRs (α, β, γ).[57] The two families of RARs and RXRs are transcriptional factors and control transcription by binding to specific retinoid response elements located in the promoter region of target genes. These will be discussed later in more details.

RXR primary sequences can be also divided into several domains from A to E and do not possess an F domain at the carboxy-terminal end, unlike RARs and other members of the thyroid/steroid hormone receptor. In addition, RXRs possess very low homology with the RARs and go back in evolution to *Drosophila*, where a gene product ultraspiracle (usp) is homologous to the RXR protein.[60] However, usp is not responsive to retinoids and its function clearly predates that of RA.[57]

The complexity of RA function is further accentuated by the discovery of several RAR isoforms (7α, 4β, 7γ)[56,61] and preliminary evidence is suggestive of isoforms for RXRs.[57,62] These isoforms are generated either by differential splicing and/or by activation via distinct promoters. This will generate isoforms that differ in their 5'UTR and the amino terminal A region that are fused to a common B–F region.

Studies have shown that all three RAR[56,63] and RXR[57] gene transcripts show specific spatio-temporal patterns of distribution in embryos and adults. In general, it is agreed that RARα is present in most tissues in embryos and adults, particularly RARα1 isoform which has the pattern of a housekeeping gene expression.[64,65] Our work[66] and the work of others[67] indicated that RARβ and RARγ expression patterns are more restricted and appear to be mutually exclusive in many tissues. RARβ is specific for tissues derived from the endoderm and is expressed preferentially in simple columnar and pseudostratified epithelia.[67] On the other hand, RARγ seems to be specific for the precartilage, cartilage, and squamous stratified epithelia. RXRs were also shown to be expressed differently from RARs and all three transcripts appear from day 10 of mouse embryogenesis.[57] Later in adult tissues RXRα is predominantly seen in the skin, liver, kidney, lung, muscle, and spleen.[57] In general, RXRβ is expressed at low levels in most tissues. RXRγ is more restricted and is mainly expressed at high levels in the heart and skeletal muscle and at lower levels in the brain, liver, and kidney. We will summarize our work on the cervical epithelium to indicate cell-type specificity for these receptor types and their modulation by vitamin A status.

Retinoid response elements

The RARs and RXRs are ligand activated transcriptional factors that bind to specific DNA response elements of RA target genes.[48,58] The recognition of these sequences by the DNA-binding domain of these receptors responds to certain rules that have been described as relatively simple.[68] It seems that all three major receptors, the vitamin D3 receptor (VDR), the thyroid hormone receptor (TR) and the RARs bind as dimers to two direct repeats of the hexameric nucleotide of ideal sequence AGGTCA.[68] In most cases, according to Evans and collaborators,[68] the specificity is imparted by the sequence of nucleotides that separates the two repeats. The '3,4,5 rule' states that a three nucleotide sequence separating the two AGGTCA motifs (AGGTCA NNN AGGTCA) imparts specificity for recognition by the VDR, a four nucleotide separation (AGGTCA NNNN AGGTCA) specifies recognition by the TR, while a separation by a five nucleotide

sequence (AGGTCA NNNNN AGGTCA) specifies recognition by RARs. Recently, Kliewer et al[69] have shown that a one nucleotide separation of AGGTCA motifs is recognized by RXR homodimers. Table 24.2 presents a summary of RA and CRA target genes and their response elements.[70]

The AGGTCA NNNNN AGGTCA motif has been found in retinoic acid response elements (RARE) present in the promoter region of several genes. The prototype for this RARE is present in the promoter of the RARβ2 gene (human and mouse) which is highly responsive to RA.[71,72] It has also been reported for the RAREs present in the RARα2 (human and mouse)[64,73] and the human RARγ2 promoters[61] and in the RARE of the human alcohol dehydrogenase (ADH-3)[74] and the mouse complement H factor (CP-H).[75] In addition to the AGGTCA NNNNN AGGTCA RARE, shorter spacings of two nucleotides have been found in the promoter region of the mouse CRBPI gene[76] and in the RARE (Table 24.2) of the rat CRABPII gene.[77] Other retinoid response elements and different spacings between the two repeats have also been reported.[78-88] Besides the direct repeat type of RAREs, palindromic RAREs have also been described as shown in Table 24.2.

Heterodimers of RXR and other receptors

An important and unique characteristic of the RXRs is that they function as auxiliary receptors for a variety of other nuclear receptors with which they form heterodimers (for reviews[51,52]) including, RARs, TR, VDR, peroxisomal proliferator activated receptor (PPAR)[68,89-91] and chicken ovalbumin upstream promoter transcription factor (COUP-TF).[92] Depending on the receptors and the response elements involved, these heterodimeric interactions may activate or suppress the target genes. When the heterodimers bind to the response element of the alternate receptor (e.g., VDR .RXR binding to the AGGTCA NNN AGGTCA motif) this interaction results in activation of transcription; this occurs for the heterodimers TR.RXR binding to AGGTCA NNNN AGGTCA, the response element specific for the TR; and for the RAR.RXR binding to the

Table 24.2 Summary of retinoid response elements*,**

Genes		Characteristics
RARE sequences		
mRARα2	5′ – (–59) GGCG**AGTTCA**GCAAG**AGTTCA**GCCGA (–34) –3′	Direct repeat of of six-base half element (ideal AGGTCA) separated by five nucleotides (DR-5).
hRARα2	5′ – (–58) GGCG**AGTTCA**GCGAG**AGTTCA**GCCGC (–33) –3′	
mRARβ2	5′ – (–57) GAAG**GGTTCA**CCGAA**AGTTCA**CTCGC (–32) –3′	
hRARβ2	5′ – (–57) GTAG**GGTTCA**CCGAA**AGTTCA**CTCGC (–32) –3′	
hRARγ2	5′ – (–401) GGCC**GGGTCA**GGAGGAG**GTGA**GCGCGC (–375) –3	
hADH3	5′ – (–280) ACAG**GGGTCA**TTCAG**AGTTCA**GTTTT (–305) –3′	
mCP-H	5′ – (–147) CAGC**AGGTCA**CTGAC**AGGGCA**TAGTA (–122) –3′	
mCRBPI	5′ – (–1015) TAGT**AGGTCA**AAA**GGTCA**GACAC (–993) –3′	Direct repeat of six-base half element (ideal AGGTCA) separated by one, two and four nucleotides (DR-1; DR-2; DR-4).
mLB1	5′ – (–432) **GAGGTGA**GCTA**GGTTAA**GCCCTTAGAAAAA**GGGTCAA** (–468) –3′	
mCRABPII	RARE1 5′ – (–1162) CCCC**AGTTCA**CC**AGGTCA**GGGCT (–1140) –3′	
	RARE2 5′ – (–638) TAGA**AGGGCA**GA**GGTCA**CAGCC (–659) –3′	
Putative RXRE sequences		
rAcyl-CoA	Ox5′ – (–558) **AGGACA** A **AGGTCA** (–570) –3′	Direct repeat of six-base half element (ideal AGGTCA) separated by one nucleotide (DR-1).
hApoAI	5′ – (–192) **AGGGCA** G **GGGTCA** (–204) –3′	
rApoCIII	5′ – (–73) **TGGTCA** A **AGGTCA** (–85) –3′	
r3-KA-CoA Thiol	5′ – (–669) **GGTTCA** A **AGGTCT** (–681) –3	
rOTC	5′ – (+178) **AGTTCA** G **AGGTTA** (+166) –3	
rPEPCK	5′ – (–439) **CGGCCA** A **AGGTCA** (–451) –3′	
rCRBPII	5′ – (–639) GTC**GTCA**C**AGGTCA**C**AGGTCA** C**AGGTCA**C**AGTTCA** (–605) –3′	
HBV Enhancer	5′ – (–1138) **TGAACC** T **TTACCC** (–1150) –3′	
cOVAL	5′ – (–85) **GTGTCA** A **AGGTCA** (–73) –3′	
Palindromic RARE		
Synthetic	**AGGTCA TGACCT**	Inverted repeat of 6-based half element (ideal AGGTCA) without spacing; mediates RAR and TR stimulation
rGH	5′ – (–185) C **AGGGAC** GTG **ACCGCA** (–170) –3′	Rat growth hormone TRE, also a RARE
hOST	5′ – (–510) **GGTGA** C **TCACC** (–500) –3′	AP-1 binding vitamin D response element and RARE

* Reproduced from Ref. 69, with permission.
** The table includes natural RAREs from mouse and human RARα2 and β2 promoters (mRARα2 (71), hRARα2 (64), mRARβ2 (70), hRARβ2 (69), human RARγ2 promoter (hRARγ2 (61), human alcohol dehydrogenase 3 promoter (hADH3 (72)), mouse complement factor H (mCP-H (73)), mouse cellular retinol binding protein I (mCRBPI (74)), mouse laminin β1 (mLB1 (75)), and mouse cellular retinoic acid binding protein II (mCRABPII (76)). Also shown are putative retinoid X response elements (RXREs) from rat fatty acyl-CoA oxidase (rAcyl-CoA Ox (77)), human Apolipoprotein AI (hApoAI (78)), rat apolipoprotein CIII (rApoCIII (79)), rat 3-ketoacyl-CoA thiolase (r3-KA-CoA Thiol (80), rat ornithine transcarbamylase (rOTC (81)), rat phosphoenolpyruvate carboxykinase (rPEPCK (82)), rat cellular retinol binding protein II (rCRBPII (75)), hepatitis B virus enhancer (HBV enhancer (83)), and chicken ovalbumin promoter (cOVAL (84)). Finally, two palindromic RAREs from rat growth hormone (rGH (85)) and human osteocalcin genes (hOST (86)) are also presented.

AGGTCA NNNNN AGGTCA motif specific for the RAR.[69] Activation is also the result of the interaction of PPAR with RXR interacting with the AGGTCA N AGGTCA motif. Inhibition, on the other hand, is the result of COUP-TF.RXR heterodimer interacting with the AGGTCA N AGGTCA motif. Equally inhibitory is the interaction of the heterodimer RAR.RXR with the motif AGGTCA N AGGTCA.[69]

In summary, it is evident that a multiplicity of pathways are likely to be influenced by the retinoids through heterodimeric interactions such as those discussed above. The RXRs may well function as the liaison between thyroid hormone, steroid hormone, vitamin D_3, and peroxisomal proliferators thereby linking together biological processes formerly thought to be independent. Similar interactions may be relevant to the cervical epithelium because it is the target of the opposing actions of retinoids and steroids.

RETINOIDS AS DETERMINANTS OF CERVICAL EPITHELIAL MORPHOLOGY

The cervical epithelium comprises two major phenotypes: the squamous stratified and the simple columnar phenotypes. These two epithelia join at the squamocolumnar junction, which can be positioned endocervically or ectocervically, dependent upon a variety of factors, including age, hormonal, and nutritional status. Because of this, both columnar and squamous phenotypes can be found in the endocervical canal or ecto-cervically. Therefore, we have introduced the terms 'suprajunctional' and 'subjunctional' to indicate the position of epithelial cells vis-à-vis the junction. The mobility of the junction throughout life probably contributes to its being the most common locus for the development of neoplastic disease due to continuous cell renewal at this site.[93,94] Just as for the epithelium of the cervix, the neoplastic lesions can have two major phenotypes; these are the adenocarcinoma and the squamous cell carcinoma, with the latter being the most common.

Mouse animal model for the histogenesis of squamous metaplasia of the cervical epithelium

Squamous metaplasia of the normally simple-columnar epithelium is a preneoplastic lesion and is preceded by the appearance of basal-like cells called reserve cells. We have recently described an animal model[96] based on dietary retinoid depletion which permits the appearance of reserve cells and the subsequent formation of the more advanced lesion squamous metaplasia. The stratified squamous subjunctional epithelium of the RA+ mice (3 μg RA/g diet) expressed keratins K5/K14, K6, K13 basally and suprabasally and K1/K10 suprabasally. At the squamocolumnar junction, the simple columnar suprajunctional epithelium did not show the presence of these keratins but specifically stained for K8.

When a mouse is fed a vitamin A-deficient diet for extended periods, i.e., for the first 10 and 14 weeks of life in nude and BALB/c mice, respectively, squamous metaplasia starts appearing in the suprajunctional epithelium. This phenomenon is shown in Fig. 24.4,[96] which also highlights keratin staining by specific antibodies to cytokeratins K5 and K8. It is immediately apparent that the suprajunctional columnar epithelium stains specifically for K8 and the squamous subjunctional epithelium for K5, under normal conditions of retinoid nutriture (Fig. 24.4A and B). However, K5-positive cells appear suprajunctionally (Fig. 24.4C) and populate large areas as squamous foci in more advanced conditions of deficiency (Fig. 24.4E). These same squamous foci are also positive for K6, K13 and K1/K10. Eventually, the entire suprajunctional columnar epithelium is replaced by a squamous-keratinizing epithelium, thereby eliminating the junction (Fig. 24.4E and F). This condition is completely reversible upon administration of physiological levels of RA provided that infection does not kill the animal.

Using specific antibodies and riboprobes for K5 we have been able to follow the appearance of single reserve cells expressing K5 mRNA and protein and find them proximal and distal from the junction, suggesting that they arise in a sub-columnar position in the simple columnar epithelium of the cervix, rather than migrating from the squamous stratified epithelium.[96] After these cells grew into a squamous focus, K1 and K13 mRNAs became expressed suprabasally. The somewhat sporadic pattern of formation of squamous loci suggests that specific cells at different sites have the potential to independently respond to the nutritional condition of vitamin A deficiency. Therefore it is obvious that retinoid status plays a key role in maintaining differentiative characteristics of the cervical and glandular epithelia.

Retinoid binding proteins in cervical epithelium

The cervical epithelium is an ideal system to study the specificity of retinoid receptor expression for each cell type, since it presents with both the squamous stratified and the simple columnar phenotypes. For this purpose we have analyzed by in situ hybridization, using ^{35}S-labeled riboprobes,

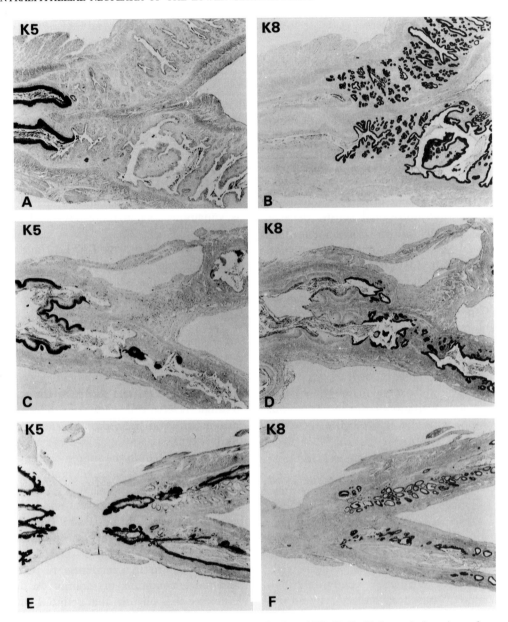

Fig. 24.4 Immunohistochemistry of keratins K5 (A, C, E) and K8 (B, D, F) in cervical sections of mice. **A,B** RA + diet; **C,D** mild vitamin-A deficiency; **E,F** severe vitamin-A deficiency. Reproduced from Ref. 95 with permission.

the distribution pattern of RARα, β and γ major isoforms and RXRα, β and γ (Table 24.3, reference 66). RARα mRNA (α1 and α2) were found to be expressed in all epithelial cells basally and suprabasally. In sharp contrast, RARβ (β2 and β3) were shown to be specifically expressed in columnar cells and RARγ (γ1 and γ2) in the squa-

mous stratified epithelium albeit to a lower level. RXRα and to a lesser extent RXRβ were mainly expressed basally in the stratified squamous and metaplastic epithelium and in columnar cells. RXRγ was undetectable in all cervical epithelia. The condition of vitamin A deficiency resulted in a down modulation of RARβ and RXRα and β

Table 24.3 Expression of RARs and RXRs in mouse cervical epithelium

	Stratified squamous[a]	Simple columnar[b]	Stratified metaplastic[c]
RARα	+ (B&S)	+	+ (B&S)
RARβ	–	+	+ (B)
RARγ	–/+ (B&S)	–	–/+ (B&S)
RXRα	+ (B)	+	+ (B)
RXRβ	+ (B)	+	+ (B)
RXRγ	–	–	–

The expression of the different receptors is indicated by the following: –, undetectable in 90% or more of the total number of sections; –/+, occasionally levels of expression above background could be observed; +, detectable in 90% or more of the total number of sections; B&S, basal and suprabasal; B, mainly basal. All sections were exposed in the dark for periods of 3–4 weeks.
[a]Stratified squamous refers to the stratified squamous subjunctional epithelium, under normal or vitamin A deficiency conditions.
[b]Simple columnar refers to the suprajunctional epithelium under normal conditions or to the residual columnar epithelium under vitamin A deficiency conditions.
[c]Stratified squamous metaplastic refers to stratified squamous non-keratinizing epithelium replacing simple columnar epithelium in vitamin A deficiency.

transcripts in the squamous metaplastic epithelium. We are presently studying the effect of cervical dysplasia and neoplasia on retinoid receptor expression.

A variety of other binding proteins, namely cellular retinol binding proteins (CRBPs) 1 and 2 and cellular retinoic acid binding proteins (CRABP) 1 and 2, regulate the function of retinoids at the cellular level.[34,97,98] CRBPs bind retinol thereby concentrating and storing it for later use[98] whereas CRABPs bind T-RA, but not C-RA, sequester it and increase its degradation, therefore making it unavailable for use.[99] Recently, Hillemanns and coworkers[100] investigated by immunofluorescence studies the localization of CRABP 1 and CRBP 1 proteins in normal, squamous metaplastic, different grades of CIN and invasive cancer of the uterine cervix. CRBP 1 was present in all layers of the cervical epithelium and showed no difference between normal, metaplastic, dysplastic or cancerous tissue. In contrast, CRABP 1 was mainly localized in basal cells of normal squamous and squamous metaplastic epithelium and low grade CIN. However, in CIN 2–3 and squamous cell carcinoma of the cervix,

CRABP 1 was diffusely expressed throughout the tissue except in squamous differentiating cells probably due to a greater abundance of basal-like cells in this tissue. It is of interest to note that RXRα and RXRβ colocalize with CRABP 1 in basal cells of normal squamous and squamous metaplastic epithelium, suggesting that C-RA may be an important regulator in these basal cells. In addition, the fact that CRABP is elevated in high grades CIN (CIN 2–3) and invasive cervical cancer suggests that advanced cases of these diseases may not be responsive to T-RA. The use of β-carotene, or of other retinoids like retinol or C-RA or retinoid analogs may be an attractive alternative for the treatment of advanced cases of CIN and cervical cancer.

The concept that retinoids may function as potent chemopreventive agents against the development of epithelial cancer was derived from the observation that the preneoplastic lesion squamous metaplasia is inhibited by RA. This may in fact have important biological consequences, if one considers that virus infection with the human papilloma virus (HPV 16 and HPV 18) and reproduction of the virus appears to be enhanced in the presence of agents that favor the formation of keratinizing squamous metaplastic cells, like the condition of vitamin A deficiency.

HUMAN PAPILLOMA VIRUS AND RETINOIDS

Premalignant and malignant disease of the cervix are frequently associated with highly transforming forms of HPV, in particular types 16 and 18,[101] and this subject will be covered in more details in other chapters.[102,103] The oncogenic potential of HPV 16 and HPV 18 is related primarily to two early genes, E6 and E7. Moreover, HPV replication has been shown to be associated with the differentiating squamous layers of the cervical epithelium and foreskin, and is strongly inhibited by RA.[104,106]

Agarwall and collaborators[105] investigated the effect of HPV on ectocervical cell differentiation and its modulation by retinoids. Towards this end they developed a clonal cell line of ectocervical epithelial cells expressing HPV 16 (ECE16-1) which had a similar keratin profile as the parent cells when grown in retinoid-free medium. Upon addition of retinoids, ECE16-1 showed an altered keratin profile and failed to differentiate. This may reduce the extent of papillomavirus replication and transcription. In addition, Pirisi et al[106] have shown that human foreskin keratinocyte cell lines immortalized by transfection with HPV 16 DNA are more sensitive than normal human keratinocytes to growth inhibition and differentiation control by RA. These authors also found a general inhibition by RA on the expression of HPV 16 early genes and a decrease of E6 and E7 protein levels, and RA inhibition of HPV-16 mediated immortalization of human keratinocytes.[107] Furthermore, Bartsch et al[108] have shown that RA inhibits the growth of HPV 18-positive Hela cervical carcinoma cells by reducing HPV 18 E6/E7 mRNA levels. The RA mediated reduction of HPV 18 E6/E7 mRNA levels was caused mainly by RAR mediated transcriptional repression via regulatory elements located in the central enhancer of the HPV 18 upstream regulatory region and interference with AP1. Furthermore, RA treatment resulted in an upregulation of RARβ mRNA levels in nontumorigenic Hela hybrid cells but not in tumorigenic ones.[108] This is particularly interesting because RARβ gene mapped to a region on the short arm of chromosome 3 that is frequently deleted in several cancers,[109,110] including those of the uterine cervix,[111] therefore suggesting it as a tumor suppressor gene. These data explained how at the molecular level retinoids are useful in the treatment of several epithelial diseases, including HPV-linked CIN.

SUMMARY AND PERSPECTIVES

It is obvious that retinoids are powerful regulators of epithelial differentiation, mainly of simple columnar epithelia like the suprajunctional cervical epithelium. In general, they prevent tumorigenesis by inhibiting squamous metaplasia which is a preneoplastic lesion in the development of squamous cell carcinoma. In addition, retinoids can act as chemopreventive agents in reversing and treating premalignant and malignant cervical lesions and have been used in phase 1 and 2 clinical trials of RA for CIN. An additional advantage of retinoids in the treatment of cervical

dysplasia and neoplasia is that they reduce the extent of HPV replication in epithelial cells.

Retinoids have also been shown to function as chemopreventive agents against the development of epithelial cancer in a variety of systems.[112] Most well known is the chemopreventive activity of topical RA against skin papillomas and carcinoma formation[113] in the two-stage system of mouse skin carcinogenesis.[114] We have also demonstrated that dietary high levels (30 μg/g diet) of RA specifically inhibits the conversion step from papilloma to carcinoma without any major effect on papilloma formation.[115] In human beings squamous or basal cell carcinoma of the head and neck are inhibited by high levels of dietary 13-cis retinoic acid.[116] Also in patients with xeroderma pigmentosum, a disease characterized by the formation of a large number of skin carcinomas, formation of new carcinomas after resection of the previous tumors is strongly inhibited by dietary RA, but resumes quickly upon withdrawal of the drug. The chemopreventive activity of the retinoids have also been conducted in mammary, lung, prostate, and buccal and esophageal epithelia.[117]

Besides its action as a chemopreventive agent, RA has also been shown to work as a potent inducer of differentiation of neoplastic cells.[70] Of particular interest has been the discovery that RA induces the differentiation of the human leukemic cell line (HL-60) to mature granulocytes.[118] This discovery was followed by the successful treatment of APL patients with RA and their complete remission, first reported by Huang et al[119] and confirmed by other investigators.[120–122] The disease was found to be associated with a chromosomal reciprocal translocation (t15;17) of the long arm of chromosome 17 to chromosome 15.[123] Remarkably, the breakpoint was characterized to occur in the A region of the RARα gene.[124] The newly formed gene was a chimera of the PML gene of unknown function and of the RARα.[125,126] Together with the responsiveness to RA, the translocation established a strong association between this neoplastic disease and retinoid function.

Therefore, treatment with retinoids constitutes a novel approach to therapy by the induction of differentiation of abnormal cells into functionally mature ones, replacing the traditional chemotherapy by cell killing. Retinoids may be useful in the management of cervical cancer through differentiation therapy in combination or in lieu of current therapeutic approaches for cervical dysplasias involving hysterectomy, surgical conization, cryosurgery, laser therapy or others. Each treatment has advantages and disadvantages and may not be as effective in progressing stages of CIN and cervical cancer. Prevention of cervical cancer and the pharmacological use of retinoids in the treatment of precancerous lesions and HPV-induced cancers should be considered in clinical settings and the focus of future research.

ACKNOWLEDGMENTS

This paper was written in part while Luigi M. De Luca was a visiting professor at the Institute of Histology and General Embryology of the University of Rome, La Sapienza, Italy. The authors would like to thank Dr. L.-C. Chen for critical review of the manuscript.

REFERENCES

1. Rosenthal D, Lancillotti F, Darwiche N, Sinha R, De Luca L M. Retinoids in epithelial differentiation and tumorigenesis. In: Blomhoff R, ed. Vitamin A in health and disease. New York: Marcel Dekker, 1994, pp 425–450.
2. De Luca L M. Retinoids and their receptors in differentiation, embryogenesis and neoplasia. FASEB J 1991; 5: 2924–2933.
3. Glass C K, DiRenzo J, Kurokawa R, Han Z H. Regulation of gene expression by retinoic acid receptors. DNA Cell Biol 1991; 10: 623–638.
4. Wolbach S B, Howe P R. Tissue changes following deprivation of fat-soluble A-vitamin. J Exper Med 1925; 42: 753–778.
5. Auerbach O, Stout A P, Hammond E C, Garfinkel L. Changes in bronchial epithelium in relation to cigarette smoking and in relation to lung cancer. New Engl J Med 1961; 265: 253–267.
6. Trump B F, McDowell E M, Glavin F et al. The respiratory epithelium. III. Histogenesis of epidermoid metaplasia and carcinoma in situ in the human. J Nat Cancer Inst 1978; 61: 563–575.
7. Lancillotti F, Darwiche N, Celli G, De Luca L M. Retinoid status and the control of keratin expression and adhesion during the histogenesis of squamous metaplasia of tracheal epithelium. Cancer Res 1992; 22: 6144–6152.
8. Correa P, Cuello C, Duque E. Carcinoma and intestinal metaplasia of the stomach in Colombian migrants. J Nat Cancer Inst 1970; 44: 297–306.
9. Ming S C, Goldman H, Freiman D G. Intestinal metaplasia and histogenesis of carcinoma in human stomach. Light and electron microscopic study. Cancer 1967; 20: 1418–1429.
10. Koss L. Tumors of the urinary bladder. In: Atlas of tumor pathology, 2nd Series, Fascile 11. Washington: Armed Forces Institute of Pathology, 1975: p 103.
11. Ferenczy A, Anatomy and histology of the cervix and cervical intraepithelial neoplasia. In: Blaustein A, ed. Pathology of the female genital tract, 2nd edn. New York: Springer, 1982: pp 126–132.
12. Ferenczy A, Richert R M, Female reproductive system. In: Dynamics of scan and transmission electron microscopy. New York: John Wiley, 1992: pp 66–68.
13. De Luca L M, Historical developments in vitamin A research. In: De Luca H F, ed. Fat soluble vitamins. New York: Plenum, 1978: pp 1–67.
14. Moon R C, McCormick D L, Mehta R G. Inhibition of carcinogenesis by retinoids. Cancer Res 1983; 43: 24696–24755.
15. Gorodesky G I, Eckert R L, Utian W H, Sheean L, Rorke E A. Cultured human ectocervical epithelial cell differentiation is regulated by the combined direct actions of sex steroids, glucocorticoids, and retinoids. J Clin Endocrinol Metab 1990; 70: pp 1624–1630.
16. Mossman B T, Ley B W, Craighead J E. Squamous metaplasia of the tracheal epithelium in organ culture. I. Effects of hydrocortisone and beta-retinyl acetate. Exper Mol Pathol 1976; 24: 405–414.
17. Kahn R H. Effect of locally applied vitamin A and estrogen on the rat vagina. Am J Anat 1954; 95: 309–335.
18. Gorodeski G I, Eckert R L, Utian W H, Sheenan L, Rorke E A. Retinoids, sex steroids and glucocorticoids regulate ectocervical cell envelope formation but not the level of the envelope precursor, involucrin. Differentiation 1989; 42: 75–80.
19. Baumann C A, Steenbock H. The vaginal smear method of determining vitamin A. Science 1932; 76: 417–420.
20. Roop D R, Regulation of keratin gene expression during differentiation of epidermal and vaginal epithelial cells. In: Sawyer R H, ed. Current topics in development biology. Orlando: Academic Press, 1987: pp 195–207.
21. Romney S L, Palan P R, Duttagupta C et al. Retinoids and the prevention of cervical dysplasias. Am J Obstet Gynecol 1981; 141: 890–894.
22. Bernstein A, Harris B. The relationship of dietary and serum vitamin A to the occurrence of cervical intraepithelial neoplasia in sexually active women. Am J Obstet Gynecol 1984; 148: 309–312.
23. La Vecchia C, Franceschi S, Decarli A et al. Dietary vitamin A and the risk of invasive cervical cancer. Int J Cancer 1984; 34: 319–322.
24. Palan P R, Mikhail M S, Basu J, Romney S L. Plasma levels of antioxidant beta-carotene and alpha-tocopherol in uterine cervix dysplasias and cancer. Nutr Cancer 1991; 15: 13–20.
25. Marshall J R, Graham S, Byers T, Swanson M, Brasure J. Diet and smoking in the epidemiology of cancer of the cervix. J Nat Cancer Inst 1983; 70: 847–851.
26. Graham V, Surwit E S, Weiner S, Meyskens F L.

Phase II trial of beta-all-trans-retinoic acid for cervical intraepithelial neoplasia delivered via a collagen sponge and cervical cap. West J Med 1986; 145: 192–195.

27. Meyskens F L, Graham V, Chvapil M, Dorr R T, Alberts D S, Surwit E A. A phase I trial of beta-all-trans-retinoic acid delivered via a collagen sponge and a cervical cap for mild or moderate intraepithelial cervical neoplasia. J Nat Cancer Inst 1983; 71: 921–925.

28. Meyskens F L, Surwit E S. Clinical experience with topical tretinoin in the treatment of cervical dysplasia. J Am Acad Dermatol 1986; 15: 826–829.

29. Weiner S A, Surwit E A, Graham V E, Meyskens F L. A phase I trial of topically applied trans-retinoic acid in cervical dysplasia–clinical efficacy. Invest New Drugs 1986; 4: 241–244.

30. Surwit E A, Graham V, Droegemueller W et al. Evaluation of topically applied trans-retinoic acid in the treatment of cervical intraepithelial lesions. Am J Obstet Gynecol 1982; 143: 821–823.

31. Romney S L, Dwyer A, Slagle S et al. Chemoprevention of cervix cancer: Phase I–II: A feasibility study involving the topical vaginal administration of retinyl acetate gel. Gynecol Oncol 1985; 20: 109–119.

32. Palan P R, Mikhail M S, Basu J, Romney S L. Beta-carotene levels in exfoliated cervicovaginal epithelial cells in cervical intraepithelial neoplasia and cervical cancer. Am J Obstet Gynecol 1992; 167: 1899–1903.

33. Goodman D S, Olson J A. The conversion of all-trans-β-carotene into retinol. Methods Enzymol 1969; 15: 463–475.

34. Blomhoff R, Green M H, Berg T, Norum K R. Transport and storage of vitamin A. Science 1990; 250: 399–404.

35. Wolf G. Multiple functions of vitamin A. Physiol Rev 1984; 64: 873–937.

36. Goodman D S, Plasma retinol binding protein. In: Sporn M B, Roberts A B, Goodman D S, eds. The retinoids, vol 2. Orlando, FL: Academic Press, 1984: pp 41–88.

37. Goodman D S, Blaner W S, Biosynthesis, absorption, and hepatic metabolism of retinol. In: Sporn M B, Roberts A B, Goodman D S, ed. The retinoids, vol 2. Orlando, FL: Academic Press, 1984: pp 1–39.

38. Thompson J N, Howell J M, Pitt G A J, McLaughlin C I. The biological activity of retinoic acid in the domestic fowl and the effects of vitamin A deficiency on the chick embryo. Br J Nutr 1969; 23: 471–490.

39. Wedden S, Thaller C, Eichele G. Targeted slow-release of retinoids into chick embryos. Methods Enzymol 1990; 190B: 201–209.

40. Tickle C, Summerbell D, Wolpert L. Positional signalling and specification of digits in chick limb morphogenesis. Nature 1975; 254: 199–202.

41. Wanek N, Gardiner D M, Muneoka K, Bryant S V. Conversion by retinoic acid of anterior cells into ZPA cells in the chick wing bud. Nature 1991; 350: 81–83.

42. Noji S, Nohno T, Koyama E et al. Retinoic acid induces polarizing activity but is unlikely to be a morphogen in the chick limb bud. Nature 1991; 350: 83–86.

43. Thaller C, Eichele G. Isolation of 3,4-didehydroretinoic acid, a novel morphogenetic signal in the chick wing bud. Nature 1990; 345: 815–819.

44. Törma H, Vahlquist A. Biosynthesis of 3-dehydroretinol (vitamin A2) from all-trans-retinol (vitamin A1) in human epidermis. J Invest Dermatol 1985; 85: 498–500.

45. Buck J, Derguini F, Levi E, Nakanishi K, Hammerling U. Intracellular signaling by 14-hydroxy-4,14-retro retinol. Science 1991; 254: 1654–1656.

46. Blomhoff R, Green M H, Green J B, Berg T, Norum K R. Vitamin A metabolism: new perspectives on absorption, transport, and storage. Physiol Rev 1991; 71: 951–990.

47. Evans R M. The steroid and thyroid hormone receptor superfamily. Science 1988; 240: 889–895.

48. Leid M, Kastner P, Chambon P. Multiplicity generates diversity in the retinoic acid signalling pathways. TIBS 1992; 17: 427–433.

49. Giguere V, Ong E S, Segui P, Evans R M. Identification of a receptor for the morphogen retinoic acid. Nature 1987; 330: 624–629.

50. Petkovich M, Brand N J, Krust A, Chambon P. A human retinoic acid receptor which belongs to the family of nuclear receptors. Nature 1987; 330: 444–450.

51. Kastner P, Leid M, Chambon P. The role of nuclear retinoic acid receptors in the regulation of gene expression. In: Blomhoff R, ed. Vitamin A in health and disease. New York: Marcel Dekker, 1994, pp 189–238.

52. Kliewer S A, Mangelsdorf D J, Umesono K, Evans R. The retinoid X receptors: modulators of multiple hormonal signaling pathways. In: Blomhoff R, ed. Vitamin A in health and disease. New York: Marcel Dekker, 1994, pp 239–255.

53. Green S, Chambon P. Nuclear receptors enhance our understanding of transcription regulation. Trends Genet 1988; 4: 309–314.

54. Schwabe J W, Rhodes D. Beyond zinc fingers: steroid hormone receptors have a novel structural motif for DNA recognition. Trends Biochem Sci 1991; 16: 291–296.

55. Allenby G, Bocquel M T, Saunders M et al. Retinoic acid receptors and retinoid X receptors: interactions with endogenous retinoic acids. Proc Nat Acad Sci USA 1993; 90: 30–34.

56. Ruberte E, Kastner P, Dolle P et al. Retinoic acid receptors in the embryo. Sem Dev Biol 1991; 2: 153–159.

57. Mangelsdorf D J, Borgmeyer U, Heyman R A et al. Characterization of three RXR genes that mediate the action of 9-cis retinoic acid. Genes Dev 1992; 6: 329–344.

58. Leid M, Kastner P, Lyons R et al. Purification, cloning, and RXR identity of the HeLa cell factor with which RAR or TR heterodimerizes to bind target sequences efficiently. Cell 1992; 68: 377–395.

59. Mattei M G, Petkovich M, Mattei J F, Brand N, Chambon P. Mapping of the human retinoic acid receptor to the q21 band of chromosome 17. Human Genet 1988; 80: 186–188.

60. Oro A E, McKeown M, Evans R M. Relationship between the product of the Drosophila ultraspiracle locus and the vertebrate retinoid X receptor. Nature 1990; 347: 298–301.

61. Lehmann J M, Zhang X K, Pfahl M. RARτ2 expression is regulated through a retinoic acid response element embedded in Sp1 sites. Molec Cell Biol 1992; 12: 2976–2985.

62. Hamada K, Gleason S L, Levi B Z, Hirschfeld S, Appella E, Ozato K. H-2RIIBP, a member of the nuclear hormone receptor superfamily that binds to both the regulatory element of major histocompatibility class I genes and the estrogen response element. Proc Nat Acad Sci USA 1989; 86: 8289–8293.

63. Ruberte E, Dolle P, Chambon P, Morriss-Kay G. Retinoic acid receptors and cellular retinoid binding proteins II. Their differential pattern of transcription during early morphogenesis in mouse embryo. Development 1991; 111: 45–60.

64. Brand N J, Petkovich M, Chambon P. Characterization of a functional promoter for the human retinoic acid receptor-α (hRAR-alpha). Nucleic Acids Res 1990; 18: 6799–6806.

65. Zelent A, Krust A, Petkovich M, Kastner P, Chambon P. Cloning of murine alpha and beta retinoic acid receptors and a novel receptor gamma predominantly expressed in skin. Nature 1989; 339: 714–717.

66. Darniche N, Celli G, De Luca L M. Specificity of retinoid receptor gene expression in mouse cervical epithelia. Endocrinology 1994; 134 2018–2025.

67. Dolle P, Ruberte E, Leroy P, Morriss-Kay G, Chambon P. Retinoic acid receptors and cellular retinoid binding proteins I. A systematic study of their differential pattern of transcription during mouse organogenesis. Development 1990; 110: 1133–1151.

68. Umesono K, Murakami K K, Thompson C C, Evans R M. Direct repeats as selective response elements for the thyroid hormone, retinoic acid, and vitamin D3 receptors. Cell 1991; 65: 1255–1266.

69. Kliewer S A, Umesono K, Mangelsdorf D J, Evans R M. Retinoid X receptor interacts with nuclear receptors in retinoic acid, thyroid hormone and vitamin D₃ signalling. Nature 1992; 355: 446–449.

70. Ross S A, Chen L C, Darwiche N, De Luca L M. Retinoids in neoplasia. In: Pusztai L, Lewis C E, Yap E, eds. Regulation of proliferation of neoplastic cells. Oxford: Oxford University Press, 1993: (in press).

71. de The H, Vivanco-Ruiz M, Tiollais P, Stunnenberg H, Dejean A. Identification of a retinoic acid responsive element in the retinoic acid receptor β gene. Nature 1990; 343: 177–180.

72. Sucov H M, Murakami K K, Evans R M. Characterization of an autoregulated response element in the mouse retinoic acid receptor type beta gene. Proc Nat Acad Sci USA 1990; 87: 5392–5396.

73. Leroy P, Nakshatri H, Chambon P. Mouse retinoic acid receptor alpha 2 isoform is transcribed from a promoter that contains a retinoic acid response element. Proc Nat Acad Sci USA 1991; 88: 10138–10142.

74. Duester G, Shean M L, McBride M S, Stewart M J. Retinoic acid response element in the human alcohol dehydrogenase gene ADH3: implications for regulation of retinoic acid synthesis. Molec Cell Biol 1991; 11: 1638–1646.

75. Munos-Canores, Vik D P, Tack B F. Mapping of a retinoic acid-responsive element in the promoter region of the complement factor H gene. J Biol Chem 1990; 265: 20065–20068.

76. Smith W C, Nakshatri H, Leroy P, Rees J, Chambon P. A retinoic acid response element is present in the mouse cellular retinol binding protein I (mCRBPI) promoter. EMBO J 1991; 10: 2223–2230.

77. Mangelsdorf D J, Umesono K, Kliewer S A, Borgmeyer U, Ong E S, Evans R M. A direct repeat in the cellular retinol-binding protein type II gene confers differential regulation by RXR and RAR. Cell 1991; 66: 555–561.

78. Vasios G W, Gold D G, Petkovich M, Chambon P, Gudas L J. A retinoic acid-responsive element is present in the 5′ flanking region of the laminin B1 gene. Proc Nat Acad Sci USA 1989; 86: 9099–9103.

79. Osumi T, Ishii N, Miyazawa S, Hashimoto T. Isolation and structural characterization of the rat acyl-CoA oxidase gene. J Biol Chem 1987; 262: 8138–8143.

80. Sastry K N, Seedorf U, Karathanasis S K. Different cis-acting DNA elements control expression of the human apolipoprotein AI gene in different cell types. Molec Cell Biol 1988; 8: 605–614.

81. Haddad I A, Ordovas J M, Fitzpatrick T, Karathanasis S K. Linkage, evolution, and expression of the rat apolipoprotein A-I, C-III, and A-IV genes. J Biol Chem 1986; 261: 13268–13277.

82. Hijikata M, Wen J K, Osumi T, Hashimoto T. Rat peroxisomal 3-ketoacyl-CoA thiolase gene. Occurrence of two closely related but differentially regulated genes. J Biol Chem 1990; 265: 4600–4606.

83. Murakami T, Nishiyori A, Takiguchi M, Mori M. Promoter and 11-kilobase upstream enhancer elements responsible for hepatoma cell-specific expression of the rat ornithine transcarbamylase gene. Molec Cell Biol 1990; 10: 1180–1191.

84. Lucas P C, O'Brien R M, Mitchell J A et al. A retinoic acid response element is part of a pleiotropic domain in the phosphoenolpyruvate carboxykinase gene. Proc Nat Acad Sci USA 1991; 88: 2184–2188.

85. Huan B, Siddiqui A. Retinoid X receptor RXRα binds to and trans-activates the hepatitis B virus enhancer. Proc Nat Acad Sci USA 1992; 89: 9059–9063.

86. Wang L H, Tsai S Y, Cook R G, Beattie W G, Tsai M J, O'Malley B W. COUP transcription factor is a member of the steroid receptor superfamily. Nature 1989; 340: 163–166.

87. Umesono K, Giguere V, Glass C K, Rosenfeld M G, Evans R M. Retinoic acid and thyroid hormone induce gene expression through a common responsive element. Nature 1988; 336: 262–265.

88. Schule R, Umesono K, Mangelsdorf D J, Bolado J, Pike J W, Evans R M. Jun-Fos and receptors for vitamins A and D recognize a common response element in the human osteocalcin gene. Cell 1990; 61: 497–504.

89. Liao J, Ozono K, Sone T, McDonnell D P, Pike J W. Vitamin D receptor interaction with specific DNA requires a nuclear protein and 1,25-dihydroxyvitamin D3. Proc Nat Acad Sci USA 1990; 87: 9751–9755.

90. Murray M B, Towle H C. Identification of nuclear factors that enhance binding of the thyroid hormone receptor to a thyroid hormone response element. Molec Endocrinol 1989; 3: 1434–1442.

91. Yu V C, Delsert C, Andersen B, et al. RXRβ: a coregulator that enhances binding of retinoic acid, thyroid hormone, and vitamin D receptors to their cognate response elements. Cell 1991; 67: 1251–1266.

92. Kliewer S A, Umesono K, Heyman R A, Mangelsdorf D J, Dyck J A, Evans R M. Retinoid X receptor-COUP-TF interactions modulate retinoic acid signaling. Proc Nat Acad Sci USA 1993;

93. Castano-Almendral A, Muller H, Naujoks H,

Castano-Almendral J L. Topographical and histological localization of dysplasias, carcinomata in situ, microinvasions and microcarcinomata. Gynecol Oncol 1973; 1: 320–329.

94. Reagan J W, Fu Y S. The uterine cervix. In: Silverberg S G, ed. Principles and practice of surgical pathology. New York: J. Wiley, 1983: p 1223.

95. Fluhmann C F. Comparative studies of squamous metaplasia of the cervix uteri and endometrium. Am J Obstet Gynecol 1992;

96. Darwiche N, Celli G, Sly L, Lancillotti F, De Luca L M. Retinoid status controls the appearance of reserve cells and keratin expression in mouse cervical epithelium. Cancer Res 1993; 53: 2287–2299.

97. Dew S E, Ong D E. Specificity of the retinol transporter of the rat small intestine brush border. Biochemistry 1994; 33: 12340–12345.

98. Perez-Castro A V, Toth-Rogler L E, Wei L N, Nguyen-Huu M C. Spatial and temporal pattern of expression of the cellular retinoic acid-binding protein and the cellular retinol-binding protein during mouse embryogenesis. Proc Nat Acad Sci USA 1989; 86: 8813–8817 [published erratum appears in Proc Nat Acad Sci USA 1990; 87(4): 1626–1627].

99. Maden M, Ong D E, Summerbell D, Chytil F. Spatial distribution of cellular protein binding to retinoic acid in the chick limb bud. Nature 1988; 335: 733–735.

100. Hillemanns P, Tannous-Khuri L, Koulos J P, Talmage D, Wright T C, Jr. Localization of cellular retinoid-binding proteins in human cervical intraepithelial neoplasia and invasive carcinoma. Am J Pathol 1992; 141: 973–980.

101. Durst M, Gissmann L, Ikenberg H, zur Hausen H. A papillomavirus DNA from a cervical carcinoma and its prevalence in cancer biopsy samples from different geographic regions. Proc Nat Acad Sci USA 1983; 80: 3812–3815.

102. Howley P M. Role of the human papillomaviruses in human cancer. Cancer Res 1991; 51: 5019s–5022s.

103. zur Hausen H Z. Viruses in human cancers. Science 1991; 254: 1167–1173.

104. Taichman L B, LaPorta R F, The expression of papillomaviruses in epithelial cells. In: Salzman N P, Howley P M, eds. The Papovaviridae. New York: Plenum Publishing, 1987: pp 109–139.

105. Agarwal C, Rorke E A, Irwin J C, Eckert R L. Immortalization by human papillomavirus type 16 alters retinoid regulation of human ectocervical epithelial cell differentiation. Cancer Res 1991; 51: 3982–3989.

106. Pirisi L, Batova A, Jenkins G R, Hodam J R, Creek K E. Increased sensitivity of human keratinocytes immortalized by human papillomavirus type 16 DNA to growth control by retinoids. Cancer Res 1992; 52: 187–193.

107. Khan M A, Jenkins G R, Tolleson W H, Creek K E, Pirisi L. Retinoic acid inhibition of human papillomavirus type 16-mediated transformation of human keratinocytes. Cancer Res 1993; 53: 905–909.

108. Bartsch D, Boye B, Baust C, zur Hausen H, Schwarz E. Retinoic acid-mediated repression of human papillomavirus 18 transcription and different ligand regulation of the retinoic acid receptor β gene in non-tumorigenic and tumorigenic HeLa hybrid cells. EMBO J 1992; 11: 2283–2291.

109. Naylor S L, Johnson B E, Minna J D, Sakaguchi A Y.
Loss of heterozygosity of chromosome 3p markers in small-cell lung cancer. Nature 1987; 329: 451–454.

110. Zbar B, Brauch H, Talmadge C, Linehan M. Loss of alleles of loci on the short arm of chromosome 3 in renal cell carcinoma. Nature 1987; 327: 721–724.

111. Yokota J, Tsukada Y, Nakajima T. Loss of heterozygosity on the short arm of chromosome 3 in carcinoma of the uterine cervix. Cancer Res 1989; 49: 3598–3601.

112. Sporn M B, Newton D L. Chemoprevention of cancer with retinoids. Fed Proc 1979; 38: 2528–2534.

113. Verma A K, Slaga T J, Wertz P W, Mueller G C, Boutwell R K. Inhibition of skin tumor promotion by retinoic acid and its metabolite 5,6-epoxyretinoic acid. Cancer Res 1980; 40: 2367–2371.

114. Yuspa S H, Tumor promotion in epidermal cells in culture. In: Slaga T, ed. Mechanisms of tumor promotion, vol III. Boca Raton: CRC Press, 1984: pp 1–11.

115. De Luca L M, Sly L, Jones C S, Chen L C. Effects of dietary retinoic acid on skin papilloma and carcinoma formation in female SENCAR mice. Carcinogenesis 1993; 14: 539–542.

116. Hong W K, Lippman S M, Itri L M et al. Prevention of second primary tumors with isotretinoin in squamous-cell carcinoma of the head and neck. New Engl J Med 1990; 323: 795–801.

117. Sporn M B, Dunlop N M, Newton D L, Smith J M. Prevention of chemical carcinogenesis by vitamin A and its synthetic analogs (retinoids). Fed Proc 1976; 35: 1332–1338.

118. Breitman T R, Selonick S E, Collins S J. Induction of differentiation of the human promyelocytic leukemia cell line (HL-60) by retinoic acid. Proc Nat Acad Sci USA 1980; 77: 2935–2940.

119. Huang M E, Ye Y C, Chen S R et al. Use of all-trans retinoic acid in the treatment of acute promyelocytic leukemia. Blood 1988; 72: 567–572.

120. Chomienne C, Ballerini P, Balitrand N et al. Retinoic acid therapy for promyelocytic leukaemia [letter]. Lancet 1989; 2: 746–747.

121. Degos L, Chomienne C, Ballerini P et al. All-trans retinoic acid: a novel differentiation therapy for acute promyelocytic leukemia. Proc ASCO 1990; 9: 207.

122. Castaigne S, Chomienne C, Daniel M T et al. All-trans retinoic acid as a differentiation therapy for acute promyelocytic leukemia. I. Clinical results. Blood 1990; 76: 1704–1709.

123. Borrow J, Goddard A D, Sheer D, Solomon E. Molecular analysis of acute promyelocytic leukemia breakpoint cluster region on chromosome 17. Science 1990; 249: 1577–1580.

124. de Thë H, Chomienne C, Lanotte M, Degos L, Dejean A. The t(15;17) translocation of acute promyelocytic leukaemia fuses the retinoic acid receptor alpha gene to a novel transcribed locus. Nature 1990; 347: 558–561.

125. de Thë H, Lavau C, Marchio A, Chomienne C, Degos L, Dejean A. The PML-RAR alpha fusion mRNA generated by the t(15;17) translocation in acute promyelocytic leukemia encodes a functionally altered RAR. Cell 1991; 66: 675–684.

126. Kakizuka A, Miller W H Jr, Umesono K et al. Chromosomal translocation t(15;17) in human acute promyelocytic leukemia fuses RAR alpha with a novel putative transcription factor, PML. Cell 1991; 66: 663–674.

25. Oncogenes in cervical neoplasia

Laure Aurelian

INTRODUCTION

Compelling evidence indicates that cancer arises via a multistep process requiring the contribution of multiple events and involving the cooperation of multiple genes. Genetic modifications found in cancer cells fall into two major categories: (i) dominant alterations, the targets of which are designated proto-oncogenes, i.e., the normal counterparts of genes that can be manipulated to a transforming allele (oncogenes), and (ii) recessive modifications, the targets of which are known as antioncogenes or tumor suppressor genes. Dominant modifications typically result in the gain of a function; recessive lesions cause the loss of a function. Mechanisms involved in the induction of cancer associated genetic alterations include mutation and amplification of specific DNA sequences. Here, I will briefly review our present understanding of these modifications as they relate to cervical carcinogenesis.

PROTO-ONCOGENES, ONCOGENES AND THEIR FUNCTIONS

The potential of proto-oncogenes to participate in carcinogenesis stems from the fact that their protein products are elements of biochemical circuitries that regulate cell replication. Signaling networks that mediate normal functions include the interaction of growth factors, cytokines and hormones with specific membrane receptors, thereby triggering a cascade of intracellular biochemical signals which result in the activation, or the repression, of various subsets of genes. The finding that progression through the cell cycle requires the coordinated action of complementary classes of growth factors led to the competence/progression model[1] schematically represented in Fig. 25.1.[2,3] Competence factors are involved in the advance of cells from the G_0 (resting) phase into the G_1 phase of the cell cycle. After the G_1 phase is traversed, the cells become committed

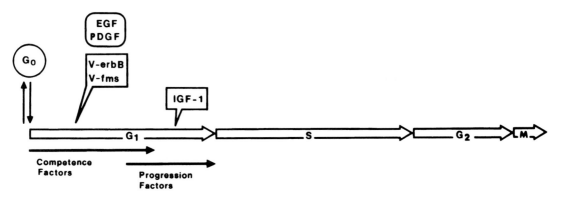

Fig. 25.1 Schematic representation of the dual signal system for progression through the cell cycle posits the coordinated action of two growth factors (that can be substituted by oncogenes) in the induction of DNA synthesis. For example, overexpression of c-*myc* can substitute for PDGF.[2] IGF-1 can be substituted by constitutive expression of c-*myc*.[3]

to DNA synthesis under the influence of progression factors. Some growth factors (e.g., epidermal growth factor (EGF)) function as competence factors. Others, such as the insulin-like growth factor 1 (IGF-1) are progression factors. The distinction between competence and progression factors does not apply to all cell types. However, a dual signal system is applicable to most.[4] Malignant cells arise in a multistep process in which these normal functions are subverted or substituted by oncogenes.

Despite their diversity,[5] the known proto-oncogenes evidence only three mechanisms of action: (i) protein phosphorylation (with serine (Ser), threonine (Thr) or tyrosine (Tyr) as the substrates),[6] (ii) signal transmission by GTPases,[7] and (iii) control of transcription from DNA (transcription factors).[8] The oncogene counterparts of the known proto-oncogenes have similar functions except that they are permanently functional (activated). As shown in Fig. 25.2,[9] oncogenic modifications include truncation (e.g., v-erbB derived from EGF receptor) and critical mutations (e.g., neu derived from erbB2).[9]

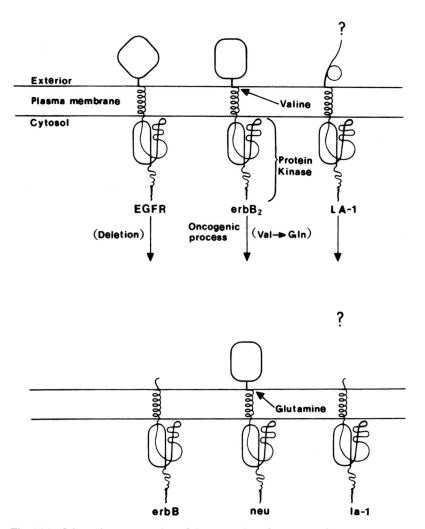

Fig. 25.2 Schematic representation of the generation of oncogenes from proto-oncogenes. Modifications include truncation, exemplified by the EGFR and mutation of a critical amino acid residue, exemplified by erbB2, the receptor for glial growth factors.[9] The LA-1 oncogene is assumed to arise from a proto-oncogene by an as yet unknown modification, possibly involving truncation of the extracellular domain.

Table 25.1 Representative oncogenes and their function

Oncogene	Function
	Extracellular
sis	PDGF (β chain) growth factor
hst	FGF-related growth factor
	Plasma membrane
erbB	Truncated EGF receptor PK (Tyr)
neu	Receptor-like PK (Tyr)
fms	Mutant CSF-1 receptor PK (Tyr)
trk	Truncated receptor-like PK (Tyr)
LA-1	Receptor-like PK (Ser/Thr)
src	Membrane associated nonreceptor PK (Tyr)
lck	Membrane associated nonreceptor PK (Tyr)
ras	Membrane associated GTP binding/GTPase
	Cytoplasmic
raf	Cytoplasmic PK (Ser)
Grb_2	SH2/SH3 protein (adaptor)
Sos	Guanine nucleotide exchange factor
	Nuclear
myc	Sequence specific DNA binding nuclear transcription factor
fos	Combines with *jun* to generate AP-1 transcription factor
jun	Sequence specific DNA binding protein, part of AP-1
erbA	Dominant negative mutant thyroxine (T3) receptor
p53	Mutant form may sequester wild type tumor suppressor

Representative oncogenes and their functions are listed in Table 25.1. Oncogenes can code for secreted proteins (growth factors) which act via autocrine loops to stimulate growth. Best studied among these is *sis*, that codes for platelet-derived growth factor (PDGF). Significantly, however, oncogenes in this category do not transform cells when added exogenously, suggesting that stimulation of their receptors may be important in their ability to transform cells.[10] Other oncogenes code for mutant forms of growth factor receptors. Most of these are derived from growth factor receptors Tyr protein kinases (PK). Ser/Thr growth factor receptor PKs and Tyr phosphatases were also identified,[10–12] suggesting that Ser phosphorylation and Tyr dephosphorylation may also be involved in growth factor receptor signaling and oncogene modification. The oncoprotein products of growth factor receptor kinase oncogenes transform by delivering a continuous, ligand-independent, mitogenic signal which is achieved by their ability to phosphorylate target proteins.[4,10,13]

Other oncoproteins that transform cells by protein phosphorylation are associated with the inner face of the cytoplasmic membranes. The best known members of this group of oncogenes are the *src* family of Tyr PKs. In normal cells, these PKs presumably deliver a mitogenic signal by binding to the cytoplasmic tails of kinase negative cell surface receptors. A good example is provided by pp56[lck] that binds to the kinase negative CD4 receptor on the surface of T-lymphocytes, thereby providing it with the ability to deliver the required signal.[14] Mutationally activated versions of this type of oncogene presumably deliver a continuous, rather than regulated, signal.

The membrane associated G proteins that function as signal transducers for cell surface growth factor receptors are best exemplified by the *ras* family of proteins which are GTP-binding GTPases. *ras* acts as a common intracellular relay point for signals initiated by a variety of growth factors. In its activated form, *ras* is bound to GTP; GDP bound *ras* is inactive.[15] *ras* activation is mediated by guanine nucleotide releasing factors (e.g., Sos) that catalyze the release of bound GDP.[16,17] Its deactivation is mediated by proteins that stimulate the GTPase activity of *ras* (GTPase activating protein (GAP).[7,18]

Most cytoplasmic oncoproteins, such as *raf*, are Ser/Thr kinases that are presumably involved in relaying the signal from the cell surface to the nucleus. Other cytoplasmic enzymes in the cascade are designated mitogen activated protein (MAP) kinases that work together in an orderly sequence forming a kinase cascade. Oncogenic forms of *raf* are deleted in the amino-terminal regulatory sequences, thereby becoming permanently activated.[19] Molecular adaptors[20] are another type of cytoplasmic oncoprotein. They contain sequences (*src* homology domains (SH2 and SH3)) that serve to facilitate protein–protein interactions. One such adaptor, Grb_2, mediates the interaction of Sos with activated growth factor receptors that leads to *ras* activation.[16,17]

The nuclear oncogenes code for transcription factors that, by virtue of increased expression or activity, can increase the expression of genes whose promoters or enhancers carry the appropriate response elements. c-*jun*, c-*fos* and c-*myc* are 'immediate early' genes that are rapidly induced when resting cells are treated with mitogens. Their targets are therefore likely to be involved in initiating or promoting growth. Indeed *myc* and *jun* participate in DNA replication[21,22] and continued expression of c-*myc* was implicated in transformation.[23] Mutations in the leucine zipper of v-*fos* that prevent its dimerization with c-*jun*[24] were shown to interfere with its transforming activity, thereby connecting the ability of c-*fos* to function in the AP-1 transcription factor with oncogenicity.[25] However, as many genes contain AP-1 target sites, it is unclear which AP-1 regulated genes are relevant to carcinogenesis. Another nuclear oncogene, v-*erbA* (a thyroid hormone receptor antagonist[26]), prevents the spontaneous differentiation of cells transformed by v-*erbB* and expands the range of conditions under which the transformed cells can propagate.[8]

MITOGENIC SIGNALING PATHWAYS

How do cells respond to extracellular growth signals? Present understanding of signaling pathways is schematically represented in Fig. 25.3, using PDGF and *LA*-1 oncogene as models. Briefly, ligand binding to the receptor (PDGF), or its constitutive (oncogenic) activation (*LA*-1), causes receptor autophosphorylation, and the transphosphorylation of substrates with which it becomes physically associated. These include phospholipase C (PLC-γ), phosphatidylinositol 3′ kinase (PI-3K), GAP, *src* and *src*-like Tyr PKs as well as the guanine release factor Sos that binds in a complex with the Grb$_2$ adaptor molecule.

PLC-γ, hydrolyzes phosphatidylinositol 4,5-biphosphate and generates inositol triphosphate that causes release of stored intracellular calcium, and diacylglycerol that activates protein kinase C (PKC). PKC is involved in the action of a number of tumor promoters.[27] Phosphorylation of PLC-γ on Tyr increases its catalytic activity in vitro.[28] PI-3K phosphorylates the inositol ring of phosphatidyl-inositol in the 3′ position. It is believed to function in the process of transformation, since v-src mutants that fail to associate with PI-3K are nontransforming. *src* and other related Tyr kinases are also activated rapidly in cells stimulated with PDGF.[4]

ras is a prominent member of the pathway and it serves as a relay point. Indeed microinjection of activated *ras* into quiescent cells induces DNA synthesis.[29] The picture that has developed so far shows that when growth factor receptors are phosphorylated they bind the Grb$_2$–Sos complex. The Sos protein then binds to *ras*-GDP, which is anchored to the cell membrane, and activates it by causing the exchange of GDP with GTP.[16,17] *ras* is inactivated by proteins such as GAP that increase its weak intrinsic GTPase activity. However, activated growth factor receptors also bind and phosphorylate GAP[30] thereby decreasing its ability to inactivate *ras*.[31,32]

The *raf* protein comes into the pathway after *ras*.[33] It may become physically associated with the activated *ras*. Presumably *raf* phosphorylates an enzyme called MAP kinase which in turn activates a MAP kinase cascade. The last member of the cascade phosphorylates nuclear transcription factors, such as c-*fos*, c-*jun* and c-*myc*,[34,35] that are required for DNA synthesis and mitogenic responses.[36-38]

As *ras* activation seems to be critical for the action of many different receptors, it is likely that specificity is achieved by unique, potentially tissue specific, signaling molecules. Indeed, while competence factors are interchangeable (Fig. 25.1), their substrates differ. The PDGF receptor interacts with all of the kinase substrates in Fig. 25.3, while the CSF-1 receptor does not phosphorylate PLC-γ or GAP[39] and the EGF receptor and *erbB*-2 phosphorylate GAP inefficiently.[40] *LA*-1 does not seem to interact with PI-3 kinase or *src* (Aurelian L, unpublished) but it binds Grb$_2$-Sos and efficiently phosphorylates GAP.[41] Similarly, while *ras* proteins are present in all cells, some guanine release factors are tissue specific.[42] From the standpoint of carcinogenesis, these findings suggest that some genetic changes are common to many types of tumors whereas others are specific to certain tumors.

ANTIONCOGENES

Presumably the presence of one normal (wild type) copy of an autosomal gene interferes with oncogenesis and the normal allele can be considered

A.

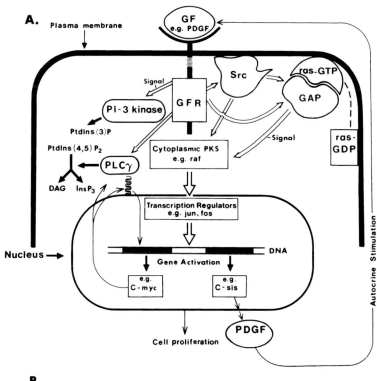

B.

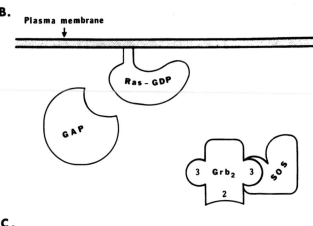

C.

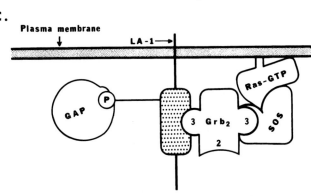

Fig. 25.3 Schematic representation of signaling pathways in growth factor receptor mediated responses. **A** The substrates of the prototype PDGF receptor include PLCγ that generates two second messengers, inositol triphosphate (InsP3) and diacylglycerol (DAG), PI-3K which phosphorylates phosphatidyl inositol [PtdIns(3)P], *src*, Grb₂-Sos and *ras*-GAP. The cytoplasmic effectors include *raf* that may react directly with *ras*-GTP and a kinase cascade that begins with MAP kinase. The final steps involve nuclear oncogenes such as c-*myc*, c-*jun* and c-*fos* that affect genes which contain AP-1. These oncogenes cause increased transcription of cellular genes involved in DNA replication and cell growth. **B** and **C** *ras* activation using *LA-1* oncogene as a model. In the absence of *LA-1*, (**B**), Grb₂-Sos travel as a cytoplasmic complex and *ras* is inactive (*ras*-GDP). In the presence of *LA-1* (**C**) the Grb₂-Sos complex and GAP bind to *LA-1* and *ras*-GAP is phosphorylated. According to this model, the Grb₂-Sos complex binds to the SH3 binding domain of *LA-1*. However, SH2 dependent binding of Grb₂-Sos at other sites in the activated *LA-1* oncogene is not excluded. Binding of Grb₂-Sos activates *ras* (*ras*-GTP), and the phosphorylated *ras*-GAP fails to inactivate it.

an antioncogene. However, relatively little is known about the function of antioncogenes. Two of them (RB and p53) are nuclear proteins.[43] They cause growth arrest of cells in G_1[36] and must be inactivated in order for cells to enter S phase. RB is inactivated by phosphorylation;[44] p53 by mutation or degradation.[45] RB and p53 have DNA binding activity and might suppress gene expression by binding to regulatory sequences. p53 has *trans*-activating function,[46] suggesting that it may have a direct role in regulating DNA synthesis or it could regulate the expression of other growth inhibitory genes.[47,48] RB appears to cause growth arrest by complexing with E2F, a transcription factor which activates cell cycle genes expressed at the G_1/S transition and encodes proteins required for DNA synthesis such as thymidine kinase and DNA polymerase. RB could also bind to other nuclear proteins,[49] thereby potentially sequestering other transcription factors. As the cell approaches the G_1/S transition, RB is phosphorylated by cdk/cyclin kinase and it remains phosphorylated through mitosis. This releases the active E2F transcription factor.

Many questions about the role of antioncogenes in carcinogenesis remain. For example, as RB is widely expressed in many cell types, it is unclear why it is only associated with retinoblastoma, a rare childhood tumor. Similarly, microinjection of anti-p53 antibody blocks serum-induced entry into S phase, suggesting that p53 is required for DNA synthesis.[50] This may reflect the unwitting use of wild type vs mutant alleles, since wild type p53 suppresses *ras*-mediated transformation,[51] while mutants of p53 cooperate with *ras* in the transformation of primary rat cells.[52] However, it is unclear why the mutant p53 behaves as an oncogene and conditions that favor this behavior are unknown. Possibly, other antioncogenes or genes regulated by RB and/or p53 have the determinant role in carcinogenesis. DCC, another candidate tumor suppressor protein has significant homology to cell adhesion molecules and presumably acts at the cell surface.[53] Seven antioncogenes have been cloned whose mutations in the germline may predispose the host to cancer. A recent review describes our present understanding of the role of antioncogenes in cancer causation.[54]

CANCER IS A MULTIFACTORIAL DISEASE: ONCOGENE COOPERATION

Experimental studies led to the conclusion that oncogenes cooperate in causing tumorigenesis. This cooperation is defined as (i) a situation in which a pair of oncogenes, acting in concert, can convert a normal cell to a tumorigenic one, and (ii) a case in which the loss of a tumor suppressor gene in conjunction with one or more oncogenes is inducing a tumorigenic phenotype.[55-57] Originally, it was thought that genetic damage associated with tumor development results from the cooperation of oncogene products that act in the nucleus with those that act in the cytoplasm. Indeed, most of the nuclear oncoproteins (*myc*, *fos*, *jun*) can cooperate with activated *ras* to transform primary rodent cells.[55] However, this is by no means a hard and fast rule. Oncogenes in the two categories (cytoplasmic and nuclear) are not always interchangeable,[56] and there are examples of cooperation between two nuclear or two cytoplasmic oncoproteins.[58]

How does genetic modification cause cancer? It is widely accepted that malignant cells arise in a multistep process in which genetic events that include the unregulated expression of growth factors, their receptors, or components of the signaling pathways, accumulate in the cancer progenitor cell over the course of many years. Immortalization, which is the prolongation of the cell's lifespan, is generally accepted as an early event in tumorigenesis.[59] In itself it constitutes an increased risk factor for the accumulation of additional mutations that are likely to be involved in the acquisition of neoplastic potential.

The sequential nature of carcinogenesis is supported by studies of mouse skin carcinoma[60] that led to the two stage model (initiation and promotion). In this system, mutagenic activation of the *ras* oncogene was shown to be a relatively early event. Tumor promotion, mediated by factors that act in an epigenetic manner, was required for outgrowth of frank carcinoma.[61] One type of tumor promoter, exemplified by the phorbol esters, activates members of the PKC family of Ser/Thr kinases.[27,62] The second type of tumor promoter, exemplified by okadaic acid, is a potent inhibitor of protein phosphatases.[63] Its net effect is to increase phosphorylation of PKC targets, thereby increasing genetic instability or stimulating the growth of the initiated cells. Ultimately, this increases the risk of cumulative mutations, or it evokes events that inactivate antioncogenes.[64]

Final conclusions about the sequential activation and cooperative interaction of oncogenes in carcinogenesis are still premature. However, genetic alterations affecting proto-oncogenes are common in human malignancies. For example, expression of PDGF and its receptors is documented in a high fraction of sarcoma and glially derived neoplasms.[65] The EGF receptor (EGFR) family of proteins is frequently implicated in human cancer. In many transformed cells, EGFR levels were shown to decrease, possibly due to the production of transforming growth factor α (TGFα). In contrast, by comparison to normal tissues, EGFR levels were significantly higher in several different squamous cell lung carcinomas, some breast cancer cells, and in brain tumors. However, in some cancers the EGFR levels were unchanged.[66] erbB-2 is often overexpressed in adenocarcinoma of the breast, stomach and ovary.[67] Among rate limiting molecules involved in mitogenic signaling, members of the ras family are among the most frequently detected oncogenes and they have been associated primarily with lung, colon and pancreatic carcinomas.[68] Some of the genetic changes that are accumulated through progression are common to many types of tumors whereas others are specific to a certain tumor. It is likely that for all tumors there is a preferred, but not obligatory, order of events. However, experimental studies with colon carcinoma suggest that it is not the temporal order in which genetic defects occur that is responsible for carcinogenesis, but rather their total accumulation.[69]

ONCOGENES AND THE CELL CYCLE

Tightly regulated decision points in the cell cycle may be the targets of oncogene activation. Quiescent fibroblasts respond only to combinations of at least two growth factors, thereby leading to the dual signal hypothesis (Fig. 25.1). Overexpression of c-myc can replace the requirement for PDGF[2] and constitutive expression of c-myb can substitute for the IGF-1 requirement.[3] An example of the connection between the cell cycle, oncogenesis, and virus infection is provided by cyclin A. This protein is expressed starting in S phase and it associates with a Ser PK designated cdc2, or with a cdc2 related PK. The exact role of this cyclin complex is unknown, but it is believed to be required for progression through the S phase.[70] cdc2 is also connected to antioncogenes RB and p53 which are phosphorylated in a cell cycle dependent manner, and the in vivo sites are phosphorylated by cdc2 in vitro.[71] RB phosphorylation occurs as the cells enter S phase.[72] Phosphorylation inactivates RB, thereby presumably allowing the cells to exit from G_1. In human hepatoma (which is associated with hepatitis virus (HBV)) a fragment of HBV integrates into the cyclin A gene[73] leading to the formation of a chimera in which the amino terminal cyclin A sequences are replaced by part of the HBV pre-S protein. Loss of amino-terminal sequences presumably stabilizes cyclin A, which in turn leads to persistent activation of the associated cdc2 related PK.

ONCOGENES AND CERVICAL CANCER

Epidemiologic studies have established that sexual activity is the major risk factor for cervical cancer[74-76] suggesting that sexually transmitted factors are involved in its development. Other risk factors include diet, hormones, contraceptive use and smoking.[74-78] Mechanistically, immortalization of the cervical cells is a likely early event. Neoplastic conversion is probably due to the accretion of additional genetic modifications. Both immortalization and neoplastic conversion could be induced by various risk factors which cause oncogene activation and/or antioncogene inactivation. Most cases of cervical cancer are probably caused by a preferred set of risk factors and order of events. Others may result from similar or different genetic modifications that are induced by different risk factors and irrespective of the order of events. Intraepithelial cervical lesions and their severity (low- vs high-grade squamous

Table 25.2 Oncogenes and cervical cancer tissues

Oncogene	Modification	Disease relation
ras	Overexpression	In 50% of high-grade SIL and invasive cancer; related to cell type; related to progression
myc	Amplification/rearrangement	In invasive cancer; conflicting results
	Overexpression	In invasive cancer; related to metastatic potential; conflicting results
EGFR	Overexpression	In invasive cancer or normal tissues or neither
LA-1	Overexpression/rearrangement	In 38% low-grade SIL; 58% high-grade SIL; 67% invasive cancer; related to progression; related to cancer relapse

intraepithelial lesions (SIL)) can be diagnosed with a high degree of accuracy. Accordingly, available information on oncogene activation and antioncogene inactivation in cervical lesions (Table 25.2) provides significant information on the various genetic modifications associated with carcinogenesis and the sequence in which they are acquired.

Growth factor receptor oncogenes

As EGFR is overexpressed in many cancers,[66] several studies considered the possibility that it is an activated growth factor receptor in cervical cancer. However, the results of these studies were conflicting. In some of them, EGFR overexpression was associated with progression from mild to severe dysplasia,[79] but not with tumor progression and metastatic potential.[80] In others, EGFR was rarely overexpressed, if at all.[81] We found that 33% of CIN 1 and 50% of invasive cancer tissues express EGFR. However, these proportions were significantly lower than those (86%) in normal cervical tissues.[82] Decreased EGFR expression in cancer tissues may reflect oncogenic activation of EGFR or its functional replacement by another activated growth factor receptor oncogene, such as *LA-1*.[82] Available evidence, discussed below, supports the latter interpretation.

The *LA-1* oncoprotein is a 60 kDa Ser/Thr specific growth factor receptor. It is fused to the large subunit of herpes simplex virus type 2 (HSV-2) ribonucleotide reductase (RR1).[12,83–85] *LA-1* causes malignant transformation of immortalized cells.[86–89] Gene expression and kinase activity are required for malignant transformation. A HSV-2 mutant that is temperature sensitive in *LA-1* oncogene expression, is transformation

negative at the nonpermissive temperature[90] and a transmembrane deleted *LA-1* mutant that does not localize to the plasma membrane is kinase negative and does not have transforming potential.[41]

LA-1 probably originated from a cellular gene, since homologous (68.6%) genomic DNA sequences were cloned from a human cervical tissue by polymerase chain reaction (PCR).[91] The entire proto-oncogene has not yet been cloned and therefore its function and the genetic modification that caused its activation remain speculative. We assume that oncogenic activation occurred through insertion of the proto-oncogene (or part thereof) into the polypeptide coding region of an ancestral HSV-2 RR1 such as suggested for the human somatomammotropin gene.[92] Presumably, the upstream (5′) recombination site is within the promoter of the HSV-2 RR1 gene thereby explaining the presence in this promoter of *cis*-response elements, such as AP-1,[91,93–95] that are characteristic of cellular, but not HSV genes. Regulation of the chimeric gene as an immediate early protein is also presumably due to the insertion of *cis*-response elements that originated with the cellular gene.[93,95] The C-terminus (3′) recombination site at the junction of PK and RR presumably occurred within the promoter region of the ancestral HSV-2 RR1, thereby giving rise to an ORF that contains enhancer core and functional promoter elements. Indeed, mathematical modeling identified the presence at the PK and RR junction of distortion patterns consistent with an enhancer region, and DNA sequence analysis revealed a consensus core enhancer element (G)–T–G–G–A(T)–(G). When cloned into expression vectors, this region had functional promoter elements and bound cellular factors.[88,91]

LA-1 is overexpressed and the gene is rearranged

in cervical tumors as compared to normal tissues. Thus, in at least five different studies using immunohistochemistry to determine *LA-1* expression, the proportion of positive tissues increased as a function of the severity of the lesion, beginning at approximately 35–46% in low-grade SIL, and increasing to 57–67% in high-grade SIL and invasive cancer. This compares to 10–14% of normal tissues.[82,96–100] The overexpression of the *LA-1* oncogene in cervical cancer tissues was also determined by immunoblotting with anti-*LA-1* antibody which revealed increased levels of the *LA-1* oncoprotein in high-grade SIL and invasive cancer, as compared to barely detectable expression in normal cervical tissues.[82] In at least three follow-up studies, *LA-1* expression predicted the persistence or progression of the disease and correlated with poor prognosis after treatment.[99–101] Finally, a recent study using PCR showed *LA-1* gene rearrangement in 44% of low grade SIL and 60% of invasive cancer, but not in normal tissues.[102] However, it remains to be determined whether *LA-1* overexpression is related to gene rearrangement. Taken in toto, these studies indicate that cervical tumor development is associated with *LA-1* oncogene overexpression/rearrangement. Significantly, *LA-1* overexpression was also observed in 33% of vulvar intraepithelial neoplasias and 67% of vulvar cancer cases.[98] It was not observed in other squamous cancers including lung, pharynx, larynx, vocal cord, tongue, floor of mouth, skin and esophagus.[82,100]

ras oncogene

As schematically represented in Fig. 25.3, *ras* is a critical component of signaling pathways in *LA-1* mediated transformation. In transformed human cells, the Grb_2–Sos complex binds to the phosphorylated *LA-1* oncoprotein thereby causing *ras* activation.[41] *ras*–GAP is also complexed with the *LA-1* oncoprotein and serves as its phosphorylation substrate. The phosphorylated *ras*–GAP has decreased GTPase stimulating activity thereby contributing to the increased amounts of activated *ras*.[41] The levels of a GTP binding protein in the *ras* family are also significantly increased in *LA-1* transformed rodent cells.[90]

When the levels of oncogene expression were evaluated as the mean staining intensity/unit area, only *ras* was overexpressed in high-grade SIL and invasive cancer as compared to normal or low-grade SIL tissues. *erbB*-2 and *myc* were not overexpressed.[103] The frequency of *ras* positive tissues increased with increased severity of the premalignant lesions from 17.9% in CIN 1 to 28.9% in CIN 2 and 53.9% in CIN 3. However, it did not increase beyond this level, remaining 50% in invasive carcinoma.[104] As CIN 1 can be considered the in vivo correlate of experimentally immortalized (but not neoplastic) cells, these findings suggest that *ras* activation occurs after immortalization and the frequency of activated *ras* is higher as cells approach a neoplastic state. We conclude that *ras* expression follows activation of the *LA-1* oncogene since 35–46% of low-grade SIL lesions were positive for *LA-1* expression as compared to 18% positive for *ras*, while similar proportions of high-grade SIL/cervical cancer were positive for both *ras* and *LA-1* expression (50–67%).

The conclusion that *ras* activation is associated with carcinogenic potential is also supported by a follow-up study in which two of 10 patients (20%) whose early lesions regressed during a 1-year follow-up period had been positive for *ras* oncogene expression. By contrast seven of 14 (50%) *ras* positive lesions progressed.[104] This conclusion cannot be accepted unequivocally, as the study groups were very small and the regressors were followed for 1 year, while the progressors were followed for 2–5 years. However, similar results were obtained in another study in which patients with *ras* positive squamous cell carcinoma had a higher incidence of lymph node metastases than *ras* negative patients.[80] Is *ras* activation associated with a specific type of cervical cancer? In one study addressing this question, *ras* overexpression, evaluated as staining intensity, was predominantly seen in keratinizing (57.1%) and large cell non-keratinizing (54.2%) tumors. Only 38.7% of small cell type carcinomas, that had a better prognosis than the other two cancer types, were positive for *ras* overexpression.[105]

Nuclear oncogenes

Reports on the association of c-*myc* with cervical neoplasia are conflicting. c-*myc* amplification and/or rearrangement was reported in 90% of cervical carcinomas[106,107] and amplification was also associated with increased severity of the carcinoma.[106] Additionally, c-*myc* overexpression (determined by immunostaining) was described in cervical carcinoma tissues,[108,109] and patients with negative lymph nodes were shown to have a 3-year disease-free survival rate of 93% when c-*myc* was expressed at normal levels whereas this rate was only 51% when c-*myc* was overexpressed.[107] c-*myc* overexpression was also associated with a 6.1-fold higher risk of distant metastases, suggesting that c-*myc* activation may lead to metastatic potential.[110] Patients negative for c-*myc* expression had a better disease-free mean (mean = 95.4 mos.) and total (mean = 118 mos.) survival than those that were c-*myc* positive (28.4 and 48.4 mos., respectively) and c-*myc* positive tumors were more likely to develop extrapelvic metastatic disease.[109] However, in three other studies c-*myc* was not amplified in cervical carcinoma tissues,[111] and its expression was rare in both cancer and normal tissues.[81,82,111] In other studies, c-*myc* was overexpressed in normal as compared to carcinoma tissues,[112] and it was expressed in a higher proportion of normal than carcinoma tissues.[113] These conflicting results are difficult to interpret. They may reflect technical difficulties arising from small and/or poorly controlled study groups, the relative instability of the c-*myc* transcript,[114] and/or the different c-*myc* activating potential of various risk factors associated with cervical cancer.

Antioncogenes

The role of antioncogenes in cervical cancer is unclear. RB and p53 are transcribed in nonmalignant and malignant cells although the amounts of p53 in cervical carcinoma cell lines are generally low.[115] We found that a small proportion (15–17%) of CIN 1 and CIN 3 tissues express p53. However, it is doubtful that p53 plays a significant role in cervical cancer, since it was expressed in a similar proportion of normal tissues.[82]

TUMOR-SPECIFIC ANTIGENS

Most tumors induced by chemical carcinogens or radiation express tumor-specific transplantation antigens (TSTA) that may be altered growth factor receptor(s) or diffusible factor(s) that mediate cell-density induced inhibition of cellular proliferation.[116] Cervical carcinoma tissues were not studied for TSTA. However, several studies have implicated a squamous cell carcinoma antigen (designated SCC) in the course of the cervical cancer. In serologic assays, the sensitivity of SCC responses after cancer treatment (percentage of positive results in patients with persistent disease) was 79% and the specificity (percentage of negative results in patients with no evidence of disease) was 91%. The incidence of elevated pretreatment serum SCC levels ranged from 37% in patients with stage 1B invasive cancer to 90% in patients with stage 4 invasive cancer. However, the positive predictive value of a single serum SCC evaluation for tumor recurrence was only 49%.[117] The association of SCC with squamous cervical carcinoma was also reported by others,[118] with a sensitivity increasing from 29% in stage 1 to 89% in stage 4 carcinomas.

The exact identity of SCC is unknown. It is one of the 14 fractions of TA4 antigen which is a 48 kDa glycoprotein located in the cytoplasm of normal squamous epithelia and in squamous carcinomas of many sites, including lung and esophagus[119] as well as in inflammatory skin disease (psoriasis).[120] The SCC positivity rate was higher in women with well differentiated (78%) than poorly differentiated (38%) cervical carcinomas suggesting that it is a differentiation related protein. In this respect it may be significant that EGF enhances SCC production by a cervical carcinoma cell line, suggesting that SCC may be an oncoprotein located downstream of EGF in signaling pathways that are activated in squamous cell carcinoma. Overexpression of heat shock protein was also reported in dyskaryotic cells from cervical smears from patients with CIN 3 but not in normal cervical cells.[121] Heat shock proteins may be involved in cell cycle regulation. However, their role in cervical cancer, if any, is unclear.

LA-1 ONCOGENE HYPOTHESIS OF CERVICAL CANCER

The *LA-1* oncogene hypothesis (Fig. 25.4) is based on the considerations reviewed above. It

LA1 Hypothesis of Cervical Cancer

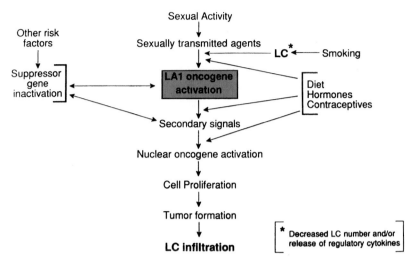

Fig. 25.4 Schematic representation of the *LA-1* oncogene hypothesis. Various risk factors, primarily sexually transmitted factors, activate *LA-1*. Other risk factors inactivate antioncogenes (tumor suppressor genes) and activate various components of the signaling pathway. Smoking is shown as reducing the density of Langerhans cells (LC) and/or causing release of regulatory cytokines, thereby contributing to *LA-1* activation. LC and/or other aspects of the immune system may also be involved at the level of immunosuppression.

assumes that the risk of cervical cancer is strongly dictated by sexual activity. Additional risk factors include smoking, diet, hormones and contraceptive use. Cellular immortalization mediated by sexually transmitted factors is posited as an early event in cervical carcinogenesis. However, the hypothesis allows for immortalization due to other factors that have immortalizing potential in vitro, including diet, hormones and contraceptives. Immortalization could also be due to the cooperation of various risk factors that could independently or simultaneously cause the conversion of proto-oncogenes to oncogenes and/or the inactivation of antioncogenes.

Activation of the *LA-1* proto-oncogene is posited as a critical event that follows immortalization. It could be an outcome of immortalization or it could be due to other risk factors that affect the immortalized cells. One or multiple risk factors associated with cervical cancer may be involved in *LA-1* activation. HSV-2 differs from all the other risk factors in that it can transform both by virtue of its ability to activate the *LA-1* proto-oncogene and due to its own, already activated, *LA-1* oncogene. Secondary messengers

involved in carcinogenesis include guanine nucleotide releasing factors and GAP, that are bound and phosphorylated by *LA-1* thereby causing *ras* activation. Transmission of the unregulated growth signal is visualized to occur through the activated *ras*, *raf* and the MAP kinase cascade, culminating in the activation of nuclear oncogenes (including c-*myc* and *fos*) and/or other genes associated with DNA replication and cell proliferation.

It seems likely that cooperating oncogenes constitutively activate distinct signaling pathways that affect transcription levels and involve both gene activation and repression. Presumably such nuclear signals initiate the same events as co-operating growth factors. However, it is unclear how many of the events needed for the genesis of cervical cancer can be explained by the activation of known oncogenes, and the inactivation of familiar antioncogenes. The *LA-1* oncogene is particularly relevant to cervical cancer since it is associated with tumor growth and connected to sexual activity. Furthermore, *LA-1* activates *ras*, *fos* and *myc*, which have also been associated with cervical cancer. Presumably other oncogenes, including some that are not yet identified, are also involved in cervical cancer.

The contribution of other risk factors is accommodated by the *LA-1* hypothesis as schematically represented in Fig. 25.4. Smoking is seen as causing Langerhans cells (LC) damage as well as decreasing their frequency in cervical tissues. This decreases local immunosurveillance and causes the release of regulatory cytokines that ultimately activate *LA-1*. Diet, hormones and contraceptives could contribute at all stages of the signaling pathway. Hormones could also induce expression of nuclear receptors that may ultimately increase cell DNA replication. As both RB and p53 are transcribed in malignant and nonmalignant cervical cells, the hypothesis invokes other, as yet unidentified risk factors, in the functional inactivation of these antioncogenes and/or the binding and inactivation of other antioncogenes.

Systematic analysis of oncogenes and anti-oncogenes altered in cervical cancer, and a better understanding of the role of oncogenic signaling pathways in cancer development will offer opportunities for improvements in diagnosis and prognosis, as well as for therapeutic intervention. For instance antisense therapy with modified oligodeoxynucleotides that target *LA-1* and/or other commonly activated oncogenes (e.g., *ras*) can be used as specific and effective means of inhibiting tumor cells the growth of which depends on *LA-1* oncogene expression.[122,123] Another strategy involves administration of monoclonal antibodies that induce *LA-1* downregulation.[84] Indeed antibodies to growth factor receptors have been shown to impair tumor cell proliferation both in vitro and in vivo.[124] Tumors that overexpress the *LA-1* oncoprotein might also be targeted with radioisotopes or toxins linked to monoclonal antibodies to the receptor. In theory, this strategy would have the advantage of being both tumor-icidal and having a high degree of specificity for the tumor cell.

REFERENCES

1. Scher C D, Shepard R C, Antoniades H N, Stiles C D. Platelet-derived growth factor and the regulation of the mammalian fibroblast cell cycle. Biochim Biophys Acta 1979; 560: 217–241.
2. Armelin H A, Armelin M C S, Kelly K et al. Functional role for c-myc in mitogenic response to platelet-derived growth factor. Nature 1984; 310: 655–660.
3. Travali S, Reiss K, Ferber A et al. Constitutively expressed c-myb abrogates the requirement for IGF-1 in 3T3 fibroblasts. Molec Cell Biol 1991; 11: 731–736.
4. Aaronson S A. Growth factors and cancer. Science 1991; 254: 1146–1153.
5. Cooper G M. Oncogenes. Boston: Jones and Bartlett, 1990.
6. Hunter T. A thousand and one protein kinases. Cell 1987; 50: 823–829.
7. Lemoine N R. The c-ras oncogenes and GAP. In: Carney D, Sikara K, eds. Genes and cancer. John Wiley 1990: pp 19–29.
8. Lewin B. Oncogenic Conversion by regulatory changes in transcription factors. Cell 1991; 64: 303–312.
9. Marchionni M A, Goodearl A D, Chen M L et al. Glial growth factors are alternatively spliced erbB2 ligands expressed in the nervous system. Nature 1993; 362: 312–318.
10. Hunter T. Cooperation between oncogenes. Cell 1991; 64: 249–270.
11. Hunter T. Protein–tyrosine phosphatases: the other side of the coin. Cell 1989; 58: 1013–1016.
12. Luo J H, Aurelian L. The transmembrane helical segment but not the invariant lysine is required for the kinase activity of the large subunit of herpes simplex virus type 2 ribonucleotide reductase (ICP10). J Biol Chem 1992; 267: 9645–9653.
13. Bishop J M. Molecular themes in oncogenesis. Cell 1991; 64: 235–248.
14. Rudd C E, Trevillyan J M, Dasgupta J D, Wong L L, Schlossman S F. The CD4 receptor is complexed in detergent lysates to a protein-tyrosine kinase (p58) from human lymphocytes. Proc Nat Acad Sci USA 1988; 85: 5190–5194.
15. Gibbs J B, Marshalll M S, Scolnick E M, Dixon R A, Vogel U S. Modulation of guanine nucleotides bound to Ras in NIH3T3 cells by oncogenes, growth factors, and the GTPase activating protein (GAP). J Biol Chem 1990; 265: 20437–20442.
16. Buday L, Downward J. Epidermal growth factor regulates p21^{ras} through the formation of a complex of receptor, Grb2 adaptor protein, and Sos nucleotide exchange factor. Cell 1993; 73: 611–620.
17. Li N, Batzer A, Daly R et al. Guanine-nucleotide-releasing factor bSos1 binds Grb2 and links receptor tyrosine kinases to Ras signalling. Nature 1993; 352: 85–88.
18. Polakis P, McCormick F. Interaction between p21ras proteins and their GTPase activating proteins. In: Cancer surveys, vol 12: Tumor suppressor genes, the cell cycle and cancer. London: Imperial Cancer Research Fund, 1992: pp 25–41.
19. Rapp U R, Cleveland J L, Bonner T I, Storm S M. The raf oncogene. In: Reddy E P, Skalka A M, Curran T, eds. The oncogene handbook. Amsterdam: Elsevier Science Publishers BV, 1988: pp 213–253.

20. Mayer B J, Hanafusa H. Association of the v-*crk* oncogene product with phosphotyrosine-containing proteins and protein kinase activity. Proc Nat Acad Sci USA 1990; 87: 2638–2642.

21. Ariga H, Imamura Y, Iguchiariga S M M. DNA replication origin and transcriptional enhancer in *c-myc* gene share the *c-myc* protein binding sequences. EMBO J 1989; 8: 4273–4279.

22. Wasylyk C, Schneikert J, Wasylyk B. Oncogene v-*jun* modulates DNA replication. Oncogene 1990; 5: 1055–1058.

23. Cole M D. The *myc* oncogene: its role in transformation and differentiation. Ann Rev Genet 1986; 20: 361–384.

24. Turner R, Tijan R. Leucine repeats and an adjacent DNA binding domain mediate the formation of functional cFos-cJun heterodimers. Science 1989; 243: 1689–1694.

25. Schuermann M, Neuberg M, Hunter J B et al. The leucine repeat motif in Fos protein mediates complex formation with Jun/AP-1 and is required for transformation. Cell 1989; 56: 507–516.

26. Damm K, Thompson C, Evans R M. Protein encoded by v-*erbA* functions as a thyroid-hormone receptor antagonist. Nature 1989; 339: 593–597.

27. Nishizuka Y. Studies and perspectives of protein kinase C. Science 1986; 233: 305–312.

28. Goldschmidt-Clermont P J, Kim J W, Machesky L M, Rhee S G, Pollard T D. Regulation of phospholipase C-gamma 1 by profilin and tyrosine phosphorylation. Science 1991; 251: 1231–1233.

29. Stacey D W, Kung H F. Transformation of NIH 3T3 cells by microinjection of Ha-*ras* p21 protein. Nature 1984; 310: 508–511.

30. Kaplan D R, Morrison D K, Wong G, McCormick F, Williams L T. PDGF β-receptor stimulates tyrosine phosphorylation of GAP and association of GAP with a signaling complex. Cell 1990; 61: 125–133.

31. Ellis C, Moran M, McCormick F, Pawson T. Phosphorylation of GAP and GAP-associated proteins by transforming and mitogenic tyrosine kinases. Nature 1990; 343: 377–381.

32. Moran M F, Polakis P, McCormick F, Pawson T, Ellis C. Protein tyrosine kinases regulate the phosphorylation protein interactions, subcellular distribution and activity of p21*ras* GTPase activating protein. Molec Cell Biol 1991; 11: 1804–1812.

33. Morrison D K, Kaplan D R, Rapp U, Roberts T M. Signal transduction from membrane to cytoplasm: growth factors and membrane-bound oncogene products increase Raf-1 phosphorylation and associated protein kinase activity. Proc Nat Acad Sci USA 1988; 85: 885–889.

34. Jamal S, Ziff E. Transactivation of c-*fos* and β-actin genes by *raf* as a step in early response to transmembrane signals. Nature 1990; 344: 463–466.

35. Rollins B J, Stiles C D. Serum-inducible genes. Adv Cancer Res 1989; 53: 1–32.

36. Diller L, Kassel J, Nelson C E et al. p53 functions as a cell cycle control protein in osteosarcomas. Molec Cell Biol 1990; 10: 5772–5781.

37. Riabowol K T, Vosaika R J, Ziff E B, Lamb N J, Feramisco J R. Microinjection of *fos* specific antibodies blocks DNA synthesis in fibroblast cells. Molec Cell Biol 1988; 8: 1670–1676.

38. Schönthal A, Gebel S, Stein B, Ponta H, Rahmsdorf H J, Herrlich P. Nuclear oncoproteins determine the genetic program in response to external stimuli. Cold Spring Harbor Symp Quant Biol 1988; 53: 779–787.

39. Downing J R, Margolis B L, Zilberstein A et al. Phospholipase C-gamma, a substrate for PDGF receptor kinase, is not phosphorylated on tyrosine during the mitogenic response to CSF-1. EMBO J 1989; 8: 3345–3350.

40. Fazioli F, Kim U H, Rhee S G, Molloy C J, Segatto O, Di Fiore P P. The erbB-2 mitogenic signaling pathway: tyrosine phosphorylation of phospholipase c-gamma and GTPase-activating protein does not correlate with erbB-2 mitogenic potency. Molec Cell Biol 1991; 11: 2040–2048.

41. Smith C C, Luo J H, Hunter J C R, Ordonez J V, Aurelian L. The transmembrane domain of the large subunit of HSV-2 ribonucleotide reductase (ICP10) is required for membrane localization, PK activity and transforming potential. (In press).

42. Shou C, Farnsworth C L, Neel B G, Feig L A. Molecular cloning of cDNAs encoding a guanine-nucleotide-releasing factor for Ras p21. Nature 1992; 358: 351–354.

43. Marshall C J. Tumor suppressor genes. Cell 1991; 64: 313–326.

44. Mihara K, Cao X R, Yen A, Chandler S et al. Cell cycle dependent phosphorylation of the human retinoblastoma gene product. Science 1989; 246: 1300–1303.

45. Crook T, Tidy J A, Vousden K H. Degradation of p53 can be targeted by HPV E6 sequences distinct from those required for p53 binding and trans-activation. Cell 1991; 67: 547–556.

46. Raycroft L, Wu H, Lozano G. Transcriptional activation by wild type but not transforming mutants of the p53 anti-oncogene. Science 1990; 249: 1049–1051.

47. Pietenpol J A, Stein R W, Moran E et al. TGF-β1 inhibition of c-*myc* transcription and growth in keratinocytes is abrogated by viral transforming proteins with pRB binding domains. Cell 1990; 61: 777–785.

48. Schneider C, King R M, Philipson L. Genes specifically expressed at growth arrest of mammalian cells. Cell 1988; 54: 787–793.

49. Robbins P D, Horowitz J M, Mulligan R M. Negative regulation of human c-*fos* by the retinoblastoma gene product. Nature 1990; 346: 668–671.

50. Mercer W E, Nelson D, DeLeo A B, Old L J, Baserga R. Microinjection of monoclonal antibody to protein p53 inhibits serum-induced DNA synthesis in 3T3 cells. Proc Nat Acad Sci USA 1982; 79: 6309–6312.

51. Finlay C A, Hinds P W, Levine A J. The p53 proto-oncogene can act as a suppressor of transformation. Cell 1989; 57: 1083–1093.

52. Lane D P, Benchimol S. p53: oncogene or anti-oncogene? Genes Devel 1990; 4: 1–8.

53. Fearon E R, Cho K R, Nigro J M et al. Identification of a chromosome 18C gene that is altered in colorectal cancers. Science 1990; 247: 49–56.

54. Knudson A G. Anti-oncogenes and human cancer. Proc Nat Acad Sci 1993; 90: 10914–10921.

55. Land H, Parada L F, Weinberg R A. Tumorigenic conversion of primary embryo fibroblasts requires at

least two cooperating oncogenes. Nature 1983; 304: 596–602.

56. Ruley H E. Transforming collaborations between *ras* and nuclear oncogenes. Cancer Cells 1990; 2: 258–268.

57. Weinberg R A. Oncogenes, anti-oncogenes, and the molecular bases of multistep carcinogenesis. Cancer Res 1989; 49: 3713–3721.

58. Reed J C, Haldar S, Croce C M, Cuddy M P. Complementation by BCL2 and c-HA-*RAS* oncogenes in malignant transformation of rat embryo fibroblasts. Molec Cell Biol 1990; 10: 4370–4374.

59. Newbold R F. Multistep malignant transformation of mammalian cells by carcinogens: induction of immortality as a key event. Carcinogenesis; a comprehensive survey 1985; 9: 17–28.

60. Balmain A, Brown K. Oncogene activation in chemical carcinogenesis. Adv Cancer Res 1988; 51: 147–182.

61. Yuspa S H, Poirier M C. Chemical carcinogenesis: from animal models to molecular models in one decade. Adv Cancer Res 1988; 50: 25–70.

62. Drinkwater N R. Experimental models and biological mechanisms for tumor promotion. Cancer Cells 1990; 2: 8–15.

63. Suganuma M, Fujiki H, Suguri H et al. Okadaic acid: an additional non phorbol-12-tetradecanoate-13-acetate type tumor promoter. Proc Nat Acad Sci USA 1988; 85: 1768–1771.

64. Ames B N, Gold L S. Too many rodent carcinogens: mitogenesis increases mutagenesis. Science 1990; 249: 970–971.

65. Nister M, Libermann T A, Betsholtz C et al. Expression of messenger RNAs for platelet-derived growth factor and transforming growth factor-alpha and their receptors in human malignant glioma cell lines. Cancer Res 1988; 48: 3910–3918.

66. Stoscheck C M, King L E Jr. Role of epidermal growth factor in carcinogenesis. Cancer Res 1986; 46: 1030–1037.

67. Slamon D J, Godolphin W, Jones L A et al. Studies of the HER-2/neu proto-oncogene in human breast and ovarian cancer. Science 1989; 244: 707–712.

68. Bos J L. The *ras* family and human carcinogenesis. Mutat Res 1988; 195: 255–271.

69. Fearon E R, Vogelstein B. A genetic model for colorectal tumorigenesis. Cell 1990; 61: 759–767.

70. D'Urso G, Marraccino R L, Marshak D R, Roberts J M. Cell cycle control of DNA replication by a homologue from human cells of the p34^{cdc2} protein kinase. Science 1990; 250: 786–791.

71. Bischoff J R, Friedman P N, Marshak D R, Prives C, Beach D. Human p53 is phosphorylated by p60-cdc2 and cyclin B-cdc2. Proc Nat Acad Sci USA 1990; 87: 4766–4770.

72. Buchovich K, Dully L A, Harlow E. The retinoblastoma protein is phosphorylated during specific phases of the cell cycle. Cell 1989; 68: 1097–1105.

73. Wang E, Chenivesse X, Henglein B, Brechot C. Hepatitis B virus integration in a cyclin A gene in a hepatocellular carcinoma. Nature 1990; 343: 555–557.

74. Franco E L. Viral etiology of cervical cancer: a critique of the evidence. Rev Infect Dis 1991; 13: 1195–1206.

75. Kessler I I. Natural history and epidemiology of cervical cancer with special reference to the role of Herpes Genitalis. In: McBrien D C H, Slater T F, eds. Cancer of the uterine cervix. Biochemical and clinical aspects. New York: Academic Press, 1984: pp 31–50.

76. Kessler I I. Cervical cancer: social and sexual correlates. In: Peto R, zur Hausen H, eds. Viral etiology of cervical cancer. New York: Cold Spring Harbor, 1986: pp 55–64.

77. Beral V, Hannaford P, Kay C. Oral contraceptive use and malignancies of the genital tract. Results from the Royal College of General Practitioners' oral contraceptive study. Lancet 1988; ii: 1331–1335.

78. Winkelstein W. Smoking and cervical cancer — current data: a review. Am J Epidemiol 1990; 131: 945–957.

79. Ueda M, Ueki M, Kitsuki K et al. Study on the management of dysplasia of the uterine cervix. Acta Obstetrica Gynecologica Japonica 1992; 44: 1165–1172.

80. Hayashi Y, Hachisuga T, Iwasaka T et al. Expression of *ras* oncogene product and EGF receptor in cervical squamous cell carcinomas and its relationship to lymph node involvement. Gynecol Oncol 1991; 40: 147–151.

81. Iwasaka T. The possibility of viral etiology in cervical carcinogenesis. Acta Obstetrica Gynecologica Japonica 1990; 42: 802–811.

82. Aurelian L, Terzano P, Smith C C et al. Amino-terminal epitope of herpes simplex virus type 2 ICP10 protein as a molecular diagnostic marker for cervical intraepithelial neoplasia. Cancer Cells 1989; 7: 187–191.

83. Chung T D, Wymer J P, Smith C C, Kulka M, Aurelian L. Protein kinase activity associated with large subunit of herpes simplex virus type 2 ribonucleotide reductase (ICP10). J Virol 1989; 63: 3389–3398.

84. Chung T D, Wymer J P, Kulka M, Smith C C, Aurelian L. Myristylation and polylysine-mediated activation of the protein kinase domain of the large subunit of herpes simplex virus type 2 ribonucleotide reductase (ICP10). Virology 1990; 179: 168–178.

85. Luo J H, Smith C C, Kulka M, Aurelian L. A truncated protein kinase domain of the large subunit of herpes simplex virus type 2 ribonucleotide reductase (ICP10) expressed in *Escherichia coli*. J Biol Chem 1991; 266: 20976–20983.

86. Hayashi Y, Iwasaka T, Smith C C, Aurelian L, Lewis G K, Ts'o P O P. Multistep transformation by defined fragments of Herpes simplex virus type 2 DNA: oncogenic region and its gene product. Proc Nat Acad Sci USA 1983; 80: 5902–5906.

87. Jariwalla R J, Aurelian L, Ts'o P O P. Immortalization and neoplastic transformation of normal diploid cells by defined cloned DNA fragments of herpes simplex virus type 2. Proc Nat Acad Sci USA 1983; 80: 5902–5906.

88. Jones C. The minimal transforming fragment of HSV-2 mtrIII can function as a complex promoter element. Virology 1989; 169: 346–353.

89. Krebs C R, Waite M, Jariwalla R J, Kucera L S. Induction of cellular functions in spontaneously immortalized Rat-2 cells transfected with cloned herpes simplex virus type 2 (HSV-2) DNA. Carcinogenesis 1987; 8: 183–185.

90. Smith C C, Kulka M, Wymer J P, Chung T D, Aurelian L. Expression of the large subunit of herpes simplex virus type 2 ribonucleotide reductase (ICP10) is required for virus growth and neoplastic transformation. J Gen Virol 1992; 73: 1417–1428.

91. Smith C C, Wymer J P, Luo J H, Aurelian L. Genomic sequences homologous to the protein kinase region of the bifunctional herpes simplex virus type 2 protein ICP10. Virus Genes 1991; 5(3): 215–226.

92. Selby M J, Barta A, Baxter J D, Bell G I, Eberhardt N L. Analysis of a major human chorionic somatomammotropin gene. Evidence for two functional promoter elements. J Biol Chem 1984; 259: 13131–13138.

93. Wymer J P, Kulka M, Chung T D, Chang Y C, Hayward G S, Aurelian L. Identification of alpha-like cis-response elements in the promoter of a HSV-2 delayed early gene. J Virol 1989; 63: 2773–2784.

94. Wymer J P, Aurelian L. Papillomavirus trans-activator protein E2 activates expression from the promoter for the ribonucleotide reductase large subunit from herpes simplex virus type 2. J Gen Virol 1990; 71: 1817–1820.

95. Wymer J P, Aprhys C M J, Chung T D, Feng C P, Kulka M, Aurelian L. Immediate early and functional AP-1 cis-response elements are involved in the transcriptional regulation of the large subunit of herpes simplex virus type 2 ribonucleotide reductase (ICP10). Virus Res 1992; 23: 253–270.

96. Costa S, Smith C C, Taylor S, Aurelian L, Orlandi C. Intracellular localization and serological identification of a HSV-2 protein in cervical cancer. Eur J Gynec Oncol 1986; 7: 1–12.

97. Costa S, D'Errico A, Grigioni W F et al. Monoclonal antibody to HSV-2 protein as an immunodiagnostic marker in cervical cancer. Cancer Detect Prevent 1987; 1: 189–205.

98. Costa S, Rotola A, Terzano P et al. Search for herpes simplex virus 2 and human papillomavirus genetic expression in vulvar neoplasia. J Reprod Med 1990; 35: 1108–1112.

99. Sainz de la Cuesta R, Reed T P, Brothman J C, Dubin N H. LA-1 oncogene: a possible new prognostic index for evaluating cervical squamous intraepithelial lesions. J Reprod Med 1993; 38: 173–178.

100. Terzano P, Martini F, Costa S, Martinelli G N. Immunohistochemistry with antibody to the *LA-1* oncogene as a prognostic marker in cervical intraepithelial neoplasia. Gynecol Oncol 1993; 48: 317–327.

101. Te Velde E R, Aurelian L. Antibodies to the herpes simplex virus type 2 induced tumor-associated antigen AG-4 as markers of recurrence in cervical cancer. Tumour Biol 1987; 8: 26–33.

102. Sharma B K, Nelson J W, Smith C C, Aurelian L. Detection of *LA-1* oncogene in paraffin embedded tissues cervical cancer tissues by polymerase chain reaction. Int J Oncol 1994; 4: 23–28.

103. Pinion S B, Kennedy J H, Miller R W, MacLean A B. Oncogene expression in cervical intraepithelial neoplasia and invasive cancer of the cervix. Lancet 1991; 337: 819–820.

104. Sagae S, Kudo R, Kuzumaki N et al. Ras oncogene expression and progression in intraepithelial neoplasia of the uterine cervix. Cancer 1990; 66: 295–301.

105. Sagae S, Kuzumaki N, Hisada T, Mugikura Y, Kudo R, Hashimoto M. Oncogene expression and prognosis of invasive squamous cell carcinomas of the uterine cervix. Cancer 1989; 63: 1577–1582.

106. Ocadiz R, Sauceda R, Cruz M, Graef A M, Gariglio P. High correlation between molecular alterations of the c-*myc* oncogene and carcinoma of the uterine cervix. Cancer Res 1987; 47: 4173–4177.

107. Riou G, Bourhis J, Lê M G. The c-*myc* proto-oncogene in invasive carcinomas of the uterine cervix: clinical relevance of overexpression in early stages of the cancer. Anticancer Res 1990; 10: 1225–1231.

108. Covington M, Sikora K, Turner M J, White J O, Moore P, Souther P W. C-myc expression in cervical cancer. Lancet 1987; 1: 1260–1261.

109. Sowani A, Ong G, Dische S et al. C-myc oncogene expression and clinical outcome in carcinoma of the cervix. Molec Cell Probes 1989; 3: 117–123.

110. Riou G, Barrois M, Lê M G, George M, Le Doussal V, Haie C. c-*myc* proto-oncogene expression and prognosis in early carcinoma of the uterine cervix. Lancet 1987; i: 761–763.

111. Di Luca D, Costa S, Monini P et al. Search for human papillomavirus, herpes simplex virus and c-*myc* oncogene in human genital tumors. Int J Cancer 1989; 40: 570–577.

112. Hendy-Ibbs P, Cox H, Evan G I, Watson J W. Flow cytometric quantitation of DNA and cmyc oncoprotein in archival biopsies of uterine cervix neoplasia. Br J Cancer 1987; 55: 275–282.

113. Hughes R G, Neill W A, Norval M. Papillomavirus and c-*myc* antigen expression in normal and Paterneoplastic cervical epithelium. J Clin Pathol 1989; 42: 46–51.

114. Rabbitts P H, Watson J V, Lamond A et al. Metabolism of c-myc gene products: c-myc mRNA and protein expression in the cell cycle. EMBO J 1985; 4: 2009–2015.

115. Scheffner M, Münger K, Byrne J C, Howley P M. The state of the p53 and retinoblastoma genes in human cervical carcinoma cell lines. Proc Nat Acad Sci USA 1991; 88: 5523–5527.

116. Prehn R T. Tumor-specific Antigens as altered growth factor receptors. Cancer Res 1989; 49: 2823–2826.

117. Duk J M, de Bruijn H W A, Groenier K H, Hollema H, ten Hoor K A, Krans M, Aalders J. Cancer of the uterine cervix: sensitivity and specificity of serum squamous cell carcinoma antigen determinations. Gynecol Oncol 1990; 39: 186–194.

118. Crombach G, Scharl A, Vierbuchen M, Würz H, Bolte A. Detection of squamous cell carcinoma antigen in normal squamous epithelia and in squamous cell carcinomas of the uterine cervix. Cancer 1989; 63: 1337–1342.

119. Ebert W, Johnson J T. Tumor markers in the management of cell carcinoma of the head, neck and lung. Princeton: Excerpta Medica, 1987.

120. Duk J M, van Voorst Vader P C, ten Hoor K A, Hollema H, Doeglas H M, de Bruijn H W A. Elevated levels of squamous cell carcinoma antigen in patients with a benign disease of the skin. Cancer 1989; 64: 1652–1656.

121. Davis J M, LaThangue N B, Taylor D L, Latchman D S, Anderson M, Tyms A S. Cellular polypeptides overexpressed after herpes simplex infection permit

virus subtyping and may help diagnose cervical cancer. Genitourinary Med 1988; 64: 321–326.

122. Kulka M, Wachsman M, Miura S et al. Antiviral effect of oligo(nucleoside methylphosphonates) complementary to the herpes simplex virus type 1 immediate early mRNAs 4 and 5. Antiviral Res 1993; 20: 115–130.

123. Ts'o P O P, Aurelian L, Chang E, Miller P S.

Non-ionic oligonucleotide analogues (Matagen™) as anticodic agents in duplex and triplex formation. Ann NY Acad Sci 1993; 660: 159–178.

124. Hudziak R M, Lewis G D, Winget M, Fendly B M, Shepard H M, Ullrich A. p185HER2 monoclonal antibody has antiproliferative effects in vitro and sensitizes human breast tumor cells to tumor necrosis factor. Molec Cell Biol 1989; 9: 1165–1172.

26. Role of the male partner in the carcinogenic process

R. Barrasso

The sexual transmission of genital warts has been known since the time of the ancient Greeks. Epidemiological studies on the sexual contacts of individuals with warts suggest an infection rate of 65%.[1] A prospective study on virgin women partners of individuals with disease showed 100% transmission.[1]

The association of cervical flat condyloma with human papillomaviruses (HPV)[2] and the detection of HPV DNA in cervical, vulvar and penile precancers[3–6] strengthens the hypothesis that cervical cancer has a venereal origin[7,8] and that there is a male reservoir of a venereal factor potentially oncogenic for the uterine cervix.

The biological link between HPV-associated lesions of external genitalia and cervical precancerous lesions has been confirmed by the detection of cervical condyloma or intraepithelial neoplasia in 76% of female partners of men with genital warts.[9] Cervical intraepithelial neoplasia (CIN) has also been found in partners of men with bowenoid papulosis[10,11] and in women with vulvar intraepithelial or invasive neoplasia.[12]

These combined epidemiological, clinical and virological findings provide justification for the introduction of the screening of the asymptomatic male partners of women with cervical HPV-associated lesions. The introduction of the colposcope and of the acetic acid test for such screening has revealed that 53–80% of the male partners of women with cervical disease present easily detectable or discrete genital lesions that mostly display histological features of HPV infection.[13–15] The use of the acetic acid also allows the detection of subclinical lesions, that are otherwise inapparent[16] and that may show histo-logical features of intraepithelial neoplasia[16] and may contain potentially oncogenic HPV types.[17–19]

We will review the diagnostic criteria for male HPV-associated genital lesions and then the epidemiological support to their role in the carcinogenic process of the uterine cervix.

DIAGNOSTIC CRITERIA

Morphology

Genital HPV-associated lesions in men may present as condylomata acuminata, papules or macules. Papules may or may not be pigmented; macules are well defined, flat, white areas appearing after the acetic acid test on a previously normal or erithematous area and should be distinguished from nonspecific acetowhitening.

Condylomata acuminata are exophytic protuberances with lobated or irregular surface, pink–reddish or white–grayish depending mainly on the location. If numerous, they become confluent (Fig. 26.1). They are prevalent on the inner aspect of the prepuce.[1,20] Extension of warts to the proximal urethra can occur. Condylomata acuminata must be distinguished from pearly papules,[21] which appear as parallel rows of discrete acuminate structures distributed circumferentially around the coronal sulcus. Their surface is smooth and they do not show the vascular pattern of mucosal condylomata.

Some genital papillomas have been found associated with HPV infection.[22] These proliferative lesions have a more papillomatous surface and are larger than condylomata acuminata. Usually pedunculated, they are darker than the surrounding skin, while some closely resemble skin warts.

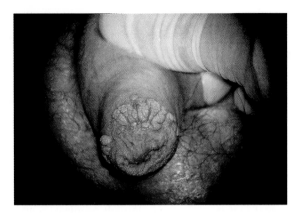

Fig. 26.1 Exophytic condylomatosis, covering the outer surface of the prepuce.

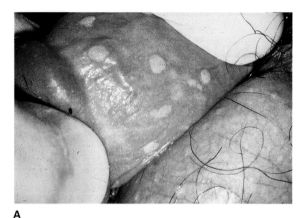

A

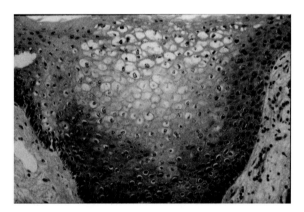

B

Fig. 26.3 **A** Slightly elevated papules of the prepuce, strongly whitening after the acetic acid test. **B** Histology shows endophytic condyloma, which was associated with HPV DNA type 42.

Papules are defined as clearly outlined lesions, variably elevated but not pedunculated, with round or dome-shaped, slightly hyperkeratotic or smooth surface. Nonpigmented papules are frequently seen on the penile shaft (Fig. 26.2). When located on mucous membranes, they are translucent, and the application of acetic acid produces a strong, well-demarcated reaction which allows easier detection (Fig. 26.3). Pigmented papules on the penile shaft and other genital areas are easily identifiable since they are brown or even blackish (Fig. 26.4). When located on mucosa, they are reddish (Fig. 26.5) or leukoplakia-like.

Macules are defined as well-demarcated flat areas showing a white reaction after acetic acid

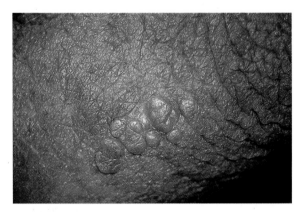

Fig. 26.2 Nonpigmented papules of the shaft, showing histologic features of condyloma and associated with HPV DNA type 6.

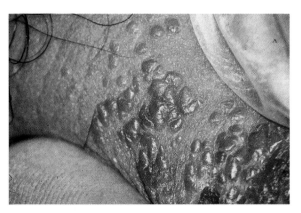

Fig. 26.4 Pigmented papules of the shaft, showing histology of intraepithelial neoplasia and associated with HPV DNA type 16.

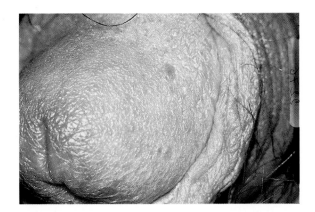

Fig. 26.5 Erythematous papule of the glans, showing histology of intraepithelial neoplasia and associated with HPV 33.

application and containing colposcopically detectable capillary loops.[17] They correspond in the case of erythematous macules to pink or reddish areas with capillary loops detected by the colposcope before the acetic acid test or otherwise to areas of epithelial sufaces that were normal on colposcopy before the test. Macules are usually found on the prepuce (Fig. 26.6) or glands or, occasionally, in the urethra. They are rarely detected on the penile skin.

Macules should be distinguished from nonspecific white reactions, mostly diffuse and ill-defined and devoid of capillary loops. These features have irritative, inflammatory or infectious origins.

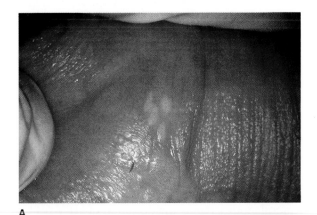

A

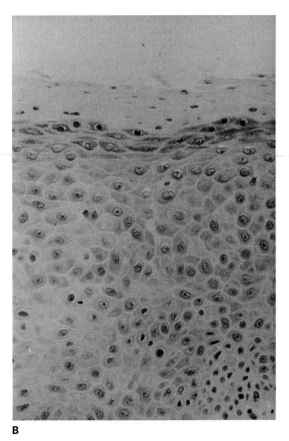

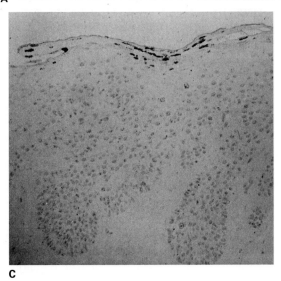

C   B

Fig. 26.6A Macules of the prepuce, only appearing after the acetic acid test. **B** Histology shows minimal changes, with pronounced parakeratosis and without koilocytosis. **C** In situ hybridization with HPV 42 probe is positive, showing possible viral replication and, thus, infectivity of such nonkoilocytotic lesions.

Histology

Condylomata acuminata invariably show histological features of condyloma (koilocytosis, papillomatosis, acanthosis, parakeratosis). Papillomas and nonpigmented papules may show the same features (Fig. 26.3B), but they may also lack koilocytosis, so that the differential diagnosis from papillomas not related to HPV infection is difficult.[22,23]

Macules usually show features of endophytic papilloma;[22] acanthosis is marked, papillomatosis and parakeratosis are discrete and koilocytosis is focal or absent (Fig. 26.6B).

Pigmented papules and erythematous macules show the histological features of penile intraepithelial neoplasia (PIN): basal/parabasal cell atypia and atypical mitotic figures, as defined for vulvar intraepithelial neoplasia.[24] Koilocytosis may be present in PIN 1 and 2. The identification of erythematous macules among subclinical lesions is thus of major relevance, since their histology may be highly atypical.[25]

Nonspecific acetowhitening is generally related to inflammatory features and/or very mild degrees of acanthosis and parakeratosis, without koilocytosis and papillomatosis. Distinction between macules and nonspecific acetowhitening is possible by careful morphological analysis and is of major relevance for epidemiological studies and for clinical protocols. In fact, these lesions are usually found in biopsies obtained from partners of women with disease; the pathologist may feel 'forced' to diagnose borderline condylomas and the clinician will consequently treat or follow men who are told they have a sexually transmitted infection. In these cases, viral testing and, particularly, in situ hybridization, could be most helpful to avoid overtreatment and psychological problems.

Cytology

Cytological examination of endourethral smears stained using Papanicolaou's method has been advocated by Krebs and Schneider,[26] but routine testing of urine specimens has produced unsatisfactory results.[13,27] Urethral scrapings for viral studies have been proposed,[28,29] in order to search for a urethral reservoir of latent HPV infection.

Our data clearly show the high false-positive rate of urethral cytology, which is due to difficulties in identifying true koilocytes and the extremely low frequency (1–2%) of HPV infection as detected by Southern blot from urethral or penile scrapes in the absence of colposcopically detected lesions.[30] Rosenberg[31] finds less than 3% HPV-positive in urethral scrapes from colposcopically normal male partners of women with disease, and Grussendorf-Conen[28] finds 6% positives in penile scrapes from men without clinically detectable lesions. Since the advent of the polymerase chain reaction (PCR) technique, it seems that the rate of HPV infection in males, as detected by penile and urethral scrapes is around 10%, thus similar to the one found in women (Bosch X, personal communication). Kataoka[32] finds 12% positives from urethral scrapes in a control group. In the author's previous experience,[30] however, less then 5% of urethral scraping in partners of women with lesions are positive when analyzed by the PCR technique when men do not present colposcopically detected lesions. Thus, our data do not confirm the existence of an urethral reservoir of infectious virus. This is of clinical relevance, since patients lesions-free can be considered as noninfectious.

As for the search of HPV in urine samples, several studies report the detection of HPV 6/11[33] or even 16.[34] However, a more recent paper[35] does not confirm these observation. HPV DNA was detected in none of 73 urine samples from men attending a sexually transmitted disease clinic using the PCR technique with consensus primers to the L1 open reading frame.

Virology

Virological findings in specimens from penile lesions analyzed by Southern blot show that condylomata acuminata, papillomas and non-pigmented papules mostly contain HPV types 6 and 11. About 20% of papillomas and papules are not associated with known HPVs, although their morphology suggests the association. This confirms that histological features of papilloma without koilocytosis are not fully specific for HPV infection.[23]

Pigmented papules and erythematous macules mostly showing histological features of PIN contain potentially oncogenic HPVs in a large proportion of cases.[22,25,36]

However, studies have pointed out that pigmented papules account for only half of detected cases of PIN[30,37] this underlying the importance of the detection of cases of clinically flat or subclinical PIN. A series[25] has clearly shown that erythematous macules are associated with histological features of intraepithelial neoplasia and contain potentially oncogenic HPVs, mostly HPV 16.

Macules whitening on a previously normal epithelium contain HPV 42 in 70% of positive cases.[22] HPV 6 and 11, as well as potentially oncogenic types are infrequently detected in such lesions. It should be stressed that 35% of macules showing histological features of endophytic papilloma and almost 100% of nonspecific acetowhitening are HPV-negative.[22,23] Recent studies by the PCR technique confirm that at least half of subclinical lesion with minimal histologic changes are HPV-positive.[38]

In situ hybridization of macules in which HPV DNA is detected by Southern blot is mostly positive (Fig. 26.6C), suggesting that virus may replicate and that these lesions may be infectious.

All these observations show that the clinical distinction among, macules, erythematous macules and nonspecific acetowhitening is most relevant. However, the average clinician can not be asked to always recognize by the naked eye, a magnifying lens or even a colposcope such subtle morphological differences. This is why we believe that a local anti-inflammatory treatment should be given to all men presenting with white areas after the acetic acid test. By this simple triage, 80% of reactions to the acetic acid test will disappear. At this point, it is important to stress that half of white areas persisting after anti-inflammatory treatment will probably turn to be PIN[25,36] and the most part of the other half will show minimal histologic changes without clear koilocytosis associated to a low-risk HPV in about 70% of cases.

SEXUAL TRANSMISSION AND ONCOGENIC POTENTIAL

When male partners of women with HPV-associated genital disease are examined by colposcopy and the acetic acid test about 40–50%

of them show HPV-associated lesions. About 20–30% of regular male partners of women with CIN have been showed to present histological features of PIN.[17,39] Among them, 9% of partners of women with CIN 3 present PIN 3.[19] The rate of PIN is much lower in studies from the USA. This may be linked to the higher diffusion of circumcision, since circumcised male partners of women with CIN present a three-fold lower rate of PIN than uncircumcised men.[25]

When the presence of HPV infection has been virologically studied by genital scrapings in both women with disease and their regular partners, one-third[40] to one-half[41] of couples have been showed to harbor the same HPV type. Correlative clinical, histological and virological studies have revealed that condylomata acuminata, when present in both partners, usually contain the same HPV type (6 or 11).[42] Concomitant CIN and PIN contain the same potentially oncogenic HPV type in only 50% of cases.[43] These data underline the difficulties encountered in the study of sexual transmission: studies performed on genital scrapings do not allow the correlation of histology and virology, since they may pick up latent infection. On the other hand, studies performed on one or two biopsy specimens do not allow the study of all HPV-associated lesions. Moreover, the biology of latent infection and the mechanisms of its reactivation are poorly understood. In our series, biopsies were performed on the first-appearing lesion and on recurrent lesions at the same site after treatment, and six out of eight men were found to harbor different HPV types. This could be due to genital infection with several HPV types, with only one or two types being activated at a time to give rise to lesions. This could explain some of the discrepancies in the viral study of lesions detected in regular partners.

High-grade PIN is detected in men who are on average 7 years older than men with low-grade lesions. These observation give rise to the hypothesis of a progression of PIN through grades as well as CIN associated with potentially oncogenic HPV infections. Moreover, the preferential location of intraepithelial neoplasia (preputial cavity in 70% of the cases) is the same as invasive cancers and the mean age of patients with cancer of the penis is about 20 years higher than the mean age of men with intraepithelial neoplastic lesions.[25]

These data would be in agreement with a slow evolution, according to the same mechanism acting for cervical cancer.

As for the risk of penile cancer, a disease of men around the age of 60, it is rare in Europe and North America. Its association with HPV infection has not been adequately studied. Durst[3] and Boshart[44] found viral DNA from oncogenic HPVs (HPV 16, 18) in 25% (1/4) and 30% (3/10) of cancers of the penis. In 1986, Villa and Lopes[45] detected HPV 18 in 39% of the cases in their series. By PCR, 63% of penile cancers contain HPV DNA, mostly type 16.[46]

The progression towards invasive cancer seems to be much more frequent in women than in men, even though in the majority of cases, HPV infection is observed in both partners. This difference between the evolutive behavior of intraepithelial neoplastic lesions may be linked to distinctive morphohistological features of the penile and female genital tract epithelia, most of all to the existence of the transformation zone on the cervix.

In relation to the role of screening and treatment of the male partner in prevention of cervical cancer, it has been shown that treatment of male partners does not decrease the failure rate of treatment for cervical dysplasia in their female partners.[47] These results underline the role of the transformation zone of the cervix in the development of dysplasia. Women in whom treatment has ablated the transformation zone seem to be at reduced risk of developing a new lesion, in spite of the existence of an HPV reservoir in their male partner. It can also be supposed that once the first lesions appear, the cycle of the infection will progress independently from possible reinfection and that women with genital HPV-associated lesions will recur or not more likely in relation with their developing immunity.

However, from the point of view of the prevention of the spread of the disease, it seems proven enough that male with genital HPV-associated risk can be considered as high-risk males: 65% of sexual contacts of patients with warts prospectively studied developed warts, and 100% of virgin women developed warts after sexual contacts with men with warts.[1] Sixty-five percent of partners of women with CIN present genital HPV-associated lesions, compared with 2% of men in a control group. Moreover, virgin women may present quickly developed CIN a few months after the first sexual contacts with men presenting lesions associated with potentially oncogenic HPVs.[48] These data, together with the finding of the co-existence of HPV 16 or 33 associated cervical and PIN in regular partners,[43] indicate strongly the role of male HPV-associated lesions in the development of cervical intraepithelial neoplasia in untreated women.

About 2% of women present cervical HPV-associated lesions. In one study,[17] about 2% of men in a control group present genital HPV-associated lesions: the prevalence of HPV-associated lesions in the general population seems thus to be the same for men and women. Since 65% of male partners of women with disease present lesions, their screening could allow detection and treatment of two thirds of all HPV-associated genital lesions in the male population. However, two important clinical questions that remain to be resolved are whether men with latent infection (10–15% of the male population) are infectious and whether they are at increased risk for developing HPV-related lesions. A positive answer to at least one of these questions would render the screening useless.

If the answer is negative, the male partner screening and treatment could be evaluated in a cervical cancer screening program; possibly giving an answer to the hypothesis of the role of men in the carcinogenic process of the uterine cervix.

REFERENCES

1. Oriel J D. Natural history of genital warts. Br J Ven Dis 1971; 47: 1–13.
2. Meisels A, Fortin R. Condylomatous lesions of the cervix and vagina. I. Cytologic patterns. Acta Cytol 1976; 20: 505–509.
3. Durst M, Gissmann L, Ikenberg H, zur Hausen H. A papillomavirus DNA from a cervical carcinoma and its prevalence in cancer biopsy samples from different geographic regions. Proc Nat Acad Sci 1983; 80: 3812–3815.
4. Ikenberg H, Gissmann L, Gross G, Grussendorf-Conen E I, zur Hausen H. Human papillomavirus type 16-

related DNA in genital Bowen's disease and in bowenoid papulosis. Int J Cancer 1983; 32: 563–565.

5. Crum C P, Mitao M, Levine R U, Silverstein S J. Cervical papillomaviruses segregate within morphologically distinct precancerous lesions. J Virol 1985; 54: 675–681.

6. Mc Cance D J, Kalashe A, Ashdown K. Human papillomavirus types 16 and 18 in carcinomas of the penis from Brazil. Int J Cancer 1986; 37: 55–59.

7. Rotkin I D. A comparison review of key epidemiological studies in cervical cancer related to current searches for transmissible agents. Cancer Res 1973; 33: 1353–1367.

8. Kessler II. Venereal factors in human cervical cancer: evidence for marital clusters. Cancer 1977; 39: 1912–1919.

9. Campion M J, Singer A, Clarkson P K, McCance D J. Increased risk of cervical neoplasia in consorts of men with penile condylomata acuminata. Lancet 1985; i: 943–946.

10. Wade T R, Kopf A W, Ackermann A B. Bowenoid papulosis of the penis. Cancer 1978; 42: 1890–1893.

11. Obalek S, Jablonska S, Beaudenon S, Walkzak S, Orth G. Bowenoid papulosis of the male and female genitalia: risk of cervical neoplasia. J Am Acad Dermatol 1986; 14: 433–444.

12. Obalek S, Jablonska S, Orth G. HPV-associated intraepithelial neoplasia of external genitalia. Clin Dermatol 1985; 3: 104–113.

13. Levine R U, Crum C P, Herman E, Silvers D, Ferenczy A, Richart R M. Cervical papillomavirus infection and intraepithelial neoplasia: a study of the male sexual partner. Obstet Gynecol 1984; 64: 16–20.

14. Sedlacek T V, Cunnane M, Carpiniello V. Colposcopy in the diagnosis of penile condyloma. Am J Obstet Gynecol 1986; 154: 494–496.

15. Sand P, Bowen L, Blischke S, Ostergart D R. Evaluation of male consorts of women with genital human papillomavirus infection. Obstet Gynecol 1986; 68: 679–681.

16. Barrasso R, Guillemotonia A, Catalan F, Siboulet A, Coupez F. Lésions génitales masculines à Papillomavirus. Ann Dermatol 1986; 113: 787–795.

17. Barrasso R, de Brux J, Croissant O, Orth G. High prevalence of papillomavirus-associated penile intraepithelial neoplasia in sexual partners of women with cervical intraepithelial neoplasia. New Engl J Med 1987; 317: 916–923.

18. Syrjånen S M, von Krogh G, Syrjånen K J. Detection of human papillomavirus DNA in anogenital condylomata in men using in situ DNA Hybridization applied to paraffine sections. Genitourinary Med 1987; 63: 32–39.

19. Campion M J, McCance D J, Mitchell H S, Jenkins D, Singer A. Subclinical penile human papillomavirus infection and dysplasia in consorts of women with cervical dysplasia. Genitourinary Med 1988; 64: 90–99.

20. von Krogh G, Syrjånen S M, Syrjånen K J. Advantage of human papillomaviruses typing in the clinical evaluation of genitoanal warts. Experience with in situ deoxyribonucleic acid hybridization technique applied on paraffine sections. J Urol 1988; 75: 717–721.

21. Ackermann A B, Kornberg R. Pearly penile papules. Acral angiofibromas. Arch Dermatol 1973; 108: 673–675.

22. Barrasso R, Jablonska S. Clinical, colposcopic and histologic spectrum of male human papillomavirus-associated genital lesions. Clin Pract Gynecol 1989; 2: 73–101.

23. Nuovo G J, Hochman H A, Eliezri Y D, Lastarria D, Comite S L, Silvers D N. Detection of human papillomavirus DNA in penile lesions histologically negative for condylomata. Am J Surg Pathol 1990; 14: 829–836.

24. Crum C P, Egawa K, Fu Y S. Intraepithelial squamous cell lesions of the vulva: biological and histological criteria for the distinction of condyloma from vulvar intraepithelial neoplasia. Am J Obstet Gynecol 1984; 82: 77–84.

25. Aynaud O, Ionesco M, Barrasso R. Penile intraepithelial neoplasia: morphologic features correlate with specific histologic and virological findings. Cancer 1994; 74: 1762–1767.

26. Krebs H B, Schneider V. Human papillomavirus-associated lesions of the penis: colposcopy, cytology and histology. Obstet Gynecol 1987; 70: 299–304.

27. Nahhas W A, Marshall M L, Ponziani J. Evaluation of urinary cytology of male sexual partners of women with cervical intraepithelial neoplasia and human papillomavirus infection. Gynecol Oncol 1986; 24: 279–284.

28. Grussendorf-Conen E I, de Villiers E M, Gissmann L. Human papillomavirus genomes in penile smears of healthy men. Lancet 1986; i: 1092 (letter).

29. Rosenberg S K, Reid R, Greenberg M. Sexually transmitted papillomaviral infection in the male. II. The urethral reservoir. Urology 1988; 32: 47–53.

30. Aynaud O, Ionesco M, Barrasso R. Lack of cytological and virological detection of papillomavirus infection in the urethra of healthy men. (Submitted for publication).

31. Rosenberg S K, Husain M, Herman G E, Elfont E A. Sexually transmitted papillomavirus infection in the male. VI. Simultaneous urethral cytology–Virapap testing of male consorts of women with genital human papillomaviral infection. Urology 1990; 36: 38–41.

32. Katakoa A, Claesson U, Hansson B G, Eriksson M, Lindh E. Human papillomavirus infection of the male diagnosed by Southern-blot hybridization and polymerase chain reaction: comparison between urethra samples and penile biopsy samples. J Med Virol 1991; 33: 159–164.

33. Mechers W J G, Schift R, Stolz E, Lindeman J, Quint W G V. Human papillomavirus detection in urine samples from male patients by the polymerase chain reaction. J Clin Microbiol 1989; 27: 1711–1714.

34. Nakazawa A, Inoue M, Fujita M, Tanizawa O, Hakura A. Detection of human papillomavirus type 16 in sexual partners of patients having cervical cancer by polymerase chain reaction. Jpn J Cancer Res 1991; 82: 1187–1190.

35. Geddy P, Wells M, Lacey C J N. Lack of detection of human papillomavirus DNA in male urine samples. Genitourinary Med 1993; 69: 276–279.

36. Lowhagen G B, Bolmstedt A, Ryd W, Voog E. The prevalence of high risk HPV types in penile condyloma-like lesions. Correlation between HPV type and morphology. Genitourinary Med 1993; 69: 87–90.

37. Barrasso R, Aynaud O. In preparation.

38. Aziz D C, Ferre F, Robitaille J, Ferenczy A. Human papillomavirus testing in the clinical laboratory. II. Vaginal, vulvar, perineal and penile squamous lesions. J Gynecol Surg 1993; 9: 9–15.

39. Zanardi C, Guerra B, Martinelli G, de Brux J, Barrasso R. Papillomavirus-related genital lesions in

male partners of women with genital condyloma or cervical intraepithelial neoplasia: diagnostic approach. Cervix 1988; 6: 127–134.

40. Gross G, Hagendorn M, Ikenberg H. Bowenoid papulosis: presence of human papillomavirus structural antigens and of HPV 16-related DNA sequences. Arch Dermatol 1985; 121: 858–862.

41. Schneider A, Sawada E, Gissmann L, Shah K. Human papillomaviruses in women with a history of abnormal Papanicolau smears and in their male partners. Obstet Gynecol 1987; 69: 554–562.

42. Wickenden C, Hanna N, Taylor-Robinson D et al. Sexual transmission of human papillomaviruses in heterosexual and male homosexual couples, studied by DNA hybridization. Genitourinary Med 1988; 64: 34–38.

43. Barrasso R, Gross G. Male HPV-associated lesions: epidemiology and diagnostic criteria. In: Gross G, Jablonska S, Pfister H, Stegner H E, eds. Genital papillomavirus infections. Berlin: Springer-Verlag, 1990: pp 23–33.

44. Boshart M, Gissmann L, Ikenberg H, Kleinheinz A, Scheurlen W, zur Hausen H. A new type of papillomavirus DNA: its presence in genital cancer biopsies and in cell lines derived from cervical cancer. EMBO J 1984; 3: 1151–1157.

45. Villa L L, Lopez A. Human papillomavirus DNA sequences in penile carcinomas in Brazil. Int J Cancer 1986; 37: 853–855.

46. Iwasawa A, Kumamoto Y, Fujinaga K. Detection of human papillomavirus deoxyribonucleic acid in penile carcinoma by polymerase chain reaction and in situ hybridization. J Urol 1993; 149: 59–63.

47. Krebs H B, Helmkamp B F. Does the treatment of genital condylomata in men decrease the treatment failure rate of cervix dysplasia in the female sexual partner? Obstet Gynecol 1990; 76: 660–663.

48. Barrasso R, Aynaud O, (in preparation).

27. Concurrent genital infections recognized at colposcopy

Jorma Paavonen

INTRODUCTION

Colposcopy is generally used to evaluate women whose cytologic findings suggest cervical neoplasia, to obtain directed biopsies from the most significant lesions. Colposcopy has not been extensively used as a screening procedure for cervical or vaginal infections. Therefore, the prevalence of various colposcopic features in different populations with or without specific genital infections is not known. Many colposcopic features are associated with specific cervical or vaginal infections, but the accuracy of specific colposcopic features for the diagnosis of various cervicovaginal infections is not well known.

COLPOSCOPIC EXAMINATION

It is important to emphasize that general physical and gynecologic examination should not be ignored despite the fact that the colposcopic examination receives the most attention. The general atmosphere in the examining room should be such that the patient can be as relaxed as possible. The examination procedure should be carefully explained to the patient. The external genitalia, lower abdominal wall, pubic area, buttocks, and inner aspects of the thighs should be inspected. During the speculum examination the appearance of the epithelial surfaces and genital secretions should be noted. Antiseptic jellies or creams should not be used to ease the introduction of the speculum into the vagina: instead sterile saline or plain water warmed to body temperature may be used.

Colposcopic terminology, as approved by the International Federation of Cervical Pathology and Colposcopy in 1990 should be used in recording the colposcopic findings.

MAJOR PATHOGENS CAUSING CERVICAL OR VAGINAL INFECTIONS AND COLPOSCOPIC FEATURES ASSOCIATED WITH SPECIFIC PATHOGENS

Chlamydia trachomatis

Genital chlamydial infections have been recognized as a major public health problem. *Chlamydia trachomatis* is the major cause of mucopurulent cervicitis (MPC) and pelvic inflammatory disease (PID).[1-3] Other clinical manifestations of chlamydial lower genital tract infection include acute urethral syndrome, bartholinitis, and proctitis. Late manifestations of genital chlamydial infection in women include tubal factor infertility and tubal pregnancy.[4]

Erythema, edema, and induced mucosal bleeding are common features of chlamydial cervicitis (Fig. 27.1). A cervicitis severity score based on these three features has proven useful in clinical studies of the response of cervicitis to antimicrobial therapy.[5] The histopathologic features of chlamydial cervicitis include severe inflammatory infiltration of the stroma leading to erythema and increased vascularity of the transformations zone.[6,7] The term 'hypertrophic follicular cervicitis' has been introduced to describe the extreme edema and friability of the ectopy and the transformation zone frequently seen in women with chlamydial cervicitis. Well-formed lymphoid follicles or germinal centers are frequently seen in the cervical stroma of women with chlamydial cervicitis.

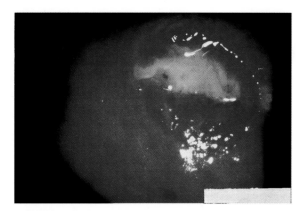

Fig. 27.1 Mucopurulent cervicitis caused by *Chlamydia trachomatis*.

Neisseria gonorrhoeae

The endocervical canal is the primary site of urogenital gonococcal infection in women. The most common symptoms are those of most lower genital tract infections in women and include increased vaginal discharge, dysuria, intermenstrual uterine bleeding, and menorrhagia, each of which may occur alone or in combination. Although the physical examination may be normal, many infected women have cervical abnormalities that include purulent or mucopurulent cervical discharge, erythema and edema of the zone of ectopy, and mucosal bleeding that is easily induced by swabbing the endocervical epithelium. The clinical assessment of women with gonorrhea is often confounded by the high prevalence of coexisting cervical or vaginal infections with *Chlamydia trachomatis*, *Trichomonas vaginalis*, *Candida albicans*, herpes simplex virus, and a variety of other organisms.

Herpes simplex virus

Herpes simplex virus (HSV) is the most common cause of genital ulcer disease. HSV causes 40–60% of genital ulcerations in patients presenting to gynecologic practices or sexually transmitted disease clinics (STD). Higher rates have been reported. Koutsky et al[8] found that on the basis of cultures, serologic testing, and clinical findings, HSV was the probable cause of the ulcers, pustules, or vesicles of the vulvar and perianal region

in 88% of women who presented with such findings. The clinical manifestations of genital herpes vary greatly, depending in part on whether the patient is experiencing the first episode of infection or has recurrent disease. The first episode of genital herpes is a disease of both systemic and local manifestations; it is associated with systemic symptoms, involves multiple genital sites, and has a prolonged duration of viral shedding and lesions. In women with primary genital HSV infection widely spaced bilateral ulcerative lesions on the external genitalia are the most frequent presenting sign. HSV infection of the cervix usually involves the squamous epithelium of the ectocervix (Fig. 27.2) in contrast to the mucopurulent endocervicitis caused by *Chlamydia trachomatis* or *Neisseria gonorrhoeae*. The high rate of isolation of HSV from the cervical lesions in the primary episode contrasts sharply with the low rate of isolation and low rate of cervical lesions in women who present with recurrent genital herpes. Local symptoms of recurrent genital herpes are mild and the duration is shorter compared to the symptoms in primary infection. The lesions are usually unilateral. Recent studies have described atypical genital HSV infection with a diverse clinical spectrum. HSV is often isolated from genital lesions not thought to be herpetic, such as small linear ulcerations, erythematous areas, fissures, or cracks.[8,9] This suggests that all genital ulcerations and fissures should be examined and evaluated for herpes. Even the most detailed

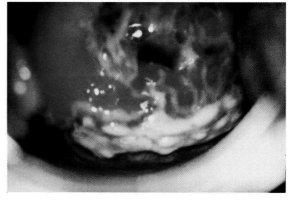

Fig. 27.2 Genital ulcer caused by herpes simplex virus type 2.

clinical or cytologic testing will identify only 65–70% of cervical HSV infections. In one study, necrotic or ulcerative areas were visible on the cervix by speculum examination in 23 women, and an additional 10 women had small ulcerative cervical lesions detectable only by colposcopy.[8] Hence, colposcopic examination increases the sensitivity of clinical examination in patients with genital HSV infection.

Cytomegalovirus

Most cytomegalovirus (CMV) infections in immunocompetent humans are asymptomatic. However, the wide spectrum of CMV-associated diseases in newborns and immunocompromised individuals clearly shows that CMV is a significant pathogen. It is of interest that some studies have linked CMV and cervical neoplasia, although the role of CMV in cervical pathology is still largely unknown.[10]

Trichomonas vaginalis

Worldwide, trichomoniasis is the most common sexually transmitted disease. Trichomoniasis accounts for approximately one-third of vaginal infections diagnosed in STD clinics. *Trichomonas vaginalis* is highly site-specific, and is capable of producing infection in the human urogenital tract only. *Trichomonas vaginalis* principally infects squamous epithelium in the genital tract causing ectocervicitis, but not endocervicitis. The spectrum of clinical manifestations of trichomoniasis in women ranges from asymptomatic infection to profuse purulent vaginitis. In symptomatic infection, the vulva shows diffuse erythema, On speculum examination, excessive discharge is observed in most cases. In severe cases the vaginal walls may present a hemorrhagic appearance caused by capillary proliferation and tiny punctate hemorrhages. Such inflammatory process results in the finding termed colpitis macularis,[11] or strawberry cervix (Fig. 27.3), The reported prevalence of colpitis macularis has varied from 2% to 92% in various studies, with the higher prevalence found by colposcopic examination.[12,13] Although many studies have found an association

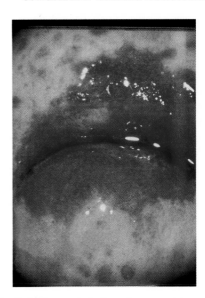

Fig. 27.3 Colpitis macularis (strawberry cervix) caused by *Trichomonas vaginalis*.

between trichomoniasis and abnormal vaginal discharge, virtually all of such studies have have had several major problems. For instance, definitions of abnormal discharge have been imprecise, and only a few studies have attempted to adjust for cervicitis as a cause of vaginal discharge, or for coinfections such as bacterial vaginosis. Women with trichomoniasis are known to be at high risk for other STDs.

Gardnerella vaginalis

Gardnerella vaginalis, formerly known as *Haemophilus vaginalis*, is highly associated with bacterial vaginosis, but can be isolated in high concentrations from women with no signs of vaginal infection. It is generally thought that *G. vaginalis* interacts with anaerobic bacteria and genital mycoplasmas to cause bacterial vaginosis.[14,15] In high concentrations, *G. vaginalis* seems to be a marker for bacterial vaginosis.

Bacterial vaginosis

Bacterial vaginosis (BV) is the most prevalent cause of vaginal symptoms among women of fertile age. BV is a clinical entity characterized by symptoms of increased quantities of malodorous vaginal discharge.[15] BV is not caused by a single microorganism. Some poorly known alterations in the vaginal environment lead to a decrease in the quantity of lactobacilli and an increase in the quantity of a variety of anaerobic and facultative bacteria and mycoplasmas. *Bacteroides* species, *Peptostreptococcus* species, *G. vaginalis*, and *Mobiluncus* species are most strongly associated with BV, although all these organisms in lower quantities also belong to the normal endogenous vaginal flora.[16] Physical examination and analysis of vaginal fluid reveals a homogenous whitish discharge adherent to the vaginal walls (Fig. 27.4), elevated pH of vaginal fluid, development of fishy odor when vaginal fluid is mixed with 10% potassium hydroxide, and clue cells on microscopic examination of vaginal fluid (wet mount).[17] There is usually no inflammation of the vaginal epithelium. BV represents a disturbance of the vaginal microbial ecosystem rather than true epithelial infection. Typically, wet mount examination does not reveal an increased number of polymorphonuclear leukocytes. Recent studies have demonstrated an increased risk of prematurity and chorionamnionitis among pregnant women with BV. BV is also a risk factor for pelvic inflammatory disease, postpartum endometritis, and postoperative infections.

Yeast

Vulvovaginal candidiasis (VVC) remains the commonest cause of vaginal infection, and is increasing in frequency. At least 75% of all women will experience at least one episode of VVC during their lifetime. Most yeasts isolated from the vagina are *Candida albicans*. Pruritus and vaginal discharge are the usual complaints. These symptoms are nonspecific and not invariably associated with VVC. Vaginal discharge can be profuse or minimal. Although typically described as cottage-cheese-like, the discharge may vary from watery to homogenously thick. Soreness, irritation, burning, dyspareunia, and external dysuria are commonly present. On examination vaginal mucosal erythema is present together with adherent whitish discharge. Erythema and swelling of the labia and vulva is frequently present. Multiple linear fissures can be present on the vulva. Vulvar involvement may extend into inguinal and perianal regions.

Other vaginal conditions recognized at colposcopy

Inflammatory vaginitis, also known as desquamative inflammatory vaginitis (DIV), is a rare cause of purulent ulcerative vaginitis not caused by candidiasis, trichomoniasis, or BV.[18] DIV occurs both in premenopausal and in postmenopausal women. However, the exact prevalence of this exudative vaginitis has not been studied. Some studies have linked inflammatory vaginitis to group B *Streptococcus*, but in most cases the cause is unknown. Typically, the vaginal discharge is extremely heavy and purulent. Wet mount examination characteristically shows high numbers of leukocytes and oval or round parabasal cells. Parabasal cells suggest epithelial exfoliation and not atrophy. Colposcopic examination reveals extensive diffuse areas of vascular petecchiae, and areas of epithelial erosion. The vaginal walls are easily traumatized during the speculum examination resulting in superficial ulcerations, fissures and petecchiae (Fig. 27.5). Acetic acid treatment shows diffuse acetowhitening involving almost the entire vagina. Biopsy shows acute and chronic inflammation involving both the mucosa and submucosa.

Vulvar conditions recognized at colposcopy

Vulvar vestibulitis, previously known as 'burning vulva syndrome,' is a common but underdiagnosed

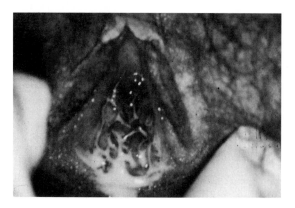

Fig. 27.4 Homogenous vulvovaginal discharge characteristic of bacterial vaginosis.

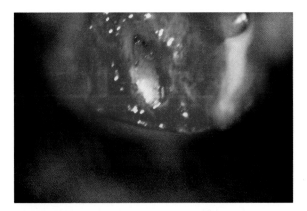

Fig. 27.5 Desquamative inflammatory vaginitis of unknown etiology.

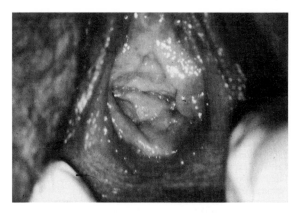

Fig. 27.6 Vulvar vestibulitis of unknown etiology.

cause of vulvodynia. Vulvodynia is chronic vulvar discomfort in patients complaining of burning, stinging, irritation, or rawness. In the vulvar vestibule are the openings of the urethra, and Skene's and Bartholin's glands. Close examination also reveals the tiny pit-like openings of the minor vestibular glands which scatter throughout the vestibule and mostly in the lower fourchette and in the base of the hymenal ring. The vulvar vestibule extends laterally from the hymenal ring to a line of more keratinized skin on the labia majora (Hart's line). Hart's line can easily be visualized by the colposcope.

Characteristic features of vestibulitis are dyspareunia, erythema of the vestibulum, and vestibular point tenderness provoked by a moist cotton-tipped swab (or by a finger). Vulvar vestibulitis can be acute or chronic, and the etiology is unknown.[19] Whereas acute vulvar vestibulitis usually resolves with the treatment of specific infection such as yeast, chronic vestibulitis can persist for months or years causing severe discomfort, frustration and fear. Besides vulvar vestibulitis, vulvar dermatoses and dysesthetic vulvodynia should also be considered in the differential diagnosis of chronic vulvodynia.[20]

Colposcopic examination greatly helps to appreciate the complex anatomy of the vulvar vestibulum, and helps in the differential diagnosis of vulvodynia. The erythema characteristically seen with the vulvar vestibulitis syndrome can be diffuse or focal, and is usually localized around the orifices of the major or minor vulvar vestibular glands (Fig. 27.6). Sometimes colposcopically directed biopsies are indicated to rule out other causes of vulvodynia. Histopathology of vulvar vestibulitis shows mild to moderate chronic inflammatory infiltration predominantly characterized by lymphocytes and plasma cells in the superficial stroma with some polymorphonuclear leukocytes present.

With the exception of a positive association between detection of vulvar fissures and yeast infection no specific vulvar colposcopic findings have been associated with bacterial vaginosis, *Chlamydia trachomatis*, or *Trichomonas vaginalis*.[21]

Significant associations of colposcopic features adjusting for coinfections

Many colposcopic features are associated with several infectious pathogens. For instance, positive associations can be found for endocervical mucopus and multiple pathogens causing endocervical or ectocervical infections. Therefore, to further examine the associations of colposcopic features with specific pathogens or diagnoses, logistic regression models should be used to adjust for coinfections. However, very few such studies have been reported. Table 27.1 shows the results of a study among 600 randomly selected women attending an STD clinic in which independent associations of several defined colposcopic features were studied, adjusting for coinfections.[22]

Table 27.1 Odds ratios for associations of specific microorganisms, koilocytosis, or bacterial vaginosis, with various colposcopic features, after adjustment for coinfections*

Colposcopic finding	CT	GC	HSV	CMV	GV	TV	K	BV
Mucopus	4.5d	2.3b	4.8d	2.0	1.3	1.7	1.7	0.9
Ulcers/necrotic areas	1.1	0.2	227.7d	1.9	2.6	1.9	4.9a	0.3
Strawberry cervix	0.2b	0.7	0.1	2.3	1.3	85.8d	0.1a	1.7
Increased surface vascularity	2.0d	0.7	22.7d	2.1	0.7	2.1a	1.7	1.1
Hypertrophic follicular cervicitis	5.4d	1.7	0.4	1.6	0.3b	0.3a	0.7	1.6
Immature metaplasia	3.0b	1.6	2.1	14.4d	0.7	0.7	1.6	0.9
Leukoplakia	0.1a	3.5	0.1	0.7	1.2	0.7	4.7a	0.6
Satellite lesions	0.7	1.0	0.4	1.5	2.3a	1.3	4.4c	0.4a
Cervical asperities	0.7	1.0	0.4	1.4	1.0	0.6	2.0a	1.5
Vaginal asperities	0.6	0.9	0.5	1.4	0.8	0.8	1.7	1.5
Atypical transformation zone	1.6	0.8	0.4	1.4	1.2	1.3	2.6c	1.3

*Odds ratios less than one indicate negative associations; a = $P < 0.05$; b = $P < 00.01$; c = $P < 0.001$; d = $P < 0.0001$. CT, *C. trachomatis*; GC, *N. gonorrhoreae*; HSV, herpes simplex virus; CMV, cytomegalovirus; GV, *G. vaginalis*; TV, *T. vaginalis*; K, koilocytosis; BV, bacterial vaginosis. Ureaplasma urealyticum and yeast showed no associations with any of the colposcopic features studied, and therefore are not listed.

Endocervical mucopus was associated with the isolation of *Chlamydia trachomatis*, HSV, and *Neisseria gonorrhoeae*. This is plausible since all three pathogens are thought to cause endocervicitis. Increased surface vascularity in the cervix was also associated with *C. trachomatis*.

Cervical ulcers or necrotic areas were strongly associated with HSV. The colposcope aids in the detection of small ectocervical ulcerations or small ulcerations occurring on the transformation zone which are often difficult to detect by examination with the unaided eye. Increased surface vascularity was also associated with HSV. Histopathologic studies have shown marked vascular changes in the subadjacent stroma associated with healing of cervical HSV infection.

Both *C. trachomatis* and CMV were independently associated with immature metaplasia. In the cervical epithelium, the metaplastic process involves permanent conversion of columnar epithelium to squamous epithelium. Immature metaplastic cells are probably the most vulnerable of the cervical epithelial cells to pathogens that might cause cervical neoplasia. It is of interest that some studies have linked both *C. trachomatis* and CMV to cervical neoplasia. Several studies have demonstrated a link between *C. trachomatis* and atypical metaplasia.

SIGNIFICANCE AND IMPLICATIONS

The colposcope is obviously not a substitute for specific microbiologic studies. However, awareness of the colposcopic features is important for colposcopists to identify patients who need specific microbiologic studies, just as awareness of cytologic or histologic manifestations of infections is important to cytopathologists. Furthermore, colposcopy is a potentially useful adjunct for research on the pathogenesis of a variety of genital infections.

As we enter the second decade of the HIV pandemic, STD control efforts must be be established and strengthened.[23] STD control has become a major health priority. Both individual programs and national policies should focus on the full spectrum of all prevalent STDs, rather than exclusively on HPV infection or cytologic atypia. It should be emphasized that most women referred for cytologic atypia are at high risk for STDs in general. Therefore, colposcopists should understand the challenges and implications of such links. Similarly, counseling of colposcopy clinic patients should include information on their risk for STDs. Furthermore, microbial, cytologic and colposcopic studies of the role of concomitant genital infections in the natural history of HPV infection and cytologic atypia are urgently needed.

REFERENCES

1. Brunham R C, Paavonen J, Stevens C E et al. Mucopurulent cervicitis — The ignored counterpart of urethritis in men. New Engl J Med 1984; 311: 1–6.
2. Mårdh P-A, Ripa T, Svensson L, Weström L. Chlamydia trachomatis infection in patients with acute salpingitis. New Engl J Med 1977; 296: 1377–1379.
3. Paavonen J, Teisala K, Heinonen P K et al. Microbiological and histopathological findings in acute pelvic inflammatory disease. Br J Obstet Gynecol 1987; 94: 454–460.
4. Cates W Jr, Wasserheit J N, Genital chlamydial infections: Epidemiology and reproductive sequelae. Am J Obstet Gynecol 1991; 164: 1771–1781.
5. Paavonen J, Roberts P L, Stevens C E et al. Randomized treatment of mucopurulent cervicitis with doxycycline or amoxicillin. Am J Obstet Gynecol 1989; 161: 128–135.
6. Kiviat N, Paavonen J, Wölner-Hanssen P et al. Histopathology of endocervical infection caused by *Chlamydia trachomatis*, herpes simplex virus, *Trichomonas vaginalis*, and *Neisseria gonorrhoeae*. Human Pathol 1990; 21: 831–837.
7. Paavonen J, Meyer B, Vesterinen E, Saksela E. Colposcopic and histologic findings of cervical chlamydial infection. Obstet Gynecol 1982; 59: 712–715.
8. Koutsky L A, Stevens C E, Holmes K K et al. Underdiagnosis of genital herpes by current clinical and viral-isolation procedures. New Engl J Med 1992; 326: 1533–1539.
9. Koutsky L A, Ashley R L, Holmes K K et al. The frequency of unrecognized type 2 herpes simplex virus infection among women. Implications for the control of genital herpes. Sex Transm Dis 1990; 17: 90–94.
10. Paavonen J, Koutsky L A, Kiviat N. Cervical neoplasia and other STD related genital and anal neoplasias. In: Holmes K K, et al eds. Sexually transmitted diseases, 2nd edn. New York: McGraw-Hill, 1990: pp 561–592.
11. Lang W R, Ludmir A. A pathognomonic colposcopic sign of Trichomonas vaginalis vaginitis. Acta Cytol 1961; 5: 390–392.
12. Wölner-Hanssen P, Krieger J N, Stevens C E et al. Clinical manifestations of vaginal trichomoniasis. JAMA 1989; 261: 571–576.
13. Krieger J N, Wölner-Hanssen P, Stevens C, Holmes K K: Characteristics of Trichomonas vaginalis isolates from women with and without colpitis macularis. J Infect Dis 1990; 161: 307–311.
14. Spiegel C A, Amsel R, Eschenbach D A, Schoenkneckt F, Holmes K K: Anaerobic abacteria in nonspecific vaginitis. New Engl J Med 1980; 303: 601–607.
15. Eschenbach D A, Hillier S, Critchlow C, Stevens C, DeRouen T, Holmes K K. Diagnosis and clinical manifestations of bacterial vaginosis. Am J Obstet Gynecol 1988; 158: 819–823.
16. Hillier S L, Holmes K K. Bacterial vaginosis. In: Holmes K K et al, eds. Sexually transmitted diseases, 2nd edn. New York: McGraw-Hill, 1990: pp 547–559.
17. Amsel R, Totten P A, Spiegel C A, Chen K C S, Eschenbach D A, Holmes K K. Nonspecific vaginitis: Diagnostic criteria and microbial and epidemiologic associations. Am J Med 1983; 74: 14–22.
18. Oates J K, Rowen D. Desquamative inflammatory vaginitis. Genitourin Med 1990; 66: 275–279
19. Marinoff S C, Turner M L C. Vulvar vestibulitis syndrome: An overview. Am J Obstet Gynecol 1991; 165: 1228–1233.
20. McKay M. Vulvitis and vulvovaginitis: Cutaneous considerations. Am J Obstet Gynecol 1991; 165: 1176–1182.
21. Paavonen J, Christiansen J K, Koutsky L et al. Colposcopic presentation of human papillomavirus infection of the vulva. 11th International Congress of the International Society for the Study of Vulvar Disease. September 22–27 1991, Oxford, UK, Abstract #8.
22. Paavonen J, Stevens C E, Wölner-Hanssen P et al. Colposcopic manifestations of cervical and vaginal infections. Obstet Gynecol Surv 1988; 43: 373–381.
23. Wasserheit J N. Epidemiological synergy. Interrelationships between human immunodeficiency virus infection and other sexually transmitted diseases. Sex Transm Dis 1991; 19: 61–77.

Index

Age
    cervical cancer and, 52–4, 205, 235
    VAIN and, 169
    vulvar cancer and, 116
    vulvar dysplasia and, 117
AIDS, 263, 264
AIS *see* Cervical adenocarcinoma-in-situ
Allergic reactions, genital, 74, 75–6
Antigens, tumor-specific, 334
Apocrine glands, 15
ASCUS, 178
    Pap smears, 213, 214–15
    secondary screening of, 210–12

Bacterial vaginosis, 352
Biopsy
    colposcopic in pregnancy, 223–4
    cone, 189–90, 237–8, 304–5
    punch, 180, 303–4
    for vulvar warts, 141–2
Bowen's disease, 37, 39, 111

Candida, 75
    albicans, 77–8, 352
Carcinogenesis
    AIS and, 254
    cervical, 83, 92
    oncogenes and, 330–1
    role of male partner in, 341–8
β carotene, 310, 311
Cervical adenocarcinoma, 31–3, 251
    CIGN and, 254–5
    colposcopy and, 303
    effect of screening on, 296
    treatment of, 289–90
Cervical adenocarcinoma-in-situ, 31–3, 251–62
    management of, 258–60
    treatment of, 289
    see also Cervical intraepithelial glandular neoplasia
Cervical cancer, 277–92
    age and, 52–4, 205, 235
    clinical staging, 281–3
    cytological follow-up and, 298
    diagnosis, 284–5

epidemiology, 49–54
HIV and, 57–8, 264–6
HPV and, 202, 204–6
immunosuppression and, 264–5
interferons for, 157–63
microinvasion, 30–1, 283–4
oncogenes and, 331–6
p53 and, 89
pathophysiology, 277–80
pregnancy and, 222, 223–4, 226, 227–8
prognosis, 280–1
screening and mortality, 295–6
small cell, 33–4
smoking and, 89–90
treatment, 286–90
treatment of male partner and, 346
vitamins and, 311
Cervical carcinoma-in-situ, 54–6
Cervical conization, 189–91, 237–8, 304–5
Cervical intraepithelial neoplasia (CIN)
    colposcopy for, 185–8
    cytological classification, 178
    distinction between low and high, 29–30
    herpes viruses and, 90–1
    high-grade, 28–9
    histological profile, 181–2
    HIV and, 58, 265, 267–74
    HPV and, 19, 85, 86–8, 201–2
    interferons for, 157–62
    lesion size, 179–80, 181
    local destruction of, 192–3
    low-grade, 23–8
    management, 188–93
    PIN and, 345
    in pregnancy, 221–9
    prevalence of, 56–7
    psychological effects of treatment, 244
    referral patterns, 180–1
    retinoic acid for, 310–11
    retrospective studies, 178–9
    surgical excision, 189–92
    VAIN and, 170
    vitamins and, 311

Cervical neoplasia, 19–36
    adenocarcinoma *see* Cervical adenocarcinoma
    CIN *see* Cervical intraepithelial neoplasia
    epidemiology of, 49–60
    HPV and, 19–30, 84–6
    in situ hybridization, 26–7
    koilocytosis, 27–8
    latent infection, 20–2
    microinvasion, 30–1
    oncogenes and, 325–40
    screening for HPV, 22–3
    small cell carcinoma, 33–4
Cervical intraepithelial glandular neoplasia (CIGN), 252–8
    carcinogenesis, 254
    cervical adenocarcinoma and, 254–5
    detection of, 256–8
    histological characteristics, 251
    HPV and, 253
    incidence, 255–6
    oral contraceptive pill and, 253
Cervical smears, 49
    accuracy of, 177
    for HIV, 271–2
    in postmenopausal women, 232–5
    in pregnancy, 221–2
    for vulvar warts, 138, 139
Cervical screening, 53, 54, 56, 61–70, 204, 205–6
    benefits, 61–3
    case-control studies, 63
    costs of, 66–9, 294
    detection of CIGN by, 256–8
    detection of CIN by, 188
    detection of VAIN by, 169
    failures, 205
    frequency, 207
    improvements, 296–7
    inaccuracies, 294–5
    mathematical modeling, 64–6
    for mild cytological disorders, 297–9
    new methods, 299–301
    of older women, 206–7, 297
    psychological aspects of, 241–4
    requirements for success, 293–6
    secondary, 208–12

Cervical screening (*contd*)
  techniques, 293–301
  testing for HPV, 301
Cerviography, 206, 207, 299–301
Cervix
  anatomy, 1–2
  changes during pregnancy, 7–8
  columnar epithelium, 3–4
  congenital transformation zone, 7
  endometriosis, 10
  epithelial metaplasia, 9–10
  glandular hyperplasia, 8–9
  histology, 2–10
  mesonephric remnants, 8–9
  squamocolumnar junction of, 4, 6
  squamous epithelium, 2–3
  squamous metaplasia, 5–6
  transformation zone, 6
Chemoimmunotherapy for VIN,
    topical, 126–7
Chlamydia trachomatis, 77, 349–50,
    354
CIGN *see* Cervical intraepithelial
    glandular neoplasia
Classification
  AIS, 252
  cervical carcinoma, 281–3
  CIN, 20
  cytological, 178
  VAIN, 170–1
  VIN, 37, 111, 121, 122
Clitoris, 12
Cold coagulation, 193
Colposcopy, 177, 179, 185–88, 209,
    297–8, 300
  for CIGN, 258
  classical, 186
  diagnostic criteria for, 187–8
  digital imaging, 187
  diploma of, 187
  genital infections recognized at,
    349–55
  for HIV, 272
  pitfalls of, 303
  in postmenopausal women,
    235–6
  in pregnancy, 222–4, 227
  psychological effects of, 244
  saline, 186–7
  technique, 302
  unsatisfactory, 304–5
Complement, 75
Computerized image analysis, 299
Condyloma acuminata, 84
  flat, 214
  interferons for, 157, 158, 164
  on male genitalia, 341, 342, 344
  mimics, 133–6
  see also Vulvar warts
Congenital transformation zone, 7
Counseling, 247
Cryocautery, 126, 161
  of CIN, 192–3, 245
  of VAIN, 172
  of vulvar warts, 147–8

Cytokines, 75
  therapy, 155–68
Cytological abnormalities, minor,
    177–83
Cytomegalovirus (CMV), 351, 354

Dermis, vulvar, 14–15
Diagnostic techniques, 302–5
Diathermy, 84, 224, 225
  for VAIN, 173
Dinitrochlorobenzene, 127, 174
DNA–DNA in situ hybridization, 199
DNA hybridization, 96–8
Dot blot, 97, 206
Dyskaryosis, 178, 179, 224, 226

Eccrine sweat glands, 14–15
Efudex *see* 5-Fluorouracil
Electrofulguration, 147, 148, 149
Endocervical curettage, 238, 258
Endocervical glandular dysplasia, 257
Endometriosis, 10
Endourethral smear, 344
Epithelium
  columnar, 3
  squamous, 2–3
  vulvar, 13–15
Epstein–Barr virus (EBV), 84, 91
Erythroplasia of Queyrat, 37, 39
Estrogen
  postmenopausal cervix and, 232
  therapy, 76, 173, 236–7
  vitamin A and, 309

Feulgen hydrolysis, 299
Filter in situ hybridization (FISH),
    97–8
  limitations of, 198–9
5-Fluorouracil, 127, 145–7, 151
  for VAIN, 173–4
Flesch Index of Reading Ease, 246

Gardnerella vaginalis, 351–2
Genital secretion, 71
Genital warts in children, 144
Glandular hyperplasia, 8–9
Gonorrhea, 78, 350
Growth factors, 326, 327, 330
  receptor oncogenes, 332–3

Herpes simplex virus, 84, 90–1, 350–1,
    354
HIV, 79
  cervical disease and, 57–8, 265–73
  HPV and, 269–71
  immunosuppression and cervical
    cancer, 264–5
  prevalence, 263–4
Hormone replacement therapy *see*
    Estrogen

Hormones, sex, 76
Human papillomavirus (HPV)
  biology, 96
  categories, 202–4
  cervical neoplasia and, 19, 84–9, 90,
    91
  CIGN and, 253–4
  diagnostic uses of testing, 212–14
  DNA–DNA ISH limitations, 199
  DNA hybridization and, 96–8
  epidemiology, 49
  E6/E7 region of, 28, 29
  expanded screening model, 207–8
  FISH limitations, 199
  HIV and, 269–71
  immune response to, 79–80
  kidney transplant patients and, 57,
    140
  male genital, 341–6
  MIN and, 128
  minor cytological abnormalities and,
    178, 181, 182
  MPL and, 135
  natural history of, 86–7
  oncogenesis, 88
  PCR and, 87–8, 95, 98–107, 200
  quality control of testing, 214
  retinoids and, 319–20
  screening older women, 206–7
  secondary screening, 208–12
  testing, 197–219, 301
  tumor suppressor genes and,
    88–9
  types, 85–6
  VAIN and, 169–70, 172
  VIN and, 37, 42–3, 44, 45, 113–14,
    116, 122
  vulvar warts and, 135–6, 137–8,
    139–40, 151
Hybrid capture, 216
Hymen, 12
Hysterectomy
  for AIS, 258–9
  for cervical cancer, 227, 228, 287,
    289–90
  for CIN, 188, 189, 191–2
  vaginal vault smears and, 239
  VAIN and, 170

Immunology of lower female genital
    tract, 71–82
  allergic reactions, 75–6
  complement, 75
  cytokines, 75
  genital secretion components, 71
  infectious agents and, 77–80
  immunoglobins, 72–4
  macrophages, 72
  polymorphonuclear leukocytes, 72
  T-lymphocytes, 74
  vaginal mileau and, 76–7
Immunosuppression, 123
  cervical cancer and, 264–5
  HPV and, 140

Immunosuppression (*contd*)
  VAIN and, 170, 171
  VIN and, 116
In situ hybridization, 998
Interferons (IFNs), 75, 127, 147, 148–50
  characteristics, 155–6
  clinical studies with, 157–63
  efficacy of, 164
  formulations, 156–7
  future role of, 164–5
  pharmacokinetics, 157
  serum neutralizing factors, 163–4
  side-effects of, 163
  for VAIN, 174, 175
Interleukin, 155
International Society for the Study of Vulvar Disease, 111, 122
Intradermal nevi, 133, 135

Kidney transplant patients and HPV, 57, 140
Koilocytosis, 27–8

LA-1 oncogen and cervical cancer, 334–6
Labia, 11–12, 14, 15
Large loop excision of the transformation zone (LLETZ), 180, 181, 191, 192, 193, 241
  psychological effect of, 245
Laser excisional conization, 190
Laser therapy
  for CIN, 193, 245
  for VAIN, 172
  for VIN, 126
  for vulvar warts, 142–3, 144, 147, 148, 150, 151, 152
Loop electro-surgical excision procedure (LEEP), 30, 150, 180, 210

Macrophages, 72
Macules, 342–4, 345
Male partner
  carcinogenic process and, 341–8
  vulvar warts and, 142
Mathematical modeling and screening, 64–6
Melanocytic dysplasia, 111, 113, 117
Melanoma, 114, 117
Menopause
  HPV testing and, 206–7
  SCJ after, 6
  see also Postmenopausal women
Menstruation and pH, 76
Mesonephric remnants, 8–9
Metaplasia
  epithelial, 9–10
  squamous, 5–6, 317, 320
Microglandular endocervical hyperplasia, 9

Micropapillomatoisis labialis, 133, 135, 139
Miller Behavioral Styles Scale, 246
MIN, 128–30
Molluscum contagiosum, 133, 134–5
MPL, 133, 135, 139
Mucus, 71
Multifocal disease, 128–30

Neisseria gonorrhoeae, 78–9, 350

Oncogenes
  antioncogenes, 328, 330, 334
  carcinogenesis and, 331
  cell cycle and, 331
  cervical cancer and, 331–6
  function, 327
  growth factor reception, 332–3
  HPV, 88
  mitogenic signaling pathways, 328, 329
  nuclear, 333–4
  proto-, 325–6
  ras, 333
  tumor-specific antigens, 334
Oral contraceptive pill and CIGN, 253

p53, 88
  cervical cancer and, 89
  vulvar dysplasia and, 114
Paget's disease of vulva, 111, 113, 114, 117
Papanicolaou (Pap) smear *see* Cervical smears
Papillomaviruses, bovine, 138
Papules, 341, 342, 343, 344
PCR *see* Polymerase chain reaction
Penile cancer, 50, 346
Penile intraepithelial neoplasia, 344, 345
pH, 76
PMN leukocytes, 72
Podofilox, 145, 147, 151
Podophyllin, 84, 144–5, 161
Polymerase chain reaction (PCR), 182
  concensus primer, 215–16
  HPV infection and, 87–8, 102–5
  quantitative, 301
  sample preparation for, 101–2
  standard method, 98–101
  variations, 105–7
Postmenopausal women, abnormal smear in, 231–40
  colposcopy for, 235–6
  cytology screening for, 235
  estrogen therapy, 236–7
  interpretation of, 233–5
  management of, 237–9
  vaginal vault, 239
Pregnancy
  biopsy in, 224

carcinoma of cervix in, 227–8
  case history, 224–6
  cervical changes during, 7–8
  cervical smears in, 221–2
  CIN in, 221–7
  colposcopy in, 222–4
  HPV and, 141
  management of microinvasion in, 226
  vulvar warts in, 143–4
Proteins, retinoid-binding, 312, 314, 317–19
Proto-oncogenes, 325–6
Psychological aspects of cervical screening, 241–8
  colposcopy examination, 244
  counseling, 247
  information provision, 245–7
  interventions, 247–8
  treatment of CIN, 244–5

Radiotherapy
  for cervical carcinoma, 287
  VAIN and, 170, 174–5, 239
Readability, 246
Recurrent laryngeal papillomatosis, 143
Reid colposcopic score, 302
Retinoic acid, 309, 310–11, 312, 320
  retinoid X receptors and, 314–15
Retinoids
  function of, 313
  heterodimers of RXR, 315–17
  HPV and, 319–20
  proteins and, 312, 314, 317–19
  receptors, 312–17
  response elements, 315, 316
  structure, 311–12, 313
Retinyl acetate, 311

Schiller test, 185, 186, 189, 236
SCJ *see* Squamocolumnar junction
SEER program, 50–1, 54–5, 121
Sexual activity and cervical cancer, 335
SIL *see* Squamous intraepithelial lesion
Smoking and cervical cancer, 89–90, 92, 335, 336
Southern blot, 96–7
  hybridization, 198, 215, 216
Spermicides, 76
Squamocolumnar junction (SCJ), 4, 6, 231, 279, 303, 304, 317
Squamous intraepithelial lesion (SIL), 178
  HGSIL, 211, 213, 215
  LGSIL, 209–10, 212, 213, 214
STD Treatment Guidelines, 272
Surgery
  for CIN, 189–92
  for VAIN, 174
  for VIN, 126, 127

T-lymphocytes, 74–5
Tamoxifen, 235
Tocopherol, 311
Trachelectomy, partial, 238–9
Trichloroacetic acid (TCA), 143, 144,
        145, 146, 147, 151
Trichomonas vaginalis, 77, 351
Tumor suppressor genes and HPV,
        88–9

Ultrasonic surgical aspiration for
        VAIN, 175
Urethra, 12
    HPV infection of, 134, 138

Vagina
    anatomy, 10–11
    histology, 11
Vaginal intraepithelial neoplasia
        (VAIN), 169–76
    classification, 170–1
    epidemiology, 169
    etiology, 169–70
    incidence, 128, 129
    natural history, 171–2
    pathology, 171
    treatment, 172–5
Vaginal vault, abnormal smear from,
        239

Vaginitis, inflammatory, 352
Vestibule, 12
VIN *see* Vulvar intraepithelial
        neoplasia
Viral infections, 83–94
    herpesviruses, 90–1
    HPV *see* Human papillomavirus
    MIN, 128
    of vulva, 123
Virapap, 209
Vitamin A, 311–2
    CIN and, 310
    derivative retinoids, 151
    estrogen and, 309
    see also Retinoids
Vulva
    anatomy, 11–13
    histology, 13–15
Vulvar atypia, 37, 40
Vulvar carcinoma, 43–4, 115–16,
        136
Vulvar carcinoma-in-situ, 40
Vulvar dysplasia, 111–19
    cervical dysplasia and, 111
    etiology, 113
    natural history, 115–17
    terminology, 111
Vulvar intraepithelial neoplasia (VIN),
        37–47
    carcinoma and, 43–4
    clinical presentation, 124

diagnosis of, 124–5
    epidemiology, 40, 121
    etiology, 122–3
    grading, 38
    histology, 112, 121–2
    HPV and, 42–3
    incidence, 128, 129
    interferons for, 157, 159
    management, 125–7
    morphology, 38
    natural history, 44–5, 123–4
    subsets of, 38–40
    terminology, 37, 111, 121, 122
Vulvar vestibulitis, 353
Vulvar warts, 133–54
    biopsy technique, 141–2
    clinical significance, 136
    condyloma mimics, 133–6
    epidemiology, 136
    immunosuppressed patient,
        140–1
    mechanism of transmission,
        137–8
    male partner and, 142
    pregnancy and, 143–4
    treatment, 144–51
    VIN and, 122
Vulvectomy, 127

Yeast, 352